ASSESSMENT OF FEIGNED COGNITIVE IMPAIRMENT

Assessment of Feigned Cognitive Impairment

A Neuropsychological Perspective

Edited by
Kyle Brauer Boone

THE GUILFORD PRESS
New York   London

©2007 The Guilford Press
A Division of Guilford Publications, Inc.
72 Spring Street, New York, NY 10012
www.guilford.com

Printed in the United States of America

This book is printed on acid-free paper.

Last digit is print number: 9 8 7 6 5 4 3 2 1

Library of Congress Cataloging-in-Publication Data

Assessment of feigned cognitive impairment : a neuropsychological perspective /
edited by Kyle Brauer Boone.
    p. ; cm.
  Includes bibliographical references and index.
  ISBN-13: 978-1-59385-464-5 (hardcover : alk. paper)
  ISBN-10: 1-59385-464-1 (hardcover : alk. paper)
  1. Neuropsychological tests. 2. Cognition—Testing. 3. Cognition disorders—
Diagnosis. 4. Factitious disorders—Diagnosis. 5. Malingering—Diagnosis.
I. Boone, K. B. (Kyle Brauer)
  [DNLM: 1. Cognition Disorders—diagnosis. 2. Cognition Disorders—
physiopathology. 3. Neuropsychology—methods. WM 204 A845 2007]
  RC386.6.N48A86 2007
  616.8'0475—dc22

                                                        2007010710

To my father-in-law,
Winston Bosworth Boone (1925–2005), who always expressed
enthusiastic interest in my projects and my career,
and to my father,
Richard Easton Brauer, MD (1927–2007), who gave me
the confidence and ability to produce this book

About the Editor

Kyle Brauer Boone, PhD, is Professor-in-Residence in the Department of Psychiatry and Biobehavioral Sciences at the David Geffen School of Medicine, University of California, Los Angeles, and Director of Neuropsychological Services and Training in the Department of Psychiatry at Harbor–UCLA Medical Center in Torrance, California. She has published over 100 peer-reviewed articles in professional journals in the area of neuropsychological assessment and is a coauthor of *Handbook of Normative Data for Neuropsychological Assessment.* Dr. Boone has also published two tests used to assess for effort on neuropsychological exams: the b Test and the Dot Counting Test. She is fortunate to have been involved in the training of many students in neuropsychological assessment, several of whom are contributing authors to this book.

Contributors

Kimberly Alfano, PhD, Rehabilitation Institute at Santa Barbara, Santa Barbara, California

Ginger Arnold, PhD, private practice, Indianapolis, Indiana

Talin Babikian, PhD, Semel Institute for Neuroscience and Human Behavior, University of California, Los Angeles, Los Angeles, California

Carla Back-Madruga, PhD, Department of Psychiatry and Behavioral Sciences, Keck School of Medicine, University of Southern California, Los Angeles, California

Kyle Brauer Boone, PhD, Department of Psychiatry and Biobehavioral Sciences, David Geffen School of Medicine, University of California, Los Angeles, Los Angeles, California; Department of Psychiatry, Harbor–UCLA Medical Center, Torrance, California

Robert L. Denney, PsyD, U.S. Medical Center for Federal Prisoners and Forest Institute of Professional Psychology, Springfield, Missouri

Daniel L. Drane, PhD, Harborview Medical Center, Regional Epilepsy Center, University of Washington, Seattle, Washington

David Fox, PhD, Consultants in Psychological Assessment, Glendale, California

David M. Glassmire, PhD, Department of Psychology, Patton State Hospital, Patton, California; Leonard Davis School of Gerontology, University of Southern California, Los Angeles, California

Hope E. Goldberg, PhD, Department of Psychiatry, Olive View–UCLA Medical Center, Sylmar, California

Paul Green, PhD, private practice, Edmonton, Alberta, Canada

Manfred F. Greiffenstein, PhD, Psychological Systems, Inc., Royal Oak, Michigan

Lisle R. Kingery, PhD, Department of Psychiatry and Behavioral Sciences, Johns Hopkins University School of Medicine, Baltimore, Maryland

Paul R. Lees-Haley, PhD, private practice, Huntsville, Alabama

Po H. Lu, PsyD, Department of Neurology, David Geffen School of Medicine, University of California, Los Angeles, Los Angeles, California

Robert J. McCaffrey, PhD, Department of Psychology, University at Albany, State University of New York, Albany, New York

John E. Meyers, PsyD, Center for Neurosciences, Orthopaedics, and Spine, Dakota Dunes, South Dakota

Nathaniel W. Nelson, PhD, University of Minnesota Neuropsychology Laboratory, Minneapolis, Minnesota

Stephen R. Nitch, PhD, Department of Psychology, Patton State Hospital, Patton, California; Department of Psychiatry, Loma Linda University, Loma Linda, California

Steven A. Rogers, PhD, Department of Psychology, Westmont College, Santa Barbara, California

Martin L. Rohling, PhD, Department of Psychology, University of South Alabama, Mobile, Alabama

Xavier F. Salazar, PsyD, Department of Psychiatry, University of Southern California, Los Angeles, California

David J. Schretlen, PhD, Department of Psychiatry and Behavioral Sciences and Department of Radiology and Radiological Sciences, Johns Hopkins University School of Medicine, Baltimore, Maryland

Brad Spickard, MPA, Department of Psychology, Ohio University, Athens, Ohio

David C. Stone, MD, Department of Psychiatry, Harbor–UCLA Medical Center, Torrance, California

Elizabeth S. Stroup, PhD, Harborview Medical Center, Regional Epilepsy Center, University of Washington, Seattle, Washington

Julie Suhr, PhD, Department of Psychology, Ohio University, Athens, Ohio

Jerry J. Sweet, PhD, Department of Psychiatry and Behavioral Sciences, Evanston Northwestern Healthcare, Evanston, Illinois

Tara L. Victor, PhD, Department of Psychology, California State University–Dominguez Hills, Carson, California

Johnny Wen, PhD, private practice, San Pedro, California

David J. Williamson, PhD, Ortho-McNeil Janssen Scientific Affairs, Mobile, Alabama

Christine L. Yantz, MA, Department of Psychology, University at Albany, State University of New York, Albany, New York

Preface

As a postdoctoral fellow in clinical neuropsychology at the University of California, Los Angeles, in the mid-1980s, I was confronted by a patient who, when I arrived to collect him in the waiting room, was wearing a string of garlic around his neck and talking to the wall (which he identified as his invisible friend, Ron). Thus began my first experience with a patient feigning cognitive (and psychotic) symptoms. Even in my very inexperienced state, I had the distinct impression during initial testing that he was not performing with his best effort. I consulted with my supervisor about what tests might be appropriate to administer to document symptom fabrication, but he could provide little guidance, aside from commenting, "Well, why don't you give the Bender and the Mini-Mental State Examination (MMSE)?" This lack of knowledge was not specific to my supervisor, however, given that very little published literature regarding procedures to document cognitive effort existed at that time. (Interestingly, administration of the Bender Gestalt Test was not such a bad idea; the patient drew some designs upside down, a phenomenon fairly pathognomonic for malingering. In addition, he showed illogical inconsistencies on the MMSE; for example, he indicated that he was unable to repeat three words, despite several trials, yet spontaneously repeated the three-step command: "You mean you want me to take it in my hand, fold it in half, and put it on the floor?")

Unsettled by the lack of testing materials and procedures to identify malingered performance, I perused neuropsychology texts to see where this topic might have already been addressed. Luckily I had on hand the initial editions of Muriel Lezak's encyclopedia of neuropsychological tests, *Neuropsychological Assessment*, which included a section on testing for functional complaints. Here I found descriptions of André Rey's 15-Item, Word Recognition, and Dot Counting Tests—measures he developed in Switzerland dur-

ing the 1940s to detect the malingering encountered during disability evaluations. I hand-constructed the test stimuli from Lezak's instructions and on
administering them to subsequent patients whom I suspected of poor effort,
found that the tests often produced results that mirrored my clinical intu-
ition. However, continued use of the tests revealed limitations (e.g., low sensitivity) and spawned hypotheses regarding how the tests might be improved,
culminating in our recently published adaptations of these measures.

Initially when I tested patients who were not applying adequate effort, I
would become irritated because I perceived them as attempting to deceive
me and circumventing my efforts to thoroughly and objectively document
their cognitive function. However, I came to realize that they were providing
me with a fabulous learning experience (i.e., private tutorials showcasing
how individuals attempt to feign). The repeating patterns I saw in the performances of these patients directly led to many of the effort tests and procedures developed in the Neuropsychology Lab at Harbor–UCLA Medical
Center. For example, some noncredible patients reported that following
their mild head injuries, they became "dyslexic" (i.e., saw letters upside down
and backwards), a symptom never reported by non-compensation-seeking
patients with moderate to severe brain injury and one that we subsequently
attempted to capture in the b Test. The observation of particularly slowed
response times and/or insertion of pauses (e.g., in forward Digit Span) in
noncredible patients led us to incorporate time scores in most of our effort
tests, thereby increasing the sensitivity of these measures. The assessment of
noncredible patients also taught me the important interplay between clinical
practice and research: the unanswered questions and dilemmas encountered
in clinical assessments illuminate which research questions should be addressed, while the resulting empirical investigations in turn inform and raise
the standard of clinical practice.

In this book, an attempt has been made to provide clinicians with a
review of the empirically tested effectiveness of the large number of freestanding effort tests and embedded effort indicators extracted from standard neuropsychological and personality measures that are currently available. More information is now accessible regarding the effectiveness and
classification accuracy of these techniques than for any other neuropsychological tests. Nevertheless, while clinicians now have a multitude of powerful
tools to assess for effort, care must be taken not to misuse these instruments—hence the importance of investigating effort test scores in patient
groups that might be at risk for being inaccurately identified as noncredible.
To this end, chapters have been included on effort testing in populations
with low intelligence and psychiatric illness, and in patients from cultural
backgrounds that differ from those of the patients on whom the tests were
primarily validated. We have also incorporated chapters regarding effort
testing in those clinical conditions and situations for which questions regarding veracity of cognitive complaints are (or should be) prominent, namely,

mild head injury, chronic pain and/or fatigue, multiple chemical sensitivity and exposure to mold, nonepileptic seizures, adult learning disability and attention-deficit/hyperactivity disorder, and in correctional settings. Recommendations regarding the future evolution of effort testing are provided, as well as a summary of recent developments in the use of functional brain imaging in the detection of deception.

This book would not have been possible without the gentle mentoring and consistent support of Rochelle Serwator at The Guilford Press. I am also grateful to the numerous chapter authors who generously contributed their time and tremendous expertise and whom I now count as friends. I also thank my husband, Rod, and children, Galen and Fletcher, who, with good cheer, tolerated my spending long hours in a stationary position at the computer.

Contents

PART I
SYMPTOM FABRICATION

CHAPTER 1

Feigning of Physical, Psychiatric, and Cognitive Symptoms

Examples from History, the Arts, and Animal Behavior

David C. Stone
Kyle Brauer Boone

This chapter introduces a number of historical examples, and cases drawn from literature and film/TV, of exaggerated medical, cognitive, or psychiatric symptoms, as well as illustrations of illness feigning and deception from the animal kingdom.

BIRDS DO IT . . .

Deception is fundamental to survival in the animal kingdom. Broken-wing displays among several species of birds have been described; the adult bird feigns injury to draw predators away from the brood nest (Byrkjedal, 1989).

Feigning of death to avoid predators is also common in many animal species. The most well known example is the opossum, hence the reference to "playing possum." The opossum lies on its side with its mouth partially open, tongue protruding, and starts to drool with eyes still open. It remains in this position for several minutes up to 6 hours and does not react to being prodded (Kimble, 1997). In addition to the opossum, several other types of animals feign death, including crustaceans, reptiles, birds, and insects, and even primates. Cut-worms curl into balls when they play dead. Beetles hold their legs close to their bodies and fall on their backs to feign the appearance of death, and walking sticks fall to the ground, becoming nearly invisible (Turpin, 2004). Turkey vultures, when disturbed in their nest, lay on their abdomens, wings outstretched, and head down, and "freeze" in position for several minutes, refusing to move, even when poked with a stick or lifted off the ground (Vogel, 1950). Foxes, when chased by dogs or caught in a trap, at first fight savagely but then drop to the ground, showing no signs of life. Once the predator leaves, the fox cautiously raises its head first, and then arises when the foe is at a safe distance.

The spider *Pisaura mirabilis* displays death-feigning behavior prior to mating with potentially cannibalistic females. Some animals feign death as a hunting strategy, such as the Central American ciclid, which mimics a rotting fish, laying on its side in the sand (Tobler, 2005).

Munchausen by proxy syndrome, in which typically a parent causes illness in a child to gain sympathy and attention from medical professionals, has also been found to occur between pets and their owners (Munro & Thrusfield, 2001; Tucker, Finlay, & Guiton, 2002).

OF SAINTS AND FEIGNTS

Even the holiest have feigned illness. St. Macarius the Great (295–392 A.D.), preferring to pursue his religious studies, is said to have feigned sickness to avoid being forced by his parents into marriage (Youssef, 2005). St. Ephrem the Syrian (306–373 A.D.) devoted himself primarily to pastoral work, teaching, writing, and music composition. Though elected to the rank of deacon, he avoided higher office and feigned madness to escape being made bishop (Robb, 1998). Prior to his conversion to Christianity, St. Maughold (Machaldus) (d. 498 A.D.) convinced his companion Garbanus to feign death in order to deceive St. Patrick. Uncovering the veil from Garbanus's body, they found that he was actually dead. Macaldus and his companions sought pardon from St. Patrick, who then performed the miracle of bringing Garbanus back to life. Female saints have feigned as well. Prior to her conversion, Our Holy Mother Pelagia (mid-5th century) accumulated a large fortune as a courtesan. She gave all her wealth to the poor when she converted, then departed to the Mount of Olives near Jerusalem, where she lived as a recluse, pretending that she was a eunuch named Pelagius. Clearly, if the sainted can malinger illness, feigning need not be viewed as a moral failing.

LITERATURE AND THE ARTS

Odysseus feigned insanity to avoid going to war. He plowed his fields with an ox and an ass, sowing salt instead of seeds. Palamedes suspected the ruse, and placed Odysseus's infant son Telemachus on the ground in the path of his plow. Odysseus was forced to turn the animals, revealing he was not mad after all.

Early Egyptian poetry also refers to the faking of illness:

> I think I'll go home and lie very still
> feigning terminal illness.
> Then the neighbors will all troop over to stare,
> my love, perhaps, among them.
> How she'll smile while the specialists
> snarl in their teeth!
> She perfectly well knows what ails me.
> (Ramessid period of ancient Egypt, ca. 1292–1070 B.C.) (Foster, 2001)

In his *Fabulae*, the Latin author Hyginus tells the story of the virgin Agnodice, who desired to learn medicine but, as a woman, was not allowed to do so. To pass as a man, she cut her hair and donned men's clothes, and after learning the healing arts from the physician, Herophilus, offered assistance to a woman in labor. Believing Agnodice was a man, the woman refused her help, at which point Agnodice lifted her tunic, showing herself to be a woman.

As word of Agnodice spread among women in the community, male doctors soon found their services refused by women. The doctors accused Agnodice of seducing the women and the women of feigning illness to receive treatments from Agnodice. When brought before the law court, Agnodice once again lifted her tunic to show that she was indeed a woman. The male doctors then shifted their criticisms to the fact she had broken the law forbidding women to study medicine, but the doctors' own wives then appeared in court. They testified in Agnodice's defense, referring to their husbands not as spouses, but as enemies who condemned the very woman who had brought them health. Athenian law was subsequently changed to allow women to study medicine.

Shakespeare frequently used feigning as a dramatic tool. In *King Lear*, Edgar, fleeing the manhunt his misinformed father Gloucester has instigated against him, disguises himself as a crazy beggar and calls himself "Poor Tom." Behaving in ways not usually tolerated in a "normal" person, Hamlet feigns mental illness to prove Claudius's guilt in the King's death. In *Romeo and Juliet*, Juliet drinks a potion which places her in a death-like coma for 42 hours, feigning death to avert her arranged marriage to

Paris. Romeo, believing her dead, drinks a truly lethal potion himself. Upon awakening, Juliet discovers Romeo dead and kills herself with his dagger.

Feigning illness forms the core of several of Aesop's fables. In one story, two travelers see a bear approaching; one traveler climbs a tree but the other, too slow, lies on the ground and pretends to be dead. After sniffing the prone traveler, the bear leaves. The traveler in the tree climbs down and asks his companion what the bear had whispered to him. His companion replies: "Don't travel with someone who abandons you at the first sign of trouble."

In another fable, old Lion can no longer chase and catch his prey, so he lies in a cave feigning illness. When the other animals enter to inquire about his health, he kills and eats them. Fox approaches the cave, and ill-appearing Lion beckons him in for a visit. Fox responds: "I should have done so, if I hadn't noticed all the footprints point toward the cave and none the other way."

In a third story, a thief, coming upon an inn, sees the innkeeper wearing an opulent coat and desires it for himself. He walks over to the innkeeper to chat, and suddenly yawns and howls. The innkeeper, concerned, asks the stranger what is wrong. The thief tells him: "When I have yawned three times I become a ravening wolf and leap at men's throats." The thief yawns a second time and the innkeeper, now afraid, attempts to flee; but the thief grabs him by the coat, pleading with him to look after his belongings until his episode has past. When the thief begins to yawn again, the innkeeper wrestles out of his coat to escape the thief's hold, runs into the inn, and bolts the door. The thief strolls quietly away with his spoil.

The animals of Kenneth Grahame's *The Wind in the Willows* provide a rich satire of post-Victorian English society. When Toad becomes overly preoccupied with his motorcars, wrecking old ones and buying new replacements, Badger, Rat, and Mole conspire to cure Toad of his automotive obsession. They forcibly remove him from his newest car, lock him in his room, and set about their deprogramming regimen. During Mole's shift to guard the detainee, Toad feigns severe illness. When Mole sets off to the village for medical help, Toad breaks free, steals their car, and takes a wild ride through the countryside. Poor Toad is later arrested and sentenced to 20 years in prison. There is no record whether Toad malingered during his trial, nor whether counsel proffered a defense of obsessional neurosis.

Joseph Heller's *Catch-22* begins with the protagonist, Yossarian, feigning illness in a hospital to avoid combat duty. In *The Crucible*, by Arthur Miller, the belief that Betty's and Ruth's symptoms are due to witchcraft is preferable to having to admit that good Puritan girls were simply feigning illness to avoid punishment for dancing in the woods and playing at casting spells. When Tom Wingfield, the narrator of *The Glass Menagerie* by Tennessee

Williams, brings home a potential suitor for his shy sister, Laura, she feigns illness to avoid having to eat dinner with the guest.

CELLULOID FAKES

Feigning has formed the plot twists of many a Hollywood blockbuster. In *Final Analysis*, Kim Basinger plays a woman accused of killing her abusive mobster husband. Richard Gere plays the "expert" psychiatrist who testifies that she suffers from pathological alcohol intoxication; however, he later discovers that she malingered the condition. In *Primal Fear*, Edward Norton, in the role of an altar boy accused of murdering a bishop, feigns multiple personality and tricks the "neuropsychologist," Frances McDormand, as well as his attorney, the again-duped Richard Gere. In *The Usual Suspects*, Kevin Spacey's character feigns physical disability to ward off suspicion that he is the criminal mastermind, Kaiser Soze.

In *Fight Club*, Edward Norton's character takes to attending support groups for persons with terminal illness—feigning his own terminal cancer. There, he meets Marla, played by Helena Bonham Carter, who, he discovers, feigns illness as well. Few portrayals about psychiatry have had the impact of Milos Forman's *One Flew over the Cuckoo's Nest*. The film's plot begins when McMurphy (played by Jack Nicholson) feigns mental illness to get out of work on a prison farm, only to find himself in a far more restrictive environment.

In other films, exaggeration and somatization provide comic effect. In *The Fortune Cookie*, Walter Matthau, as an ambulance-chasing attorney, convinces his brother-in-law, Jack Lemmon, a cameraman knocked unconscious while covering a football game, to feign paralysis to obtain insurance compensation. Robert DeNiro, in *Analyze That*, plays a mafia boss, who, fearing he will be killed if he remains in prison, alternately feigns psychosis (including singing songs from *West Side Story* and misidentifying his psychiatrist, Billy Crystal, as Maria) and catatonia (he does not flinch when stabbed with a syringe) to secure early release. His charade includes taking 1 hour and 12 minutes to reproduce a simple block design when undergoing neuropsychological testing. In *The Royal Tenenbaums*, Royal Tenenbaum (Gene Hackman), when evicted from his hotel residence, is allowed to return to his estranged family's home when he falsely claims that he has terminal stomach cancer (although he does die of a heart attack by the movie's end).

Corporal Klinger, in the long-running television show *M*A*S*H*, maneuvered to be discharged from the military by feigning mental illness, the symptoms of which included dressing as a woman: "I'm section 8, head to toe. I'm wearing a Warner bra. I play with dolls. My last wish is to be buried in my mother's wedding gown. I'm nuts. I should be out!" In the first season's episode entitled "Bananas, Crackers, and Nuts," even Hawkeye Pierce feigns insanity to earn a leave.

FAKE STYLES OF THE RICH AND FAMOUS

Celebrated writers, scientists, and philosophers have feigned illness. The German novelist Heinrich Böll was born in 1917, a year before Germany's defeat in World War I. His studies at the University of Cologne were interrupted when Böll was forced to serve in Hitler's army in World War II, where he was stationed in Poland and France. An episode of dysentery allowed him to return home to Germany where he married his wife in March 1942. But he was returned to service in the Soviet Union and later Romania. He was wounded twice, but feigned illness and used forged papers to avoid extensive time on the battlefields.

Philosopher Jean Michel Atlan (1913–1960) was arrested in 1942 as a member of the French Resistance. He feigned mental illness and was sent for 2 years of treatment at the Hôpital Saint-Anne.

Even Einstein faked being sick. In 2004, curators at Princeton University's Firestone Library uncovered a 62-page manuscript, "Gespräche mit Einstein" ("Conversations with Einstein"), written by former Firestone librarian Johanna Fantova. Fantova first met Einstein in Berlin in 1929 and eventually became Einstein's closet woman friend. Einstein moved to Princeton, New Jersey, in 1933 to join the Institute for Advanced Studies, and Fantova arrived in the United States in 1939. The manuscript represents Fantova's firsthand account of life with Einstein in Princeton from October 1953 until a few days before Einstein's death on April 12, 1955, when he suffered a ruptured abdominal aortic aneurysm. The only diary kept by someone close to Einstein during his final years, Fantova's work seldom shrinks from portraying the physicist's opinions and idiosyncracies. Receiving a live parrot on his 75th birthday, Einstein fretted that the bird had been traumatized during shipment and spent many days telling it bad jokes to cheer it up. But Einstein also frequently feigned illness, hiding in his bed to avoid the many strangers who showed up at 112 Mercer Street to be photographed with the celebrated physicist ("Diary Sheds Light," 2004).

CRIMINAL CASES

Exaggeration of symptoms, including cognitive dysfunction, among criminal defendants awaiting trial is common. The first and most common psychiatric question for Western courts regards the defendant's capacity to stand trial. The distinction between the defendant's current trial capacity and the defendant's capacity to form criminal intent at the time of the crime—an issue at the heart of the insanity defense—is sometimes poorly represented in media accounts, and even less well understood by the public. However, successful malingering during the evaluation of trial capacity accrues many benefits: detention in a safer, more comfortable mental health facility; the accumulation of a body of evidence that could later undermine prosecutions assertions of criminal intent; and general prolonging of the trial.

Many cases of malingering appear obviously contrived. Ilse Koch, the "Bitch of Buchenwald," rose quickly among Nazi leadership through her flirtations with high-ranking officers. At Heinrich Himmler's recommendation, Ilse and Himmler's assistant Karl Otto Koch began dating, and soon after their marriage, the Koch couple were awarded command of the newly constructed Buchenwald camp near Weimar. Among the countless atrocities committed, Ilse collected the tattoos of inmates, turning their skin into lampshades, gloves, and other household decor for the Koch's villa nearby. In her second trial in Augsburg in 1950, Ilse feigned epileptic seizures. She confessed the charade to her doctor, calling it a "first-class comedy act." She hanged herself in her cell in 1967 at the age of 61.

In other criminal cases, the deception is less obvious, but the malingerer eventually unmasks him- or herself. On September 15, 1963, a bomb destroyed the Sixteenth Street Baptist Church in Birmingham, Alabama, killing Cynthia Wesley, Addie Mae Collins, Denise McNair, and Carole Robertson, ages 11 to 14. On May 22, 2002, 40 years after the bombing, Bobby Frank Cherry was finally convicted for his participation in the attack.

Early in his trial, defense attorneys for Cherry argued that he was incompetent to stand trial due to dementia. Four experts testified that he was suffering from vascular dementia, and Judge James Garrett made a finding of incompetence. After 10 weeks of medical observation at Taylor Hardin Secure Medical Facility in Tuscaloosa, evaluators finally determined that Cherry was indeed faking dementia, and he was returned to trial.

Among other factors, Cherry claimed he could not remember events from earlier decades. But Kathleen Ronan, director of psychology at Taylor Hardin, testified that Cherry gave a full personal history dating to his childhood, including details of five prior marriages, the reason he was court-martialed and discharged from the Marines in 1949, and corroborated details of his work history. She further reported that when Cherry knew he was under observed conditions, he would perform poorly but would then perform well on memory evaluations when not aware he was being tested.

When administered the Test of Memory Malingering, Cherry scored ≤ chance (trial 1 = 22, trial 2 = 22, trial 3 = 20), suggesting he was intentionally selecting the wrong answer. Psychologist Alwyn Whitehead testified that Cherry often started to pick the correct answer but then would point to the wrong answer.

Cherry had originally denied involvement in the attack, claiming he was at home watching wrestling on television when the bomb was planted. However, reporter Jerry Mitchell of the Jackson, Mississippi, *Clarion-Ledger* debunked Cherry's alibi in 1999, citing television listings from the period that proved no wrestling shows were on the night of the bombings in Jackson. Cherry expired in prison in 2004.

Another case drew considerable media attention, that of Vincent "the Chin" Gigante. Gigante's history of prior psychiatric treatment was well documented. He had been under treatment with psychiatrist Michael Scolaro, MD, as early as 1966, and was later under the care of Louis D'Adamo, MD, from the mid-1980s onward. In the context of a 1970s case, in which it was alleged Gigante bribed police officers, Scolaro wrote to prosecutors, recounting that Gigante had expressed fears his neighbors might think he was homosexual, and that this may have contributed to his bizarre interaction with police. Scolaro noted that Gigante was being treated with a number of antipsychotics. The charges in this case were eventually dropped.

It was a subsequent case, however, ultimately leading to 1997 convictions on federal charges of racketeering, extortion, labor payoff, and conspiracy to murder, that created an ongoing controversy over the quality and nature of forensic evaluations.

Judge Eugene Nickerson presided over the earliest hearings regarding trial competency. Four psychiatrists initially testified that Gigante was incompetent to stand trial. However, the prosecution presented testimony from former members of the Mafia suggesting that Gigante had sustained a "crazy act" for years. The prosecution withheld testimony by Gigante's Mafia peers until after the psychiatrists' testimony. Judge Nickerson then asked the psychiatrists, accepting the facts of the Mafia testimony as true, whether the facts changed their opinions about competency.

Two of the four psychiatrists changed their opinions, one stating he was clearly competent, one stating he was quite possibly competent. The other two held to their previous opinions. Based on the new weight of the medical evidence, Nickerson certified Gigante as competent to stand trial.

Gigante later renewed his claim of trial incompetence, this time due to Alzheimer's disease. Nickerson recused himself (his wife had been diagnosed with Alzheimer's) and the case was reassigned to Judge Jack Weinstein.

While under treatment at St. Vincent's Hospital in 1990, Andrew Kelly, PhD, attempted assessment of Mr. Gigante several times. Gigante allegedly stated that dots made him "nervous" and that "God told me that it is hot outside. . . . I don't want to draw and God told me not to . . ." Kelly eventually abandoned efforts to test Gigante. In 1991, Mr. Gigante was administered the Wechsler Adult Intelligence Scale—Revised, obtaining a Verbal IQ of 65, Performance IQ of 75, and Full Scale IQ of 69, by Rolland Parker, PhD. Apparently, these represented a considerable improvement in scores from 1971, in which Gigante achieved IQ scores in the 50s.

With the renewed objections of incompetence, now due to Alzheimer's, defense neuropsychologist Wilfred van Gorp, PhD, tested Gigante. IQ scores were again in the impaired range. Some measures to detect malingering were administered, such as the Rey 15-Item Test, the California Verbal Learning Test recognition trial, the Portland Digit Recognition Test (PDRT), and the Warrington Memory Test. The patient did not perform significantly below chance on the forced-choice measures, which was used by the defense to argue that Mr. Gigante was not malingering. However, subsequent to the trial, Larry Binder, PhD, the developer of the PDRT, has commented that Mr. Gigante did in fact perform below cutoffs indicative of malingering on 1 of 2 PDRT scales, and that inconsistency in other test scores (e.g., markedly low scores on a word-retrieval task [Boston Naming Test] but low average performance on story recall [Logical Memory] were nonsensical. Judge Weinstein ultimately found the defendant competent. Gigante was sentenced and sent to prison, where he died in 2005. Debate about his competency and malingering during the federal trial has persisted in expert circles and on the Internet.

SUMMARY

As this brief tour of animal behavior, history, and the arts illustrates, feigning is not a rare phenomenon, may indeed be integral to survival, and is prominent in the stories we tell ourselves. The examples illustrate core aspects of feigned symptomatology. First, noncredible illness behaviors are ubiquitous—across species and within our human specie. In spite of this, medical and psychology graduate school curricula traditionally devote little time to the topic.

Second, as common as feigned illness is, it is rarely helpful to see noncredible performance as a moral failing. Feigning should instead be viewed as a fascinating behavior worthy of continued, collaborative, and enthusiastic research. For the clinician who is uncomfortable with the reality that most patients engage in deception at some time or the other, detecting and then confronting feigning can be disquieting, if not fraught with countertransference. Clinicians who have accepted the mind-set that patients frequently dupe us are better prepared for the issue when it arises. Moral overtones merely encourage the clinician to overlook obvious clues to exaggeration, which in turn precludes the clinician from asking *why* the deception is occurring. Recognition of feigning behaviors may prove to be the first therapeutic step to understanding the patient's actual needs. At its extreme, a clinician's blindness to clues of exaggeration equals collusion, with the potential to reinforce the patient's maladaptive illness strategies.

REFERENCES

Analyze That. (2002). Dir. Harold Ramis. Warner Bros. Pictures.

Bergstrom, P. W. (1988). Breeding displays and vocalizations of Wilson's plovers. *Wilson Bulletin, 100*, 36–49.

Byrkjedal, I. (1989). Nest defense behavior of lesser golden-plovers. *Wilson Bulletin, 101*, 579–590.

Diary sheds light on Einstein's final years. (2004, April 26). *MSNBC Science*. Retrieved April 29, 2005, from *www.msnbc.msn.com/id/4829521/*

Fight Club. (1999). Dir. David Fincher. Twentieth Century-Fox Film Corporation.

Final Analysis. (1992). Dir. Phil Joanou. Warner Home Video.

The Fortune Cookie. (1966). Dir. Billy Wilder. United Artists.

Foster, J. L. (trans.). (2001). *Ancient Egyptian literature*. Austin: University of Texas Press.

Grahame, K. (1983). *The wind in the willows*. New York: Oxford University Press.

Gregory, P., & Gregory, J. (1984). *The fables of Aesop*. Harvard: Harvard Common Press.

Heller, J. (1961). *Catch-22*. New York: Simon and Schuster.

Homer. (1975). *The odyssey*. (R. Lattimore, trans.). New York: Harper and Row.

Hyginus, Gaius Julius. *Fabulae*, CCLXXIV.

Kimble, D. P. (1997). Didelphid behavior. *Neuroscience and Biobehavioral Reviews, 21*, 361–369.

Kuperman, V. (2006). Narratives of psychiatric malingering in works of fiction. *Medical Humanities, 32*, 67–72.

M*A*S*H. (1972–1983). 20th Century Fox Home Entertainment.

McKaye, K. R. (1981). Field observation on death feigning, a unique hunting behavior by the predatory cichlid Haplochromis livingstoni of Lake Malawi Malawi. *Environmental Biology of Fishes, 6*, 361–366.

Munro, H. M., & Thrusfield, M. V. (2001). "Battered pets": Features that raise suspicion of non-accidental injury. *Journal of Small Animal Practice, 42*, 218–226.

One Flew over the Cuckoo's Nest. (1975). Dir. Milos Forman. Pioneer Entertainment.

Primal Fear. (1996). Dir. Gregory Hoblit. Paramount Hove Video.

Proudfoot, R., Thompson, A., & Kastan, D. S. (Eds.). (1998). *The Arden Shakespeare complete works*. Walton-on-Thames, UK: Thomas Nelson.

Robb, M. M. (1998). St. Ephrem the Syrian. *The CyberDesert*. Retrieved April 29, 2005, from *agrino.org/cyberdesert/ephrem.htm*

The Royal Tenenbaums. (2001). Dir. Wes Anderon. Buena Vista Pictures.

Tobler, M. (2005). Feigning death in the Central American cichlid *Parachromis friedrichsthalii*. *Journal of Fish Biology, 66*, 877–881.

Tucker, H. S., Finlay, F., & Guiton, S. (2002). Munchausen syndrome involving pets by proxies. *Archives of Disease in Childhood, 87*, 263.

Turpin, T. (2004, December 22). Do insects sleep or are they just feigning it? *On Six Legs*. Retrieved July 22, 2006, from *www.agriculture.purdue.edu/agcomm/newscolumns/archives/OSL/2004/December/041222OSL.htm*

The Usual Suspects. (1995). Dir. Bryan Singer. Image Entertainment.

Vogel, H. H. (1950). Observations on social behavior in turkey vultures. *The Auk, 67*, 210–216.

Youssef, H. G. B. (2005). St. Macarius the Great: Clothed with the Holy Spirit. Retrieved April 29, 2005, from *www.coptic.org.au/modules/resources_ literature/article.php?articleid=189*

CHAPTER 2

Functional Neuroimaging of Deception and Malingering

Lisle R. Kingery
David J. Schretlen

Neuroimaging techniques such as functional magnetic resonance imaging (fMRI) and positron emission tomography (PET) are powerful, noninvasive tools that can provide unique insights into the neurobiological underpinnings of complex neuropsychological processes. A rapidly emerging application of these methods involves the study of deception and malingering. These studies are predicated on the assumption that engaging in deception requires the participation of specific cerebral circuits whose activation will yield a recognizable "signature." In the case of fMRI, this signature appears as blood oxygenation level dependent (BOLD) activation of specific brain regions while a person engages in deceptive behavior in the scanner. In PET imaging this signature typically is measured by alterations in regional cerebral blood flow (rCBF) following injection of a radiotracer, such as ^{15}O-labeled water, while a person responds deceptively in the scanner. In this chapter we review all 13 known neuroimaging studies of deception and malingering. The novelty of using these methods is demonstrated by the fact that not a single one of these was published before 2001, and most were published since 2004. Only two reported investigations of simulated malingering; the rest involved studies of deception. In this chapter we review the findings of all 13 studies because malingering involves deception, and studies of deception therefore might shed light on the neural underpinnings of malingering.

What accounts for the recent interest in using functional neuroimaging to study deception and malingering? One reason is that functional neuroimaging has the potential to advance our scientific understanding of the neurobiology of deceptive behavior. Another is the hope that further development of these methods ultimately will yield tools that can reliably and accurately detect deceptive behavior in individual cases (Ford, 2006). As demonstrated by other chapters in this volume, many psychological tests are sensitive to symptom distortion and deceptive behavior. The use of electrophysiological measures of peripheral nervous system activity, such as galvanic skin response, blood pressure, and heart or respiration rate to detect other forms of deception, also has been the subject of extensive research (Yankee, 1995). Recent advances in the analysis of evoked response potentials (ERPs) have renewed interest in the search for an electroencephalographic signature of deceptive behavior in the central nervous system (Johnson, Barnhardt, & Zhu, 2003, 2005). Like ERPs, functional neuroimaging assesses processes that are more "proximal" to the neural mechanisms of deception than are assessed by cognitive, behavioral, and electrophysiological measures. Perhaps because of this, there is growing optimism that unique patterns of cerebral activation ultimately will enable investigators to detect deception in individual cases. For example, referring to the use of fMRI, Langleben recently stated, "We can't say whether this person will one day use a bomb. But we can use fMRI to find concealed information. We can ask: is X involved in terrorist organization Y?" (cited in Wild, 2005, p. 457). On the other hand, some researchers have warned that such conclusions are premature based on the current state of their scientific support. For example, Kozel, Revell, et al. (2004) argued that current applications of fMRI are "neither sensitive nor specific for detecting deception" in individual cases (p. 302). Farah (2002), among others, also argued that using functional neuroimaging for lie detection raises ethical issues, especially concerning the privacy of an individual's mental life. However, because lying is a ubiquitous behavior that occurs in virtually every setting and can result in substantial harm (DePaulo, Kashy, Kirkendol, Wyer, & Epstein, 1996), recent successful applications of functional neuroimaging to investigate and detect deception guarantee that these methods will play an increasingly prominent role in research on deception over time (Ford, 2006).

The aims of this chapter are threefold. After describing the methodology of the current review, we first summarize the methodological features of previously reported functional neuroimaging studies of deception and malingering. Second, we review the findings of these studies as a function of the activation paradigm used, attempt to draw preliminary conclusions about patterns of brain activation they reveal, and link these findings with conceptualizations of the cognitive operations involved in deception. Third, we discuss recommendations for future research that are suggested by limitations of the existing evidence. Although Spence et al. (2004) reviewed functional neuroimaging studies of deception, several additional studies have been published since then and that review did not summarize the studies quantitatively. There are now enough studies to support a semiquantitative summary of findings reported to date.

METHODOLOGY OF THE CURRENT REVIEW

The research summarized in this review was compiled by searching the Medline (Pubmed) and PsycInfo databases using search terms including "deception," "lying," "malingering," "neuroimaging," "fMRI," and "PET." Reference sections of all relevant published reports also were reviewed to locate other studies. Reports included in the review were retrieved from peer-reviewed journals but not abstracts or conference presentations. Altogether, 13 published studies were found. These included reports of 14 independent sample results. Once compiled, we recorded from each study the sample size, sex distribution, and mean age (or age range) of participants; the experimental procedure (described below); experimental design (i.e., block design, where similar stimuli/conditions are grouped within distinct time periods, vs. event design, where stimuli are randomly or quasi-randomly presented); magnet field strength (for fMRI studies); and whether reaction time was measured.

One critical methodological challenge of any neuroimaging review is how to summarize results in a consistent manner given that studies employ varied data analysis and reporting conventions (Brett, Johnsrude, & Owen, 2002; Fox, Parsons, & Lancaster, 1998). Because studies vary in the coordinate system used to localize brain activation patterns, it is necessary to transform study findings into a common system. Most studies included in this review used x-, y-, and z-coordinates according to the Talairach system (Talairach & Tournoux, 1988). Findings reported in the Montreal Neurologic Institute (MNI) coordinate system were transformed into Talairach space (Brett et al., 2002). Following transformation, coordinates of significant activation loci were translated into verbal descriptions of the corresponding cortical regions using the Talairach Daemon (*ric.uthscsa.edu/projects/talairachdaemon.html*). Because activation of thalamic, basal ganglia, and cerebellar regions were rare, they were excluded from the analyses. Significant activations reported with a value of 0 for the x or y coordinates were also excluded because these coordinates preclude classification by hemisphere or anterior versus posterior location. Finally, patterns of cerebral activation can be examined by subtracting the BOLD signal obtained during one activity (e.g., responding truthfully) from the BOLD signal obtained during another activity (e.g., responding deceptively). In this review, only results

obtained from the subtraction of honest from deceptive responding (lie >
truth) are reported because most studies did not find significant BOLD signal changes in truth > lie comparisons and because many investigators did
not even report the latter comparison.

Using these data, we calculated the number of areas of significant activation by hemisphere and by anterior versus posterior brain regions. In the
Talairach system, x-coordinates localize points from right to left, and y-coor-
dinates localize points from anterior to posterior. Thus, large positive values
of x refer to lateral aspects of the right hemisphere, and large negative values
refer to lateral aspects of the left hemisphere. Likewise, large positive values
of the y-coordinate refer to the frontal poles, while large negative values
refer to the occipital poles. Binomial tests were used to test for significant
differences according to hemisphere and anterior vs. posterior cortical
regions, and chi-squared tests were used to determine whether there was any
evidence for an interaction between these two general regional classifications. We also summarize the percentage of studies that revealed significant
activations in more specific cortical regions, based on the verbal descriptions
of brain regions derived using the Talairach Daemon.

SUMMARY OF EXPERIMENTAL PROCEDURES
USED TO INDUCE DECEPTION

Deception can be conceptualized in many different ways. Courts of law
require witnesses to "tell the truth, the whole truth, and nothing but the
truth" because deception not only includes the telling of lies but also the
withholding of truth and the commingling of truth with deception. Because
deception refers to a variety of behaviors, previous neuroimaging studies
have employed different strategies to elicit deception. Most adapted the
"guilty knowledge test" (GKT). In this paradigm, the examinee is asked a
series of yes–no questions with instructions to answer "no" to every question
(Lykken, 1960). However, some of the questions are "relevant" in that they
involve actual features of the crime under investigation, and others are "neutral" in that their contents are irrelevant to the crime under investigation,
but they are worded so that an innocent suspect would not be able to discriminate them from "relevant" questions. Many studies have shown that
people demonstrate stronger psychophysiological responses to relevant than
neutral questions using this paradigm (Ben-Shakhar & Elaad, 2003).

As shown in Table 2.1, six studies involved adaptations of the GKT paradigm. Using ordinary playing cards, Langleben et al. (2002) gave each participant a 5 of clubs prior to scanning. Then, during a brain fMRI scan, participants were shown the 5 of clubs, 2 of hearts, and other cards one at a time
and asked whether or not they were holding each one. Because they were
told to deny holding all cards, their responses to the 5 of clubs were decep-

TABLE 2.1. Study Characteristics

Year	First author	Procedure[a]	No. of participants (male–female)	Age[b]	Magnet (tesla)	Analytic design	Coordinate system[c]	Reaction time
2004	Kozel (pilot)	GKT	8 (8–0)	18–40	1.5	Block	TT	No
2004	Kozel (replication)	GKT	10 (NA)	27.8	3.0	Event	MNI	No
2005	Kozel (exp. 1)	GKT	30 (17–13)	30.4	3.0	Event	MNI	Yes
2005	Kozel (exp. 2)	GKT	31 (12–19)	33.4	3.0	Event	MNI	Yes
2002	Langelben	GKT	18 (11–7)	32	4.0	Event	TT	No
2005	Langleben	GKT	26 (26–0)	19.36	3.0	Event	TT	Yes
2004	Phan	GKT	14 (7–7)	32	4.0	Event	MNI	No
2002	Lee	Malinger	5 (5–0)	33.5	1.5	Block	TT	No
2005	Lee (sample 1)[d]	Malinger	8 (8–0)	23.8	1.5	Block	TT	No
2005	Lee (sample 2)[d]	Malinger	15 (7–8)	22	1.5	Block	TT	No
2005	Lee (sample 3)[d]	Malinger	6 (NA)	26.9	1.5	Block	TT	No
2006	Abe	Other	14 (14–0)	20	N/A	Event	MNI	Yes
2003	Ganis	Other	10 (3–7)	25	1.5	Block	TT	Yes
2005	Nunez	Other	20 (10–10)	26	1.5	Block	MNI	Yes
2001	Spence	Other	10 (10–0)	24	1.5	Block	TT	Yes
2006	Mohamed	Other	11 (6–5)	28.9	1.5	Block	TT	No

[a] GKT, guilty knowledge test.
[b] Reported as mean or range.
[c] TT, Talairach and Tournot; MNI, Montreal Neurological Institute.
[d] Although three samples were tested, the results were reported in a single conjunction analysis.

tive (guilty knowledge), whereas their denials of having other cards were truthful. Phan et al. (2005) and Langleben et al. (2005) used nearly identical stimuli in replications of this study. In a series of three investigations (one of which included two independent samples), Kozel and colleagues had participants "steal" either a wristwatch or a ring from a desk in the laboratory and then answer a series of yes–no questions about the objects ("Did you take the ring?") while undergoing an fMRI scan (Kozel et al., 2005; Kozel, Padgett, & George, 2004; Kozel, Revell, et al., 2004). Because subjects were instructed to deny taking the "stolen" item, their responses to these questions were deceptive (guilty knowledge), whereas their denials of taking the other object were truthful.

Five other studies involved deception but differed from the GKT paradigm. For example, prior to scanning, Spence et al. (2001) asked each participant 36 questions, such as whether he made his bed that day. Then, during an fMRI scan, the investigators posed the same 36 questions twice, and cued participants to answer truthfully once and deceptively once in response to each question. Nunez, Casey, Egner, Hare, and Hirsch (2005) generated 72 yes–no autobiographical ("Do you own a laptop computer?") and non-autobiographical ("Is a laptop computer portable?") questions. Like Spence et al. (2001), these investigators presented each question twice, once with instructions to lie and once with instructions to tell the truth, while subjects were scanned with brain fMRI. In a procedurally complicated study, Ganis, Kosslyn, Stose, Thompson, and Yurgelun-Todd (2003) obtained detailed information about two personal experiences from each subject, and constructed alternative, fictional details for one of their experiences. Then, while subjects underwent a brain fMRI scan, they answered a series of questions about both the veridical and fictional experiences. Their deceptive responses varied according to whether or not they were memorized and whether or not they fit into the context of the experimentally determined veridical or personal stories. The data analysis aimed to identify BOLD correlates of these two dimensions. Most recently, Mohamed et al. (2006) employed perhaps the most dramatic experimental design to date. In this study, 6 of 11 subjects participated in a "mock shooting." After being instructed in handgun safety, each subject fired blank shots from a handgun in a testing room in the functional neuroimaging center. All subjects also underwent an interview that used a "forensic assessment interview technique" and then an fMRI and a polygraph assessment. All subjects completed two separate fMRI scans. During one they were instructed to lie to all questions, and during the other one they were instructed to tell the truth to all questions. Questions were either about the shooting (e.g., Did you shoot the gun?) or were irrelevant (e.g., Is today Sunday?). Based on this design, three lie contrasts were examined. The most important of these compared the BOLD signal when subjects denied shooting the gun versus told the truth to control questions.

Abe et al. (2006) conducted the only PET study of deception to date. Their procedure was developed to contrast two distinct types of lies: either pretending to know or pretending not to know. They accomplished this by first exposing all participants to 20 real-world events prior to the PET scan. The events included experiences such as coloring a picture, playing a musical instrument, and consulting a dictionary. Each event involved 1 of 10 actions (coloring, solving puzzles, etc.) and 20 implements (musical instrument, dictionary, etc.). This design therefore allowed these experiences to be classified according to task and implement used. During the PET scan, participants were shown 40 pictures, half of which were of implements they had previously used and half of which were of implements they had not used. Based on this design, data analysis was conducted using two lie and two truth conditions. In two conditions the participants were instructed to deny previously engaging in each task, and in two conditions they were told report engaging in each task.

Lee and colleagues (2002, 2005) published two reports of feigned memory impairment. The most recent of these combined results of three fMRI studies. Their procedures are most similar to studies of simulated malingering in that participants were told to purposefully do poorly on an experimental forced-choice recognition task. The first report (Lee et al., 2002) included two sets of stimuli: a three-digit, same/different, recognition memory task and yes–no autobiographical memory task in which the questions (e.g., "where were you born") were paired with predetermined answers (e.g., "London"). In both conditions, participants were instructed to deliberately do poorly on the task by imagining that a "bad result" on the memory test would result in "an attractive sum of money" (p. 159). Following the feigned memory condition, participants also completed three additional independent conditions for each task during which they were instructed to respond honestly, incorrectly, and randomly. In the second report by this group of investigators (Lee et al., 2005), participants were given the same instructions and underwent a similar three-digit forced-choice memory test as well as a forced-choice test for Chinese words. In both studies, the primary results reported were based on the comparison of BOLD signal changes in the feigned memory impairment condition minus answering correctly condition.

SUMMARY OF RESULTS

Table 2.1 summarizes the basic features of the studies included in this review. As shown, more men than women have been studied, most subjects were young adults (mean age = 27), and all participants were healthy and free of psychiatric or neurological illness. Nine of the 16 studies that were based on unique samples employed a block design. Most studies were conducted at a field strength of 1.5 tesla, although some acquired data at 3T or 4T. Seven studies included measures of choice reaction time.

Table 2.2 summarizes the brain activation foci grouped by task type (Guilty Knowledge, Malingering, Other), hemisphere, and anterior/posterior brain region. A total of 133 independent foci of activation was reported. As shown in Table 2.2, greater activation in anterior regions was observed across studies, regardless of task type. Binomial tests comparing anterior versus posterior activations were significant for each task type individually and for all studies combined ($p < .001$). In contrast, there was no evidence of hemispheric differences within the different types of task or across all studies combined ($p = .62$). A binomial test comparing the left- and right-hemisphere activations within anterior brain regions also failed to reveal significant differences ($p = .33$). Chi-square analyses were used to test for an association between cerebral hemisphere and anterior versus posterior regions. This revealed significant results only for the GKT ($x^2_{(1)} = 6.1, p < .05$), where relatively fewer activations in the right posterior region of the brain compared to the other three brain regions.

Figure 2.1 summarizes the percentage of all studies that reported significant activations in the lie > truth contrasts according to specific cortical regions within each hemisphere. The most consistent finding across all studies is that deceptive responding most consistently activates the middle and inferior frontal gyri, bilaterally. In addition, the superior frontal, cingulate, and medial frontal gyri appear to be commonly invoked when subjects engage in deceptive responses, though fewer than 50% of all studies reported this finding. Other regions of activation that were found less consistently (often in only a single study) included middle and superior temporal, inferior parietal, precentral, and postcentral gyri.

TABLE 2.2. Number of Activations Coded According to Task, Hemisphere, and Brain Region

Study type	Number of samples	Brain region	Left hemisphere	Right hemisphere
Guilty Knowledge Test	7	Anterior	16	23
		Posterior	15	5
Malingering	2	Anterior	11	11
		Posterior	6	6
Other	5	Anterior	14	17
		Posterior	3	6
Combined	14	Anterior	41	5
		Posterior	24	17

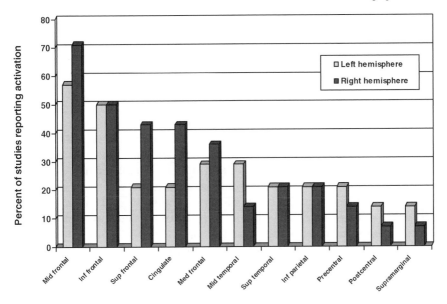

FIGURE 2.1. Percent of studies reporting significant activation in specific cortical regions.

COGNITIVE OPERATIONS INVOLVED IN DECEPTIVE BEHAVIOR

Almost all of the investigators whose research is reviewed here conceptualize the cognitive operations required by deception as involving some type of "executive" function. Their conceptualizations refer to cognitive inhibition (e.g., of the "prepotent" tendency to respond honestly) (Lee et al., 2005), conflict monitoring and resolution (Nunez et al., 2005), and generativity (e.g., of falsehoods) (Nunez et al., 2005; Spence et al., 2001, 2004), among others. A common underlying notion is the idea that responding deceptively, whether by telling a lie or withholding the truth, requires more complex cognitive processing or greater mental control than responding honestly. The finding that lying usually is characterized by increased response times in behavioral studies supports this notion (Johnson et al., 2003, 2004, 2005). In any case, deception generally is thought to recruit executive processes that are believed to be controlled by anterior brain circuits, particularly involving the dorsolateral, ventromedial, or cingulate cortex.

Previous neuroimaging research has consistently shown that prefrontal brain regions are differentially engaged during tasks involving response inhibition and cognitive interference (Szameitat, Schubert, Muller, & Von Cramon, 2002). A meta-analysis of neuroimaging studies of working memory led Wager and Smith (2003) to conclude that tasks involving executive demands produce reliable activation largely in the frontal cortex, and that working memory tasks involving inhibition and switching particularly engage the inferior frontal cortex. Taken together, the findings of this review offer qualified support of the hypothesis that experimentally induced deception is associated with the relative activation of prefrontal brain regions, particularly the middle and inferior frontal gyri. Thus, the findings of studies reported to date support the view that engaging in experimentally induced deceptive behavior does differentially engage those brain regions known to be involved in executive control.

While neuroimaging studies of deception and malingering consistently point to the involvement of prefrontal cortices, they do not suggest greater recruitment of the left or right cerebral hemisphere. That is, findings reported to date provide little support for the notion that lying draws disproportionately on the right hemisphere (Keenan, Rubio, Racioppi, Johnson, & Barnacz, 2005). Some data (Ganis et al., 2003) suggest a relatively greater right-hemisphere activation, particularly in the cingulate cortex, but bilateral activation of anterior brain regions is more common (Abe et al., 2006; Kozel et al., 2005; Langleben et al., 2005; Lee et al., 2002, 2005; Spence et al., 2001).

LIMITATIONS AND SUGGESTIONS FOR FUTURE RESEARCH

While the studies reviewed here yielded some fairly consistent results, several limitations deserve note. First, the extent to which these findings generalize to contexts outside the laboratory is unknown, as the methods used to date are characterized by "low ecological relevance and risk" (Langleben et al., 2005). All participants included thus far have been young, healthy, and cooperative. Second, even when group differences in BOLD activation are robust, there is very little evidence to support the view that fMRI methods can accurately detect specific instances of deceptive behavior, although new approaches to data analysis eventually might overcome these limitations (Davatzikos et al., 2005). Third, although most studies have not revealed significant BOLD activation in truth > lie contrasts, two recent studies using the same dataset but different data analytic techniques did (Davatzikos et al., 2005; Langleben et al., 2005). Surprisingly, in this analysis, more voxels and clusters were activated by the contrast of truth telling minus lying than by the more conventional lying minus truth telling contrast. These researchers noted that their findings argue against truthful responses being conceptualized as a "default" or routine cognitive process that does not require additional cognitive resources. However, they hypothesize that because the majority of activations in the lie > truth contrast were rostral to those found in the truth > lie comparison, lying involves more complex (i.e., "executive") cognitive operation than truth telling.

Given that simple choice response times consistently are slower during deceptive than honest responding (Johnson et al., 2003), it is notable that less than half of the studies included measures of response time (RT). In fact, of those that reported RT, not all found that the lying was accompanied by increased RT. Given that RT can be relatively easily measured in the fMRI environment, it is recommended that RT measures be included in neuroimaging studies of deception to serve as an additional validation measure of the experimental design.

Because several brain regions were activated in only one or two studies, accurate interpretation of the role and nature of activation in these regions requires further research. Presumably, some of these differences were due to study-specific experimental procedures. Further research is required to fully understand the effect of specific methodological features. For example, the brain neural circuits that process auditory and visual material differ in important structural and functional ways. Consequently, it is possible that the neural correlates of deception involving visual versus auditory stimuli may differ in important ways (Spence et al., 2001) and further research in this area is needed. In addition, only one study has examined the role of autobiographical versus nonautobiographical information (Nunez et al., 2005) and these findings suggest that the more self-relevant the material, the more cognitive control is required during lying. This study is also unique in that it is the only one to date that included measures of personality traits that theoretically may impact the relationship between brain activity and deceptive cognition. Their preliminary results suggest that self-report measures from the Psychopathic Personality Inventory (Lilienfeld & Andrews, 1996) correlate in meaningful ways with activity in the brain regions that are implicated in deceptive responding. For example, two personality traits, "carefree nonplanfulness" and "alienation," were correlated with significantly greater activation in mesial prefrontal and anterior cingulate regions during autobiographical conditions (regardless of truth or lie condition) than during nonautobiographical trials. In addition, in a deceptive condition comparison, relatively less activation was seen in posterior cingulate regions for subjects who scored higher on the "coldheartedness" scale, suggesting that individuals prone to be unemotional, guiltless, and detached evidence less activation during deceptive responding to false nonautobiographical material. Including other theoretically relevant measures of individual differences or diagnostic groups (e.g., personality disorders) will lead to a further refined understanding of the neurobiological correlates of deceptive behavior.

As outlined in this review, the application of functional neuroimaging techniques is in a very early stage of development and the findings described previously tend to support the broad conclusion that simple laboratory tasks designed to induce deceptive responses often engage prefrontal brain regions bilaterally. However, the argument that fMRI methods are capable of reliably identifying deceptive responding in individual cases, in our view, is not supported at present by the available data.

REFERENCES

Abe, N., Suzuki, M., Tsukiura, T., Mori, E., Yamaguchi, K., Itoh, M., et al. (2006). Dissociable roles of prefrontal and anterior cingulate cortices in deception. *Cerebral Cortex, 16*, 192–199.

Ben-Shakhar, G., & Elaad, E. (2003). The validity of psychophysiological detection of information with the Guilty Knowledge Test: A meta-analytic review. *Journal of Applied Psychology, 88*(1), 131–151.

Brett, M., Johnsrude, I. S., & Owen, A. M. (2002). The problem of functional localization in the human brain. *Nature Reviews Neuroscience, 3*(3), 243–249.

Davatzikos, C., Ruparel, K., Fan, Y., Shen, D. G., Acharyya, M., Loughead, J. W., et al. (2005). Classifying spatial patterns of brain activity with machine learning methods: application to lie detection. *Neuroimage, 28*(3), 663–668.

DePaulo, B. M., Kashy, D. A., Kirkendol, S. E., Wyer, M. M., & Epstein, J. A. (1996). Lying in everyday life. *Journal of Personality and Social Psychology, 70*(5), 979–995.

Farah, M. J. (2002). Emerging ethical issues in neuroscience. *Nature Neuroscience, 5*(11), 1123–1129.

Ford, E. B. (2006). Lie detection: Historical, neuropsychiatric and legal dimensions. *International Journal of Law and Psychiatry, 29,* 159–177.

Fox, P. T., Parsons, L. M., & Lancaster, J. L. (1998). Beyond the single study: Function/location metanalysis in cognitive neuroimaging. *Current Opinions in Neurobiology, 8*(2), 178–187.

Ganis, G., Kosslyn, S. M., Stose, S., Thompson, W. L., & Yurgelun-Todd, D. A. (2003). Neural correlates of different types of deception: An fMRI investigation. *Cerebral Cortex 13*(8), 830–836.

Johnson, R., Jr., Barnhardt, J., & Zhu, J. (2003). The deceptive response: effects of response conflict and strategic monitoring on the late positive component and episodic memory-related brain activity. *Biology Psychology, 64*(3), 217–253.

Johnson, R., Jr., Barnhardt, J., & Zhu, J. (2004). The contribution of executive processes to deceptive responding. *Neuropsychologia 42*(7), 878–901.

Johnson, R., Jr., Barnhardt, J., & Zhu, J. (2005). Differential effects of practice on the executive processes used for truthful and deceptive responses: an event-related brain potential study. *Brain Research Cognitive Brain Research, 24*(3), 386–404.

Keenan, J. P., Rubio, J., Racioppi, C., Johnson, A., & Barnacz, A. (2005). The right hemisphere and the dark side of consciousness. *Cortex, 41*(5), 695–704.

Kozel, F. A., Johnson, K. A., Mu, Q., Grenesko, E. L., Laken, S. J., & George, M. S. (2005). Detecting deception using functional magnetic resonance imaging. *Biological Psychiatry, 58*(8), 605–613.

Kozel, F. A., Padgett, T. M., & George, M. S. (2004). A replication study of the neural correlates of deception. *Behavioral Neuroscience, 118*(4), 852–856.

Kozel, F. A., Revell, L. J., Lorberbaum, J. P., Shastri, A., Elhai, J. D., Horner, M. D., et al. (2004). A pilot study of functional magnetic resonance imaging brain correlates of deception in healthy young men. *Journal of Neuropsychiatry and Clinical Neurosciences, 16*(3), 295–305.

Langleben, D. D., Loughead, J. W., Bilker, W. B., Ruparel, K., Childress, A. R., Busch, S. I., et al. (2005). Telling truth from lie in individual subjects with fast event-related fMRI. *Human Brain Mapping, 26*(4), 262–272.

Langleben, D. D., Schroeder, L., Maldjian, J. A., Gur, R. C., McDonald, S., Ragland, J. D., et al. (2002). Brain activity during simulated deception: an event-related functional magnetic resonance study. *Neuroimage, 15*(3), 727–732.

Lee, T. M., Liu, H. L., Chan, C. C., Ng, Y. B., Fox, P. T., & Gao, J. H. (2005). Neural correlates of feigned memory impairment. *Neuroimage, 28*(2), 305–313.

Lee, T. M., Liu, H. L., Tan, L. H., Chan, C. C., Mahankali, S., Feng, C. M., et al. (2002). Lie detection by functional magnetic resonance imaging. *Human Brain Mapping, 15*(3), 157–164.

Lilienfeld, S. O., & Andrews, B. P. (1996). Development and preliminary validation of a self-report measure of psychopathic personality traits in noncriminal populations. *Journal of Personality Assessment, 66*(3), 488–524.

Lykken, D. T. (1960). The validity of the guilty knowledge technique: The effects of faking. *Journal of Applied Psychology 44*, 258–262.

Mohamed, F. B., Faro, S. H., Gordon, N. J., Platek, S. M., Ahmad, H., & Williams, J. M. (2006). Brain mapping of deception and truth telling about an ecologically valid situation: Functional MR imaging and polygraph investigation—Initial experience. *Radiology, 238*(2), 679–688.

Nunez, J. M., Casey, B. J., Egner, T., Hare, T., & Hirsch, J. (2005). Intentional false responding shares neural substrates with response conflict and cognitive control. *Neuroimage 25*(1), 267–277.

Phan, K. L., Magalhaes, A., Ziemlewicz, T. J., Fitzgerald, D. A., Green, C., & Smith, W. (2005). Neural correlates of telling lies: A functional magnetic resonance imaging study at 4 Tesla. *Academic Radiology, 12*(2), 164–172.

Spence, S. A., Farrow, T. F., Herford, A. E., Wilkinson, I. D., Zheng, Y., & Woodruff, P. W. (2001). Behavioural and functional anatomical correlates of deception in humans. *Neuroreport, 12*(13), 2849–2853.

Spence, S. A., Hunter, M. D., Farrow, T. F., Green, R. D., Leung, D. H., Hughes, C. J., et al. (2004). A cognitive neurobiological account of deception: Evidence from functional neuroimaging. *Philosophical Transactions of the Royal Society of London B Biological Sciences, 359*(1451), 1755–1762.

Szameitat, A. J., Schubert, T., Muller, K., & Von Cramon, D. Y. (2002). Localization of executive functions in dual-task performance with fMRI. *Journal of Cognitive Neuroscience, 14*(8), 1184–1199.

Talairach, J., & Tournoux, P. (1988). *Co-planar stereotaxic atlas of the human brain. 3-Dimensional proportional system: An approach to cerebral imaging.* New York: Thieme Medical.

Wager, T. D., & Smith, E. E. (2003). Neuroimaging studies of working memory: A meta-analysis. *Cognitive, Affective and Behavioral Neuroscience, 3*(4), 255–274.

Wild, J. (2005). Brain imaging ready to detect terrorists, say neuroscientists. *Nature 437*(7058), 457.

Yankee, W. J. (1995). The current status of research in forensic psychophysiology and its application in the psychophysiological detection of deception. *Journal of Forensic Science, 40*(1), 63–68.

PART II

COGNITIVE EFFORT ASSESSMENT TECHNIQUES AND STRATEGIES

CHAPTER 3

A Reconsideration of the Slick et al. (1999) Criteria for Malingered Neurocognitive Dysfunction

Kyle Brauer Boone

Until 15 years ago, the issue of detection of noncredible performance on cognitive testing was rarely addressed in the field of clinical neuropsychology. However, since that time, over 300 publications have appeared on this topic. In 1999, Slick and colleagues provided a comprehensive integration of this new information into well-reasoned guidelines for the diagnoses of malingered neurocognitive dysfunction (MND). They outline three categories of MND: (1) definite (characterized by external incentive to malinger and definite negative response bias [i.e., below-chance performance on one or more forced choice effort tests]); (2) probable (external incentive plus two or more effort test failures [excluding below-chance performance on forced-choice tests] or one effort test failure and one instance of noncredible self-reported symptom or test data discrepancy); and (3) possible (external incentive plus discrepant evidence from self-report).

However, before diagnostic algorithms are formally adopted, it is important that the field engage in continuing dialogue and refinement of issues in this controversial area. In particular, there are three aspects of the Slick, Sherman, and Iverson (1999) recommendations that are problematic in clinical practice: (1) the diagnosis of "malingering" per se, (2) the use of forced-choice measures as the only index of "definitive" suboptimal effort, and (3) the procedure of warning patients that effort measures will be administered.

29

SHOULD WE BE DIAGNOSING "MALINGERING"?

Slick et al. (1999) suggested that through use of their criteria, the presence of "malingered" neurocognitive deficits can be accurately diagnosed. According to their algorithm, patients who have "psychiatric, neurologic, or developmental factors" which could "fully account" for noncredible test performances and symptoms, such as "psychological need to play the sick role," are excluded from a diagnosis of MND. In the latter case, it is recommended that the patient be diagnosed with "feigned cognitive deficits secondary to [specify psychiatric/developmental/neurological disorder]" (p. 555). However, no further guidance is provided as to how to determine whether other conditions are in fact "fully" responsible for the suspect performances. Further, the authors assert that MND is "the volitional exaggeration or fabrication of cognitive dysfunction for the purpose of obtaining substantial material gain, or avoiding or escaping formal duty or responsibility" (p. 552), but no instruction is provided regarding how to determine whether the malingering behavior is truly "volitional."

Slick et al. (1999) do not specify the potential psychiatric, neurological, or developmental diagnoses which might serve as alternative diagnoses to MND. Research indicates that depression (see Goldberg, Back-Madruga, & Boone, Chapter 13, this volume), schizophrenia (see Goldberg, Back-Madruga, & Boone, Chapter 13, this volume), brain injury (Boone, Lu, & Herzberg, 2002a, 2002b; Slick, Hopp, Strauss, Hunter, & Pinch, 1994; Tombaugh, 1997), learning disability (Boone, Lu, & Herzberg, 2002a, 2002b), aphasia (Tombaugh, 1997), and epilepsy (Grote et al., 2000) are not typically associated with "failures" on effort tests. Thus, the presence of these disorders would not account for poor performance on effort tests.

In contrast, the most problematic differential diagnosis would appear to be between somatoform disorder and malingering. In somatoform disorder, "physical" symptoms are thought to be created unconsciously by the patient for psychological reasons and do not have a true "organic" basis. In both malingering and somatoform presentations the symptoms are not credible, but what theoretically differs between the two is whether the symptoms are consciously (i.e., malingering) or unconsciously (i.e., somatoform) created. Although the presence of fabricated cognitive symptomatology is underappreciated in current thought regarding somatoform disorders (e.g., there is no reference to fabricated cognitive complaints in the DMS-IV criteria for conversion disorder), examination of Freud's original writings on conversion disorder reveals that noncredible cognitive symptoms were an integral part of this condition; for example, "Freud's remarks about Frau Cecile von M indicate that her hysterical attacks and neuralgias were accompanied by reversible amnesia and clouding of consciousness" (Mace, 1994, p. 186). More recently, Liberini, Faglia, and Salvi (1993) described six patients with cognitive impairment which they determined to be "probably related to hysterical conversion reaction" (p. 325.) Similarly, Cicerone and Kalmar (1995) suggested that their subgroup of persistent postconcussive patients with "gross neuropsychological impairment and a level of functional disability that is strikingly disproportionate to their injury . . . may best be characterized as exhibiting a conversion pseudodementia" (p. 11). Finally, Bierley et al. (2001) described four patients who demonstrated chance or below-chance performance on recognition memory testing; none of the patients had external incentive to feign and test scores were associated with elevated somatic scores on a depression rating scale. Clearly, somatoform disorder needs to be ruled out before a diagnosis of malingered cognitive dysfunction can be made. However, we have no effective tools with which to accomplish this task.

Although forced-choice paradigms are frequently claimed to identify "malingering" (Bianchini, Mathias, & Greve, 2001), this technique was in fact originally used to identify conversion disorder (Pankratz, 1979). Denney (1999) recognized this dilemma: "As symptom validity testing was originally designed to detect conversion syndromes, one cannot automatically cry malingering when suppressed scores occur" (p. 16). Further, in hypnotized individuals, whose behavior is presumed not to be under conscious control, below-chance performance occurs in over 25% of those instructed to produce amnesia (Spanos, James, & de Groot, 1990). Erickson notes: "Ingenious procedures like Symptom Validity Testing . . . can establish the likelihood of motivated wrong answering but not conscious intent" (Pankratz & Erickson, 1990, p. 382). Miller (1999) elaborates: "The fact that those with hysterical sensory symptoms perform at below chance levels on forced choice testing does not necessarily mean that they are deliberately faking. It is conceptually possible that the same unconscious mechanisms that induce a subjective impression of, say, blindness, also unconsciously dispose the same individuals to opt for the incorrect stimulus on most trials" (p. 186).

By way of further example, it makes little conceptual sense that the act of producing a pseudoseizure (which can involve several minutes of thrashing and jerking in the absence of any abnormal electrical discharge) is generally accepted as a nonconscious behavior associated with conversion disorder (Stone, Sharpe, & Binzer, 2004), while offering a preponderance of incorrect answers on a forced-choice test is considered definitive evidence of "conscious" and deliberate symptom production. It has been argued that in the latter situation, the patient "knows" the correct answer and "chooses" not to provide it, but this could be the same type of "choice" a pseudoseizure patient makes when throwing him- or herself to the floor in a "seizure."

Other authors have recognized that cognitive effort tests in fact serve "double duty" in identifying symptom fabrication associated not only with malingering but also with care-seeking in somatoform conditions. Sweet and King (2002) recommend that cognitive effort tests be administered not just in "adversarial situations" (i.e., medical legal, disability seeking) but "in any clinical case in which motivation may be problematic ... [such as when] incredible or rare symptoms appear to have garnered sympathy or attention from family or significant others" (p. 263).

The reason for failed-effort test performance in both malingering and conversion disorder is addressed by Randolph (personal communication, December 13, 2006): "malingering and conversion behaviors must draw from the same pool of knowledge about what brain injury is like. That is, there is no reason to suspect that the subconscious ... has any special pool of knowledge about how to 'act brain-injured' that the conscious mind is not also privy to."

To use cognitive effort tests as indicators of malingering, empirical research would have to show that in fact only malingerers fail the measures. However, no such research exists, precisely because there are no verified, objective criteria available to assign subjects to malingering versus somatoform groups.

Unfortunately, personality inventories are similarly unhelpful in reliably differentiating between malingering and somatoform conditions. While the 1-3/3-1 Minnesota Multiphasic Personality Inventory (MMPI)/MMPI-2 codetype has been traditionally viewed as a "conversion" profile, Larrabee (1998) indicated that this codetype can also be indicative of "somatic malingering," or the deliberate feigning of physical symptoms, such as fatigue and malaise. According to DSM-IV, individuals engaging in malingering tend to have antisocial personality disorders, which suggests that malingering and somatoform presentations could be separated on the basis of antisocial characteristics in the former. However, the presence of noncredible performance on cognitive effort tests has not been found to be related to elevations on the antisocial scales of the MMPI (Greiffenstein, Gola, & Baker, 1995; Temple, McBride, Horner, & Taylor, 2003; Youngjohn, Burrows, & Erdal, 1995), the Millon Clinical Multiaxial Inventory (MCMI; Boone et al., 1995), and the Personality Assessment Inventory (PAI; Sumanti, Boone, Savodnik, & Gorsuch, 2006), casting doubt on the widespread presence of antisocial behavior in malingered cognitive symptoms. Gerson (2002) concludes that "the presence of antisocial personality disorder is neither necessary nor sufficient for consideration of malingering which may occur in any clinical or forensic context" (p. 61).

Similarly, brain imaging data have also not been able to discriminate somatoform/conversion behavior from deliberate feigning. Preliminary functional brain imaging studies have identified activation of an inhibitory role of the right anterior cingulate and/or right orbitofrontal cortex in the manifestation of conversion phenomena (Halligan, Athwal, Oakley, & Frackowiak, 2000; Marshall, Halligan, Fink, Wade, & Frackowiak, 1997; Tiihonen, Kuikka, Viinamaki, Lehtonen, & Partanen, 1995) and in hypnotic paralysis (Halligan et al., 2000), while anterior cingulate and frontal cortex have been found to show increased activity when subjects provide deceptive responses (Ganis, Kosslyn, Stose, Thompson, & Yurgelun-Todd, 2003; Kozel, Padgett, & George, 2004; Kozel, Revell, et al., 2004; Langleben et al., 2002). (Of interest, given that activation of right anterior cingulate and right prefrontal and orbitofrontal cortex is also observed during completion of the Stroop interference paradigm [Bench et al., 1993; Liddle, Friston, Frith, & Frackowiak, 1992; Pardo, Pardo, Janer, & Raichle, 1990], it would seem that the anterior cingulate is involved in overriding automatized/default behavior, of which "telling the truth" would be a subset.)

The aforementioned commonalities between malingering and somatoform/conversion presentations and the fact that no objective techniques are available to differentiate the two raise the obvious possibility that they are one and the same phenomenon. However, accumulated clinical experience indicates that there is at least a qualitative difference between patients who only "don" their symptoms when expedient (e.g., when undergoing medical evaluations) but otherwise engage in a symptom-free lifestyle, versus patients who adopt a chronic "patient role" as they navigate through life and who appear to believe in their symptoms.

Traditional psychoanalytic thought views somatoform conditions as a process of "conversion" of psychological conflict into physical symptoms; however, many authors criticize this formulation because the actual mechanism by which the conversion occurs is not specified and/or cannot be merged with current knowledge in cognitive science (Sierra & Berrios, 1999); "the notion that a psychological state directly causes an apparently physical symptom which the patient truly experiences as real (i.e., unfeigned) is very difficult to translate into an underlying mechanism" (Miller, 1999, p. 188). Alternatively, some authors have suggested that the nonconscious generation of nonorganic physical symptoms (and cognitive symptoms) could occur:

1. Within currently understood functions of the supervisory attention system (SAS) or central executive control system which allow an "autosuggestive disorder" (Oakley, 1999), or secondary to a dysfunction of an attentional-awareness system (Sierra & Berrios, 1999).

2. Due to an inhibitory mechanism, based in prefrontal physiology, which activates at an advanced stage of information processing (Sierra & Berrios, 1999).

3. In the presence of a dissociation between semantic and episodic representations of sensory perceptions (Kihlstrom, 1984, 1994).

4. With active use of cognitive strategies, or "constructive cognitions," which allow patients to integrate and resolve conflict between reality information and their beliefs in their supposed illness (Bryant & McConkey, 1999).

5. In a "cognitive-psychologically informed account of self-deception" based on a "failure to accurately appraise the subjectively available evidence (Turner, 1999, p. 193).

6. In social role taking in which perceptions, judgments, and memories tend to be biased in ways that benefit the self (Meridyth & Wallbrown, 1991).

7. Due to actions (or *in*actions) which the patient disavows, when faced with some overwhelming situation, which threatens the identify of the self (Spence, 1999).

8. In association with a "nocebo" effect (i.e., that the expectation of illness in fact causes illness) (Hahn, 1997) which emerges due to a combination of suggestion, somatization, rationalization, and contingent financial reward as one advocates for one's illness in the course of litigation (Bellamy, 1997).

9. In a "symptom magnification syndrome" which involves a "self-destructive pattern of behavior . . . learned and maintained through social reinforcement . . . the effect of which is to control the life circumstances of the sufferer" (Matheson, 1991, p. 45).

Even if malingering and somatoform disorders independently exist, the DSM-IV belief that they do not overlap is disputed. Many authors have in fact argued that "the distinction between conscious and unconscious symptom production is not clear" (Nies & Sweet, 1994), and that malingering and somatoform conditions are not mutually exclusive or dichotomous (Swanson, 1985) but instead lie on a continuum or gradient (Nadelson, 1979) anchored on one end by unconscious motivation and "self" deception, and on the other end by conscious and voluntary behavior associated with "other" deception (Cunnien, 1997; Ford, 1986; Ford & Smith, 1987; Gerson, 2002; Haines & Norris, 1995; Rohling, Langhinrichsen-Rohling, & Miller, 2003). Alternatively, self-deception and other-deception may lie on separate continua, with malingering related to low self-deception and high other-deception, somatoform conditions tied to high self-deception and low other-deception, and mixed malingering and somatoform conditions associated with at least moderate self- and other-deception. Even within a "pure" malingering category, feigning likely occurs on a graded continuum from mild to extreme (Rogers, 1988).

Some authors have elaborated on the complex interrelationships between conscious and nonconscious feigning. Travin and Potter (1984) assert:

> To the degree that the malingering act is an intact coping mechanism, and more closely related to the external world, it may be placed in the other deceiver category. When the malingering-like act, though adaptive to the external world, concordantly serves an unconscious need or defense in the intrapsychic world, it falls into the range of mixed or self-deceivers.

> . . . Malingering or malingering-like behavior is enmeshed in personalities with variegated elements of intact and disordered functioning with varying voluntary and involuntary components. (p. 196)

Others have also suggested that conscious misbehavior may be motivated by unconscious factors (Schenck, 1970; Folks, Ford, & Houck, 1990). Tombaugh (2002) comments: "Even when conscious deception occurs, it may not be possible to rule out that the fabrication served, at least in part, to preserve the person's psychological integrity by unconsciously serving other psychological needs" (p. 88). As Ensalada (2000) explains, "The determination of voluntariness does not establish intentionality; i.e., consciousness of actions and consciousness of motives are not necessarily related" (p. 744).

In addition, a patient's position on continuua may not necessarily be static over time. Stevens (1986) notes: "conscious and nonconscious elements are often commingled and vary in time and degree" (p. 249). Likewise, Gerson (2002) asserts: "a given patient may simultaneously demonstrate features of both disorders, or may shift from one to another over time" (p. 61). For example, some patients may appear more "somatoform" at the beginning of litigation but gradually shift into an apparent malingering presentation, initially providing an accurate and complete medical history to examiners but during subsequent examinations, "censoring" information perceived to be harmful to their case.

Even within the "nonconscious" category, there appear to at least two types of patients: (1) patients with likely conversion disorder who fabricate symptoms, as shown in some lowered cognitive scores and failed effort measures, and (2) a second group, more "hypochondriacal" in orientation, who pass effort indicators and show normal performance on cognitive tests but perceive that they are performing poorly on the tasks. For example, the latter group, when administered the Rey Auditory Verbal Learning Test (RAVLT), may spontaneously comment, "See, I told you I could not do this!" and actually start crying, although examination of objective scores reveals intact performance. (See Williamson, Drane, & Stroup, Chapter 15, this volume, for a further illustration of somatoform subgroups).

An additional problem with the DSM-IV view that somatoform disorders and malingering are nonoverlapping and mutually exclusive is that patients are precluded from carrying both diagnoses simultaneously, leading to some rather nonsensical possibilities. According to the DSM-IV, somatoform disorders are not diagnosed if a tangible external goal as a possible impetus for symptom creation is present. Using this reasoning, if a patient with a preexisting somatoform condition subsequently is involved in an accident and files a lawsuit involving the same symptoms as reflected in the somatoform condition, he or she would be instantly "cured" of the premorbid somatoform disorder. Conversion symptoms are not rare, with prevalence estimates of 20–25% for patients admitted to a general medical setting (Ford, 1983). There is no reason to believe that these individuals are any less likely to be involved in accidents or other types of litigated injuries than the general population. Greiffenstein and Baker (2001) in fact report that a sample of persistent postconcussive disorder patients showed a somatoform orientation (as evidenced by elevations on MMPI scales 1 and 3) *prior to* their injuries. Kay, Newman, Cavallo, Ezrachi, and Resnick (1992) argued that "conscious malingering is probably much less common than motivated but unconscious holding onto symptoms, which can be influenced by the very process of being in litigation" (p. 380). Thus, the co-occurrence of somato-form symptoms and presence of external gain clearly is not unusual. Berry (personal communication, April 27, 2002) drew attention to this issue through the use of the following table, which argues for the conceptual via-bility of the intersection of "external goal" and "unconscious" determinants of behavior:

	External goal	Internal goal
Conscious	Malingering	Factitious
Unconscious	X	Somatoform

Slick et al. (1999) assert that the clinician only has to determine whether a psychiatric, neurological, or developmental disorder "fully accounts" for the noncredible symptoms; if it does not, the diagnosis would be malinger-ing. But how is this assessment made and is it realistic? It would be reason-able to assume that any patient in litigation spends at least some time dis-cussing with his or her attorney the issue of monetary compensation. Would a several-minute conversation prompted by the attorney regarding financial reparations constitute enough of an "external incentive" to classify the patient as less than "fully" somatoform? According to the Slick et al. (1999) criteria, if we somehow determine a patient to be 99% somatoform and only 1% malingering, he or she would be consigned to the MND category. Con-versely, even a patient who is a "pure" malingerer at the outset of litigation could be expected to develop some "unconscious" maintenance of his or her symptoms due to the operation of such psychological processes as "diagnosis threat" (e.g., cognitive "deficits" are produced in a form of self-fulfilling prophecy in individuals who are told that the group of which they are a member [e.g., postconcussion] has such deficits; Suhr & Gunstad, 2002) and misattribution (e.g., postconcussive individuals "recall" their postconcussive symptoms as only occurring after the head injury and they mistakenly attri-bute the symptoms to the injury when in fact they experience the symp-toms at the same rates as nonconcussed individuals; Ferguson, Mittenberg, Barone, & Schneider, 1999).

In summary, despite the fact that somatoform/conversion phenomena have been described for over 100 years, we do not have data showing that they exist separately and are dichotomous from malingering, nor do we have objective techniques to objectively differentiate somatoform conditions from malingering. Thus, we are unable to follow the Slick et al. (1999) recommendation when diagnosing MND to rule out other psychiatric conditions including nonconscious impetuses to symptom production. As a result, to attempt to diagnose malingering is highly problematic. Miller (1999) concludes:

> Whether a true underlying distinction between hysteria and malingering exists or not, the fact that the two cannot at present be distinguished with reliability means that the issue of whether the symptom is genuinely experienced as opposed to being feigned is a highly unsatisfactory criterion to be used for diagnostic or classificatory purposes. (p. 186)

However, it is questionable whether in fact we even need to make a determination as to whether feigned symptoms are due to malingering or somatoform mechanisms. As clinical neuropsychologists, our mandate is to determine whether patients have objectively verified (i.e., credible) cognitive dysfunction. Using standard neuropsychological measures and currently available effort tests, we can do this well. In a litigation or disability setting, it is incumbent upon patients to provide evidence of cognitive dysfunction. If they fail effort tests, they have not done this. Whether or not patients believe in their symptoms is not particularly relevant. The core issue is symptom credibility; the "reason" for the lack of credibility may be a moot point.

It might be argued that if no determination is made between malingering and somatoform disorder, even if the claim of brain injury is discounted, all noncredible plaintiffs could still be awarded compensation for a somatoform disorder claimed to be caused by the accident. However, there is no literature documenting that somatoform conditions emerge in response to accidents or injuries. Instead, somatoform presentations appear to reflect a chronic characterological predisposition, and whether or not the full somatoform disorder develops seems not to be dictated by the presence of trauma but rather by the "need" for symptoms. Many somatoform patients experience various injuries in their lives but do not become symptomatic in terms of development of pseudophysical symptoms until a life situation emerges which the symptoms help solve; for example, the development of postaccident "physical" symptoms can enable a patient to exit a job that was associated with significant preaccident stress. Case in point, I evaluated a patient who recovered well from a moderate brain injury, quickly returning to a new job he enjoyed, but 9 years later, following an equivocal brain injury with no loss of consciousness, he failed to return to the occupation he now viewed as "boring" and a "dead-end" job.

If the field of clinical neuropsychology decides that it is important to determine to what extent cognitive symptoms are deliberately feigned, then a major research focus will need to be expended on developing techniques that can in fact do this. Our currently available "effort" tests only measure behavior, not the intention behind the behavior. As Tombaugh (2002) notes: "One potential solution to this problem in forensic assessments is to circumvent the entire issue of intentionality by viewing a low score as an indication that the person failed to put forth his/her best effort without attributing this motivational bias to any particular source" (p. 88).

In conclusion, we need to discard the terms "malingering" in all but the most rare circumstances in which there is incontrovertible evidence of malingering (asymptomatic behavior on surveillance tapes, patient admission of malingering, etc.). Instead, terms that describe behavior, not intent, such as "noncredible symptoms/performance," "negative response bias," and "nonphysiological, suspect or suboptimal effort," should be substituted.

Recommendations

It is recommended that the Slick et al. (1999) terminology be changed from "diagnosis of malingered neurocognitive function" to "determination of noncredible neurocognitive function."

USE OF FORCED-CHOICE MEASURES AS DEFINITIVE PROOF OF NONCREDIBLE PERFORMANCE

Slick et al. (1999) suggest that "definitive" malingered neurocognitive performance can only be determined by below-chance performance on forced-choice measures. Without below-chance scores, a patient can at most be diagnosed as displaying "probable" malingering.

However, these criteria are problematic, as discussed below, because they assume that below-chance performance is only found in malingerers, and that definitive noncredible performance can be based on results from a single measure. Further, they limit the diagnosis of definite noncredible performance to only "unsophisticated" patients.

Slick et al. (1999) view significantly below-chance performance on forced-choice measures as close to a "gold standard" for identifying malingering as we have aside from patient confession. Reynolds (1998) further argues that a below-chance score is "not a random or chance occurrence but represents a purposive distortion by the examinee" (p. 272). The assumption is that a patient can only perform significantly below chance is if he or she *consciously* provides incorrect answers. However, given that "significantly below chance" is defined as $p < .05$, a significantly below-chance performance theoretically could occur in 5 of 100 credible patients.

I am aware of three patients with severe, unequivocal cognitive impairment and no motive to feign who in fact scored significantly below chance on forced measures. The first patient was an inpatient whom I tested who had confusion secondary to vascular dementia, and who obtained a score of 20 of 50 on the Warrington Recognition Test—Faces subtest. The second patient had dementia secondary to mitrochondrial neurogastrointestinal encephalomyopathy and received a score of 11/50 on the Warrington Recognition Memory Test—Faces subtest, although he passed all other effort indicators (Wen, Boone, Sherman, & Long, 2005). Similarly, Ladowsky-Brooks and Fischer (2003) reported a case of frontotemporal dementia in which below-chance performance (0 of 50!) was observed on the Test of Memory Malingering (TOMM). These patients were not in litigation and had no motive to feign impairment and thus would not in fact be diagnosed as being malingerers using the Slick et al. (1999) criteria. However, the fact that actual patients with marked brain dysfunction can perform significantly below chance on a forced-choice paradigm is problematic for the Slick et al. (1999) algorithm.

Even if significantly below-chance performance on forced-choice testing was specific to malingering, there is evidence that it only detects a particular type of malingerer. Binder and Willis (1991) reported below-chance performance in only 2 of 13 simulators, while Wiggins and Brandt (1988) indicated that none of their 48 stimulators scored significantly below chance. Slick et al. (1994) documented that only 15% of feigning subjects scored below chance. In fact, most authors have found that most subjects feigning cognitive symptoms show above-chance levels of accuracy on forced-choice paradigms (Bianchini et al., 2001; Guilmette, Hart, & Giuliano, 1993; Guilmette, Hart, Giuliano, & Leninger, 1994; Greiffenstein, Baker, & Gola, 1994; Martin, Gouvier, Todd, Bolter, & Niccolls, 1992; Martin, Hayes, & Gouvier, 1996; Prigatano & Amin, 1993; Tombaugh, 1997). Cercy, Schretlen, and Brandt (1997) observed that significantly below-chance performance only occurs in "unsophisticated" individuals who do not intuit that significantly below-chance performance is not credible. Thus, using the Slick et al. (1999) algorithm, only "unsophisticated" suspect effort patients would ever be determined to be definitively noncredible.

Fortunately, there is an alternative to relying on a single, imperfect measure to determine "definitive" noncredible performance, namely, the administration of several, well-validated effort indices, as is currently recommended for clinical practice (Ashendorf, O'Bryant, & McCaffrey, 2003; Bush et al., 2005; Iverson & Binder, 2000; Spreen & Strauss, 1998; Thompson, 2002). If a patient fails several freestanding effort tests and exhibits a noncredible pattern on standard cognitive tests sensitive to feigning (as described in Chapters 6, 7, 8, and 9, this volume), and shows inconsistency between test scores within and across testing sessions and with performance on activities of daily living, it can be argued that this is definite noncredible performance.

If the false-positive rate on the effort techniques is set at 10% (by choosing cutoffs that have at least 90% specificity), and if the tests are uncorrelated, the chance that three abnormal scores could have occurred by "chance" would be 1 in 1,000 (i.e., $1/10 \times 1/10 \times 1/10$), while four abnormal scores would be associated with a probability of 1 in 10,000, and so on. Effort measures are at least modestly correlated with each other (Nelson et al., 2003); thus, the probability of several failed-effort indicators in a credible subject is higher than that for uncorrelated measures. However, Larrabee (2003) reported three-way combinations of effort indicators derived from standard neuropsychological measures which were associated with 100% specificity (no false positives), while our lab has found high specificity (96%; excluding patients with dementia and IQ < 70) associated with failure on two indicators (92% sensitivity; Victor & Boone, 2006). We have observed noncredible patients to fail as many as 8–12 such indicators, an extremely unlikely finding if due to chance. It can be argued that the use of several effort indicators in combination is more reflective of "definite" noncredible performance than any single effort test, including forced-choice measures, particularly when the former are supplemented by behavioral criteria (improbable injury outcome such as dementia following uncomplicated mild traumatic brain injury, inconsistency between scores and actual daily life functioning, etc.). Further, it is problematic to hinge our ability to diagnosis "definitive" noncredible performance on only one technique (i.e., forced choice) in which patients, unfortunately, can be readily coached.

Recommendations

It is recommended that the criteria for definite noncredible performance be determined by failure on at least three validated effort measures with minimal shared variance and with cutoffs set to ≥ 90% specificity, and behavioral evidence of noncredible symptoms (i.e., dramatic inconsistency between test scores and activities of daily living (ADLs) [e.g., very low scores but normal ADLs] and/or claimed diagnosis [e.g., dementia after mild traumatic brain injury], and/or across sequential exams).

SHOULD PATIENTS BE WARNED ABOUT THE ADMINISTRATION OF EFFORT TESTS?

Slick et al. (1999) suggest that patients be warned that effort tests will be included in the neuropsychological assessment. No rationale is provided for the directive; however, the recommendation appears to rest on the belief that (1) warnings are successful in reducing symptom fabrication, (2) warnings do not compromise standard testing procedures, and (3) it is improper and deceptive to administer effort tests without prior warning. However, these assumptions are problematic.

Youngjohn, Lees-Haley, and Binder (1999) have argued that warning subjects regarding the presence of effort measures within a test battery does not stop subjects from feigning but, instead, makes them more "savvy" in their approach and therefore more difficult to detect. They note that the performance of warned simulators was still below that of controls on memory indices, and in posttest interviews, warned simulators revealed that they still attempted to feign despite being alerted to the presence of effort measures. Gervais, Green, Allen, and Iverson (2001) found an initial failure rate of 41–42% on the CARB (Computerized Assessment of Response Bias) in pain patients, but when patients were told that pain does not have effect on the test, that the test is easy and they should not get much below 100%, and that if they did score much below 100% the examiner would question whether they were making an adequate effort, failure rate on the CARB dropped to 6%, although 34% of patients still failed the Word Memory Test (WMT), indicating that the patients were still faking, just not on the CARB. Gunstad and Suhr (2001) also observed that 80% of unwarned simulators were detected by an abbreviated version of the Portland Digit Recognition Test (PDRT), while only 35% of warned simulators were identified. In a previous study, a 32% detection rate for unwarned subjects versus 7% in warned malingerers was documented (Suhr & Gunstad, 2000). These findings emerged even though the warning was nonspecific and a full battery of cognitive tests was administered, not just the PDRT. Of particular concern was their finding that the only measure in the test battery which was associated with significantly better performance in the warned versus unwarned simulators was the forced-choice measure, "suggesting that the warned subjects recognized forced choice as a malingering test" (p. 415). They conclude: "individuals who receive a warning about malingering detection may suppress the tendency to do devastatingly poor on measures they perceived to be easy, and thus may better escape detection" (Gunstad & Suhr, 2001, p. 402). Other investigators have likewise failed to document a significant deterrent effect of warning (Johnson, Bellah, Dodge, Kelley, & Livingston, 1998; Sullivan, Keane, & Deffenti, 2001; Sullivan & Richer, 2002; Wong, Lerner-Poppen, & Durham, 1998). Thus, it would appear that warning may simply alert malingerers to be "on the lookout" for the effort tests and to raise their performance disproportionately on these measures as compared to the standard cognitive tasks, thereby increasing their chances of feigning successfully.

In addition, while warning does not appear to have the intended effect of diminishing feigned test performance, it may also render the examination nonstandard; that is, administration no longer conforms to that under which the tests comprising the battery were developed. Further, could there be a negative effect on patient–examiner rapport if credible patients are warned that they will be administered tests to confirm the veracity of their test responses? As Youngjohn et al. (1999) note, some patients may be offended if told that tests will be administered to see if they are faking.

It could be argued that we are "deceiving" patients by not warning them about the presence of effort measures in the neuropsychological test battery. However, in other professions within the medical field, no such warnings are given. For example, neurologists conduct tests during their exam to determine whether motor weakness is credible (e.g., "give-way" weakness), but neurology texts do not instruct neurologists to warn patients that these tests will be done. Similarly, specialized audiological tests can determine whether reported hearing loss is credible or feigned, but audiologists are not told to warn their patients of the existence of these checks. Further, occupational therapy literature recommends examination of grip strength patterns to assess for malingered symptoms, but there are no accompanying instructions informing patients that this will be implemented.

Even within the field of clinical psychology, there is no precedent for warning patients that efforts will be taken to determine the veracity of reported symptoms. Specifically, the MMPI-2 and MCMI-III include validity indices, but none of the test manuals or major reference texts recommend that patients be forewarned of the presence of these scales. The Structured Interview of Reported Symptoms specifically assesses for feigned psychotic symptoms, but patients are not informed of this fact. In fact, some have argued that providing patients with information regarding validity scales is in violation of ethical principles regarding test security (Wetter & Corrigan, 1995).

The recommendation that patients be warned specifically about the administration of "effort" tests may stem from the fact that traditionally these have been freestanding, single-purpose measures added to the neuropsychological battery, rather than a priori being built into standard neuropsychological tests such as was the case for the MMPI/MMPI-2. However, now several effective techniques for identifying suspect effort can be gleaned from standard neuropsychological instruments, such as Digit Span (see Chapter 6, this volume), Wisconsin Card Sorting Test (see Chapter 8, this volume), RAVLT recognition trial (see Chapter 7, this volume), RAVLT/RO discriminant function (Sherman, Boone, Lu, & Razani, 2002), finger tapping (see Chapter 9, this volume), and the Rey–Osterreith figure (Lu, Boone, Cozolino, & Mitchell, 2003), among others, making it possible to assess for effort without relying on specific effort tests. The field of clinical neuropsychology may well shift to relying on indices of effort from standard tests to circumvent the coaching by attorneys on freestanding effort tests (e.g., it is likely harder to coach a patient to perform credibly on a RAVLT/RO discriminant function than the TOMM). In the situation in which the same tests are used to measure effort but also cognitive skills, would the psychologist still be encouraged to warn about embedded effort indices?

Perhaps the impetus to warn about the presence of measures of effort arises from the ethical mandate to obtain informed consent from patients prior to evaluation, which may include informing patients regarding the potential risks from participating in the testing (Johnson-Greene, 2005). Various negative consequences can accompany the finding that a patient was not credible on neuropsychological testing, including reduced monetary compensation in personal injury litigation. However, it can be argued that patients do not have to be specifically warned regarding the risks of providing fraudulent data. There is an understood social contract that when one is queried by medical professionals regarding injuries from an accident or deficits that interfere with one's ability to work, one is to provide truthful responses. In fact, there are numerous circumstances in our society in which citizens can be punished for fraudulent or otherwise untruthful behavior, the consequences of which they are not specifically warned about a priori. For example, when witnesses are placed under oath prior to testifying, they are instructed to "tell the truth, the whole truth, and nothing but the truth" but are not specifically warned regarding the consequences of perjury, which can include incarceration. Why should a psychologist be held to a different standard of disclosure? Further, if we are to warn patients regarding the possible negative consequences of being caught if they feign symptoms, should not we also warn them of the unanticipated ramifications if they in fact successfully feign symptoms? For example, if examiners accept dementia-level scores as valid, patients' driver's licenses can be taken away, children could be removed from their care, they might not be allowed to handle their own finances or sign legal documents, and so on.

The desire to forewarn may arise from the observation that some patients who likely have credible injuries are found to be feigning on effort testing. This subset of patients may be motivated by the concern that the examiner will not detect their very real problems, and they may exaggerate cognitive deficits in an attempt to ensure that their difficulties are in fact documented by the examiner. In response to this concern, it is recommended that the following admonition, or one similar, be included in the informed consent process:

> "The importance of performing with my best effort on the testing has been explained to me. While some patients might be disposed to exaggerate problems on testing as way of making sure their problems are well-documented, I have been informed that this, rather than helping my case, may actually make my test profile more problematic to interpret."

Ideally, this will stop the essentially truthful patient from attempting to "stack the deck" without directly informing about the presence of effort tests. If patients fail effort tests after receiving this caution, it can be reasonably assumed that (1) they themselves do not believe that they have detectable cognitive problems that would be documented on objective testing if they applied their best effort (e.g., if one truly has a fractured leg, would one malinger on physical exam?), and (2) they do not in fact want the examiner to accurately document their cognitive abilities (i.e., that their skills are intact).

Recommendations

Due to concerns regarding the impact of warnings on effort test performance, several authors are recommending that clinicians should not including warnings in their evaluations of patients (Youngjohn et al., 1999; Victor & Abeles, 2004; Wong et al., 1998). Although it would be prudent that the neuropsychologist encourage patients to perform with their best efforts on testing, patients should not be warned regarding the presence of effort indices within the battery.

REFERENCES

Ashendorf, L., O'Bryant, S. E., & McCaffrey, R. J. (2003). Specificity of malingering detection strategies in older adults using the CVLT and WCST. *The Clinical Neuropsychologist, 17*, 255–262.

Bellamy, R. (1997). Compensation neurosis: Financial reward for illness as nocebo. *Clinical Orthopaedics and Related Research, 336*, 94–106.

Bench, C. J., Frith, C. D., Grasby, P. M., Friston, K. J., Paulsen, E., Frackowiak, R. S. J., et al. (1993). Investigations of the functional anatomy of attention using the Stroop test. *Neuropsychologia, 31*, 907–922.

Bianchini, K. J., Mathias, C. W., & Greve, K. W. (2001). Symptom validity testing: A critical review. *The Clinical Neuropsychologist, 15*, 19–45.

Bierley, R. A., Drake, A. I., Ahmed, S., Date, E. S., Rosner, M., Warden, D., et al. (2001). Biased responding: A case series demonstrating a relationship between somatic symptoms and impaired recognition memory performance for traumatic brain injured individuals. *Brain Injury, 15*, 697–714.

Binder, L. M., & Willis, S. C. (1991). Assessment of motivation after financially compensable minor head trauma. *Psychological Assessment, 3*, 175–181.

Boone, K., Lu, P., & Herzberg, D. (2002a). *The b Test: Manual.* Los Angeles: Western Psychological Services.

Boone, K., Lu, P., & Herzberg, D. (2002b). *Rey Dot Counting Test: A handbook.* Los Angeles: Western Psychological Services.

Boone, K. B., Savodnik, I., Ghaffarian, S., Lee, A., Freeman, D., & Berman, N. (1995). Rey 15-item memorization and dot counting scores in a "stress" claim workers' compensation population: Relationship to personality (MCMI) scores. *Journal of Clinical Psychology, 51*, 457–463.

Bryant, R. A., & McConkey, K. M. (1999). Functional blindness: A construction of cognitive and social influences. *Cognitive Neuropsychiatry, 4*, 227–242.

Bush, S. S., Ruff, R. M., Troster, A. I., Barth, J. T., Koffler, S. P., Pliskin, N. H., et al. (2005). Symptom validity assessment: Practice issues and medical necessity (NAN Policy and Planning Committee). *Archives of Clinical Neuropsychology, 20*, 419–426.

Cercy, S. P., Schretlen, D. J., & Brandt, J. (1997). Simulated amnesia and the pseudo-memory phenomena. In R. Rogers (Ed.), *Clinical assessment of malingering and deception* (2nd ed., pp. 85–107). New York: Guilford Press.

Cicerone, K. D., & Kalmar, K. (1995). Persistent postconcussion syndrome: The structure of subjective complaints after mild traumatic brain injury. *Journal of Head Trauma Rehabilitation, 10,* 1–17.

Cunnien, A. (1997). Psychiatric and medical syndromes associated with deception. In R. Rogers (Ed.), *Clinical assessment of malingering and deception* (2nd ed., pp. 23–46). New York: Guilford Press.

Denney, R. L. (1999). A brief symptom validity testing procedure for Logical Memory of the Wechsler Memory Scale–Revised which can demonstrate verbal memory in the fact of claimed disability. *Journal of Forensic Neuropsychology, 1,* 5–26.

Ensalada, L. H. (2000). The importance of illness behavior in disability management. *Occupational Medicine, 15,* 739–754.

Ferguson, R. J., Mittenberg, W., Barone, D. F., & Schneider, B. (1999). Post-concussion syndrome following sport-related head injury: Expectation as etiology. *Neuropsychology, 13,* 582–589.

Folks, D. G., Ford, C. V., & Houck, C. A. (1990). Somatoform disorders, factitious disorders, and malingering. In A. Stoudemire (Ed.), *Clinical psychiatry for medical students.* New York: Lippincott.

Ford, C. V. (1983). *The somatizing disorders: Illness as a way of life.* New York: Elsevier.

Ford, C. V. (1986). The somatizing disorders. *Psychosomatics, 27,* 327–337.

Ford, C. V., & Smith, G. R. (1987). Somatoform disorders, factitious disorders, and disability syndromes. In A. Stoudemire & B. S. Fogel (Eds.), *Principles of medical psychiatry.* New York: Grune & Stratton.

Ganis, G., Kosslyn, S. M., Stose, S., Thompson, W. L., & Yurgelun-Todd, D. A. (2003). Neural correlates of different types of deception: An fMRI investigation. *Cerebral Cortex, 13,* 830–836.

Gerson, A. R. (2002). Beyond DSM-IV: A meta-review of the literature on malingering. *American Journal of Forensic Psychology, 20,* 57–69.

Gervais, R. O., Green, P., Allen, L. M., & Iverson, G. L. (2001). Effects of coaching on symptom validity testing in chronic pain patients presenting for disability assessments. *Journal of Forensic Neuropsychology, 2,* 1–19.

Greiffenstein, M. F., & Baker, J. W. (2001). Descriptive analysis of premorbid MMPI-2 profiles in chronic postconcussive patients. *Journal of the International Neuropsychological Society, 7,* 181.

Greiffenstein, M. F., Baker, J. W., & Gola, T. (1994). Validation of malingered amnesic measures with a large clinical sample. *Psychological Assessment, 6,* 218–224.

Greiffenstein, M. F., Gola, T., & Baker, J. W. (1995). MMPI-2 validity scales versus domain specific measures in detection of factitious traumatic brain injury. *The Clinical Neuropsychologist, 9,* 230–240.

Grote, C. L., Kooker, E. K., Garron, D. C., Nyenhuis, D. L., Smith, C. A., & Mattingly, M. L. (2000). Performance of compensation seeking and non-compensation seeking samples on the Victoria Symptom Validity Test: Cross-validation and extension of a standardization study. *Journal of Clinical and Experimental Neuropsychology, 6,* 709–719.

Guilmette, T. J., Hart, K. L., & Giuliano, A. J. (1993). Malingering detection: The use of a forced-choice method in identifying organic versus simulated memory impairment. *The Clinical Neuropsychologist, 7,* 59–69.

Guilmette, T. J., Hart, K. L., Giuliano, A. J., & Leninger, B. E. (1994). Detecting simulated memory impairment: Comparison of the Rey Fifteen-Item Test and the Hiscock Forced-Choice Procedure. *The Clinical Neuropsychologist, 8,* 283–294.

Gunstad, J., & Suhr, J. A. (2001). Efficacy of the full and abbreviated forms of the Portland Digit Recognition Test: Vulnerability to coaching. *The Clinical Neuropsychologist, 15,* 397–404.

Hahn, R. A. (1997). The nocebo phenomenon: Concept, evidence, and implications for public health. *Preventive Medicine, 26,* 607–611.

Haines, M. E., & Norris, M. P. (1995). Detecting the malingering of cognitive deficits: An update. *Neuropsychology Review, 5,* 125–148.

Halligan, P. W., Athwal, B. S., Oakley, D. A., & Frackowiak, R. S. (2000). Imaging hypnotic paralysis: implications for conversion hysteria. *The Lancet, 355,* 986–987.

Iverson, G. L., & Binder, L. M. (2000). Detecting exaggeration and malingering in neuropsychological assessment. *Journal of Head Trauma Rehabilitation, 15,* 829–858.

Johnson, J. L., Bellah, C. G., Dodge, T., Kelley, W., & Livingston, M. M. (1998). Effect of warning on feigned malingering on the WAIS-R in college samples. *Perceptual and Motor Skills, 87,* 152–154.

Johnson-Greene, D. (2005). Informed consent in clinical neuropsychology practice. Official statement of the National Academy of Neuropsychology. *Archives of Clinical Neuropsychology, 20,* 335–340.

Kay, T., Newman, B., Cavallo, M., Ezrachi, O., & Resnick, M. (1992). Toward a neuropsychological model of functional disability after mild traumatic brain injury. *Neuropsychology, 6,* 371–384.

Kihlstrom, J. F. (1984). Commentary: Psychodynamics and social cognition—Notes on the fusion of psychoanalysis and psychology. *Journal of Personality, 62,* 681–696.

Kihlstrom, J. F. (1994). One hundred years of hysteria. In S. J. Lynn & J. W. Rhue (Eds.), *Dissociation: Clinical and theoretical perspectives* (pp. 365–394). New York: Guilford Press.

Kozel, F. A., Padgett, T. M., & George, M. S. (2004). A replication study of the neural correlates of deception. *Behavioral Neuroscience, 118,* 852–856.

Kozel, F. A., Revell, L. J., Lorberbaum, J. P., Shawstri, A., Elhia, J. D., Horner, M. D., et al. (2004). A pilot study of functional magnetic resonance imaging brain correlates of deception in healthy young men. *Journal of Neuropsychiatry and Clinical Neurosciences, 16,* 295–305.

Ladowsky-Brooks, R. L., & Fischer, C. E. (2003). Ganser symptoms in a case of frontal-temporal lobe dementia: Is there a common neural substrate? *Journal of Clinical and Experimental Neuropsychology, 25,* 761–768.

Langleben, D. D., Schroeder, L., Maldjian, J. A., Gur, R. C., McDonald, S., Ragland, J. D., et al. (2002). Brain activity during simulated deception: An event-related functional magnetic resonance study. *Neuroimage, 15,* 727–732.

Larrabee, G. (1998). Somatic malingering on the MMPI and MMPI-2 in personal injury litigants. *The Clinical Neuropsychologist, 12,* 179–188.

Larrabee, G. (2003). Detection of malingering using atypical performance patterns on standard neuropsychological tests. *The Clinical Neuropsychologist, 17,* 410–425.

Liberini, P., Faglia, L., & Salvi, F. (1993). Cognitive impairment related to conversion disorder: A two-year follow-up study. *Journal of Nervous and Mental Disease, 181,* 325–327.

Liddle, P. F., Friston, K. J., Frith, C. D., & Frackowiak, R. S. J. (1992). Cerebral blood flow and mental processes in schizophrenia. *Journal of the Royal Society of Medicine, 85,* 224–227.

Lu, P., Boone, K. B., Cozolino, L., & Mitchell, C. (2003). Effectiveness of the Rey-Osterrieth Complex Figure Test and the Meyers and Meyers Recognition Trial in the detection of suspect effort. *The Clinical Neuropsychologist, 17,* 426–440.

Mace, C. J. (1994). Reversible cognitive impairment related to conversion disorder. *Journal of Nervous and Mental Disease, 182,* 186–187.

Marshall, J. C., Halligan, P. W., Fink, G. R., Wade, D. T., & Frackowiak, R. S. (1997). The functional anatomy of a hysterical paralysis. *Cognition, 64,* B1–B8.

Martin, R. C., Gouvier, D., Todd, M. E., Bolter, J. F., & Niccolls, R. (1992). Effects of task instruction on malingered memory performance. *Forensic Reports, 5,* 393–397.

Martin, R. C., Hayes, J. S., & Gouvier, W. D. (1996). Differential vulnerability between postconcussion self-report and objective malingering tests in identifying simulated mild head injury. *Journal of Clinical and Experimental Neuropsychology, 18,* 265–275.

Matheson, L. N. (1991). Symptom magnification syndrome structured interview: Rationale and procedure. *Journal of Occupational Rehabilitation, 1,* 43–56.

Meridyth, S. P., & Wallbrown, F. H. (1991). Reconsidering response sets, test-taking attitudes, dissimulation, self-deception, and social desirability. *Psychological Reports, 69,* 891–905.

Miller, E. (1999). Conversion hysteria: Is it a viable concept? *Cognitive Neuropsychiatry, 4,* 181–191.

Nadelson, T. (1979). The Munchausen syndrome: Borderline characterological features. *General Hospital Psychiatry, AP, 1,* 11–17.

Nelson, N. W., Boone, K., Dueck, A., Wagener, L., Lu, P., & Grills, C. (2003). Relationship between eight measures of suspect effort. *The Clinical Neuropsychologist, 17,* 263–272.

Nies, K. J., & Sweet, J. J. (1994). Neuropsychological assessment and malingering: A critical review of past and present strategies. *Archives of Clinical Neuropsychology, 9,* 501–552.

Oakley, D. (1999). Hypnosis and conversion hysteria: A unifying model. *Cognitive Neuropsychiatry, 4,* 243–266/

Pankratz, L. (1979). Symptom validity testing and symptom retraining: Procedures for the assessment and treatment of functional sensory deficits. *Journal of Consulting and Clinical Psychology, 47,* 409–410.

Pankratz, L., & Erickson, R. C. (1990). Two views of malingering. *The Clinical Neuropsychologist, 4,* 379–389.

Pardo, J. V., Pardo, P. J., Janer, K. W., & Raichle, M. E. (1990). The anterior cingulate cortex mediates processing selection in the Stroop attentional conflict paradigm. *Proceedings of the National Academy of Sciences, USA, 87,* 256–259.

Prigatano, G. P., & Amin, K. (1993). Digit memory test: Unequivocal cerebral dysfunction and suspected malingering. *Journal of Clinical and Experimental Neuropsychology, 15,* 537–546.

Reynolds, C. R. (1998). Common sense, clinicians, and actuarialism. In C. R. Reynolds (Ed.), *Detection of malingering during head injury litigation* (pp. 261–286). New York: Plenum Press.

Rogers, R. (1988). *Clinical assessment of malingering and deception.* New York: Guilford Press.

Rohling, M. L., Langhinrichsen-Rohling, J., & Miller, L. S. (2003). Actuarial assessment of malingering: Rohling's interpretive In R. Franklin (Ed.), *Prediction in forensic and neuropsychology.* Hillsdale, NJ: Erlbaum.

Schneck, J. M. (1970). Pseudomalingering and Leonid Andreyeus' "The Dilemma"? *Psychiatric Questions*, *44*, 49–54.

Sherman, D. S., Boone, K. B., Lu, P., & Razani, J. (2002). Re-examination of a Rey Auditory Verbal Learning Test/Rey Complex Figure discriminant function to detect suboptimal effort. *The Clinical Neuropsychologist*, *16*, 242–250.

Sierra, M., & Berrios, G. E. (1999). Towards a neuropsychiatry of conversive hysteria. *Cognitive Neuropsychiatry*, *4*, 267–287.

Slick, D., Hopp, G., Strauss, E., Hunter, M., & Pinch, D. (1994). Detecting dissimulation: Profiles of simulated malingerers, traumatic brain-injury patients, and normal controls on a revised version of Hiscock and Hiscock's forced-choice memory test. *Journal of Clinical and Experimental Neuropsychology*, *16*, 472–481.

Slick, D. J., Sherman, E. M., & Iverson, G. L. (1999). Diagnostic criteria for malingered neurocognitive dysfunction: Proposed standards for clinical practice and research. *The Clinical Neuropsychologist*, *13*, 545–561.

Spanos, N., James, B., & de Groot, H. (1990). Detection of simulated hypnotic amnesia. *Journal of Abnormal Psychology*, *99*, 179–182.

Spence, S. A. (1999). Hysterical paralyses as disorders of actions. *Cognitive Neuropsychiatry*, *4*, 203–226.

Spreen, O., & Strauss, E. (1998). *A compendium of neuropsychological tests: Administration, norms, and commentary* (2nd ed.). New York: Oxford University Press.

Stevens, H. (1986). Is it organic or is it functional? Is it hysteria or malingering? *Psychiatric Clinics of North American*, *9*, 241–254.

Stone, J., Sharpe, M., & Binzer, M. (2004). Motor conversion symptoms and pseudoseizures: A comparison of clinical characteristics. *Psychosomatics*, *45*, 492–499.

Suhr, J. A., & Gunstad, J. (2000). The effects of coaching on the sensitivity and specificity of malingering measures. *Archives of Clinical Neuropsychology*, *15*, 415–424.

Suhr, J. A., & Gunstad, J. (2002). "Diagnosis threat": The effect of negative expectations on cognitive performance in head injury. *Journal of Clinical and Experimental Neuropsychology*, *24*, 448–457.

Sullivan, K. A., Keane, B., & Deffenti, C. (2001). Malingering on the RAVLT: Part 1. Deterrence strategies. *Archives of Clinical Neuropsychology*, *16*, 627–641.

Sullivan, K., & Richer, C. (2002). Malingering on subjective complaint tasks: An exploration of the deterrent effects of warning. *Archives of Clinical Neuropsychology*, *17*, 691–708.

Sumanti, M., Boone, K. B., Savodnik, I., & Gorsuch, R. (2006). Noncredible psychiatric and cognitive symptoms in a Worker's Compensation "Stress" claim sample. *The Clinical Neuropsychologist*, *20*, 754–765.

Swanson, D. A. (1985). Malingering and associated syndromes. *Psychiatric Medicine*, *2*, 287–293.

Sweet, J., & King, J. (2002). Category test validity indicators: Overview and practice recommendations. *Journal of Forensic Neuropsychology*, *3*, 241–274.

Temple, R. O., McBride, A. M., Horner, M. D., & Taylor, R. M. (2003). Personality characteristics of patients showing suboptimal cognitive effort. *The Clinical Neuropsychologist*, *17*, 402–409.

Thompson, G. B. (2002). The Victoria Symptom Validity Test: An enhanced test of symptom validity. *Journal of Forensic Neuropsychology*, *2*, 43–67.

Tiihonen, J., Kuikka, J., Viinamaki, H., Lehtonen, J., & Partanen, J. (1995). Altered cerebral blood flow during hysterical paresthesia. *Biological Psychiatry, 37,* 134–135.

Tombaugh, T. N. (1997). The Test of Memory Malingering (TOMM): Normative data from cognitively intact and cognitively impaired individuals. *Psychological Assessment, 9,* 260–268.

Tombaugh, T. N. (2002). The Test of Memory Malingering (TOMM) in forensic psychology. *Journal of Forensic Neuropsychology, 2,* 69–96.

Travin, S., & Protter, P. (1984). Malingering and malingering-like behavior: Some clinical and conceptual issues. *Psychiatric Quarterly, 56,* 189–197.

Turner, M. (1999). Malingering, hysteria and the factitious disorders. *Cognitive Neuropsychiatry, 4,* 193–202.

Victor, T. L., & Abeles, N. (2004). Coaching clients to take psychological and neuropsychological tests: A clash of ethical obligations. *Professional Psychology, 35,* 373–379.

Victor, T., & Boone, K. (2006). *Using multiple measures of effort: Certain test combinations yield the most accurate results.* Poster presented at the International Neuropsychological Society Annual Conference.

Wen, J., Boone, K., Sherman, D., & Long, A. (2005). *Neuropsychological sequelae of mitochondrial neurogastrointestinal encephalomyopathy (MNGIE): Case report.* Poster presented at the International Neuropsychological Society Annual Conference.

Wetter, M. W., & Corrigan, S. K. (1995). Providing information to clients about psychological tests: A survey of attorneys' and law students' attitudes. *Professional Psychology: Research and Practice, 26,* 474–477.

Wiggins, E. C., & Brandt, J. (1988). The detection of simulated amnesia. *Law and Human Behavior, 12,* 57–78.

Wong, J. L., Lerner-Poppen, L., & Durham, J. (1998). Does warning reduce obvious malingering on memory and motor tasks in college samples. *International Journal of Rehabilitation and Health, 4,* 153–165.

Youngjohn, J. R., Burrows, L., & Erdal, K. (1995). Brain damage or compensation neurosis? The controversial post-concussion syndrome. *The Clinical Neuropsychologist, 9,* 112–123.

Youngjohn, J. R., Lees-Haley, P. R., & Binder, L. M. (1999). Comment: Warning malingerers produces more sophisticated malingering. *Archives of Clinical Neuropsychology, 14,* 511–515.

CHAPTER 4

Spoiled for Choice

Making Comparisons between Forced-Choice Effort Tests

Paul Green

The widespread acceptance of the need for objective tests of symptom validity in clinical neuropsychology is reflected in a recent position paper from the National Academy of Neuropsychology (Bush et al., 2005). The authors state that *"an adequate assessment of response validity is essential in order to maximize confidence in the results of neurocognitive and personality measures"* (p. 419). It is stated that measures of symptom validity are "medically necessary" if the assessment itself is medically necessary. However, the authors do not attempt to provide guidance on the selection of methods for determining symptom validity. This is understandable because there is limited empirical research in which one method has been compared with another in the same groups of patients.

According to the Slick, Sherman, and Iverson (1999) criteria for malingered neurocognitive dysfunction, the use of at least one symptom validity test (SVT) or effort test is central to the definition of both definite and probable malingering. The authors stipulate that such tests must be well validated. On the other hand, SVTs differ from each other in their levels of sensitivity to poor effort, sometimes to a major degree, as we see later, and the meaning of "well-validated" is not obvious. The use of SVTs with different levels of sensitivity to poor effort and specificity could result in differences of opinion about the validity of the data in many cases (Green, 2001). In fact, differences in understanding of what it is that SVTs measure can also lead to differences of opinion. This chapter explores the problem, using large datasets from actual patients given more than one SVT.

THE EFFECTS OF EFFORT

It is now widely accepted that we need SVTs to measure effort (Iverson & Binder, 2000) because *the amount of effort a person makes has been shown to affect neuropsychological test scores* to a major degree. Research has documented that the Word Memory Test (WMT; Green & Astner, 1995; Green, 2003b) is failed more often by people with mild than with severe brain injury (Green, Iverson, & Allen, 1999). Cases with mild head injury failing the WMT score far lower across a large test battery than those with genuinely severe brain injury whose effort was good (Green, Rohling, Lees-Haley, & Allen, 2001). In the latter study, 50% of test battery variance in 904 patients of various diagnoses was explained by effort, whereas education explained only 11% of the variance and brain injury severity explained less than 5%. Equally large effects of effort were found in patients with seizures or psychological nonepileptic seizures by Drane et al. (2006), leading them to conclude that effort, as measured by the WMT, had a far greater effect on test scores than did diagnosis. Similarly, Constantinou, Bauer, Ashendorf, Fisher, and McCaffrey (2005) reported that effort measured by the Test of Memory Malingering (TOMM; Tombaugh, 1996) explained 47% of the variance in a summary score from the Halstead–Reitan battery in groups of litigators with mild head injuries. One implication of such findings is that the mean group scores from many past studies, particularly of mild brain injury, were probably erroneous because of unidentified poor effort.

Effort tests are used today mainly because *they help us to determine whether effort is sufficient to produce valid data and, hence, whether other test data are likely to be valid*. Much rests on the validity of neuropsychological test data and thus it is necessary to ask how well one effort test compares with another in predicting whether or not other test data are valid. There are some studies in which several effort tests have been used with the same subjects, ensuring that sample characteristics cannot explain differences between results on one SVT versus the other. For example, Tan, Slick, Strauss, and Hultsch (2002), in a study comparing three well-known effort tests (TOMM, WMT, Victoria Symptom Validity Test; Slick, Hopp, Strauss, & Thompson, 1996), observed that the WMT was the most accurate, achieving 100% effectiveness in discriminating between simulators and good-effort volunteers. Merten, Green, Henry, Blaskewitz, and Brockhaus (2005) compared several methods for evaluating effort, including German adaptations of the Amsterdam Short-Term Memory Test (ASTM; Schmand & Lindeboom, 2005) and the Medical Symptom Validity Test (MSVT; Green, 2004), and found both the ASTM and MSVT to be highly accurate and approximately equivalent in differentiating between known simulators and good-effort cases. However, other methods, such as the ratio of Trailmaking A to B, were no better than chance at identifying the known poor-effort volunteers.

Such simulator studies have an important role to play because they allow us to assess the accuracy of effort tests in classifying effort in cases known to be making either a good or a poor effort. However, comparative data on SVTs are also needed in clinical and forensic settings. In the following sections, the WMT, the TOMM, the MSVT, and the Computerized Assessment of Response Bias (CARB; Conder, Allen, & Cox, 1992; Allen, Conder, Green, & Cox, 1997) are compared with each other.

COMPARING TOMM AND WMT

Gervais, Rohling, Green, and Ford (2004) studied 519 consecutive compensation-seeking cases given the TOMM, the WMT, and the CARB. The failure rates in their sample were 11% on the TOMM, 17% on the CARB, and 32% on the WMT effort subtests. These differences are important because, in clinical assessments, it would usually be concluded that a person's neuropsychological test results are of doubtful validity if an effort test is failed. If so, should we assume that unreliable test data were present in 32% of cases, as suggested by the WMT failure rate, or in only 11% of cases, as suggested by the TOMM?

Gervais et al. (2004) concluded that the differences in SVT failure rates were best explained by the WMT being more sensitive to poor effort than the TOMM. The distinction was not between *either* those failing the TOMM *or* those failing the WMT because *all those failing the TOMM also failed the WMT*, apart from one case. Yet there were 109 cases who failed the WMT but who did not fail the TOMM (i.e., 21% of all cases). Gervais et al. (2004) pointed out that, in those cases passing the TOMM but failing the WMT, the results from the CARB independently suggested poor effort. Also, *there were significant decrements in the overall neuropsychological test scores in those who passed the TOMM but failed the WMT*, compared with cases passing all three effort tests. There were even greater decrements in those who failed both the WMT and the TOMM, suggesting that poor effort in that study was a matter of degree.

A later database kindly provided for analysis by Dr. Roger Gervais (private practice, Edmonton, Alberta, Canada) contained data from over a thousand consecutive patients given both the TOMM and the WMT ($n = 1,046$, including the original 519 cases). Table 4.1 shows agreement between the TOMM and the WMT in this enlarged sample. A failing score on the TOMM was defined by a score on trial 2 of less than 45 correct out of 50 (i.e., < 90% correct). A failure on the WMT was determined when any one of the primary effort scores (immediate recognition, delayed recognition, or consistency between the two) was 82.5% or lower.[1]

TABLE 4.1. Agreement between TOMM and WMT in 1,315 Patients Given Both Tests

| | WMT | | | | | |
| | Gervais data, Canada | | Moss data, England | | Samples 1 and 2 combined | |
TOMM	Pass	Fail	Pass	Fail	Pass	Fail
Pass	698	240	122	90	820	330
Fail	6	102	2	55	8	157

Agreement between the two tests with regard to good versus poor effort in the Gervais sample was 76%. That is, they disagreed in 24% of cases or roughly a quarter of the sample. *In particular, 240 (23% of all cases) passed the TOMM and failed the WMT.* In contrast, less than 1% of cases (6 of 1,046) passed the TOMM but failed the WMT.

Very similar results were independently obtained by Alan Moss of Birmingham, England (personal communication, March, 2006), despite minimal overlap between the diagnoses of patients in these two studies. His sample was composed of 269 people making personal injury claims, almost entirely for traumatic brain injury. In contrast, only 3% (*n* = 35) of the Gervais sample had a diagnosis of traumatic brain injury; the majority were diagnosed with major depression (*n* = 151), anxiety-based disorders, including posttraumatic stress disorders (*n* = 273), pain disorders, including fibromyalgia (*n* = 337) and orthopedic injuries (*n* = 166). However, nearly all had some financial incentive to exaggerate their symptoms, in that they had claims for disability of one sort or another.

In both samples combined (Table 4.1), fewer than 1 of every 186 cases (8 of 1,315) failed the TOMM and passed the WMT. However, 25% of all cases failed the WMT and passed the TOMM (330 of 1,315). I argue later that these results are best explained by "false negatives" for the TOMM (i.e., TOMM scores suggesting good effort, when poor effort and invalid test data may be proven by other means).

For example, Table 4.2 shows the percentage of failures on the TOMM for each level of effort on the WMT in the Gervais sample. The lowest WMT scores were *at or below the chance mean score of 50%, with an average of only 44% correct.* It is striking that 30% of this group passed the TOMM! Similarly, in the Moss sample, there were 12 subjects with WMT scores below 50% (mean 39% correct) and 3 of them (i.e., 25%) passed the TOMM. These are clear examples of false-negative classifications by the TOMM. No one could reasonably argue that mean scores below 50% on WMT immediate recognition (IR) or delayed recognition (DR) could have resulted from good effort in the sample in question. Instead, those who passed the TOMM but whose mean WMT scores were at or below 50% correct were almost certainly cases of poor effort, as indicated by grossly deficient scores on the WMT, but they

TABLE 4.2. Percentage Failing TOMM by Level of Effort on the WMT (Gervais Data)

WMT mean effort score[a]	% failing WMT	% failing TOMM	n	Mean WMT % correct[a]	SD	Mean CVLT short-delay recall	SD
91–100%	0%	0%	620	97%	3	11.1	3.1
81–90%	60%	0%	201	87%	3	8.9	3.3
71–80%	100%	20%	93	76%	3	8.8	3.3
61–70%	100%	40%	66	67%	3	6.9	2.6
51–60%	100%	70%	43	56%	3	6.8	2.5
50% or lower	100%	70%	23	44%	4	4.3	2.6

[a] The WMT mean effort score is the mean of immediate recognition, delayed recognition, and consistency between the two.

went undetected by the TOMM. The opposite pattern did not occur (i.e., scores of 50% correct or lower on the TOMM but passing the WMT).

Table 4.2 shows that none of 821 patients scoring in the top two WMT effort ranges failed the TOMM. However, when WMT effort scores were 80% or lower, some cases did fail the TOMM and the lower the WMT effort scores, the higher the TOMM failure rates. Why should they fail either the TOMM or the WMT? Based on their diagnoses, very few of the Gervais sample would be expected to have any cognitive impairment. Yet there were 66 nonneurological, non-head-injured, nondemented patients in the Gervais sample with WMT scores of 60% or lower. *For many reasons, poor effort is the only reasonable explanation for such extremely low scores, but, nevertheless, 30% of all the latter cases passed the TOMM.*

The following findings cited in the WMT Windows program and manual (Green, 2003b), and as described in a review of the WMT (Green, Lees-Haley, & Allen, 2002), are of relevance in judging the specificity (i.e., true negative identification rate) of the WMT: (1) testable mentally handicapped adults scored over 95% correct on the WMT effort measures; (2) children with an average Verbal IQ of 64 scored a mean of 89% correct on the three primary WMT effort measures; (3) disabling diseases of the brain do not cause failure on the WMT, except in some extremely severe cases who need 24 hours a day care; (4) mean scores of approximately 95% correct were found in neurological patients tested in Holland and Spain with translations of the WMT and no neurological patient in the latter study failed the primary WMT effort subtests (Gorissen, Sanz, & Schmand, 2005); (5) the mean WMT score was 68% in patients with advanced dementia, who averaged 78 years of age and were residing in a long-term care institution; and (6) patients asked to fake memory impairment on the WMT scored a mean of 62% on the primary WMT effort subtests (Green, 2003b). Hence, those in the Gervais sample with WMT scores below 60% were clearly not making a valid effort, but 30% of them passed the TOMM.

TABLE 4.3. WMT Effort Scores in People with Various Levels of Effort on the TOMM (Gervais Data)

TOMM trial 2	% failing TOMM	% failing WMT	n	Mean WMT effort scores	SD
45–50	0%	30%	938	91	10.20
40–44	100%	90%	41	69	11.99
35–39	100%	90%	26	71	10.95
30–34	100%	100%	16	58	7.53
25–29	100%	100%	14	56	12.09
<25	100%	100%	11	49	9.49

The reverse perspective is shown in the top row of Table 4.3, in which there were 938 cases passing the TOMM with trial 2 scores between 45 and 50. *It is remarkable that 30% of these cases failed the WMT.* When the TOMM trial 2 score was 34 of 50 or below, all cases failed the WMT. In the range 35–44 on the TOMM, 90% of cases failed the WMT. *Hence, when TOMM was failed, there was a high level of agreement between the TOMM and the WMT*, but there was major discrepancy between these two tests when the TOMM was passed.

Investigating WMT–TOMM Discrepancies

In clinical and forensic assessments, it is not unusual to find that one neuropsychologist uses the TOMM and concludes good effort whereas another uses the WMT with the same patient and concludes that effort was insufficient to produce valid test data. What should we conclude when WMT results suggest poor effort but TOMM scores suggest good effort, as in 25% of the 1,315 patients in Table 4.1?

The bottom row of Table 4.4 shows that those who failed the TOMM and the WMT (group 4) had a mean score of only 62% on WMT IR, DR, and consistency. This is identical to the *patient simulator* group in the WMT test manual (Green, 2003b). It is important to recognize that the WMT does not just yield a "pass" or "fail" result. It produces a profile of at least six scores, which reflect the relative difficulty levels of each subtest, assuming that the person makes good effort, as in the dementia patients in Figure 4.1 below. The actual mean scores and standard deviations in the fail both TOMM/WMT cases (reported first) versus the patient simulators (reported second) were IR (immediate recognition) = 63% (SD = 15) versus 63% (SD = 13); DR (delayed recognition = 60% (SD = 14) versus 62% (SD = 12); CNS (consistency between the two) = 64% (SD = 11) versus 63% (SD = 9); MC (multiple choice) = 41% (SD = 16) versus 40% (SD = 14); PA (paired associates) = 40% (SD = 16) versus 41% (SD = 17); FR (free recall) = 24% (SD = 12) versus 22% (SD = 10). It is clear that the profiles of the simulators and the fail both TOMM/WMT cases are almost identical; there was a mean difference of less than 1% (0.3%) in these six scores.

TABLE 4.4. Mean Effort Scores on the WMT and TOMM Trial 2 in Four Subgroups

Pattern of effort test failure	n	Mean WMT[a]	SD	Mean TOMM trial 2 of 50	SD	% of group failing CARB
Pass both	698	96%	4	50	1	0%
Fail only TOMM	6	93%	4	40	3	20%
Fail only WMT	240	77%	10	49	1	30%
Fail both	102	62%	12	35	8	70%

[a] The mean WMT is the mean of WMT immediate recognition, delayed recognition, and consistency.

The extreme similarity across all six WMT scores is important because we know with near certainty that the "simulator" patients were faking memory impairment, as requested by the tester. No other group, apart from simulators, has ever scored that low. A score of 62% in the fail both the TOMM and WMT is even lower than the mean score of 68% from institutionalized patients with advanced dementia with a mean age of 78 years (Brockhaus's data in Green, 2003b). It is far lower than the mean of 95% from neurological patients selected for having impaired memory on the California Verbal Learning Test (CVLT) and far lower than the mean score of 95% from children of various diagnoses tested clinically (Green & Flaro, 2003). Hence, it seems that TOMM failure in the Gervais sample occurred almost entirely in those with *grossly* deficient effort, as indicated by abysmally low WMT scores, matched only by known simulators. Consistent with the interpretation of poor effort, 70% of those failing both the TOMM and the WMT also failed the CARB. This is very significant because CARB is extremely easy for adults, with the exception of some patients with dementia.

In those who failed the WMT and passed the TOMM (group 3, Table 4.4), the WMT score of 77% was significantly higher than that of the fail both TOMM/WMT group (Mann–Whitney U test, $p < .0001$). A mean of 77% is, nevertheless, considerably lower than the mean score from young children with clinical conditions (Green & Flaro, 2003) and not much higher than the mean from subjects who were asked to simulate memory impairment. It is far lower than the mean from neurological patients and it is lower than the mean of 82.3% from people with confirmed early dementia who averaged 74 years of age (Green, 2003b). Based on their diagnoses, it is not plausible that the patients in the Gervais sample scored so low on WMT compared with the latter groups *while making an effort to do well*. In support of this conclusion, 30% of the cases in the pass-TOMM/fail-WMT group also failed the CARB. It is hard to argue that a group in which 30% of cases failed such an extremely easy effort test as the CARB, as well as failing the WMT, could be making sufficient effort to produce valid test results.

Effects of Effort on CVLT and IQ Scores

From the basic WMT validation studies (e.g., Green et al., 2002), we would question the effort of the people in both groups 3 (pass-TOMM/fail-WMT) and 4 (fail both TOMM/WMT) in Table 4.4, who scored either 77% or 62% correct on the mean of the WMT effort measures, despite having no neurological diagnosis. Examination of their neuropsychological test scores further reinforces this conclusion. Tables 4.5 and 4.6 allow us to examine scores from other neuropsychological tests in the four subgroups and especially the group of most interest, group 3. On the CVLT (Delis, Kramer, Kaplan & Ober, 1987), the four effort subgroups in Table 4.5 differed to a highly significant level in terms of both their short-delayed free recall (SDFR) scores (F = 44; df = 3, 639; p < .0001) and their long-delayed free recall (LDFR) scores (F = 57; df = 3, 639; p < .0001). Thus, failure on effort tests predicts lowered scores on other tests, at least in this instance.

Post hoc analysis shows that *group 1, who passed both effort tests, scored significantly higher on CVLT SDFR (p < .001) and LDFR (p < .001) than group 3, who failed the WMT but passed the TOMM.* This would be consistent with poor effort in the latter subgroup. In support of this conclusion, a mean score of 8.8 of 16 (SD = 3) on CVLT short delayed free recall was found in patients with a severe traumatic brain injury and a mean Glasgow Coma Scale score of 5 (patients from the writer's outpatient database). Therefore, even though they had no brain injury or disease, those in the pass-TOMM/fail-WMT group had slightly lower mean CVLT FR scores than cases of severe brain injury (Table 4.5). This is best explained by poor effort in group 3.

The CVLT recognition hits score is often used as an indicator of effort. The mean CVLT recognition hits score of 11.6 (SD = 3) in group 3 was markedly lower than the mean of 14.8 (SD = 1.6) in group 1 (F = 12; df = 4, 900; p < .0001). Another indicator that the suppressed CVLT scores in group 3 arose from poor effort is that their mean score on another effort test, the CARB (91%, SD = 12), was significantly lower than that of group 1 (pass both TOMM/WMT; 98%, SD = 4, Mann–Whitney, Z = 8.6, p < .0001). A score of 91% would be a "fail" within the current CARB program, indicating poor effort.

TABLE 4.5. CVLT Short- and Long-Delay Free-Recall Scores in Subgroups with Various Patterns of Effort Test Failure

Pattern of effort test failure	n	Mean short-delay free recall/16	SD	Mean long-delay free recall/16	SD
Pass both	698	10.9	3.2	11.3	3.2
Fail only TOMM	6	8.4	4.9	9.0	5.4
Fail only WMT	240	8.4	3.2	8.5	3.3
Fail both	102	7.0	3.2	6.6	3.3

Table 4.6 shows that intelligence test scores are also significantly affected by effort ($F = 18$, $df = 3$, 798, $p < .0001$). There is almost a standard deviation difference between the mean Full Scale IQ scores of those who failed both the WMT and the TOMM and those who passed both effort tests. *The group which failed the WMT but passed the TOMM produced intermediate Full Scale IQ scores, which were significantly lower than the mean score from group 1* (pass both; Bonferroni, $p < .0001$) *but significantly higher than group 4* (fail both; $p < .04$). This is consistent with the fact that the mean WMT effort score of 77% in group 3 was intermediate between those of groups 1 and 4 (Table 4.4). WMT effort varies along a continuum. The lower the WMT scores, the lower the scores we find on tests such as the CVLT and intelligence tests.

Although the mean WMT effort score correlated only very weakly with years of education ($r = .1$), it was correlated significantly and positively with most of the ability tests in the Gervais sample, including CVLT recall ($r = .5$), verbal IQ ($r = .25$), delayed story recall ($r = .42$), Wide Range Achievement Test–3 Arithmetic ($r = .26$) and Wisconsin Card Sorting Test categories achieved ($r = -0.16$). TOMM trial 2 scores also correlated with the latter variables, respectively, at r values of 0.35, 0.2, 0.25, 0.17, and 0.14, all significant correlations but somewhat lower than those for the WMT.

As predicted by the WMT, the IQ and CVLT data suggest low effort in group 3 and even lower effort in group 4. The argument that the group differences in IQ or CVLT scores could reflect actual differences in ability may be rejected because, above the age of 7, years of education are not generally correlated with WMT effort scores (Green & Flaro, 2003). Also, although the three effort groups in Table 4.6 differed slightly and statistically in years of education, all groups had a mean education with a very narrow range between 11 and 12 years, which cannot account for large differences in scores on the TOMM or the WMT.

TABLE 4.6. IQ Scores by Levels of Effort

Pattern of effort test failure	FSIQ mean	SD	VIQ mean	SD	PIQ mean	SD	Years of education mean	SD
Pass both ($n = 698$)	99	14	97	13	102	15	11.8	2.4
Fail only WMT ($n = 240$)	93	14	92	13	95	15	11.3	2.6
Fail TOMM and WMT ($n = 102$)	86	14	86	13	88	15	11.2	2.5

Note. IQ measured using either the Wechler Adult Intelligence Scale–III or the Multidimensional Aptitude Battery; group 2 not shown because $n = 2$.

Relationships with Memory Complaints

Reduced effort on cognitive tests is thought to be associated with an underlying *exaggeration of symptoms*, especially memory complaints. Therefore, we would expect to find an inverse relationship between effort scores and memory complaints on a standardized questionnaire. In the Gervais sample, 984 cases were given the Memory Complaints Inventory (MCI) (Green, 2003a; Green, Gervais, & Merten, 2005), on which there are nine scales representing different types of subjective memory complaints, such as inability to work because of memory problems. Scores are expressed as percentages of the maximum possible score per scale. As predicted, the mean overall scores on the MCI varied substantially by effort level ($F = 94$; $df = 3, 977$; $p < .0001$; Table 4.7).

Consistent with symptom exaggeration, *those who failed the WMT and passed the TOMM had significantly more memory complaints on the MCI than those passing both effort tests* (Mann–Whitney, Z = 7.8, $p < .0001$). To put this in perspective, the mean score of 32% in subgroup 3 is above the mean MCI score of 25% ($SD = 20$) from 56 cases of severe traumatic brain injury with a mean Glasgow Coma Scale score of 6, all of whom had abnormal brain scans on CT or MRI. (Note: The latter cases were drawn from the writer's consecutive outpatient series of 1,549 cases.) *Thus, there were more memory complaints in the pass-TOMM/fail-WMT group than in people with severe brain injuries.* Consistent with a continuum of symptom exaggeration and effort, there was an even higher mean MCI score of 50% in group 4, which failed both the WMT and TOMM (Table 4.7).

The data in Tables 4.8 and 4.9 are consistent with the conclusion that lowered WMT or TOMM scores are indicative of exaggerated memory complaints. The correlation between overall memory complaints on the MCI and scores on WMT effort subtests in the Gervais sample was –.5 (significant at $p < .0001$; Table 4.8). The correlation between overall memory complaints on the MCI and TOMM trial 2 scores was –.42 (also significant at $p < .0001$; Table 4.9). In 1,107 cases I tested, the correlation between the mean MCI score and the mean WMT effort score was –.43, replicating the relationship in samples of patients of very different diagnostic mixtures. Low effort and high memory complaints go together. *Those failing WMT and passing TOMM show poor effort and high memory complaints.*

TABLE 4.7. MCI Scores and Effort

Pattern of effort test failure	n	Mean MCI score as % of maximum	SD
Pass both	658	21%	15
Fail only TOMM	6	51%	28
Fail only WMT	228	32%	19
Fail both	98	50%	19

TABLE 4.8. Memory Complaints on the MCI versus Level of Effort on WMT

WMT mean effort score[a]	n	Mean MCI memory complaints (% of max.)	SD
91–100%	616	20%	15
81–90%	199	29%	17
71–80%	93	35%	17
61–70%	66	44%	20
51–60%	43	51%	19
≤ 50%	23	50%	24

[a] The mean WMT effort score is the mean of immediate recognition, delayed recognition, and consistency.

Simulators Contrasted with Patients Suffering from Dementia

Independent studies of persons asked to simulate impairment on the WMT have revealed exceptionally high levels of accuracy in classifying good versus poor effort, using the failure criterion of IR, DR or consistency is less than or equal to 82.5%. The classification accuracy was 100% in a study of patients who were asked to fake memory impairment (Green et al., 2002) and it was 97% in sophisticated volunteer simulators, mainly psychologists and physicians (one false negative, Iverson, Green, & Gervais, 1999). In an independent replication study, the WMT was 100% accurate in differentiating good effort from simulated impairment (Tan et al., 2002). In a German study with 100 good-effort volunteers and 29 simulators (Brockhaus & Merten, 2004), the classification accuracy of the WMT was 100%. Further, it was between 99% and 100% in two Turkish studies (Brockhaus, Peker, & Fritze, 2005) and it was 100% in a Russian study (Tydecks, Merten, & Gubbay, in press).

In the latter studies, the simulators produced mean profiles across the first six WMT scores which were distinctively characteristic of poor effort and, in important ways, different from the profiles found in dementia. Figure 4.1 reveals the typical pattern of WMT scores from simulators (Iverson et al., 1999) contrasted with data from groups of patients with early or advanced dementia, provided for use in the WMT Windows program by Dr. Robbi Brockhaus (Krefeld, Germany).

TABLE 4.9. Memory Complaints on the MCI versus Level of Effort on TOMM

TOMM 2 score	n	Mean MCI memory complaints (% of max.)	SD
45–50	938	24%	17
40–44	37	46%	16
35–40	24	40%	17
30–34	16	60%	19
25–30	14	53%	21
< 25/50	11	63%	18

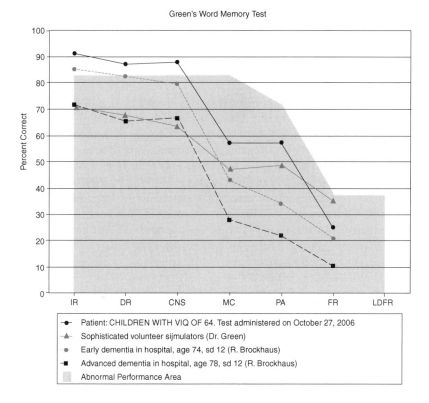

FIGURE 4.1. WMT profiles in patients with early or advanced dementia and children of very low IQ, contrasted with known simulators. Copyright 1995–2003 by Paul Green. Reprinted by permission.

The mean scores in the early and advanced dementia groups shown in Figure 4.1 reflect the objective differences in subtest difficulty, in which IR and DR are the easiest subtests, MC and PA are intermediate, and the FR and LDFR subtests are the most difficult. When IR and DR scores or the consistency between the two (CNS) are 82.5% or lower, the availability of multiple WMT subtests assists in differentiating between: (1) WMT scores which are invalid owing to poor and/or fluctuating effort and (2) scores from a person with such extreme impairment that he or she is incapable of passing the effort subtests, which happens in some patients with dementia.

The broken lines of the early and the advanced dementia patients in Figure 4.1 differ in the overall level of scores, but they are parallel to each other. They both slope down steeply to the right, revealing the good-effort pattern, in which the scores steadily decrease as the subtests become harder. In both Figure 4.1 and Table 4.10, we can see that the ratio of the mean IR score to the mean FR score in early-dementia patients is about 4:1 (85% to 21%), showing that FR is much harder than recognition in those with actual severe impairment. Similarly, children with a mean Verbal IQ of 64 had a mean IR score of 91% and a mean FR score of 25% (3.6 to 1). The mean IR score in the advanced-dementia patients in Figure 4.1 is about seven times greater than the mean FR score.

Psychologists and physicians who were asked to simulate memory impairment and to avoid being detected ("sophisticated simulators" in Figure 4.1) did not show this pattern. They scored lower than the children with a Verbal IQ of 64 on IR and DR, and they scored just as low as the advanced-dementia patients on these extremely easy subtests. *However, the simulators scored higher than the dementia patients on the most difficult measures, the PA and FR subtests.* The ratio of their scores on the easiest to the hardest subtests was only 2:1 (IR = 71% vs. FR = 35%). Such data reveal internal inconsistencies within known simulators' WMT profiles, as well as discrepancies with dementia patients' scores. The simulator profiles are best explained by fluctuating and generally low effort.

The WMT "simulator profile" is directly relevant when considering the implications of passing TOMM while failing WMT (see Figure 4.2). Figure 4.2 and Table 4.10 both show that the pass-TOMM/fail-WMT group from Dr. Gervais's sample had a WMT profile very similar to that of known simulators and quite unlike that of dementia patients. Their mean IR score was 79%, which is lower than the early-dementia group's mean score. However, they scored higher than early-dementia patients on the most difficult WMT subtests (MC, PA and FR)! Such a pattern of scores would *not* suggest verbal memory impairment similar to that of dementia patients. *Instead*, the overall pattern of WMT subtest scores in those passing TOMM and failing WMT

TABLE 4.10. Mean WMT Scores (and *SD*) in Cases Failing WMT but Passing TOMM, Compared with Simulators and Patients with Dementia

Group	Easier subtests			Harder subtests		
	IR	DR	CNS	MC	PA	FR
a. Early dementia	85% (11)	82% (15)	79% (12)	43% (20)	34% (15)	21% (16)
b. Sophisticated simulators	71% (12)	67% (16)	64% (12)	47% (18)	48% (20)	35% (19)
c. Gervais's cases failing WMT and passing TOMM	79% (13)	80% (12)	73% (11)	58% (17)	53% (17)	30% (12)
Groups a–b	+14%	+15%	+15%	−4%	−14%	−14%
Groups a–c	+6%	+2%	+6%	−15%	−19%	−9%

Note. IR, immediate recognition; DR, delayed recognition; CNS, consistency between IR and DR; MC, multiple choice; PA, paired-associate recall; FR, free recall of the word pairs.

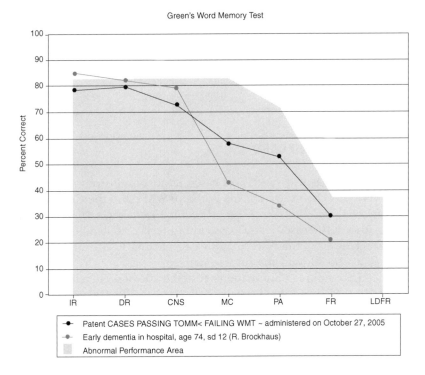

FIGURE 4.2. Contrast between the pass-TOMM/fail-WMT group (the flatter line) and patients aged 74 years with early dementia. Copyright 1995–2003 by Paul Green. Reprinted by permission.

resembles that found in simulators, presumably because their effort fluctuates and is suboptimal, leading to unreliable scores.

Summary

The evidence considered above all points in one direction: Those cases passing the TOMM and failing the WMT were false-negative classifications for the TOMM. They had a WMT profile most similar to that of known simulators. Their WMT profiles were very dissimilar to those of people with genuinely severe cognitive deficits, including neurological patients with brain diseases, dementia patients, and children with a very low IQ. The pass-TOMM/fail-WMT cases had elevated memory complaints, compared with those passing both effort tests. They had scores on other effort measures (CARB and CVLT recognition hits) strongly indicating poor effort. They showed an implausible suppression of performance across various neuropsychological tests. In some cases, the WMT effort scores were below 50% correct and yet they still passed the TOMM. Thus, poor effort was not accurately identified by the TOMM in these cases, but it was detected by the WMT.

TABLE 4.11. Agreement between CARB and WMT or TOMM in 1,524 Patients (Gervais Data)

	Pass WMT	Fail WMT	Pass TOMM	Fail TOMM
Pass CARB	1,019	275	916	45
Fail CARB	52	178	105	91

COMPARING WMT AND CARB

In the database of Dr. Gervais, 1,524 cases, almost exclusively with compensation or disability claims, were given both the WMT and the CARB. *The failure rate for the WMT (30%) was twice the failure rate on CARB (15%).* Table 4.11 shows that 1,197 cases either passed both tests or failed both tests (78% agreement). However, there were 178 cases passing CARB and failing the WMT and 52 who showed the reverse pattern.

In a separate sample of outpatients tested by the writer, 1,191 cases were given both the CARB and WMT (Green data, Table 4.12); 31% failed the WMT and 15% failed CARB. The majority of cases in the latter database had suffered a head injury ($n = 627$) or had a firm diagnosis of a brain disease such as stroke, tumor, multiple sclerosis, or aneurysm ($n = 113$), the remainder representing cases with major depression or bipolar disorder ($n = 122$), chronic pain ($n = 73$), orthopedic injuries ($n = 83$), chronic fatigue syndrome ($n = 35$), or miscellaneous diagnoses ($n = 138$). Despite the fact that the Gervais group contained almost no cases with brain injury or disease, the rates of WMT and CARB failure were almost identical in the two samples. What both samples had in common was that nearly all cases had compensation or disability claims.

Investigating CARB–WMT Discrepancies

One way to study the discrepancies between the CARB and the WMT is to examine the scores on neuropsychological tests in groups passing or failing the CARB and WMT, just as we did with the TOMM. Table 4.13 shows that FR of the CVLT word list differs significantly, depending on the pattern of effort test failure. The difference between the four subgroups is significant for both the CVLT SDFR and LDFR scores ($F = 84$; $df = 3, 1074$; $p < .0001$ for short delay, and $F = 106$; $df = 3, 1073$; $p < .0001$ for long delay).

TABLE 4.12. Agreement between CARB and WMT in 1,191 Patients Given Both Tests (Green Data)

	Pass WMT	Fail WMT
Pass CARB	787	221
Fail CARB	35	148

TABLE 4.13. Mean CVLT FR Scores by CARB and WMT Effort Test Results (Green Data)

Effort subgroup	n	SDFR mean	SD	LDFR mean	SD	Recognition hits mean	SD
Pass both	787	10.3	3.2	10.9	3.2	14.4	1.7
Fail only CARB	35	10.4	3.0	10.6	3.6	14.1	1.8
Fail only WMT	221	7.2	3.4	7.6	3.7	12.5	3.0
Fail both	148	6.5	3.2	6.0	3.6	10.5	3.5

Post hoc Bonferroni comparisons show that there is no significant difference between the CVLT recall scores or recognition hits scores in those who failed only the CARB versus those who passed both CARB and WMT (subgroups 1 and 2, n = 787 vs. n = 35). However, the 221 cases that failed the WMT and passed the CARB scored significantly lower on both CVLT FR trials than those who passed both effort tests ($p < .0001$).

Failing WMT thus implies poor effort on the CVLT, whether or not CARB is failed, but the reverse is not true. In the independent Gervais database, there were 776 cases given the CVLT, in addition to the CARB and the WMT. The results replicate exactly what has just been presented, with no significant difference between CVLT SDFR or LDFR scores or recognition hits in those who failed the CARB and passed the WMT, compared with those who passed the CARB and the WMT effort tests. Yet, those who failed only the WMT scored significantly lower on CVLT FR than those who passed both effort tests.

It could be argued that the latter results indicate particular sensitivity of the WMT to poor effort on *verbal memory* tasks. In theory, the CARB might be a better predictor of poor effort than WMT on tasks that do not involve verbal memory. However, in practice, this is not the case. The differences between groups 1 (pass both) to 4 (fail both) in Table 4.14 were highly significant both for Category Test errors ($p < .0001$, $F = 16.3$, $df = 3,874$) and for Trailmaking B ($p < .0001$, $F = 42.2$, $df = 3,913$). Once again, effort test scores predict neuropsychological test scores.

Post hoc tests show that although they failed CARB, group 2 *did not* score significantly differently from group 1 on the Category Test or on the

TABLE 4.14. CARB Failure without WMT Failure Is Not Linked with Reduced Performance on the Category Test or Trailmaking Test

Effort subgroup	n	Mean Category Test errors	SD	n	Mean Trailmaking B (sec)	SD
Pass both	638	57	30	625	79	53
Fail only CARB	22	57	32	22	87	31
Fail only WMT	151	70	27	173	123	92
Fail both	67	78	32	97	157	128

Trailmaking Test. However, those failing only the WMT (group 3) *did* score significantly lower than group 1. This is another example of how two effort tests may not be equivalent, and it shows that failing one effort test does not necessarily have the same implications for neuropsychological test validity as failing another effort test. *It cannot be assumed that poor scores on a specific effort test will necessarily be reflected in lowered scores on neuropsychological tests. This needs to be demonstrated empirically.* For identifying poor effort on neuropsychological tests, the above data suggest that the CARB is of little or no incremental value when used in addition to the WMT.

CARB versus TOMM

Table 4.11 shows that, out of 1,157 cases given both the TOMM and the CARB, there were differences in classification between the two tests in 13% of cases. Of the latter, 723 cases were given the CVLT, in addition to the CARB and the TOMM. There were significant differences in CVLT SDFR ($F = 26.4$; $df = 3,719$; $p < .0001$) and LDFR ($F = 33$, $df = 3,719$, $p < .0001$) between four groups, which were those passing both CARB and TOMM (group 1, $n = 573$ cases), those failing the CARB and passing the TOMM (group 2, $n = 69$), those passing the CARB and failing the TOMM (group 3, $n = 31$), and those failing both effort tests (group 4, $n = 50$). The failure rates on the WMT were as follows: group 1, 20%; group 2, 70%; group 3, 90%; group 4, 100%.

The corresponding mean CVLT FR scores were: group 1, mean of SDFR and LDFR = 10.5 ($SD = 3.2$); group 2, mean = 9 ($SD = 3.3$); group 3, mean = 7.8 ($SD = 3.2$); group 4, mean = 6.5 ($SD = 3.1$). There was no significant difference in CVLT scores between the two groups in which only one of the two tests was failed (groups 2 and 3). Both of the latter groups scored higher on the mean CVLT FR score than group 4, which failed both effort tests, but they scored lower than group 1, which passed both effort tests. Thus, failure on the CARB or the TOMM, overall, was linked with decreases in verbal memory scores, as indicated by the CVLT, once again revealing an underlying continuum of effort, from the most effort in group 1 to the least effort in group 4.

COMPARING MSVT TO WMT, TOMM, AND CARB

The MSVT was designed to be much shorter and easier than the WMT, requiring only 5 minutes of administration time in most cases (Green, 2003b; Merten et al., 2005; Richman et al., 2006). The basic test structure of the MSVT (previously known as the MACT) is somewhat similar to the WMT but the MSVT consists of only 10 word pairs instead of 20, which makes it easier and cuts testing time in half. Testing time is decreased further because there is only a 10-minute delay period instead of the 30 minutes required for the

WMT, and the MSVT also has no multiple-choice or long-delayed recall trial. The MSVT is easier because each word pair represents one concept, such as "soccer-ball," whereas there are two concepts per pair in the WMT, such as "tree–lake." The list of word pairs is presented twice on the computer screen, followed by an IR and a DR trial 10 minutes later, after which there is a PA recall trial and a FR trial.

The MSVT subtests have been shown to be even easier than the WMT subtests in children with very low intelligence and in elderly people with dementia (Green, 2003b). In a recent study by Dr. Lloyd Flaro (personal communication, September, 2006), the mean score on the MSVT recognition memory trials in healthy children in grade 2 was 98% correct. In the test manual (Green, 2003b), it is shown that children with a Verbal IQ below 70 scored a mean of 97% on the recognition trials. Children who spoke no French but who were administered the test in French scored a mean of 98% correct on IR and DR. Yet, in a sample of adults seeking compensation for soft tissue injuries and undergoing independent medical examinations by physicians, 42% of cases failed the MSVT, producing mean recognition scores of approximately 70% correct (Richman et al., 2006). Those failing the MSVT scored as low as patients with dementia on the very easy subtests (IR and DR) but much higher than dementia patients on the harder subtests (PA and FR). This is the same pattern shown by simulators, whether tested in German (Merten et al., 2005), French (Gervais, Chapter 6, in the manual by Green, 2003b) or Portuguese (Courtney, Appendix B, in the manual by Green, 2003b).

As part of a large normative data gathering and simulator study with the MSVT in Brazil, Dr. John Courtney (Appendix B, in the manual by Green, 2003b) recently found that the MSVT was 97% accurate in identifying poor effort in over 300 cases. Sixty-eight of 70 cases that were asked to simulate memory deficits were identified as feigning impairment, using simple cutoff scores on the IR and DR trials. In the 229 volunteers who were asked to make a good effort, 96% of cases scored above the cutoffs. In the few who failed the MSVT, an analysis of the pattern of scores suggested that their data were not valid owing to inconsistent effort, evident in the "simulator profile." For example, they obtained approximately the same score on FR as on the much easier IR trial. An accuracy level of approximately 97% in discriminating between good-effort and poor-effort cases was also found in a simulator study by Merten et al. (2005) using the German translation of the MSVT.

WMT versus MSVT

The MSVT and the WMT were compared in 279 consecutive subjects tested by me, all of whom were involved in disability or compensation claims. In Table 4.15, it may be seen that despite the fact that the MSVT is an extremely easy test, 29% of adults failed the MSVT and 37% failed the WMT.

TABLE 4.15. Agreement between MSVT and WMT (Green and Gervais Data)

	Green		Gervais		Combining samples 1 and 2	
	Pass WMT	Fail WMT	Pass WMT	Fail WMT	Pass WMT	Fail WMT
Pass MSVT	159	39	76	22	235	61
Fail MSVT	16	65	9	22	21	87

There was agreement between the WMT and MSVT in 80.3% of cases. In 14% of cases, the MSVT was passed and the WMT was failed, which is understandable because the MSVT is objectively easier than the WMT. However, 5.7% of cases showed the opposite pattern by failing the easier of the two tasks (the MSVT) and passing the relatively difficult, although still objectively extremely easy, WMT. How can this be explained? It seems likely that inconsistent effort is present in cases passing one effort test but failing an easier test. Table 4.15 includes similar data from an independent sample tested by Gervais, all of whom were also involved in disability or compensation claims.

We may apply the same test to the MSVT as we did to the TOMM and the CARB by examining the neuropsychological test scores in those who pass the MSVT and fail the WMT or vice versa. An analysis of variance shows that there are highly significant differences between the four groups in Table 4.16 in terms of their scores on the CVLT, Category Test and Trailmaking Test. *The scores of group 2 (failing only MSVT) were significantly lower than the scores of group 1 (passing both MSVT and WMT) for both the CVLT* ($p = .04$) *and the Trailmaking Test* ($p = .002$). The comparison was not significant for the Category Test but the sample size was small. Thus, unlike the CARB, we find

TABLE 4.16. Lowered Scores in Cases Failing Effort Subtests of Either MSVT or WMT

Effort subgroup	n	Mean CVLT recall out of 16[a]	SD	n	Mean Trailmaking B in (sec)	SD	n	Mean Category Test errors	SD
Pass both	159	12.2	3	159	77	28	158	55	31
Fail only MSVT	16	9.8	3	16	173	208	13	68	31
Fail only WMT	39	8.9	3	39	139	115	35	80	33
Fail both	65	7.1	3	65	174	149	59	87	31
		$p < .0001$			$p < .0001$			$p < .0001$	

[a] The mean of short- and long-delay free recall is shown.

that those who fail the MSVT generally score lower across other neuropsy-chological tests than those who pass the MSVT, whether or not the WMT is also failed.

TOMM versus MSVT

One hundred ninety-five consecutive cases tested as outpatients by Dr. Gervais were given the MSVT, the TOMM, the CARB, and the WMT. Table 4.17 shows 80% agreement between the TOMM and the MSVT. *However, there were 33 cases, or 17% of the whole sample, who passed the TOMM and failed the MSVT.*

The mean MSVT profile in such cases was most similar to that of sub-jects asked to simulate impairment. Their mean scores on the easy subtests (IR = 80%, DR = 77%, consistency = 73%, mean = 77%) were similar to and slightly lower than those of patients with early dementia (IR = 83%, DR = 89%, consistency = 81%, mean = 84%). However, on the more difficult subtests, the cases failing MSVT and passing TOMM scored much higher than the early-dementia patients on PA (71% vs. 53%) and FR (47% vs. 31%). This gives one indication that those who passed the TOMM and failed the MSVT were performing inconsistently and making less than sufficient effort.

The mean FR score from the CVLT on SDFR and LDFR was calculated. Table 4.18 shows that there was a highly significant difference between CVLT recall scores and recognition hits across the four groups representing combinations of passing or failing the TOMM and the MSVT. Post hoc com-parisons showed that the mean recall score of 8.6 in those passing the TOMM but failing the MSVT was significantly lower than the mean score of 10.8 in those passing both tests (p = .005). Thus, failing the MSVT implies reduced effort on the CVLT, even if the TOMM is passed. The number of cases failing the TOMM and passing the MSVT is too small for testing of the significance of group differences, although the mean CVLT FR score in this group (8.8, n = 5) suggests that failing the TOMM is also linked with poor effort on the CVLT, even if the MSVT is passed. The main impression from comparing the MSVT with the TOMM is that the MSVT is much more sensi-tive to poor effort than the TOMM.

TABLE 4.17. Failures on TOMM and MSVT in Patients Given Both Tests (Gervais Data)

	Pass MSVT	Fail MSVT	Total
Pass TOMM	142	33	175
Fail TOMM	5	15	20
Total	147	48	195

TABLE 4.18. Mean Free-Recall Scores on CVLT in Groups Passing or Failing MSVT/TOMM

	n	Mean CVLT free recall	SD	Mean CVLT recognition hits	SD
Pass TOMM and MSVT	132	10.8	3.3	15	1.6
Fail only TOMM	5	8.8	2.5	13	1.9
Fail only MSVT	30	8.6	2.9	13	2.5
Fail both	14	7.1	2.8	13	2.8
		$p < .001$		$p < .001$	

CARB versus MSVT

The MSVT is also more sensitive than the CARB. In 198 cases, 138 cases passed both tests, 17 failed both tests, 7 failed only the CARB and not the MSVT, but 30 failed the MSVT and passed the CARB. Using similar methods to those used earlier, when comparing other effort tests with each other, it is clear that those failing the MSVT and passing the CARB were false negatives for the CARB, but the details are not presented here because of space limitations.

SUMMARY OF AVAILABLE DATA

Combining together my clinical outpatient series ($n = 1,549$) and those of Gervais ($n = 2,237$) and Moss ($n = 269$), we have data from almost 4,000 cases of various diagnoses involved in compensation claims in which at least two separate tests of effort were administered. From the analyses discussed earlier, it appears that the WMT is a more sensitive measure of effort than either the CARB or the TOMM.

It is possible to make a simple table comparing each method for evaluating effort with the results of the WMT (Table 4.19). Cross-tabulations allow us to study how well each method predicts failure on the WMT. We may then calculate the sensitivity and specificity, as well as positive predictive power (PPP) and negative predictive power (NPP), for each test as a predictor of poor effort as measured by the WMT. In Table 4.19, the external criterion is WMT failure and calculations assume a 30% base rate of WMT failure. Tests are ranked from least (0) to most sensitive (0.71) relative to the WMT. This method has some flaws. For example, it ignores the fact that effort is a continuous variable and it forces results from all tests into a "pass" or a "fail." It omits consideration of whether, in fact, effort is poor on neuropsychological tests and whether symptom complaints are high in those failing each effort test. On the other hand, it allows us to rate all the effort measures against a single criterion, which, in this case, is WMT failure. Table

TABLE 4.19. Sensitivity, Specificity, PPP, and NPP for Various Effort Tests versus WMT

Tests	Cutoff	Tester	n	Sensitivity	Specificity	PPP	NPP
1-in-5	< 29	Green	16[a]	0.0	1.0	Na	0.50
Finger-Tap sum	< 63	Green	858	0.17	0.93	0.53	0.73
TOMM	< 45	Gervais	1,046	0.29	0.99	0.93	0.77
WRMT-F	< 33	Green	1,193	0.31	0.94	0.7	0.76
TOMM	< 45	Moss	269	0.37	0.98	0.91	0.78
WRMT-W	< 33	Green	465	0.37	0.98	0.91	0.78
CARB	< 90	Green	1,452	0.40	0.96	0.80	0.78
CARB	< 90	Gervais	1,532	0.40	0.95	0.77	0.78
21-item	< 13	Green	132	0.38	0.94	0.73	0.78
MSVT	< 85	Gervais	129	0.50	0.89	0.67	0.81
RDS-7	< 7	Green	153	0.56	0.83	0.59	0.81
ASTM	< 94	Green	272	0.59	0.84	0.62	0.82
MSVT	< 80 = low	Green	279	0.57	0.96	0.85	0.84
MSVT	< 85 = usual	Green	279	0.62	0.91	0.75	0.85
MSVT	< 90 = high	Green	279	0.71	0.84	0.66	0.87

Note. Sensitivity = proportion of WMT failures correctly classified as poor effort by each one of the other effort tests; specificity = proportion of WMT passers who were correctly classified as good effort by the other effort tests.
[a] Use of the 1-in-5 test was stopped after no case failed it. No case scored below 32. Several complained that it was too obvious and too simple. PPP could not be calculated because of a division by zero error.

4.19 includes data from the TOMM, Warrington's Recognition Memory Test–Words (WRMT-W) and WRMT–Faces (WRMT-F; Warrington, 1984), the CARB, the MSVT, the ASTM (Schmand & Lindeboom, 2005), the Reliable Digit Span (Greiffenstein, Baker, & Gola, 1994), the 21-item test (Iverson & Franzen, 1996), the sum of right and left finger tapping (Larrabee, 2003), and the 1-in-5 test (Tydecks et al., in press).

As an example of how to read the data in the table, take the example of the TOMM in the third line from the top. Sensitivity is 0.29 (true positive rate) and specificity is .99 (true negative rate). This may be read as indicating that in 99% of cases in which the TOMM was failed, the WMT was also failed; that is, there are very few false positives for the TOMM in that sense. However, when the WMT was failed, the TOMM was failed in only 30% of cases, indicating a very high false-negative rate for the TOMM relative to the WMT. NPP is 0.77, meaning that in general there is a 77% probability that the person predicted by the TOMM to have good effort on the WMT will actually pass the WMT if the base rate of WMT failure is 30%. PPP is 0.93, meaning that there is a 93% probability that a person predicted by the TOMM to fail the WMT will actually fail it if the base rate of WMT failure is 30%.

It was shown above that as a group, those who failed the WMT and passed the TOMM were undoubtedly *false negatives for the TOMM (i.e., misclassifications)* because their effort was shown to be poor using several different methods. The TOMM's failure to detect between 62% and 70% of WMT failures in two large samples, including some with lower-than-chance WMT scores, might be argued to be an unacceptably high error rate for the TOMM if it were intended for use as the sole effort test. The specificity was relatively high, however, for the TOMM as well as for most of the effort tests in Table 4.19.

CHOOSING A COMBINATION OF EFFORT TESTS

Within the Slick et al. (1999) criteria for malingering, failing "*one or more well-validated SVTs*" is evidence of exaggeration or faking of cognitive deficits, but we are left wondering what "well validated" really means. No two effort tests are identical and often one is failed while the other is passed. Therefore, the use of any single effort test in isolation is probably not advisable, but what is the best combination of SVTs to use? It is self-evident that choosing more sensitive effort tests is desirable, as long as specificity is comparable, because this decreases the error rate in determining whether test data are unreliable because of suboptimal effort. For example, the use of a low-sensitivity test, such as the sum of finger-tapping scores being below 63, may be justified, as long as it is appreciated that passing the test does not imply good effort. Most cases of poor effort will actually pass such tests and hence, will not be identified, whereas failure implies poor effort in most cases.

This chapter has shown that, generally, as effort test scores decrease, the scores on neuropsychological tests decline and memory complaints increase, consistent with a presumed underlying variable of symptom exaggeration. Within this approach, it has been shown using various methods that some effort tests (e.g., the WMT or the MSVT) are considerably more sensitive to reduced effort than others (e.g., the TOMM or the CARB). The lowest neuropsychological test scores are typically found in those who fail two effort tests, such as the TOMM and the WMT. However, this is not because combining two effort tests adds to their sensitivity. It is because those failing the least sensitive of the two effort tests (e.g., the TOMM) are also those who score at the lower end of the continuum on the more sensitive of the two effort tests (e.g., the WMT; see Table 4.4). Failing one effort test but not the other usually indicates an intermediate level of reduced effort, and the best effort is present in those passing both effort tests.

Where effort falls on a continuum cannot be decided based on a "democratic show of hands" or on an average from several effort tests, because this assumes that all tests are equally sensitive and specific. Even if several low-sensitivity effort tests are passed, what might seem superficially to be quite small drops in scores on just one effort test could indicate that neuropsychological test scores significantly underestimate true abilities. For example, in my outpatient series, 826 cases scored 91% or above on the mean WMT effort score and 228 cases scored between 81% and 90%. Their mean WMT effort scores were 97% (*SD* = 3) and 86% (*SD* = 3) respectively. The mean SDFR CVLT score of 10.4 (*SD* = 3) in the former was significantly greater than the mean of 8.3 (*SD* = 3) in the latter (*F* = 85, *df* = 5,1347, *p* < .0001). *Thus, even a drop in WMT effort scores from 97% to 86% was associated with a statistically and clinically significant drop in CVLT scores.* Yet no case who scored between 81% and 100% correct on the WMT failed the TOMM (Table 4.2).

As shown earlier, failure on the WMT or the MSVT while passing the TOMM is a frequent finding and it implies that effort is probably insufficient to produce valid results. *It follows logically that if a person passes the TOMM, then good effort on other tests cannot be assumed, even if the TOMM trial two score is 50 of 50.* Similarly, other investigations reveal that the WMT is often failed by people who have passed the CARB and yet such cases have other clear hallmarks of poor effort (e.g., lowered scores on other neuropsychological tests and WMT profiles similar to those of known simulators). In the relatively few cases in which the WMT is passed and the CARB is failed, generally reduced scores on neuropsychological tests are not observed. This means that CARB failure in some cases does not tap the presumed underlying variable of effort.

Perhaps the criteria of Slick et al. (1999) for malingered neurocognitive dysfunction need to be developed further to incorporate some benchmark standard for validity, such that only tests proven to have minimally acceptable levels of sensitivity and specificity should be used. A good place to start would be to rate the sensitivity of effort tests in simulator studies, which employ solid and universally applicable markers to define who is making a poor effort and who is not. Ideally, simulator studies should incorporate several different effort tests, so that their relative sensitivity to each other can be calculated, as in the study of Merten et al. (2005). The WMT and the MSVT have already been shown to be approximately 100% accurate in classifying good or poor effort in such simulator studies, as noted earlier. In addition, it would be highly desirable if simulator studies incorporated effort tests within the context of a comprehensive neuropsychological assessment, using two subgroups of healthy volunteers, who are asked either to make a systematically good effort or to simulate impairment on testing. Then, it would be possible to study the effectiveness of various effort tests in predicting neuropsychological battery performance. In such an approach, *central importance is attached to the ability of specific effort tests to predict whether or not other neuropsychological test scores are accurate.* This aspect of effort test validity emphasizes something that we can measure objectively (neuropsychological test scores), while minimizing the need for controversial and hard-to-measure variables, such as the person's intent or motivation for failing effort tests. Interpretations about intent and volitional behavior may be required by most definitions of "malingering," but, in research as in clinical practice, such inferences may be separated from the question of whether effort is sufficient to produce valid neuropsychological test data. Whether or not data are invalid can be treated separately from why.

Just as major projects have attempted to document "dose–response" relationships between severity of head injury and neuropsychological test battery scores (Dikmen, Machamer, Winn, & Temkin, 1995, Rohling, Meyers, & Millis, 2003), we need to establish the "dose–response" relationship between effort levels on specific effort tests and neuropsychological test battery scores. Tables resembling extended versions of Tables 4.4 to 4.6 in this chapter might be created, using many neuropsychological tests. What makes this task imperative is that effort has such a large effect on test scores (Green et al., 2001; Constantinou et al., 2005).

In the absence of such comprehensive and objective comparative data on effort tests, clinicians need to make their choices of SVTs carefully, paying attention to the published data on the validity of their chosen effort tests, in as many samples as possible, clinical as well as experimental. Bearing in mind that some effort tests differ greatly from others, especially in sensitivity, it is probably wise to use several effort tests routinely for several reasons. First, this allows the clinician to gather comparative data and to appreciate how effort tests differ very significantly from each other. Ideally, all effort and neuropsychological data would be entered routinely into a spreadsheet for later analysis, so that we can study the effects on all neuropsychological tests of passing or failing each effort test. Second, effort might vary over time, even within the same test session, necessitating continuous sampling of effort. Finally, some effort tests might have been coached and the more effort tests that are employed, the less likely it is that coaching will be effective.

When the ASTM, the WMT, the MSVT, the RDS, the TOMM or other tests in Table 4.19 are failed, it is likely that effort is poor and that other neuropsychological test data will underestimate the person's actual abilities, *assuming that we can rule out dementia.* For relatively low sensitivity effort tests such as the TOMM or the CARB, on the other hand, failing marks imply poor effort but passing marks do not guarantee good effort.

There are special advantages to the use of tests such as the WMT and the MSVT, which employ not only very easy tasks but also multiple subtests of varying degrees of difficulty, for which there are data from many comparison groups, including people with dementia. The fact that simulators and dementia patients produce different profiles of test results on the WMT and the MSVT can assist us in ruling out "false positives." If someone with dementia scores below 82.5% on the WMT (i.e., a fail) and produces a profile across all other subtests which is typical of dementia, they might not be a "false positive" but could be performing in keeping with their diagnosis. In fact, such a profile is helpful in diagnosing truly severe cognitive impairment.

NOTE

1. WMT cutoffs: In the WMT Windows program, the word "warning" appears if MC (multiple choice) is 70 or lower or if PA (paired associates) is 50% or lower. This is because, except in cases of extremely severe impairment (e.g., dementia), such scores would be so low as to be of questionable validity. Interpretation of such scores is left to the judgment of the clinician. However, if we were, in addition, to classify as WMT failures those with scores on MC of 70% or below or PA scores of 50% or below, there would be an extra 142 cases failing the WMT and passing the TOMM in Table 4.2. This would leave only two cases failing the TOMM and passing the WMT.

REFERENCES

Allen, L., Conder, R. L., Green, P., & Cox, D. R. (1997). *CARB '97 manual for the computerized assessment of response bias*. Durham, NC: CogShell.

Brockhaus, R., & Merten, T. (2004). Neuropsychologische Diagnostik suboptimalen Leistungsverhaltens mit dem Word Memory Test. *Nervenartz, 75*, 882–887.

Brockhaus, R., Peker, O., & Fritze, E. (2005). *Testing effort in Turkish speaking subjects: Validation of a translation of the Word Memory Test*. Poster presented at the International Neuropsychological Society, Dublin.

Bush, S., Ruff, M., Troster, I., Barth, J., Koffler, S., Pliskin, N., Holmes, M. D., Jung, M., Koerner, E., et al. (2005). NAN position paper. Symptom validity assessment: Practice issues and medical necessity. NAN policy and planning committee. *Archives of Clinical Neuropsychology, 20*, 419–426.

Conder, R., Allen, L., & Cox, D. (1992). *Manual for the computerized assessment of response bias*. Durham, NC: CogShell.

Constantinou, M., Bauer, L., Ashendorf, L., Fisher, J., & McCaffrey, R. J. (2005). Is poor performance on recognition memory effort measures indicative of generalized poor performance on neuropsychological tasks? *Archives of Clinical Neuropsychology, 20*(2), 191–198.

Delis, D. C., Kramer, J. H., Kaplan, E., & Ober, B. A. (1987). *California Verbal Learning Test, Adult Version*. San Antonio, TX: Psychological Corporation.

Dikmen, S. S., Machamer, J. E., Winn, H. R., & Temkin, N. R. (1995). Neuropsychological outcome at one year post head injury. *Neuropsychology, 9*, 80–90.

Drane, D. L., Williamson, D. J., Stroup, E. S., Holmes, M. D., Jung, M., Koerner, E., et al. (2006). Cognitive impairment is not equal in patients with epileptic and psychogenic nonepileptic seizures. *Epilepsia, 47*(11), 1879–1886.

Gervais, R., Rohling, M., Green, P., & Ford, W. (2004). A comparison of WMT, CARB and TOMM failure rates in non-head injury disability claimants. *Archives of Clinical Neuropsychology, 19*(4), 475–487.

Gorissen, M., Sanz, J. C., & Schmand, B. (2005). Effort and cognition in schizophrenia patients. *Schizophrenia Research, 78*, 2–3, 199–208.

Green, P. (2001). Why clinicians often disagree about the validity of test results. *Neurorehabilitation, 16*, 231–236.

Green, P. (2003a). *Memory Complaints Inventory.* Edmonton, Alberta, Canada: Author.

Green, P. (2003b). *Word Memory Test for Windows: User's manual and program.* Edmonton, Alberta, Canada: Author. (Revised 2005)

Green, P. (2004). *Medical Symptom Validity Test for Windows: User's manual and program.* Edmonton, Alberta, Canada: Author.

Green, P., & Astner, K. (1995). *Manual for the Oral Word Memory Test.* Durham, NC: Cognisyst. (Out of print)

Green, P., & Flaro, L. (2003). Word Memory Test performance in children. *Child Neuropsychology, 9*(3), 189–207.

Green, P., Gervais, R., & Merten, T. (2005). Das Memory Complaints Inventory (MCI): Das Memory Complaints Inventory (MCI): Gedächtnisstörungen, Beschwerdenschilderung und Leistungsmotivation [The Memory Complaints Inventory (MCI): Memory impairment, symptom presentation, and test effort.] *Neurologie & Rehabilitation, 11*(3), 139–144.

Green, P., Iverson, G. L., & Allen, L. M. (1999). Detecting malingering in head injury litigation with the Word Memory Test. *Brain Injury, 13*, 813–819.

Green, P., Lees-Haley, P. R., & Allen, L. M. (2002). The Word Memory Test and the Validity of Neuropsychological Test Scores. *Journal of Forensic Neuropsychology, 2*, 97–124.

Green, P., Rohling, M. L., Lees-Haley, P. R., & Allen, L. M. (2001). Effort has a greater effect on test scores than severe brain injury in compensation claimants. *Brain Injury, 15*(12), 1045–1060.

Greiffenstein, M. F., Baker, W. J., & Gola, T. (1994). Validation of malingered amnesia measures with a large clinical sample. *Psychological Assessment, 6*, 218–224.

Iverson, G. L., & Binder, L. M. (2000). Detecting exaggeration and malingering in neuropsychological assessment. *Journal of Head Trauma Rehabilitation, 15*, 829–858.

Iverson, G., & Franzen, M. (1996). *21-item test.* Unpublished manuscript.

Iverson, G., Green, P., & Gervais, R. (1999). Using the Word Memory Test to detect biased responding in head injury litigation. *The Journal of Cognitive Rehabilitation, 17*(2), 4–8.

Larrabee, G. J. (2003). Detection of malingering using atypical performance patterns on standard neuropsychological tests. *The Clinical Neuropsychologist, 17*, 410–425.

Merten, T., Green, P., Henry, M., Blaskewitz, N., & Brockhaus, R. (2005). Analog validation of German language symptom validity tests and the influence of coaching. *Archives of Clinical Neuropsychology, 20*(6), 719–727.

Richman, J., Green, P., Gervais, R., Flaro, L., Merten, T., Brockhaus, R., et al. (2006). Objective tests of symptom exaggeration in independent medical examinations. *Journal of Occupational and Environmental Medicine, 48*(3), 303–311.

Rohling, M. L., Meyers, J. M., & Millis, S. R. (2003). Neuropsychological impairment following traumatic brain injury: A dose–response analysis. *The Clinical Neuropsychologist, 17*(3), 289–302.

Schmand, B., & Lindeboom, J. (2005). *Amsterdam Short-Term Memory Test. Manual.* Leiden, The Netherlands: PITS.

Slick, D., Hopp, G., Strauss, E., & Thompson, G. (1996) *The Victoria Symptom Validity Test.* Lutz, FL: Psychological Assessment Resources.

Slick, D. J., Sherman, E. M. S., & Iverson, G. L. (1999). Diagnostic criteria for malingered neurocognitive dysfunction: Proposed standards for clinical practice and research. *The Clinical Neuropsychologist, 13*, 545–561.

Tan, J., Slick, D., Strauss, E., & Hultsch, D. F. (2002). Malingering strategies on symptom validity tests. *The Clinical Neuropsychologist, 16*(4), 495–505.

Tombaugh, T. N. (1996). *Test of Memory Malingering.* Toronto, Ontario, Canada: Multi-Health Systems.

Tydecks, S., Merten, T., & Gubbay, J. (in press). The Word Memory Test and the One-in-Five Test in an analogue study with Russian-speaking participants. *International Journal of Forensic Psychology.*

Warrington, E. (1984). *Recognition Memory Test.* Windsor, UK: NFER Nelson.

CHAPTER 5

Non-Forced-Choice Measures to Detect Noncredible Cognitive Performance

Stephen R. Nitch
David M. Glassmire

In recent years, two-alternative forced-choice testing has become one of the most popular methods of detecting suboptimal effort during neuropsychological evaluations. For example, in a recent survey of experts in the area of cognitive malingering, 25% of respondents indicated that they used the Test of Memory Malingering (TOMM) "always" and another 20.8% reported that they used this instrument "often" (Slick, Tan, Strauss, & Hultsch, 2004). In a more recent survey of assessment practices among neuropsychologists, Rabin, Barr, and Burton (2005) found that the TOMM was ranked 19th among the most commonly used instruments employed in memory assessments. Interestingly, the TOMM was the only validity measure to appear in the top 20 instruments used in memory assessments among practicing neuropsychologists. With the increasing use of forced-choice effort testing in neuropsychological evaluations, examinees with incentive to appear disabled are likely becoming more sophisticated about the purpose of such tests. In addition, attorneys who are familiar with the concept of forced-choice testing might coach examinees on how to recognize such tests and on how to perform so as not to raise suspicion regarding their level of effort. For example, Youngjohn (1995) described a case in which an attorney admitted during an administrative judicial hearing that he had educated his client about the purposes of various neuropsychological tests prior to a neuropsychological evaluation. Thus, it is important to have a wide variety of validated effort techniques that do not all rely on a forced-choice paradigm.

This chapter focuses on four non-forced-choice measures of malingering: (1) the Rey 15-Item Test, (2) the Dot Counting Test, (3) the Rey Word Recognition Test, and (4) the b Test. All these measures rely on the floor-effect principle (Rogers, Harrell, & Liff, 1993), as they use tasks that are sufficiently easy that most individuals with neuropsychological deficits can complete them successfully. The Dot Counting Test also allows for performance curve analysis, as it contains a number of items that can be ordered by level of difficulty, thus allowing the clinician to compare performances across easy and difficult items. For each of these four tests, we briefly describe the history and development of the measure. Where available, we also provide administration and scoring information, cutoff scores recommended in the literature, classification accuracy statistics, interpretive caveats, and published alternative scoring methods.

REY 15-ITEM TEST

The Rey 15-Item Test (FIT)[1] was developed by Andre Rey (1964) and has been described in prominent neuropsychology texts (e.g., Lezak, 1995; Spreen & Strauss, 1998). Survey data show that it is one of the most commonly administered effort measures. In their survey of experts in the assessment of cognitive malingering, Slick et al. (2004) found that the FIT was used "always" by 12.5% of respondents and was used "often" by an additional 20.8% of the individuals surveyed. In addition, in Rabin et al.'s (2005) survey of practicing neuropsychologists, the FIT was the only effort measure other than the TOMM in the list of the 40 most commonly administered instruments in memory assessment. The FIT has likely maintained its popularity due to its ease of administration and scoring, as well as its quick administration time. The FIT was developed as a technique for assessing the validity of visual memory complaints and consists of 15 simple, highly redundant items presented in five rows of three characters each. The examinee is shown the stimulus sheet for 10 seconds, after which the sheet is removed and the examinee is asked to reproduce as many of the 15 items as he or she can remember on a blank sheet of paper.

The FIT uses the floor-effect principle (Rogers et al., 1993) as it is thought to be so simple that "all but the most severely brain damaged or retarded patients can perform [the task] easily" (Lezak, 1995, p. 802). Although 15 items are significantly above the short-term memory buffer of 7 plus or minus 2 items (Miller, 1956), the FIT really only requires memorization of five ideational units, as items can be chunked into conceptually meaningful categories (i.e., uppercase letters, lowercase letters, Arabic numbers, Roman numerals, and shapes). Despite this fact, the FIT is presented explicitly to the examinee as a memorization task of 15 *different* items. It is thought that these instructions will make the FIT appear harder than it actually is, thereby enticing examinees who are malingering to suppress their performance out of a belief that poor performance will not raise suspicion regarding their level of effort. Several empirical investigations have suggested that individuals with incentive to appear disabled perform more poorly on the FIT than do individuals without such incentive (Bernard, Houston, & Natoli, 1993; Lee, Loring, & Martin, 1992; Simon, 1994; Griffin, Normington, & Glassmire, 1996).

The simplest and most common method of scoring the FIT is to add up the total number of items that were correctly reproduced to arrive at a single quantitative score. Different cutoffs have been suggested for detecting malingering based on the total number of items recalled, although the most commonly reported cutoff is fewer than nine items. Lezak (1995) suggested that "anyone who is not significantly deteriorated can recall at least three of the five character sets, or nine items" (p. 802). A cutoff of fewer than nine items correct makes conceptual sense, as it capitalizes on the fact that each row of three items actually requires memorization of only one concept in order to recall all three of the items from that particular row. Therefore, when the clinician uses a cutoff of fewer than nine items, the examinee needs only to remember three ideational units to be classified as putting forth a valid effort.

Tables 5.1 and 5.2 present published sensitivity and specificity values for a cutoff of fewer than nine items; sensitivity levels average slightly less than

TABLE 5.1. Summary of Previously Published Sensitivity Values for the FIT Using a Free-Recall Cutoff of < 9

Sensitivity (%)	n	Sample	Author
		Studies employing simulators	
12	69	Normals and inpatient substance abusers	Schretlen et al. (1991)
15	20	College students	Guilmette, Hart, Giuliano, & Leininger (1994)
61	49	College students	Arnett et al. (1995)
72	25	First-year medical students	Arnett et al. (1995)
7	32	College students	Griffin et al. (1997)
		Studies employing suspected malingerers in clinical settings	
43	7	Civil litigation/suspected malingerers	Schretlen et al. (1991)
43	14	Malingerers in forensic inpatient setting	King (1992)
38	16	Litigating neurological outpatients	Lee et al. (1992)
16	56	Neuropsychology clinic referrals with motive to exaggerate symptoms	Frederick et al. (1994)
70	18	Suspected forensic malingerers	Frederick, Sarfaty, Johnston, & Powel (1994)
62	43	Probable malingerers	Greiffenstein et al. (1994)
86	14	Forensic/criminal malingerers	Simon (1994)
5	154	Workers' compensation "stress" claimants	Boone et al. (1995)
71	7	Workers' compensation "stress" claimants	Millis & Kler (1995)
8	233	Suspected malingerers	Sumanti, Boone, Savodnick, & Gorsuch (2006)

TABLE 5.2. Summary of Previously Published Specificity Values for the FIT Using a Free-Recall Cutoff of < 9

Specificity (%)	n	Sample	Author
		Patients with dementia	
13	15	Mild dementia	Philpott (1992)
0	22	Moderate dementia	Philpott (1992)
0	12	Moderate/severe dementia	Philpott (1992)
64	14	Dementia (severity unspecified)	Spiegel (2006)
		General neuropsychology referrals	
80	60	Nonlitigating patients with mild memory impairment	Morgan (1991)
73	148	Mixed patient group (neuropsychiatric, brain injured, mixed dementia, severe psychiatric, and genuine amnesics)	Schretlen et al. (1991)
92	40	Nonlitigating neurological outpatients	Lee et al. (1992)
97	49	Neuropsychology clinic referrals without motive to malinger	Frederick et al. (1994)
55	20	Moderate to severe brain-damaged inpatients in rehab (CVA, HI, Hypoxia, Dementia with HI, PSP)	Guilmette et al. (1994)
76	34	Mixed neuropsychology referrals with radiological or electrophysiological evidence of neurological damage	Arnett et al. (1995)
84	25	Mixed neuropsychology referrals with radiological or electrophysiological evidence of neurological damage	Arnett et al. (1995)
		Patients with cerebrovascular accident	
60	20	Stroke patients (location unspecified)	Shamieh (1996)
		Patients with seizure disorder	
93	100	Temporal lobe seizure patients	Lee et al. (1992)
		Patients with head injury	
89	18	Brain-damaged inpatients in rehabilitation	Bernard & Fowler (1990)
56	16	Forensic inpatients with moderate to severe "organic" disorders	King (1992)
88	33	Traumatic brain injury	Greiffenstein et al. (1994)
100	7	Traumatic brain injury	Millis & Kler (1995)
90	20	Severe head trauma patients	Shamieh (1996)
		Individuals with learning disabilities	
100	40	College students	Warner-Chacon (1994)

(continued)

TABLE 5.2. *(continued)*

Specificity (%)	n	Sample	Author
		Individuals with low intelligence	
62	16	Patients with mental retardation	Goldberg & Miller (1986) Spiegel (2006)
77	49	Borderline IQ (70–79)	Spiegel (2006)
98	40	Low average IQ (80–89)	Spiegel (2006)
		Nonclinical samples	
100	16	Normal controls	Bernard & Fowler (1990)
100	80	Normal controls	Schretlen et al. (1991)
98	47	Normal middle-age/older controls	Philpott (1992)
100	32	College students	Griffin et al. (1997)
		Psychiatric patients	
100	50	Inpatients	Goldberg & Miller (1986)
90	18	Forensic patients referred for psychiatric treatment	Frederick et al. (1994)
90	20	Affective disorder (major depression with and without psychosis)	Guilmette et al. (1994)
86	14	Severe psychiatric disturbance (schizophrenia, schizoaffective, delusional)	Simon (1994)
87	30	Outpatients and inpatients with schizophrenia	Back et al. (1996)
34	37	Board-and-care residents with schizophrenia or other major mental illness, developmental disability, or advanced age	Griffin et al. (1997)
95	64	Older outpatients with major depression	Lee et al. (2000)
95	91	Affective disorder outpatients	Spiegel (2006)
88	51	Psychotic disorder outpatients	Spiegel (2006)

Note. CVA, cerebrovascular accident; HI, head injury; PSP, progressive supranuclear palsy.

50%, while specificity values are typically above 90% (Boone, Salazar, Lu, Warner-Chacon, & Razani, 2002; Vickery, Berry, Inman, Harris, & Orey, 2001). However, there are notable exceptions to the latter. An examinee's FIT performance may be adversely affected by the presence of genuine memory disorders (Schretlen, Brandt, Krafft, & van Gorp, 1991), dementia (Schretlen et al., 1991; Spiegel, 2006), stroke (Shamieh, 1996), low intelligence (i.e., borderline or lower IQ; Goldberg & Miller, 1986; Spiegel, 2006), reduced educational level (Back, Boone, Edwards, & Park, 1996; Spiegel, 2006), psychosis (Back et al., 1996; Griffin, Glassmire, Henderson, & McCann, 1997; Simon, 1994; Spiegel, 2006), and older age (Griffin et al., 1997; Schretlen et al., 1991; Spiegel, 2006). Therefore, clinicians should be cautious in making determinations of suspect effort based on the FIT among individuals with the aforementioned conditions).

Alternative Administration/Scoring Procedures

A number of investigators have developed alternative scoring methodologies that can potentially provide useful information in addition to the quantitative total-free-recall score on the FIT. Arnett, Hammeke, and Schwartz (1995) examined a number of quantitative and qualitative indices in two different simulation studies. In the first study, they compared FIT performances of college students instructed to malinger to those of a mixed group of neuropsychology patients with radiological (i.e., magnetic resonance imaging [MRI] or computed tomography [CT] scan) or electrophysiological (i.e., EEG) evidence of neurological damage. In a second study, they compared the FIT performances of first-year medical students instructed to feign to those of a different group of mixed neuropsychology patients using the same selection criteria. Arnett et al. (1995) found that a cutoff of less than two correct rows in the proper sequence was associated with a sensitivity (i.e., percentage of simulators correctly identified) of 47% and a specificity (i.e., percentage of nonsimulators correctly identified) of 97% in the first study, and a sensitivity of 64% and a specificity of 96% in the second study. The authors noted that due to the low sensitivity of this cutoff across their two studies, performance above the cutoff does not necessarily provide strong evidence to rule out malingering. However, because of the high specificity obtained across both studies, they concluded that recall of less than two rows strongly suggests malingering.

Griffin et al. (1996) recommended altering the FIT's instructions by requesting that examinees reproduce the 15 items "just as they appear on the card" (p. 387). Griffin et al. (1996) developed a qualitative scoring system that did not penalize examinees for omitting items but did subtract for other types of errors, such as within-row sequencing errors (e.g., 132) or embellishments of the stimulus figures, among others. Possible malingerers (i.e., individuals attempting to secure disability compensation for psychiatric symptoms) performed significantly worse than controls on quantitative score but equal to psychiatrically disabled nonmalingerers in residential placement. However, the controls and psychiatrically disabled individuals scored comparably on qualitative errors, and when combined, this larger group committed significantly fewer qualitative errors than the possible malingerer group; in particular, the possible malingerers generated more "dyslexic" (e.g., "d" for "b"), embellishment (an elaboration or adornment of a stimulus figure or elaborate drawing in lieu of the stimuli), gestalt (failure to reproduce a 3×5 configuration), and row sequence (rows not reproduced in correct sequence) errors.

Greiffenstein, Baker, and Gola (1996) evaluated four different scoring methods for the FIT in a comparison of mild traumatic brain injury (TBI) examinees who were suspected to be malingering and a group of moderate to severely injured TBI patients with dense amnesiacs removed from their sample. A score that considered the spatial placement of the recalled characters had higher classification accuracy than the standard score consisting of the total number of items recalled. The "spatial" score was calculated by summing the number of symbols accurately placed *within* a row. For example, a row consisting of the sequence "A C B D" would receive a spatial score of only one because only the "A" is placed in the correct spatial position. Although the "D" in the previous example was placed in the correct spatial position, it would not be given credit due to the fact that it was not part of the original FIT stimulus. Only correct items placed in the correct spatial position receive credit. A row consisting of the sequence "1 3 3 2" would receive a spatial score of two because the "1" and the second "3" are located in the correct spatial positions. A spatial score of less than 9 resulted in a sensitivity of 69% and a specificity of 82%, whereas the traditional quantitative scoring system (using a cutoff of less than 10 items) resulted in a sensitivity of 64% and a specificity of 78%. The authors did not provide information regarding the sensitivity and specificity values of the more commonly used quantitative cutoff of fewer than nine items.

Griffin et al. (1997) developed a modified version of the FIT (the Rey II) that was intended to be easier, but to appear more difficult, than the original FIT. To make the Rey II easier, these authors increased the internal logic of the test by removing the row of shapes, which did not have an inherent logical progression. The Rey II was made to appear harder by adding two-part figures to the stimulus card (e.g., a row of three circles, each surrounding a character in the A–B–C sequence). A group of college students in fact rated the Rey II as appearing significantly more difficult than the original FIT. The two-part figures in the Rey II also allowed for a larger number of potential qualitative errors. For example, examinees are penalized for production of only one part of a two-part figure.

Using a combination of differential prevalence and simulated malingering designs, Griffin et al. (1997) found that the qualitative scoring system for the Rey II demonstrated improved sensitivity and specificity for detection of noncredible performance in comparison to the original quantitatively scored FIT. In this study, the sensitivity of the quantitatively scored FIT using a cutoff of 9 was only 7% among college students instructed to malinger. In comparison, in the same sample, a qualitative error cutoff of 2 on the Rey II resulted in an improved sensitivity of 58%. The specificity of the quantitatively scored FIT among individuals from board-and-care homes with various psychiatric diagnoses was 34%. In contrast, the qualitative error cutoff of 2 on the Rey II resulted in a specificity of 73% in the same psychiatric sample.

The improved specificity of the qualitatively scored Rey II in comparison to the quantitatively scored FIT likely resulted from lower correlations between the Rey II qualitative score and performance on ability measures that may be compromised by various psychiatric and neuropsychological disorders. Griffin et al. (1997) calculated correlations between the quantitatively scored FIT, the Rey II qualitative score, and the total score for the Mini-Mental State Examination (MMSE; Folstein, Folstein, & McHugh, 1975), the Figural Memory subtest from the Wechsler Memory Scale–Revised (WMS-R; Wechsler, 1987), and the Altus Information Inventory, which is a brief measure of intellectual ability that has been found to be predictive of Wechsler Adult Intelligence Scale–Revised (WAIS–R; Gorsuch & Spielberger, 1965; Moon & Gorsuch, 1988) scores. Among the sample of psychiatric patients, the original quantitatively scored FIT correlated significantly with the MMSE total score ($r = .43$), the WMS-R Figural Memory subtest score ($r = .56$), and the Altus Information Inventory score ($r = .40$). In contrast, correlations between the Rey II qualitative system and these variables were nonsignificant (i.e., $r = .03$, $r = -.06$, and $r = -.16$, respectively). Although qualitative scoring indices may be less sensitive to genuine neuropsychological and intellectual deficits than the quantitative FIT score, none of the qualitative scoring indices discussed earlier have been cross-validated. Therefore, although these qualitative scoring indices show promise in identifying suspect effort on the FIT, they should be used cautiously until more data are available regarding the generalizability of the findings.

Boone, Salazar, et al. (2002) developed a recognition trial for the FIT in an effort to improve the test's sensitivity to suspect effort while concurrently retaining a high level of specificity. By employing a recognition trial following the traditional free-recall portion of the test, these authors effectively lowered the "floor" of the test by making it easier. It is a generally accepted neuropsychological principle that recognition memory tasks are simpler than free-recall tasks due to the fact that recognition tasks provide a cue to aid the examinee in remembering the previously presented information. In particular, visual recognition has been found to be a relatively well-preserved ability among amnesic patients and patients with traumatic brain injury (Freed, Corkin, Growden, & Nissen, 1989; Glassmire et al., 2003; Hart & O'Shanick, 1993; Tombaugh, 1997). In addition, recognition memory paradigms have been found to be particularly sensitive to noncredible cognitive symptoms (Boone, Salazar, et al., 2002; Greiffenstein et al., 1996; Glassmire et al., 2003; Iverson & Franzen, 1994; Tombaugh, 1997). This finding may be due to a misconception in the general public that recognition and free-recall tasks are equally difficult.

The Boone, Salazar, et al. (2002) recognition task consists of a page with 15 items from the standard FIT stimulus sheet interspersed with 15 foils that are similar to the target items (see Boone, Salazar, et al., 2002, for a reproduction of the recognition stimulus page). In this version of the FIT, the free-recall task is first presented in a standard format. At the conclusion, the examinee's reproductions are removed from view and the recognition form is then placed in front of the examinee with the following instructions: "On this page are the 15 things I showed you as well as 15 items that were not on the page. I want you to circle the things you remember from the page I showed you." Four different scores can be calculated including (1) recall correct, (2) recognition correct, (3) false-positive recognition errors, and (4) a combination score derived from the following equation: Total Score = recall correct + (recognition correct–false positives).

Boone, Salazar, et al. (2002) compared the performances of a suspect effort group with those of three groups: (1) neuropsychology clinic referrals not in litigation or seeking disability, (2) college students with learning disabilities, and (3) an older nonclinical control sample. The suspect effort group included neuropsychological examinees with documented noncredible cognitive symptoms who were referred for assessments in the context of litigation or disability evaluation. Criteria for inclusion in the suspect effort group included noncredible performance on at least two measures other than the FIT, as well as the presence of at least one other behavioral criterion associated with suspect effort (e.g., a pattern or severity of neuropsychological scores not consistent with medical or psychiatric condition, marked inconsistency between neuropsychological scores and activities of daily living, etc.). Boone, Salazar, et al. (2002) found that the use of the free recall + recognition combination score (cutoff < 20) increased FIT sensitivity from 47% (for the standard administration format) to 71%. Moreover, the combination score retained a high a specificity of 92% or above (i.e., an 8% or less false-positive rate in detecting suspect effort) across the three comparison groups.

In summary, when using the FIT, clinicians can take advantage of a number of indices. First, if a free-recall cutoff of fewer than nine items is used, clinicians can refer to Table 5.1 for sensitivity values and to Table 5.2 for specificity values that most closely match their clinical setting. The clinician should keep in mind that due to the relatively low sensitivity values obtained in many studies, the FIT in isolation cannot be used to *rule out* the presence of suboptimal effort. In contrast, due to the generally high specificity values across studies, the FIT is an effective tool in *ruling in* suspect effort. That is, when scores < 9 are observed, such scores are highly specific to the presence of inadequate effort except in select patient groups (e.g., borderline to mentally retarded IQ, stroke, dementia, low educational level, marked memory impairment, low-functioning psychotic patients, older patients). Alternatively, the concomitant use of the recognition trial developed by Boone, Salazar, et al. (2002) appears to increase test sensitivity to acceptable levels (i.e., 71%) without sacrificing specificity, although cross-validation data for this technique are needed. Finally, clinicians can examine for the presence of the various qualitative errors that may suggest the presence of suspect effort. However, these data are preliminary and should be used cautiously. Although the Rey II demonstrated promise in the detection of suboptimal effort, this instrument requires cross-validation before adoption into mainstream clinical practice. Due to the success of the FIT recognition trial observed by Boone, Salazar, et al. (2002), it is recommended that future research on either the FIT or the Rey II include a recognition trial.

DOT COUNTING TEST

André Rey (1941) originally developed the Dot Counting Test (DCT) as a technique to detect malingered cognitive symptoms. In its original design, a varied number of ungrouped dots were presented with the instructions to count the dots as quickly as possible. The key determinant of valid effort was a "linear progression" of response time as the number of dots increased (Frederick, 1997), referred to as performance curve analysis (Rogers et al., 1993). The test was later modified to its current format, which includes separate sets of grouped and ungrouped dots. The standardized version of the test (Boone, Lu, & Herzberg, 2002a) consists of 12 5″ × 7″ cards with varying numbers of dots. On the first set of six cards (ungrouped), there is a random arrangement of dots (ranging from 7 to 27 dots), whereas on the second set of six cards, the dots are arranged in clear visual patterns that facilitate a quick count (ranging from 8 to 28 dots). Patients are instructed to count the dots as quickly as possible and then verbalize their answers aloud. Responses and response times are then recorded for each card.

Until recently, there has been a paucity of empirical research examining the utility of the DCT despite the fact that it has been in existence for over 60 years. In addition, the studies that have examined its effectiveness have varied in terms of their methodology. For instance, many "analogue" studies have employed simulators instructed to malinger rather than groups of suspect-effort patients identified through independent criteria (Boone, Lu, Back, et al., 2002). Also, past researchers have followed different interpretive rules, particularly with regard to the types of scores that define suspect performance.

Traditionally, there have been two main approaches to the interpretation of the DCT version incorporating grouped and ungrouped dots (Lezak, 1995). The first, also originally employed by Rey, is that patients should (theoretically) take more time to count increased numbers of dots; more than one deviation from this linear pattern is considered suspect. The second interpretative strategy advises that suspect effort should be considered when the time taken to count grouped dots is equal to or greater than the time required to count ungrouped dots. However, more recently additional interpretation strategies have been adopted in an attempt to maximize the predictive ability of the DCT in the detection of suspect effort.

Most studies examining the effectiveness of the DCT in the identification of suspect effort have employed simulators (i.e., subjects instructed to feign), typically college students. Martin, Hayes, and Gouvier (1996) reported that students coached on how to avoid detection of malingering and uncoached college student simulators made significantly more errors on the DCT than did college students with or without a reported history of mild head injury. Based on this finding, the authors concluded that the student simulators were unable to portray brain impairment realistically on the DCT. Similarly, Paul, Franzen, Cohen, and Fremouw (1992) found that community and psychiatric simulators committed significantly more counting errors on the DCT than did patients with documented brain injury. However, the simulators did not differ from the patient group in terms of grouped or ungrouped dot counting time. In a study conducted by Beetar and Williams (1995), coached student simulators made counting errors on approximately one-third of the trials on a computer-modified version of the DCT, while the student control group committed errors on only 10% of the trials. Further, the simulators in this study also had significantly longer response times than the control sample.

Binks, Gouvier, and Waters (1997) conducted one of the most comprehensive studies using multiple subject groups and six dependent variables derived from the DCT. The authors reported that the number of total errors was best able to discriminate college undergraduate simulators (naïve and coached) from student controls and actual neuropsychological patients. Other variables that had some effectiveness in this regard were the total time for ungrouped dots minus the total time for grouped dots and the slopes of the response latency curves for the ungrouped and grouped dot counting trials, respectively. The authors concluded that the DCT represents an attractive and "less transparent" alternative in the detection of noncredible performance than do traditional forced-choice tests.

Recently, Erdal (2004) analyzed the effects of different types of motivation (e.g., compensation vs. avoiding punishment) and coaching (e.g., instruction regarding postconcussive symptoms) on DCT performance in college student simulators. She found that those simulators motivated by compensation made more "sequencing errors" (e.g., took longer to count cards with fewer dots) and required more time to count dots than simulators not offered compensation, simulators motivated to fake in order to avoid blame, and controls (nonsimulators). Those simulators who were coached on symptoms of postconcussion only, or coached and warned against appearing "too obvious," still took significantly longer to count both grouped and ungrouped cards than did the control group. However, those receiving coaching and warning were better in sequencing time patterns than the other simulation groups, with the exception of those subjects who were offered compensation; compensation appeared to negate the effect of the warning. These results suggest that different motivations uniquely affect DCT performance and that coached or warned malingerers can still be detected by the presence of delayed response times.

The effectiveness of the DCT has also been documented in clinical and forensic settings using actual noncredible patients identified via independent criteria. Hayes, Hale, and Gouvier (1998) reported that the DCT, in combination with the FIT and the M Test which measures malingering of schizophrenic symptoms (Beaber, Marston, Michelli, & Mills, 1985), correctly identified 60% of suspected malingerers in a forensic population. Youngjohn, Burrows, and Erdal (1995) documented that 26% of patients with reported symptoms of postconcussive syndrome did not show the usual pattern of taking more time to count larger groups of dots. Notably, all these patients were in litigation or were seeking monetary compensation for their injuries (and many had performed poorly on other tests of effort including the Portland Digit Recognition Test). Youngjohn et al. (1995) also found that 11% of their sample required as much time to count grouped as ungrouped dots, leading the authors to speculate that "variable attention, motivation, and/or cooperation" was present in this subset.

Despite the encouraging results of the foregoing studies, some investigators have questioned the predictive ability of the DCT in identifying noncredible cognitive symptoms. Rose, Hall, and Szalda-Petree (1998) compared four groups of participants (coached and uncoached college student simulators, moderately to severely head-injured patients, and normal controls) on multiple measures of the DCT. They found that the brain-injured participants made more grouped trend reversals (i.e., deviation from linear pattern of increased counting time as number of dots increased) but were comparable to the other groups, including simulators, on all other scores derived from the DCT (grouped and ungrouped counting time and number correct; ungrouped trend reversals). The control group showed significantly faster counting times for grouped dots as compared to all other groups of participants, who did not differ. Rose et al. also noted that the use of standardized cutoff scores (> 130 seconds counting time for grouped dots; > 180 seconds counting time for ungrouped dots) correctly classified only 9% of the simulated malingerers but resulted in 96% specificity.

In another study, Hiscock, Branham, and Hiscock (1994) reported that DCT performance (i.e., ungrouped dot counting time minus grouped dot counting time) was less effective than standard neuropsychological measures in detecting college students and prison inmates instructed to malinger. Finally, Greiffenstein et al. (1994) reported no significant group effect for either grouped or ungrouped dot counting times when comparing probable malingerers with TBI patients. However, the authors suggested that the lack of significant findings could be attributed to the use of percentile scores as the dependent measure rather than the more common use of time to completion.

Thus, although some promising data had emerged on the potential effectiveness of the DCT in the detection of suspect effort, other studies had raised significant questions regarding the usefulness of the DCT. Vickery et al. (2001), in a meta-analysis of six studies, noted that the DCT was less effective than other effort measures, separating honest responders and dissimulators by only three-quarters of a standard deviation, and recommended that other effort measures with higher demonstrated ability to differentiate groups be employed rather than the DCT.

In an attempt to provide more comprehensive and definitive data regarding the DCT as a measure of effort, Boone, Lu, Back, et al. (2002) recently undertook the most extensive study of the DCT to date. In it, they compared two suspect effort groups with various clinical groups of patients (e.g., head injury, learning disabled, stroke, schizophrenia, dementia, elderly normal, and depressed groups). All the participants in the first suspect-effort group were in litigation or seeking to obtain/maintain disability benefits, showed signs of noncredible performance on independent measures of effort, and met specific behavioral criteria (e.g., markedly inconsistent performances within or across test sessions). Patients in the second suspect-effort group were recruited from an inpatient forensic setting had been determined to be malingering by the consensus of hospital staff. Sensitivity of cutoff scores for various DCT variables (e.g., mean grouped dot counting time, ratio of mean grouped to ungrouped dot counting time, and errors) differed markedly between the civil and forensic suspect effort groups (ranging from 28% to 100%).

The variability in prediction in different suspect-effort groups found by Boone, Lu, Back, et al. (2002) indicates that individuals with noncredible symptoms drawn from different settings may choose differing approaches when attempting to fake deficits on the DCT. For example, some may exhibit very slow response times, whereas others may demonstrate counting errors. Also, in our experience, some may display suboptimal performance across both portions of the DCT (i.e., ungrouped and grouped dot cards), whereas others may restrict their fabricated poor performance to the counting of either grouped or ungrouped dots. Still others may feign signs of confusion/disorientation (e.g., claim that there are no dots on the cards!).

Boone, Lu, Back, et al. (2002) reported that the following combination formula was most sensitive in detecting individuals exerting suspect effort: mean ungrouped dot counting time + mean grouped counting time + number of errors. In later publications, this formula is referred to as an Effort Index, or "E-score" (Boone, Lu, & Herzberg, 2002a). Boone, Lu, and Herzberg (2002a) recommend adjustment of E-score cutoffs, depending on the differential diagnosis, in order to maintain adequate specificity (i.e., ≥90%) (see Table 5.3). For instance, the E-score cutoff for patients with depression is 12 (94% specificity), while for patients with schizophrenia, the cutoff must be raised to 19 to achieve comparable specificity (93%). This interpretive flexibility mitigates the confounding effects that various clinical conditions can have on DCT performance and limits false-positive identifica-

TABLE 5.3. Recommended DCT Cutoffs and Interpretive Ranges

Normal effort group	E-score cutoff	Interpretive range		Sensitivity (%)	Specificity (%)
		Normal effort	Suspect effort		
Nonclinical	11	≤ 10	≥ 11	94.1	90.2
Depression	12	≤ 11	≥ 12	91.8	93.8
Schizophrenia	19	≤ 18	≥ 19	71.8	92.9
Head injury	19	≤ 18	≥ 19	71.8	90.0
Stroke	22	≤ 21	≥ 22	62.4	88.9
Learning disability	13	≤ 12	≥ 13	88.2	90.3
Mild dementia	22	≤ 21	≥ 22	62.4	93.8
Normal effort groups combined	17	≤ 16	≥ 17	78.8	90.4

Note. Data taken from Boone, Lu, and Herzberg (2002a). Cutoff scores for Table 5.3 were selected to correspond to specificity values of approximately 90%. The formula for computing the DCT E-score is available in the test manual published by Western Psychological Services.

tions. However, DCT sensitivity in detecting suboptimal effort fluctuates with adjustments to the cutoff scores; for example, a cutoff of 12 is associated with detection of 92% of noncredible subjects, but with a cutoff of 19, sensitivity drops to 72%. Importantly, Boone et al. advised against the use of the DCT in the differential diagnosis of feigned versus actual moderate dementia, as the DCT demonstrated an approximately 50% misidentification rate in this group. In addition, more recent data have revealed unacceptably low specificity levels in populations of people with mental retardation (21%, Marshall & Happe, 2005; see also Victor & Boone, Chapter 14, this volume); DCT performance in these individuals is usually characterized by equal ungrouped and grouped dot counting times. However, for most clinical groups (e.g., head injury, learning disability, depression, schizophrenia, and older age), cutoffs can be selected that maintain specificity at ≥ 90% but also result in adequate sensitivity (i.e., ≥ 70%). Also, scores on the DCT are minimally influenced by gender, age, and education, thus avoiding the need to "correct" for these variables.

In conclusion, although the DCT has existed for over a half century, it has only recently begun to receive widespread interest in clinical and research settings. While initial research examining its effectiveness was contradictory, this was likely an artifact of the choice of scores studied and the use of simulating rather than "real world" noncredible subjects. Development of a combination score incorporating both response times and errors shows adequate sensitivity in detecting suspect effort (averaging 78.8%), with detection rates likely higher in a correctional setting. However, specificity rates vary considerably across clinical comparison groups, and in its current form, the DCT appears contraindicated for use in the determination of actual versus feigned mental retardation and moderate dementia presentations.

REY WORD RECOGNITION TEST

The Rey Word Recognition Test (WRT) was also developed by André Rey in the 1940s in his attempt to develop a systematic process to detect noncredible performance on cognitive-based tests (Frederick, 2002). It has since been used as a measure of malingering of memory complaints (Greiffenstein et al., 1994; Lezak, 1983), primarily because it represents a quick and efficient assessment tool (i.e., under 5 minutes) that has good face validity as a test of memory. However, published research regarding its effectiveness as a tool for detecting feigned memory complaints has been limited.

In its traditional format (Frederick 2002; Lezak, 1983), the patient is instructed to listen carefully and remember a list of words that is read aloud. The examiner then proceeds to read a list of 15 unrelated words at a rate of one word per second.[2] After a very brief delay (i.e., 5 seconds), the patient is given a page listing the 15 test words as well as 15 foils and is instructed to circle only those words that were from the list just presented. Patients complete the test at their own pace and typically finish within 1–2 minutes.

It should be noted that other researchers have modified the original administration, substantially changing the nature of the test. For instance, Greiffenstein et al. (1996) read both the target stimuli and the 30-word recognition list aloud to the subset of patients in their study who had reading difficulties and instructed them to say "yes" or "no" to each test item. Frederick et al. (1994) and Frederick (1997) also used this approach because they desired to present both the target stimuli and test items in the same (oral) modality. In the oral format patients must immediately make a choice for each test item in isolation. In contrast, in the original version, they can scan all 30 items at once (i.e., original list words plus foils) and systematically decide which ones to endorse as previously heard items. The magnitude of the potential impact of differences in instructional set on the predictive utility of the Rey WRT has not been empirically studied.

Rey proposed that the WRT should be administered prior to a list learning task such as the Rey Auditory Verbal Learning Test (RAVLT), in which the patient is given five trials to learn a list of 15 unrelated words. Because recognition is an easier memory task than free recall, if the patient recognizes an equal number or fewer words than recalled on the first trial of the Rey RAVLT, performance is judged to be noncredible (Lezak, 1983). This strategy has met with limited success in terms of its sensitivity in detecting suboptimal effort, although it has been noted to have very good specificity (see Table 5.4). Frederick found that only 6.4% of criminal defendants with

TABLE 5.4. Proposed Cutoffs in the Literature for the Rey Word Recognition Test

Study	Target group	Contrast group	Cutoff	Sensitivity (%)	Specificity (%)
Greiffenstein et al. (1994)	PM (*n* = 43)	TBIn (*n* = 33)	Correct < 5	59	88
			Correct < 6	81	80
	PM (*n* = 43)	PPCS (*n* = 30)	Correct < 5	61	93
			Correct < 6	86	80
Greiffenstein et al. (1995)	PM (*n* = 68)	TBIn (*n* = 56)	Correct – FP ≤ 6	79	74
	PM (*n* = 68)	PPCS (*n* = 53)	Correct – FP ≤ 6	92	61
Greiffenstein et al. (1996)	PM (*n* = 90)	TBIn (*n* = 60)	Correct ≤ RAVLT 1	58	96
			Correct – FP ≤RAVLT 1	62	86
			Correct < 6	80	93
			Correct – FP < 5	72	84
Frederick et al. (1994)			Correct – FP ≤ RAVLT 1	62	86
			Correct < 6	80	93
			Correct – FP < 5	72	84
Frederick et al. (1994)	SIM (*n* = 117)	NC (*n* = 92)	Correct ≤ RAVLT 1	4	97
	FORm (*n* = 17)	FORn (*n* = 18)	Correct ≤ RAVLT 1	23	100
Nitch et al. (2006)	PMf (*n* = 41)	MC (*n* = 41)	Correct ≤ 7	81	90
			Correct – FP + (1st 8 words) ≤ 10	68	95
				63	95
	PMm (*n* = 51)	MC (*n* = 41)	Correct ≤ 5	63	95
			Correct – FP + (1st 8 words) ≤ 7	67	95
	PM (TBI) (*n* = 38)	MC (*n* = 82)	Correct – FP ≤ 5	76	90
			Correct – FP + (1st 8 words) ≤ 9	82	90

Note. Frederick et al. (1994) modified the test administration into a forced-choice procedure. PM, probable malingerers; PMf, female probable malingerers; PMm, male probable malingerers; PM (TBI), probable malingerers reporting traumatic brain injury; TBIn, traumatic brain injury with no indication of compensation-seeking status; PPCS, persistent postconcussive syndrome; SIM, malingering simulators; MC, mixed clinical; NC, normal controls; FORm, forensic psychiatric patients with motive to fake bad; FORn, forensic psychiatric patients with no identified motive to fake bad; FP, false-positive errors; RAVLT 1, number correct on first trial of Rey Auditory Verbal Learning Test.

motive to feign showed a RAVLT trial 1 recall > Rey Word Recognition (orally administered forced choice paradigm with a range of scores from –15 to +15). Further, below-chance responding (i.e., score < –5) was found in fewer than 1%, whereas 16.9% obtained scores below the normative floor (i.e., a score of < +5).

Nitch, Boone, Wen, Arnold, and Alfano (2006) recently conducted a comprehensive study of the WRT with noncredible patients (as determined by failed psychometric and behavioral criteria and external motive to feign) and a heterogeneous neuropsychology clinic sample and a group of college students with learning disabilities. In examining various scores and score combinations derived from the WRT, these researchers reported that a combination variable (recognition correct minus false positive errors + number of words recognized from the first eight words on the list) had the best predictive utility in detecting patients in the suspect effort group. The finding that double-weighting of the first eight words from the list may increase test effectiveness suggests that patients who are attempting to feign memory deficits fail to display expected primacy effects on list-learning tasks (i.e., fail to recognize items presented earlier in the sequence).

Another primary finding from the Nitch et al. (2006) study was the need for separate gender-based cutoff scores, likely due to the better performance of women on verbal-based tasks in general (Kimura, 1999). Table 5.4 lists the predictive values for the WRT variables divided by gender. With specificity set at 90% or higher, a cutoff score of 10 or less on the combination variable was associated with 68% sensitivity in detecting noncredible women; however, this same cutoff score was associated with only 78% specificity in men. In males, the cutoff score for the combination variable had to be lowered to 7 or less in order to achieve acceptable specificity (i.e., ≥90%), although sensitivity to detection of noncredible male subjects was comparable to sensitivity in female subjects (i.e., 67%). However, use of this cutoff for detection of suspect-effort women would have lowered sensitivity to only 44%. These results indicate that failure to consider gender when interpreting the WRT can increase the probability of making a Type I error or "false alarm" in prediction for male examinees. Conversely, use of combined gender cutoff scores can increase the risk of making a Type II error or "miss" in prediction for female examinees.

Given that a common differential diagnosis is between credible versus noncredible symptoms in the context of TBI, Nitch et al. (2006) also examined the sensitivity values in the subset of suspect-effort patients who reported head trauma (primarily mild). Unfortunately, due to a small sample size, the group could not be subdivided by gender. However, the results suggested that the WRT has particular sensitivity within this subgroup. For instance, using a cutoff score of 9 or less for the combination variable, approximately 82% of suspect-effort patients were accurately detected (with 90% specificity). These data suggest that individuals feigning cognitive dysfunction in the context of mild TBI may target memory tasks in particular to illustrate their feigned disability, and thus the WRT may have particular utility in this population.

In conclusion, the Rey WRT has been in existence for decades but only a handful of publications regarding its validity have appeared. However, recent research suggests that the test has excellent sensitivity (particularly in a mild head injury population) and specificity (even in a population with learning disabilities), despite its extreme brevity. Incorporation of primacy effect data, as well as the use of gender-specific cutoffs, appear to enhance test effectiveness.

b TEST

The b Test (Boone et al., 2000; Boone, Lu, & Herzberg, 2002b) was developed to measure feigned difficulties in recognizing overlearned information and processing speed. Letter recognition and discrimination are overlearned skills; that is, they are practiced and used so frequently that they become routine and automatic. A number of studies indicate that such overlearned skills are relatively well preserved following acquired brain deficits. This is the rationale underlying the use of word pronunciation tasks, such as the North American Adult Reading Test (Blair & Spreen, 1989) and the Wechsler Test of Adult Reading (Wechsler, 2001), to predict premorbid functioning among individuals who have sustained various neurological injuries, as such tasks are relatively unaffected by such injuries.

The b Test requires examinees to circle all of the lowercase *b* letters that are interspersed with similar-appearing letters (e.g., *p*, *q*, *d*) and figures in a booklet containing 15 stimulus pages. Some distractor *b*'s are rotated to a 45-degree angle, and others have double stems. The authors hypothesized that the use of distractors similar to the letter *b* or incorporating/distorting the letter *b* would lower the b Test's face validity as a measure of effort and increase its apparent difficulty. In addition, in each successive presentation of the stimulus pages, the array of symbols becomes progressively smaller; this was anticipated to make the test appear to become harder while actually maintaining a consistently low level of difficulty throughout. Another strength of the b Test is that successful performance does not require intact memory ability, thereby lowering its sensitivity to bona fide memory deficits and increasing its specificity to noncredible symptoms.

Validation of the b Test was similar to that of the DCT, employing a real-world suspect-effort group as identified by failed performance on other effort indicators and behavioral criteria, and various clinical comparison groups (e.g., moderate/severe brain injury, depression, schizophrenia, learning disability, stroke, and normal aging). The performance of the non-credible group was characterized by slowed completion time, omission

TABLE 5.5. Recommended b Test Cutoffs and Interpretive Ranges

Normal effort group	E-score cutoff	Interpretive range		Sensitivity (%)	Specificity (%)
		Normal effort	Suspect effort		
Nonclinical	90	≤ 89	≥ 90	76.9	88.5
Depression	120	≤ 119	≥ 120	73.6	89.5
Schizophrenia	190	≤ 189	≥ 190	53.8	89.3
Head injury	90	≤ 89	≥ 90	76.9	90.0
Stroke	170	≤ 169	≥ 170	56.0	94.4
Learning disability	140	≤ 139	≥ 140	65.9	90.3
Normal effort groups combined	150	≤ 149	≥ 150	63.7	88.8

Data were taken from Boone, Lu, and Herzberg (2002b). Cutoff scores for Table 5.5 were selected to correspond to specificity values at approximately 90%. The formula for computing the b Test E-score is available in the test manual published by Western Psychological Services.

errors (i.e., b's that were not circled), and commission errors (i.e., stimuli other than b that were circled), especially circling of d's. Boone, Lu, and Herzberg (2002b) found that an equation which included mean time per page, number of total omission errors, and number of total commission errors (including double-weighting of d errors) was the most sensitive measure to the presence of suspect effort; a cut-score of ≥ 90 identified third-quarters of noncredible subjects while limiting false-positive identifications in the head injury comparison group to ≤ 10% (see Table 5.5). Similar sensitivity rates (at ≥ 90% specificity) were observed for the depressed and learning disability comparison groups. However, the substantial raising of cutoffs necessary to maintain adequate specificity in the stroke and schizophrenia groups reduced sensitivity to approximately 50%. These findings suggest that the b Test, while effective in the differential diagnosis of actual versus feigned depression, head injury, and learning disability, would not be an optimal choice for use in distinguishing real versus feigned stroke and schizophrenia. This observation is not entirely unexpected given that the b Test is a continuous performance test, and psychotic patients often perform poorly on such measures (Saykin et al., 1994).

CONCLUSION

In the past several years, there has been a dramatic rise in the use of stand-alone measures, indices, and assessment strategies used to detect malingering and other forms of insufficient effort during neuropsychological evaluations. A recent survey by Slick et al. (2004) indicated that nearly 80% of practitioners use at least one such technique in every evaluation they conduct. Given the strong research support for the forced-choice measures, it is not surprising that many of the most commonly used effort instruments in the field today adopt this format. However, there has also been an increased use of non-forced-choice measures to detect malingering. The field cannot rely solely on forced-choice techniques as a measure of effort due to the relative ease with which patients can be educated as to how to pass these measures. Of concern, there have been reports in the literature that examinees have been "coached" by others on how to pass tests of effort and motivation (Victor & Abeles, 2004; Youngjohn, 1995).

One potential advantage of non-forced-choice measures is that they are potentially less identifiable as effort tests and thus can more easily "blend in" with the other tests that are included in a comprehensive neuropsychological battery. In addition, the "typical" performance by a person with authentic brain impairment on these measures is less obvious as well. For instance, on the DCT, a potential malingerer has to quickly decide among the potential strategies of feigning mental slowing, inaccurate responding across the board, or relative impairment in counting ungrouped versus grouped dots. Given this complexity, the odds are increased that persons exerting insufficient effort will produce rare and/or unbelievable response patterns.

One of the greatest advantages of the measures reviewed in this chapter is their brevity and ease of use. Unlike forced-choice measures that require a larger number of items in order to increase their statistical reliability, most of the non-forced-choice measures are time efficient yet provide valid quantitative and qualitative data. Three of the tests reviewed here (i.e., FIT, WRT, and DCT) take less than 5 minutes to administer and all of them can be scored and interpreted in approximately the same amount of time. Current recommended practice is to administer multiple effort indicators interspersed through the test battery to continuously sample effort and to provide converging evidence of noncredible performance, thereby increasing confidence in the accuracy of the determination of suboptimal effort. In this context, the availability of multiple, brief effort measures becomes invaluable.

A note of caution is in order with regard to the use of effort measures in certain specific populations that tend to have consistently lowered specificity rates (patients with psychotic-spectrum disorders, mental retardation, dementia, stroke, etc.). In addition, the influence of clinical diagnosis, demographic variables, and the interactions among them have not been adequately explored for a number of measures, although increased attention has been given to these issues in the recent past (Arnold et al., 2005; Nitch et al., 2006, and reviewed in Salazar, Lu, Wen, and Boone, Chapter 18, this volume). Because of the predictive limitations inherent in even the most well-researched instruments, each case must be evaluated based on multiple factors, including the assessment context, behavioral observations, tests results, and collateral information (Bush et al., 2005).

NOTES

1. The FIT has been referred to by a number of names in the literature, including the Rey 15-Item Visual Memory Test, the Rey 15-Item Memorization Test, the Rey Visual Memory Test of Malingering, and the FIT, among others. For consistency and ease of reading, the test is referred to as the FIT throughout this chapter. Specific modifications of the test that have been given other names are referred to by the specific names that appear in the literature for such modifications (e.g., the Rey II).
2. Original words used by Rey (in French) differ from those used by modern researchers (Lezak, 1983) due to the outdated nature of Rey's stimuli (e.g., chamois and countryman).

REFERENCES

Arnett, P. A., Hammeke, T. A., & Schwartz, L. (1995). Quantitative and qualitative performance on Rey's 15-Item Test in neurological patients and dissimulators. *The Clinical Neuropsychologist, 9*, 17–26.

Arnold, G., Boone, K. B., Lu, P., Dean, A., Wen, J., Nitch, S., et al. (2005). Sensitivity and specificity of Finger Tapping Test scores for the detection of suspect effort. *The Clinical Neuropsychologist, 19*, 105–120.

Back, C. L., Boone, K. B., Edwards, C. T., & Parks, C. (1996). The performance of schizophrenics on three cognitive tests of malingering: Rey 15-Item Memory Test, Rey Dot Counting, and Hiscock Forced-Choice Method. *Assessment, 3*, 449–457.

Beaber, R. J., Martson, A., Michelli, J., & Mills, M. J. (1985). A brief test for measuring malingering in schizophrenic individuals. *American Journal of Psychiatry, 142*, 1478–1481.

Beetar, J. T., & Williams, J. M. (1995). Malingering response style on the memory assessment scales and symptom validity tests. *Archives of Clinical Neuropsychology, 10*, 57–72.

Bernard, L. C., & Fowler, W. (1990). Assessing the validity of memory complaints: Performance of brain-damaged and normal individuals on Rey's task to detect malingering. *Journal of Clinical Psychology, 46*, 432–436.

Bernard, L. C., Houston, W., & Natoli, L. (1993). Malingering on neuropsychological memory tests: Potential objective indicators. *Journal of Clinical Psychology, 49*, 45–53.

Binks, P. G., Gouvier, W. D., & Waters, W. F. (1997). Malingering detection with the Dot Counting Test. *Archives of Clinical Neuropsychology, 12*, 41–46.

Blair, J. R., & Spreen, O. (1989). Predicting premorbid IQ: A revision of the National Adult Reading Test. *The Clinical Neuropsychologist, 3*, 129–136.

Boone, K. B., Lu, P., Back, C., King, C., Lee, A. Philpott, L., et al. (2002). Sensitivity and specificity of the Rey Dot Counting Test in patients with suspect effort and various clinical samples. *Archives of Clinical Neuropsychology, 17*, 625–642.

Boone, K., Lu, P., & Herzberg, D. S. (2002a). *The Dot Counting Test Manual*, Los Angeles: Western Psychological Services.

Boone, K., Lu, P., & Herzberg, D. S. (2002b). *The b Test Manual*, Los Angeles: Western Psychological Services.

Boone, K. B., Lu, P., Sherman, D., Palmer, B., Back, C., Shamieh, E., et al. (2000). Validation of a new technique to detect malingering of cognitive symptoms: The b Test. *Archives of Clinical Neuropsychology, 15,* 227–241.

Boone, K. B., Salazar, X., Lu, P., Warner-Chacon, K., & Razani, J. (2002). The Rey 15-Item recognition trial: A technique to enhance sensitivity of the Rey 15-Item Memorization Test. *Journal of Clinical and Experimental Neuropsychology, 24*(5), 561–573.

Boone, K. B., Savodnik, I., Ghaffarian, S., Lee, A., Freeman, D., & Berman, N. (1995). Rey 15-Item Memorization and Dot Counting scores in a "stress" claim worker's compensation population: Relationship to personality (MCMI) scores. *Journal of Clinical Psychology, 51,* 457–463.

Bush, S. S., Ruff, R. M., Tröster, A. I., Barth, J. T., Koffler, S. P., Pliskin, N. H., et al. (2005). Symptom validity assessment: Practice issues and medical necessity. *Archives of Clinical Neuropsychology, 20*(4), 419–426.

Erdal, K. (2004). The effects of motivation, coaching, and knowledge of neuropsychology on the simulated malingering of head injury. *Archives of Clinical Neuropsychology, 19*(1), 73–88.

Folstein, M. F., Folstein, S. E., & McHugh, P. R. (1975). Mini mental state: A practical method for grading the state of patients for the clinician. *Journal of Psychiatric Research, 12,* 189–198.

Frederick, R. I. (1997). *Validity Indicator Profile Manual*, Minneapolis, MN: National Computer Systems.

Frederick, R. I. (2002). A review of Rey's strategies for detecting malingered neuropsychological impairment. *Journal of Forensic Neuropsychology. Special Issue: Detection of response bias in forensic neuropsychology: Part I, 2,* 1–25.

Frederick, R., Sarfaty, S., Johnston, J. D., & Powel, J. (1994). Validation of a detector of response bias on a forced-choice test of nonverbal ability. *Neuropsychology, 8,* 118–125.

Freed, D. M., Corkin, S. Growden, J. H., & Nissen, M. J. (1989). Selective attention in Alzheimer's Disease: Characterizing cognitive subgroups of patients. *Neuropsychology, 27,* 325–339.

Glassmire, D. M., Bierley, R. A., Wisniewski, A. M., Greene, R. L., Kennedy, J. E., & Date, E. (2003). Using the WMS-III Faces subtest to detect malingered memory impairment. *Journal of Clinical and Experimental Neuropsychology, 25,* 465–481.

Goldberg, T. O., & Miller, H. R. (1986). Performance of psychiatric inpatients and intellectually deficient individuals on a task that assesses the validity of memory complaints. *Journal of Clinical Psychology, 42,* 792–795.

Gorsuch, R., & Speilberger, C. (1965). Predictive and concurrent validity of the Altus Information Inventory with high school students. *Psychological Reports, 16,* 633–636.

Greiffenstein, M. F., Baker, W. J., & Gola, T. (1994). Validation of malingered amnesia measures with a large clinical sample. *Psychological Assessment, 6*(3), 218–224.

Greiffenstein, M. F., Baker, W. J., & Gola, T. (1996). Comparison of multiple scoring methods for Rey's malingered amnesia methods. *Archives of Clinical Neuropsychology, 11*(4), 283–293.

Greiffenstein, M. F., Gola, T., & Baker, W. J. (1995). MMPI-2 validity scales versus domain specific measures in detection of factitious traumatic brain injury. *The Clinical Neuropsychologist, 9*, 230–240.

Griffin, G. A., Glassmire, D. M., Henderson, E. H., & McCann, C. (1997). Rey II: Redesigning the Rey Screening Test of Malingering. *Journal of Clinical Psychology, 53*, 757–766.

Griffin, G. A., Normington, J. M., & Glassmire, D. M. (1996). Qualitative dimensions in scoring the Rey Visual Memory Test of Malingering. *Psychological Assessment, 8*, 383–387.

Guilmette, T. J., Hart, K. J., Giuliano, A. J., & Leininger, B. E. (1994). Detecting simulated memory impairment: Comparison of the Rey Fifteen-Item Test and the Hiscock Forced-Choice Procedure. *The Clinical Neuropsychologist, 8*, 283–294.

Hart, R. P., & O'Shanick, G. J. (1993). Forgetting rates for verbal, figural, and pictorial stimuli. *Journal of Clinical and Experimental Neuropsychology, 15*, 245–265.

Hayes, J. S., Hale, D. B., & Gouvier, W. D. (1998). Malingering detection in a mentally retarded forensic population. *Applied Neuropsychology, 5*, 33–36.

Hiscock, C. K., Branham, J. D., & Hiscock, M. (1994). Detection of feigned cognitive impairment: The two-alternative forced-choice method compared with selected conventional tests. *Journal of Psychopathology and Behavioral Assessment, 16*, 95–110.

Iverson, G. L., & Franzen, M. D. (1994). The Recognition Memory Test, Digit Span, and Knox Cube Test as markers of malingered memory impairment. *Assessment, 1*, 323–334.

Kimura, D. (1999). *Sex and cognition*. Cambridge, MA: MIT Press.

King, C. (1992). *The detection of malingering of cognitive deficits in a forensic population*. Unpublished doctoral dissertation, California School of Professional Psychology, Los Angeles.

Lee, A., Boone, K. B., Lesser, I., Wohl, M., Wilkins, S., & Parks, C. (2000). Performance of older depressed patients on two cognitive malingering tests: False positive rates for the Rey 15-Item Memorization and Dot Counting Tests. *The Clinical Neuropsychologist, 14*, 303–308.

Lee, G., Loring, D., & Martin, R. (1992). Rey's 15-Item visual memory test for the detection of malingering: Normative observations on patients with neurological disorders. *Psychological Assessment, 4*, 43–46.

Lezak, M. D. (1983). *Neuropsychological assessment* (2nd ed.). New York: Oxford University Press.

Lezak, M. D. (1995). *Neuropsychological assessment* (3rd ed.). New York: Oxford University Press.

Marshall, P., & Happe, M. (2005). *Performance of mentally retarded patients on five common tests of malingering*. Poster presented at the annual meeting of the International Neuropsychological Society, St. Louis, MO.

Martin, R. C., Hayes, J. S., & Gouvier, W. D. (1996). Differential vulnerability between postconcussion self-report and objective malingering tests in identifying simulated mild head injury. *Journal of Clinical and Experimental Neuropsychology, 18*, 265–275.

Miller, G. A. (1956). The magical number seven, plus or minus two: Some limits on our capacity for processing information. *Psychological Review, 63*, 81–97.

Millis, S. R., & Kler, S. (1992). Limitations of the Rey Fifteen-Item Test in the detection of malingering. *The Clinical Neuropsychologist, 9*, 421–424.

Moon, C., & Gorsuch, R. (1988). Information inventory: The quicker test for intelligence. *Journal of Clinical Psychology, 44*, 248–251.

Morgan, S. F. (1991). Effect of true memory impairment on a test of memory complaint validity. *Archives of Clinical Neuropsychology, 6*, 327–334.

Nitch, S., Boone, K.B., Wen, J. Arnold, G., & Alfano, K. (2006). The utility of the Rey Word Recognition Test in the detection of suspect effort. *The Clinical Neuropsychologist, 20*(4), 873–887.

Paul, D. S., Franzen, M. D., Cohen, S. H., & Fremouw, W. (1992). An investigation into the reliability and validity of two tests used in the detection of dissimulation. *International Journal of Clinical Neuropsychology, 14*, 1–9.

Philpott, L. M. (1992). *The effects of severity of cognitive impairment and age on two malingering tests: An investigation of the Rey Memory Test and Rey Dot Counting Test in Alzheimer's patients and normal middle aged/older adults.* Unpublished doctoral dissertation, California School of Professional Psychology, Los Angeles.

Rabin, L. A., Barr, W. B., & Burton, L. A. (2005). Assessment practices of clinical neuropsychologists in the United States and Canada: A survey of INS, NAN, and APA Division 40 members. *Archives of Clinical Neuropsychology, 20*, 33–65.

Rey, A. (1941). L'examen psychologie dans las cas d'encephalopathie traumatique. *Archives de Psychologie, 28*, 286–340.

Rey, A. (1964). *L'examen clinique en psychologie.* Paris: Presses Universitaires de France.

Rogers, R., Harrell, E. H., & Liff, C. D. (1993). Feigning neuropsychological impairment: A critical review of methodological and clinical considerations. *Clinical Psychology Review, 13*, 255–274.

Rose, F. E., Hall, S., & Szalda-Petree, A. D. (1998). A comparison of four tests of malingering and the effects of coaching. *Archives of Clinical Neuropsychology, 13*, 349–363.

Saykin, A. J., Shtasel, D. L., Gur, R. E., Kester, D. B., Mozley, L. H., Stafiniak, P., et al. (1994). Neuropsychological deficits in neuroleptic naïve patients with first-episode schizophrenia. *Archives of General Psychiatry, 51*, 124–131.

Schretlen, D., Brandt, J., Krafft, L., & van Gorp, W. (1991). Some caveats in using the Rey 15-Item Memory Test to detect malingered amnesia. *Psychological Assessment, 3*, 667–672.

Shamieh, E. W. (1996). *The effects of severe brain damage on three malingering tests: An investigation of the Rey Memory Test, Rey Dot Counting Test, and b Test in head trauma and stroke patients.* Unpublished doctoral dissertation, California School of Professional Psychology, Los Angeles.

Simon, M. J. (1994). The use of the Rey Memory Test to assess malingering in criminal defendants. *Journal of Clinical Psychology, 50*, 913–917.

Slick, D. J., Tan, J. E., Strauss, E. H., & Hultsch, D. F. (2004). Detecting malingering: A survey of experts' practices. *Archives of Clinical Neuropsychology, 19*(4), 465–473.

Spiegel, E. (2006). *The Rey 15-Item Memorization Test: Performance in under-represented populations in the absence of obvious motivation to feign neurocognitive symptoms.* Unpublished doctoral dissertation, Fuller Theological Seminary.

Spreen, O., & Strauss, E. (1998). *A compendium of neuropsychological tests: Administration, norms, and commentary* (2nd ed.). London: Oxford University Press.

Sumanti, M., Boone, K. B., Savodnick, I., & Gorsuch, R. (2006). Noncredible psychiatric and cognitive symptoms in a workers' compensation "stress" claim sample. *The Clinical Neuropsychologist, 20,* 754–765.

Tombaugh, T. N. (1997). The Test of Memory Malingering (TOMM): Normative data from cognitively intact and cognitively impaired individuals. *Psychological Assessment, 9,* 260–268.

Vickery, C. D., Berry, D. T. R., Inman, T. H., Harris, M. J., & Orey, S. A. (2001). Detection of inadequate effort on neuropsychological testing: A meta-analytic review of selected procedures. *Archives of Clinical Neuropsychology, 16,* 45–73.

Victor, T. L., & Abeles, N. (2004). Coaching clients to take psychological and neuropsychological tests: A clash of ethical obligations. *Professional Psychology: Research and Practice, 35,* 373–379.

Warner-Chacon, K. R. (1994). The performance of adult students with learning disabilities on cognitive tests of malingering. Unpublished doctoral dissertation. California School of Professional Psychology, Los Angeles.

Wechsler, D. (1987). *Wechsler Memory Scale–Revised: Manual.* San Antonio, TX: Psychological Corporation.

Wechsler, D. (2001). *Wechsler Test of Adult Reading Manual.* San Antonio, TX: Psychological Corporation.

Youngjohn, J. R. (1995). Confirmed attorney coaching prior to neuropsychological evaluation. *Assessment, 2,* 279–283.

Youngjohn, J. R., Burrows, L., & Erdal, K. (1995). Brain damage or compensation neurosis? The controversial post-concusssion syndrome. *The Clinical Neuropsychologist, 9,* 112–123.

CHAPTER 6

Intelligence Tests as Measures of Effort

Talin Babikian
Kyle Brauer Boone

Neuropsychologists' role in forensic evaluations has become increasingly more prevalent in recent years. Among the major publications in neuropsychology, such as *The Clinical Neuropsychologist, Archives of Clinical Neuropsychology*, and the *Journal of Clinical and Experimental Neuropsychology*, publications in forensic neuropsychology increased from 4% in 1990 to 14% in 2000, with 86% of these articles addressing issues related to malingering (Sweet, King, Malina, Bergman, & Simmons, 2002). The base rates of malingering likely vary depending on the patient population, with the following estimates reported: mild head injury (39%), fibromyalgia or chronic fatigue (35%), pain or somatoform disorder (31%), neurotoxic disorders (27%), electrical injury (22%), depressive disorders (15%), anxiety (14%), dissociative disorders (11%), seizure disorders (9%), moderate or severe head injury (9%), and vascular dementia (2%) (Mittenberg, Patton, Canyock, & Condit, 2002).

Although intelligence tests date back to the early 20th century, the use of intelligence measures or their components in detecting suspect effort has been a more recent endeavor. The use of tests specifically designed and dedicated to measure effort adds to battery length and such measures are likely targets of coaching attempts. Thus, many investigators have recently recommended that standard cognitive tasks serve "double duty" to detect non-credible test performance instead of, or in addition, to freestanding effort measures (Meyers & Volbrecht, 2003; Sherman, Boone, Lu, & Razani, 2002). Because intelligence tests are among the most commonly administered measures in a neuropsychological battery, components of such measures have recently been a focus of study in the detection of suspect effort.

The issue of feigned deficits in overall intelligence has recently become particularly salient in criminal cases, given the Supreme Court's recent ruling (*Atkins v. Virginia*, 2002) prohibiting the use of the death penalty in individuals with mental retardation. Evaluation of cognitive function is often central to sentencing decisions, thereby making it imperative for clinicians to differentiate true mental retardation from deliberate suboptimal performance. Innovative and effective measures of effort in this population are, however, lacking (see Victor and Boone, Chapter 14, this volume).

This chapter reviews the efficacy of various intelligence measures and associated subtests in detecting suboptimal effort. An effort was made to include all intelligence tests used as measures of suspect performance, however, only studies using the Wechsler Adult Intelligence Scales (WAIS-R [Wechsler, 1981] and WAIS-III [Wechsler, 1997]) were found in the literature. Investigations employing simulation designs in which subjects were instructed to feign cognitive impairment are reviewed first, following by studies examining test performance in real-world noncredible populations. The chapter concludes with a summary of studies in which test cutoffs have been evaluated in nonmalingering clinical populations. Sensitivity and specificity data are reported when available.

The lay public appears to view the Digit Span subtest of the WAIS-III as a measure of memory (Trueblood & Schmidt, 1993), when in fact it measures attention span. As a result of this misconception, individuals intent on feigning memory dysfunction appear to target the Digit Span when displaying their memory "deficits." However, patients with profound memory impairment, such as those with Alzheimer's disease, perform normally or near normal on the Digits Forward (Iverson & Franzen, 1994; Sterne, 1969). Digit Span performance is also intact in nondemented individuals with severe amnesia (Butters & Cermak, 1980), although low scores can be observed in aphasic individuals (Shallice & Warrington, 1977). Various authors have reported that Digit Span is not impaired even in severe brain injury cases (Capruso & Levin, 1992), and while an injury dose–response relationship is observed with most WAIS-III subtests, it is not seen in the Digit Span (Langeluddecke & Lucas, 2003). Because the Digit Span subtest has been a particular area of focus in malingering detection literature, separate subsections of the chapter are devoted to studies evaluating the Digit Span as a measure of effort. Included in this review are studies using the Digit Span subtest administered as part of the Wechsler Memory Scales (WMS; Revised and III). Although the WMS itself is not a measure of intelligence, the Digit Span subtest is identical to that given as part of the WAIS.

SIMULATION STUDIES

Although some concerns exist regarding the generalizability of simulation studies in determining cutoffs for clinical populations, simulation studies are more controlled and the data generally easier to collect compared to real-world samples (Demakis, 2004), and thus such investigations can be a useful starting point to help determine or guide research used to evaluate clinical cutoffs. However, there are difficulties specific to the use of simulated malingerers, which include (1) the "malingering-simulator paradox" (i.e., "asking participants to comply with instructions to fake in order to study participants who fake when asked to comply" [Rogers & Cavanaugh, 1983, p. 447]); (2) only test performance is examined whereas clinical and behavioral observations, often used in the diagnostic process, are ignored; (3) volunteers who are asked to malinger differ from real-life malingerers in such demographic variables as age and/or educational level; (4) small monetary incentive provided in simulating studies are not equivalent to large settlements at stake in forensic evaluations; and (5) actual malingerers may also have genuine brain-based impairment, which complicates the diagnostic process (Demakis, 2004).

Individuals instructed to malinger can produce a deficient IQ profile. In a study of incarcerated young offenders (n = 30; estimated IQ = 85) and postgraduate psychology students (n = 15; estimated IQ = 119) asked to feign a "mental handicap" on the WAIS-R, both groups reduced their Full Scale IQs into the mentally retarded range (mean of 57 and 61, respectively), with essentially equal Verbal and Performance IQs (Johnstone & Cooke, 2003). In addition, both groups employed similar tactics when simulating cognitive deficits, including minimal responding (zero or very low scores), which included nonbizarre incorrect responses (e.g., "I don't know"), absurd responses (bizarre, illogical, and nonsensical), or opposite responses (e.g., on Block Design, rendering the design in opposite colors, i.e., red for white and vice versa); magnitude of error (near misses in responses); noncompliance (refusal to complete a test); and honest responding. Although the authors concluded that individuals can deliberately lower their IQ scores, the authors suggest that qualitative indicators can be useful in identifying noncredible cognitive performance.

Prewarning about possible detection of malingering may not reduce production of feigned deficits on intellectual measures. Johnson, Bellah, Dodge, Kelley, and Livingston (1998) observed that undergraduate students instructed to malinger on the WAIS-R and students instructed to malinger but warned that techniques would be employed to detect malingering performance scored comparably to each other and significantly more poorly than students not instructed to feign (total sample of 45; n's in each group unreported).

A number of studies have also used real-world patient groups and compared their performance to simulated malingerers. In one study, Bernard, McGrath, and Houston (1993) instructed 89 undergraduate students to simulate head injury in a nonobvious manner on the WMS-R. Performances were compared to those of 44 closed head injury patients with verified injuries, including positive brain CT (computed tomography) or MRI (magnetic resonance imaging) scans; litigation status was not reported. The simulating group scored significantly lower than the patient group on the Digit Span subtest, and Digit Span was included in a discriminant function composed of seven subtests which was associated with 79% sensitivity and 80% specificity. Separate sensitivity/specificity data for the Digit Span are not provided.

Mittenberg, Theroux-Fichera, Zielinski, and Heilbronner (1995) compared simulating volunteers ($n = 67$) with mild to severe head injury patients not in litigation or pursuing disability compensation ($n = 67$). Groups did not significantly differ in Full Scale IQ, Verbal IQ, or Performance IQ, and 9 of 11 subtests. Only Digit Span and Similarities were statistically different between the two groups, with Digit Span lower in the simulating malingering group and Similarities higher. The age-corrected scaled scores from all the subtests were entered in a discriminant function analysis, which accurately classified 79% of the subjects (76% true positives and 82% true negatives). Further, the head-injured subjects obtained comparable scores on the Digit Span and Vocabulary subtests; however, the simulating malingering group demonstrated a lower Digit Span versus Vocabulary performance. The discriminant function incorporating Vocabulary minus Digit Span difference score accurately categorized 71% of the subjects (63% true positives and 79% true negatives). A Vocabulary minus Digit Span difference score of 5 was associated with a 70% probability of malingering, a difference of score of 7 had an 80% probability of malingering, and a difference score of 9 was demonstrated to have a 95% probability of malingering.

Inman and Berry (2002) investigated the efficacy of three WAIS-R subtests (Digit Span, Information, and Digit Symbol), in addition to a group of other commonly administered neuropsychological and effort tests. Students from a college introductory psychology class with a self-reported history of head injury (non-compensation seeking) were assigned to either the head injury control group ($n = 24$) or a head injury malingering group ($n = 21$). From a pool of students without history of head injury, 24 students were assigned to a control group and 23 students were assigned to a control malingering group. The malingering groups were instructed to feign symptoms for compensation, while the control groups were instructed to perform to the best of their abilities. Reliable Digit Span (RDS) scores were calculated (the sum of the longest string of digits repeated without error over two trials under both forward and backward condition; Greiffenstein, Baker, & Gola, 1994). The control groups (both head injured and normal) scored significantly higher on the Digit Span and Digit Symbol subtests and RDS compared to the malingering groups (head injured and normal). An RDS cutoff of < 8 was associated with 100% specificity but only 27% sensitivity. Use of Trueblood's (1994) Digit Symbol scaled score cutoff of < 5 resulted in specificity of 100% but sensitivity of only 2%.

Similarly, Demakis (2004) evaluated WAIS-R Digit Span and Vocabulary score cutoffs recommended for detection of suspect effort (Vocabulary minus Digit Span > 2, Millis, Ross, & Ricker, 1998; Digit Span < 5, Suhr, Tranel, Wefel, & Barrash, 1997; Vocabulary < 7, Digit Span < 7, Trueblood, 1994) in a sample of control (n = 27) and coached and compensated simulating (n = 26) undergraduate introductory psychology students. Simulating malingerers performed significantly worse than controls on all the measures. Specificity was adequate (93–100%) for the individual Digit Span and Vocabulary cutoffs; however, sensitivity was poor for the Suhr et al. (1997) Digit Span cutoff (27%) and Trueblood's (1994) Vocabulary cutoff (15%), although the latter's Digit Span cutoff was associated with 73% sensitivity. Specificity for the Millis et al. (1998) Vocabulary minus Digit Span cutoff was unacceptably low (74%) with moderate sensitivity (69%).

Digit Span Scores in Isolation

Heaton, Smith, Lehman, and Vogt (1978) obtained Digit Span data on 13 moderate to severe head injury patients not in litigation or attempting to obtain disability compensation, and 16 simulators paid $30 to feign effects of head injury in a nonobvious manner. Malingerers scored significantly poorer, averaging a scaled score of 7.0 (SD = 2.9), in comparison to the average performance obtained by the head injured sample (9.5, SD = 2.5). The investigators were examining the ability of neuropsychologists examining complete test protocols to identify the presence of feigning, and no data are provided regarding sensitivity/specificity rates for the Digit Span in isolation.

Iverson and Franzen (1994) compared 20 nonlitigating head injury patients (severe = 80%; moderate = 15%; mild = 5%) with memory impairment against 40 male inmates and 40 undergraduate students with no neurological injury or memory impairment on various WAIS-R Digit Span measures. The inmate and undergraduate groups were either randomly assigned to a control group or instructed to simulate malingering in the context of a lawsuit. The student and inmate control groups and the head injury group scored significantly higher than the simulators on all Digit Span variables (total score, scaled score, age-corrected scale score [ACSS], forward span, backward span). An ACSS < 5 and a forward span < 5 identified 90% to 95% of simulators, while allowing a 10% false-positive rate in head injury patients, and no false positives in nonsimulating controls and inmates. However, a backward span of < 3, while associated with acceptable specificity (100%), only detected 53% of simulators; raising the cutoff to < 4 increased sensitivity to 88% but dropped specificity in the head injury group to an unacceptable 65%.

In a subsequent study (Iverson & Franzen, 1996), WAIS-R Digit Span ACSSs, as well as maximum span for the forward and backward trials, were obtained on 20 memory-impaired patients asked to perform to the best of their abilities, and in 20 undergraduate students and 20 psychiatric patients who completed the task in both control and simulating malingering conditions in a counterbalanced design. When performing with best effort, the students and psychiatric patients and the memory-impaired patients obtained significantly higher scores than the students and psychiatric patients under the simulating condition. A Digit Span ACSS of < 4 identified 75% of simulators, with no false-positive identifications in memory-impaired individuals or students and psychiatric patients taking the test under the best-effort condition. Similarly, a forward digit span of < 4 and a backward span of < 3 were associated with 60% and 58% sensitivity, respectively, and 98–100% specificity in students and psychiatric patients performance at best effort and 95% specificity in memory-disordered individuals

Klimczak, Donovick, and Burright (1997) administered several common neuropsychological measures, including the Digit Span, to college students asked to simulate either multiple sclerosis ($n = 28$) or head injury ($n = 27$). Another 14 students were included as nonmalingering controls. Approximately half of the simulating subjects from each group were given information about their "disorder" prior to testing. Both simulating groups performed significantly poorer than the control subjects on the Digit Span total raw score; simulating groups did not differ from each other and no differences were found between simulators provided with information regarding their disorder versus those not. The authors concluded that prior knowledge of the disease had little effect on test performance and they noted that simulators used the same strategy when feigning head injury and multiple sclerosis (i.e., both groups presented with a global deficit across all cognitive domains). Sensitivity/specificity data were not reported.

Strauss et al. (2002) obtained RDS scores on three testing sessions approximately 2 weeks apart, in addition to two traditional measures of malingering (computerized dot counting test and Victoria Symptom Validity Test), on 26 naïve controls, 21 professionals working with head injury populations (experienced controls), and 27 head-injured patients who were not in litigation. Half of the sample in each group was asked to feign believable injury while the rest were asked to perform to the best of their abilities. Regardless of experience level, simulators performed worse than nonsimulators, and simulators were more inconsistent in RDS scores across three testing sessions than were nonsimulators. RDS scores correctly identified 90% of the control group, while 79.4% of the simulating sample was correctly classified. Using a cutoff of < 7, specificity was 95%, although sensitivity was only 47%.

In a study by Shum, O'Gorman, and Alpar (2004), a group of 80 undergraduate students was administered the WMS-R Digit Span subtest in addition to other measures of effort. All the students were instructed to feign memory impairments due to a traumatic brain injury. The students were divided into four groups: with and without incentive ($20 reward if they were convincing), and delayed versus immediate preparation for the simulation. In addition, 15 non-compensation-seeking patients with a history of severe head injury in a community rehab program were tested. Presence of incentive did not have a significant impact on performance, although those who had 1 week to prepare did not exaggerate memory impairment to the same extent as those who were given only 10 minutes. Sensitivity (with cutoffs set to maintain specificity at 100%) for Digit Span forward < 6 and Digit Span backward < 5 was 74% for those individuals with minimal feigning preparation time; sensitivity for forward span dropped to 62% in those simulators who had a week to prepare, although backward span sensitivity was still 72%.

Etherton, Bianchini, Ciota, and Greve (2005) examined RDS performance in 60 undergraduate college students randomly assigned to a control condition, simulating pain-related memory impairment, and a pain condition (completed task with forearm in bucket of ice water). Subjects experiencing acute pain did not differ from controls, and no acute pain subject obtained an RDS < 8. In contrast, 65% of simulators obtained an RDS of ≤ 7.

KNOWN GROUPS/REAL-WORLD MALINGERERS

In contrast to simulation studies, using real-world noncredible patients to help determine cutoffs for identifying suspect effort improves external validity (Trueblood & Binder, 1997).

Rawling and Brooks (1990) administered the WAIS-R among other measures to a head injury sample with posttraumatic amnesia of at least 2 weeks and to a probable malingerer group with posttraumatic amnesia of less than 24 hours (n = 16). Subjects from both groups were in litigation, claiming subjective significant impairments in mental functioning. The probable malingering group was on average 47.3 months postinjury; therefore, the authors concluded little likelihood of the presence of genuine neuropsychological impairment. No significant group differences were detected in subtest ACSSs or summary IQ scores, and within each group, no consistent patterns of strengths and weaknesses were observed. On the Digit Span, both groups showed a nearly equal frequency of errors in digit order, in addition or omission of digits, and in errors involving the last number of a sequence. However, initial errors (errors in first or second digit in sequence of five or less) were more common in probable malingerers, while precriterion errors (missing one of two items of equal length but getting one or both of a longer string) were more common in the head injury group. The authors further suggest that > 2 "one-off" and "impossible" errors on the Arithmetic subtest, and > 0 "dubious sequence" errors on Picture Arrangement were specific to simulators. Cross-validation data are presented for groups of 10 probable malingerers and 10 credible patients. The authors conclude that probable malingerers were more likely to make errors of commission involving gross distortions of correct responses and errors in overlearned information, while errors of omission were more common in the head injury group.

Trueblood and Schmidt (1993) reported WAIS-R data on eight individuals with mild traumatic brain injury (TBI) identified as malingering (based on significantly below-chance performance on the Hiscock and Hiscock [1989] forced-choice measure) and eight with questionable validity (i.e., individuals who passed the symptom validity test but who nonetheless demonstrated improbable performance on neuropsychological tests [e.g., zero grip strength]), along with two separate groups of age-, education-, and gender-matched mild TBI (Glasgow Coma Scale [GCS] = 13–15) patients who did not meet the foregoing criteria; all 32 subjects were in litigation or disability seeking. Both the malingering and questionable validity groups scored significantly below their controls on Digit Span, and the questionable validity group was significantly lower on WAIS-R Full Scale IQ. Examination of seven different effort indices revealed that no controls failed more than two. Sensitivity and specificity data are not reported for the experimental groups, however, in a separate sample of 74 litigating patients with mild TBI who did not meet criteria for the malingering and questionable validity group, a Digit Span ACSS < 7 was associated with 85% specificity.

A year later, Trueblood (1994) published WAIS-R data on three groups extracted from a litigating/disability-seeking mild head injury sample: 12 malingerers who performed significantly below chance on forced-choice testing, 10 patients with implausible neuropsychological data (e.g., zero grip strength) but who did not score significantly below chance on forced-choice testing, and 22 demographically matched patients (10 for comparison with the malingering group and 12 for comparison with the questionable validity group) with plausible neuropsychological performance. The malingerers and questionable validity patient scored significantly lower than their controls on Full Scale IQ, Performance IQ, Digit Span, Vocabulary, Picture Completion, and Digit Symbol. In addition, Verbal IQ was higher in controls compared to patients with questionable validity, and Picture Arrangement and Object Assembly were higher in controls compared to malingerers. The malingering and questionable validity groups also obtained more absurd responses, as determined by the author (e.g., a color other than blue for the American flag, or the shape of a ball described as a triangle; multiple reversals and substitutions on the Digit Span subtest), in contrast to controls, who obtained none. Similarly, malingerers underperformed on easy items of Picture Completion (two or more errors on items 1 through 5) and Object Assembly (any error on item 1 or 2) relative to credible patients. Three-quarters of malingerers fell below cutoffs on more than one of five WAIS-R indicators (Digit Span < 7, Vocabulary < 7, Picture Completion < 7, Digit Symbol < 5, Estimated minus obtained IQ > 18), while only 1 of 12 controls showed this profile (92% specificity).

Youngjohn, Burrows, and Erdal (1995) collected WAIS-R data on 54 litigating or disability-seeking mild TBI (≤ 30 minutes loss of consciousness, < 24 hours posttraumatic amnesia, no brain-imaging abnormalities) patients with persisting symptoms at 6 months postinjury. The worst WAIS-R performance was found on the Digit Span and the Digit Symbol ACSSs (average of 8.71 ± 3.21 and 8.60 ± 2.52, respectively).

Millis et al. (1998) reported sensitivity and specificity values for discriminant function score (DFS) coefficients derived on the WAIS-R Digit Span, Vocabulary, Arithmetic, Comprehension, Similarities, Picture Completion, and Digit Symbol subtests (Mittenberg et al., 1995), as well as the difference between Vocabulary and Digit Span (V-DS) subtest scaled scores. Litigating mild head injury patients ($n = 50$) who were presenting with incomplete effort (≤ chance on the Warrington Recognition Memory Test, i.e., less than 32 correct of 50) and moderate to severe head injury patients (litigation status not reported; $n = 50$) were administered the WAIS-R as part of a routine neuropsychological protocol. Both DFS and V-DS were significantly lower in the litigating mild head injury group compared to the moderate to severe cases, with large effect sizes reported, however, the DFS outperformed the V-DS with regard to diagnostic accuracy. Specifically, a discriminant function of ≥ .10536 correctly classified 92% of moderate/severe head-injured patients and 88% of the mild TBI patients, while a Vocabulary minus Digit Span difference of > 2 correctly identified 86% of moderate/severe TBI and 72% of mild TBI.

In a subsequent study employing the WAIS-III, Mittenberg et al. (2001) compared performance of simulating malingerers recruited from graduate-level continuing education courses ($n = 36$), litigating or disability compensation-seeking probable malingerers ($n = 36$), and nonlitigating head injury patients ($n = 36$; mild = 19%, moderate = 28%, severe = 53%), 92% of whom had imaging abnormalities. The probable malingering group attained IQ scores at least 15 points lower than would be expected based on estimates of premorbid functioning, which was considered unlikely due to their head injury characteristics (no loss of consciousness, minimal hospitalization course, and negative imaging findings). Discriminant function analyses accurately classified 83% of the nonlitigating head trauma patients, 72% of the simulating malingerers, and 44% of the probable malingerers. Further, the V-DS difference score previously published for the WAIS-R (Mittenberg et al., 1995) correctly identified 71% of the subjects (86% of the nonlitigating subjects, 56% of the simulators, and 25% of the probable malingerers). Positive predictive values for cutoff scores of 0, 1, and 2 for the DFS coefficients and 2, 3, and 4 for the V-DS difference were reported for varying base rates of malingering.

Greve, Bianchini, Mathias, Houston, and Crouch (2003) obtained WAIS-R data in a sample of 151 patients referred for neuropsychological assessments post-brain injury (mild to severe). Thirty-seven patients had no incentive to feign (referral was for treatment planning) and did not fail the Test of Memory Malingering (TOMM) or the Portland Digit Recognition Test (PDRT), and were assigned to the control group, whereas 28 of the remaining patients who were referred in the context of litigation met criteria for at least probable malingered neurocognitive disorder (MND; Slick, Sherman, & Iverson, 1999). Only 21% of the probable malingering group had sustained a moderate or severe brain injury, as compared to 51% of the control group. Despite less severe injuries, the MND group obtained significantly lower Verbal IQ, Performance IQ, and Full Scale IQ on the WAIS-R or WAIS-III than the control group. Using a DFS cutoff of > 0, sensitivity was 53% while specificity was 83%; raising the cutoff to .212 improved specificity to 89% while maintaining sensitivity of 50%. Interestingly, slightly higher sensitivity (58–59% vs. 45–36%) and specificity (89–94% vs. 78–84%) were obtained with use of the WAIS-III as compared to the WAIS-R; sensitivity and specificity rates did not differ in individuals with IQ $\leq$ 85 versus > 85. For Vocabulary minus Digit Span, using a cutoff of > 4, sensitivity was only 14% with specificity of 86%. Of note, sensitivity was 50% in the higher IQ group with specificity of 84%; however, in the lower IQ group, specificity was excellent (92%) although sensitivity was negligible (5%). Comparison of the V-DS differences scores from the WAIS-IIII versus the WAIS-R revealed higher sensitivity but lower specificity for the WAIS-III (18% and 83%, respectively) as compared to the WAIS-R (9% and 89%, respectively). The predictive accuracy of DFS was higher than V-DS, and because of their significant intercorrelation, the inclusion of both indices did not improve the predictive efficacy when compared to DFS alone.

Demakis et al. (2001) used three different methods of obtaining premorbid IQs (demographic approach, Barona; demographic and performance approach, Oklahoma Premorbid Intelligence Estimate; OPIE; and demographic and best performance approach, Best-3) in a sample of head injury patients. The patients were divided into two groups: a litigating/disability-seeking insufficient-effort group who failed at least one non-WAIS-R effort indicator and who were primarily presenting with mild TBI ($n = 27$) and a moderate to severe TBI group (litigating status not reported; $n = 48$). The insufficient-effort group performed overall lower on the WAIS-R compared to the moderate/severe TBI group. Further, both groups scored significantly below their premorbid IQs (estimated by the Barona, OPIE, and Best-3 methods); however, the insufficient-effort group had a larger discrepancy between estimated premorbid IQs and obtained IQs compared to the moderate/severe TBI group. Specifically, the IQs of the moderate to severe TBI patients were 5.6 to 11.9 points lower than premorbid estimates (depending on the method used to generate estimates), while the insufficient-effort patients exhibited as much as a 23-point IQ loss. Premorbid IQ estimates were similar across groups when only demographic data were used to generate IQ estimates; however, the insufficient-effort subjects had lowered predicted IQ scores when methods employed both demographic and performance measures, illustrating that equations employing WAIS-R subtests had been compromised by poor effort (particularly for the OPIE Performance IQ estimates). Sensitivity and specificity data are reported for nine cutoffs (which can be obtained from the authors) for discrepancies between actual and predicted Verbal IQ, Performance IQ, and Full Scale IQ for each method of predicting IQ; specificity levels were comparable across predictor methods and ranged from 73% to 88%; sensitivity levels were comparable for the Best-3 and OPIE methods (i.e., 41% to 56%) and were slightly higher for the Barona method (59% to 63%). The authors conclude that examination of the discrepancy between actual and predicted IQ may be useful in the identification of insufficient effort.

Etherton, Bianchini, Greve, and Heinly (2006) examined scores on the Working Memory Index (WMI) of the WAIS-III in a malingering chronic pain group (determined by significantly below-chance performance on a forced-choice effort test; $n = 32$), a nonmalingering pain group (based on no evidence of symptom inflation on cognitive effort tests or Minnesota Multiphasic Personality Inventory [MMPI] scales; $n = 49$), a moderate to severe TBI group with no evidence of poor effort ($n = 36$), and a memory-disorders group (no incentive to feign; $n = 39$). The malingering group scored significantly poorer on the WMI and on the three subscales (Digit Span, Letter–Number Sequencing, Arithmetic) than the other three groups, with the exception of no difference in performance as compared to the memory-disorders group for letter–number sequencing. WMI scores ≤ 70 identified almost half of the malingerers and only misidentified 4% of the credible pain patients, 8% of the TBI patients, and 10% of the memory-disordered patients; a score of ≤ 65 was associated with 100% specificity in the credible pain group while still detecting a third of malingerers. A Digit Span ACSS of ≤ 5 was found to result in no false positive identification in the credible pain group, and an 11% and 8% false-positive rate in the TBI and memory-disorders groups, respectively, while detecting 47% of malingerers. An Arithmetic subtest score of ≤ 4 was associated with specificity of $\geq 95\%$ in all credible groups while detecting 47% of malingerers. However, letter–number sequencing scores were problematic, with comparable numbers of malingerers and TBI and memory-disordered patients obtaining scaled scores of 1 (3% to 6%) and 2 (6% to 16%). In a separate sample of 64 college students randomly assigned to a control group, simulator group (feigning pain-related memory difficulties) and a group exposed to a cold pain condition while completing the WMI, simulators scored significantly below the other two groups, which did not differ from each other; no subject experiencing pain during the testing obtained a Digit Span ACSS ≤ 6, an Arithmetic ACSS ≤ 4, or letter–number sequencing ACSS ≤ 5.

Etherton, Bianchini, Heinly, and Greve (2006), again studying a noncredible pain population, investigated the use of the WAIS-III Processing Speed Index (PSI) and its subscales (Digit Symbol, Symbol Search) as measures of effort. Among patients referred for psychological pain evaluation, 32 patients scored significantly below chance on a forced-choice effort test, while 48 showed no evidence of poor effort; comparison samples of 34 moderate to severe TBI patients with good effort and 38 patients with memory impairment and no incentive to feign were obtained. The noncredible pain group scored significantly below the three other groups on the PSI and its two subscales (Digit Symbol, Symbol Search). A PSI cutoff of ≤ 75 and a Digit Symbol ACSS cutoff of ≤ 4 were associated with 92% and 96% specificity, respectively, in the credible pain patients while detecting 66% to 69% of the noncredible patients; however, specificity was unacceptable in the two other comparison groups (71% to 79% in moderate/severe TBI; 76% to 89% in memory disorder). To achieve acceptable specificity in the latter two groups, the cutoff for PSI required lowering to ≤ 65, but this dropped sensitivity to only 28%. Lowering the Digit Symbol cutoff to ≤ 3 resulted in acceptable specificity across all groups (≥ 91%), while detecting 50% of noncredible subjects. Symbol Search fared the worst; an ACSS of ≤ 4 identified 56% noncredible subjects, while only misidentifying 6% of credible pain patients; however, this cutoff misidentified 18% of TBI patients and 37% of memory-disordered patients. Even lowering the cutoff to ≤ 1 still misassigned 11% of memory-disorder patients and only flagged 19% of malingerers.

Digit Span Scores in Isolation

Greiffenstein et al. (1994) investigated RDS in a sample of consecutive referrals for neuropsychological evaluations post head injury (mild, moderate, and severe). Referrals for mild injuries were from insurance companies and attorneys while major head trauma referrals were from physicians and rehabilitation nurses. Three groups of patients were identified: (1) TBI (GCS scores of ≤ 14, positive neuroimaging findings, and hospital stay of more than 48 hours; n = 33); (2) persistent postconcussive syndrome; PPCS (posttraumatic amnesia of ≤ 20 minutes, emergency room GCS score of 15, a hospital stay of ≤ 48 hours, no positive neuroimaging findings, and three or fewer postconcussive symptoms present at 1 year postinjury; n = 30) and (3) probable malingerers; PM (n = 43) who were PPCS patients with two or more of the following: two or more improbable scores on neuropsychological measures, improbable symptom history compared to surveillance findings, total disability in at least one major area of their life 1 year postinjury, and claims of remote memory loss. RDS scores were significantly lower in the PM group compared to both the TBI and PPCS groups. An RDS cutoff of ≤ 8 was associated with high sensitivity (82%) but unacceptable specificity (54% in moderate/severe TBI, 69% in PPCS); a cutoff of ≤ 7 identified 68% to 70% of probable malingerers, with adequate specificity in the PPCS group (89%) but still excessive false-positive identifications in the moderate/severe TBI group (73%).

In a subsequent study by the same authors (Greiffenstein, Gola, & Baker, 1995), the efficacy of RDS was evaluated in a larger but comparable sample of patients, with similar findings: the TBI (≥ 48 hours of dense amnesia or coma, GCS of < 12, and positive neurological or brain imaging findings; n = 56) and persistent postconcussive patients with relatively low incentive to malinger and who had fully returned to their preaccident social and occupational roles (n = 53) scored comparably to each other on RDS and significantly higher as compared to the probable malingerer group (as defined by criteria specified above; n = 68). A cutoff score of ≤ 7 was associated with 86% to 89% sensitivity, but only 57% specificity in the TBI group and 68% specificity in the PPCS group.

Suhr et al. (1997) examined Digit Span performance in six patient groups: 31 probable malingerers (mild head injury patients seeking compensation who exhibited at least two of the following: < 75% accuracy on a forced-choice test, reported remote memory loss or other implausible symptoms, reported personal history information at variance with independent records, or showed total disability in a major social role), 31 head injury patients seeking compensation but who did not meet the foregoing criteria, 20 mild/moderate head injury patients (GCS ≥ 9, loss of consciousness or posttraumatic amnesia < 24 hours, could have positive imaging findings) not seeking compensation; 15 severe head injury patients (loss of consciousness/ posttraumatic amnesia > 24 hours, positive brain imaging findings, GCS < 9) not seeking compensation; and patients who were diagnosed with a somatization disorder (n = 29) or depression (n = 30). The probable malingerers performed significantly worse than all other groups on Digit Span ACSS. Further, the probable malingering group performed more poorly on the Digit Span forward raw score compared to the nonmalingering head injury patients seeking compensation and the non-compensation-seeking mild/ moderate head injury groups; no significant groups differences were noted for the Digit Span backward. Examination of four independent effort indices, including Digit Span, revealed that none of the non-compensation-seeking subjects failed more than two, while none of the mild/moderate head injury subjects failed any, and 3% of depressed subjects, 13% of somatization, and 15% of severe head injury patients failed one.

Meyers and Volbrecht (1998) studied RDS performance in patients with TBI with < 1 hour of loss of consciousness; 47 were in litigation and 49 were nonlitigating. All the participants reported cognitive difficulties and chronic pain. Litigating participants performed significantly more poorly on RDS and other neuropsychological measures (including Full Scale IQ) compared to nonlitigating participants. Correlations between Reliable Digits and a forced-choice measure were .38 for the litigating group and .26 for the nonlitigating group. Using a cutoff of ≤ 7, specificity was 96% and sensitivity was 49%.

Mathias, Greve, Bianchini, Houston, and Crouch (2002) reported RDS data in a group of patients with TBI referred for neuropsychological testing in the context of workers' compensation or personal injury evaluations and/ or treatment planning. Twenty-four patients (6 moderate/severe TBI; 18 mild TBI) were judged to be probable malingerers (based on Slick et al., 1999, criteria), and 30 were judged to be credible (66% moderate/severe TBI). The credible group scored significantly higher than the probable malingering group. No significant correlations were noted between RDS and either age, education, or GCS. A cutoff of ≤ 7 was associated with 67% sensitivity and 93% specificity, while sensitivity dropped to 38% at a cutoff of ≤ 6 (97% specificity); a cutoff of ≤ 5 led to no false positives but only detected 21% of probable malingerers. The authors concluded that an RDS score of ≤ 5 at any base rate can be attributed to malingering with fairly high degree of confidence.

Duncan and Ausborn (2002) provided RDS data on 188 male pretrial/ presentence detainees with no diagnosis of neurological impairment: 134 nonmalingering patients and 54 malingering patients (malingering status was based on clinical judgment of various evaluators as determined by record review, psychological test results not including the WAIS-R [e.g., MMPI, MMPI-2, Personality Assessment Inventory, Structured Interview of Reported Symptoms, Rey 15-Item Memory Test], and interviews with, and extended observations of, detainees). Mean IQ of the nonmalingering group was 87.67 while the mean IQ of the malingering group was 70.69, and the latter group had significantly less education (8.86 vs. 10.51). RDS was significantly higher in the nonmalingering group. Use of a cutoff of ≤ 6 was associated with 90.3 specificity and 56.6 sensitivity. The authors support the use of RDS; however, they did express concern that low IQ might result in low RDS given the significant correlation between WAIS-R Full Scale IQ and RDS ($r = .86$ for malingering group; $r = .56$ for nonmalingering group).

Larrabee (2003) compared 24 litigants (19 with mild TBI, 1 with alleged hypoxia, and 4 with alleged neurotoxic brain injury) who met criteria for definite malingered neurocognitive impairment (including < chance performance on the PDRT) with 31 moderate/severe closed head injury patients (some of whom were in litigation; litigants and nonlitigants did not significantly differ on standard cognitive measures and were collapsed). RDS of ≤ 7 was associated with 50% sensitivity and 94% specificity. Examination of all possible pair-wise failures of the five measures (Benton Visual Form Discrimination, Finger Tapping, WAIS-R RDS, Wisconsin Card Sorting Test—Failure to Maintain Set, Lees–Haley Fake Bad Scale from the MMPI-2) resulted in a combined hit rate of 88.2%, which was higher than the 82.4% detected by all five variables entered as continuous variables into a logistic regression.

Meyers and Volbrecht (2003) examined RDS performance in 15 groups of real-world patients (nonlitigating mild TBI = 56, nonlitigating moderate TBI = 10, nonlitigating severe TBI [LOC ≥ 1 day and ≤ 8 days] = 29, nonlitigating severe TBI [LOC ≥ 9 days], nonlitigating chronic pain = 38, depressed = 25, litigating or disability-seeking mild TBI = 84, litigating or disability-seeking moderate TBI = 19, litigating or disability-seeking chronic pain = 64, normal controls = 10, institutionalized patients = 160, noninstitutionalized and failed ≤ 1 validity check = 211, nonlitigating noninstitutionalized and failed ≥ 2 validity checks = 19, litigating noninstitutionalized and ≥ 2 failed validity checks = 17), and 21 actors instructed to play the role of a malingerer. A total of nine effort indicators were administered, including RDS. The authors note that none of the control, depressed, nonlitigating TBI or chronic pain patients failed two or more malingering tests, whereas the litigating/disability-seeking and institutionalized subjects frequently failed two or more. All the members in the group specifically instructed to malinger failed at least one test, while 83% failed two or more. The authors conclude that failure on more than one test is rare in noninstitutionalized or nonlitigating groups. Specific RDS data in isolation are not provided.

Etherton et al. (2005) obtained RDS data in a moderate to severe TBI group with no evidence of feigning (39 were compensation seeking; total $n = 69$) and two groups of chronic pain patients: (1) unambiguous spinal injuries and no evidence of exaggeration or response bias ($n = 53$), and (2) met criteria for definite MND (i.e., scored statistically below chance on TOMM or PDRT; $n = 35$). Using a cutoff of ≤ 7, sensitivity was 60% with specificity > 90%, thus providing support for expansion of use of RDS to assess credibility of cognitive complaints in patients reporting chronic pain.

Heinly, Greve, Bianchini, Love, and Brennan (2005) investigated Digit Span performance in 1,063 non-compensation-seeking general neuropsychological patients (nearly half of whom had a cerebrovascular accident (CVA), and five groups of TBI patients: no incentive (15 mild, 30 moderate/severe); incentive only (62 mild, 39 moderate severe); suspect effort, such as testing positive on any single indicator of effort (71 mild, 56 moderate severe); probable malingerer as defined by meeting Slick et al. (1999) criteria for probable MND (36 mild, 17 moderate/severe); and definite as determined by meeting criteria for Slick et al. (1999) definite MND (12 mild, 6 moderate severe). Various Digit Span scores were examined including RDS, ACSS, and maximum span forward with both trials correct, maximum span forward, combined maximum span forward and maximum span backward, maximum span backward with both trials correct, and maximum span backward. In comparisons across the TBI groups, the no-incentive and incentive-only groups did not differ from each other, nor did the probable and definite MND groups. An RDS cutoff of ≤ 6 was associated with 39% sensitivity and specificity of 96% in credible TBI patients (no incentive and incentive only), although false-positive rates of 30% were found in stroke patients, 32% in memory-disorder patients, and 12% in psychiatric patients. Similarly, an ACSS cutoff of ≤ 5 had a 36% sensitivity, and a 7% false-positive rate in the credible TBI patients, with 14% false-positive identifications in stroke, 10% in memory disorders, and 7% in psychiatric patients. Using a cutoff of maximum span backward both trials correct ≤ 2, sensitivity of 42% was obtained, with specificity in the credible TBI patients of 92%, but only 54% in stroke patients, 53% in memory-disorder patients, and 74% in psychiatric patients. Sensitivity values at acceptable specificity values (≥ 90%) for the remaining scores ranged from 16% to 30%. Thus, ACSS had the best specificity values with sensitivity rates comparable to RDS and maximum backward span correct both trials. The data for memory-disorder patients would appear to suggest that Digit Span scores may not be appropriate for use in the differential between actual versus feigned memory impairment, which is in fact the most common use for effort measures. However, as noted in the Iverson and Tulsky (2003) data, patients with serious memory impairment (Korsakoff's syndrome, temporal lobectomy, Alzheimer's disease) did not show high rates of false-positive identifications on Digit Span scores. Thus, the Heinly et al. (2005) data on unspecified "memory disorder" patients are difficult to reconcile with existing literature. Similarly, the "psychiatric disorder" group was not further described making interpretation of specificity values in this group problematic; as discussed by Goldberg, Back-Madruga, and Boone (Chapter 13, this volume), a subset of psychotic individuals do perform poorly on effort tests, although literature consistently shows that depression does not lower effort test performance.

Babikian, Boone, Lu, and Arnold (2006) examined the efficacy of suggested cutoffs for Digit Span ACSS and RDS and reported on the effectiveness of other measures derived from the Digit Span subtest, including time scores, in a sample of real-world suspect-effort patients (n = 66) as determined by incentive to feign (in litigation or attempting to obtain disability for cognitive symptoms) and failure on at least two other effort indicators and one behavior criterion (e.g., implausible self-reported symptoms); noncredible patients were compared to clinic patients with no motive to feign (n = 56) and controls (n = 32). Sensitivity of the Digit Span scaled score increased from 32% to 42% when a ≤ 5 cutoff was used instead of the previously published cutoff of ≤ 4, while maintaining specificity at ≥ 90%. However, the recommended RDS cutoff of ≤ 7 was associated with an unacceptable specificity rate (76%). Lowering the RDS cutoff from ≤ 7 to ≤ 6 raised the specificity to 93%, but sensitivity fell from 62% to 45%. Forward span time scores (average time for completing a three-digit string, average time for completing a four-digit string, and average time per digit for all items attempted) were associated with sensitivity rates of 38%, 37%, and 50%, respectively, at specificity ≥ 89%. Sensitivity and specificity rates for cutoffs for other derived Digit Span scores, including Digital Span forward raw, total number of trials attempted, longest string with one item correct, longest string with both items correct, are provided. The highest sensitivities were found for ACSS ≤ 5 *or* RDS ≤ 6 (51% sensitivity; 91% specificity) and RDS ≤ 6 *or* longest string with at least one item correct ≤ 4 (54% sensitivity; 88% specificity).

Axelrod, Fichtenberg, Millis, and Wertheimer (2006) investigated Digit Span as a measure of effort in 36 mild head injury litigants who met Slick et al. (1999) criteria for probable or definite MND as compared with 29 nonlitigating patients with documented brain injury and 22 mild brain injury patients (the majority of whom were in litigation) with no evidence of poor effort. Among various scores examined (ACSS, digit span forward, digit span backward, RDS, and Vocabulary minus Digit Span), ACSS was found to be the best discriminator between groups. An ACSS ≤ 5 was associated with 97% specificity and 36% sensitivity; use of a cutoff of ≤ 6 resulted in unacceptable specificity (83%).

NONMALINGERING CLINICAL COMPARISON GROUPS

Axelrod and Rawlings (1999) examined the Mittenberg et al. (1995) WAIS-R effort formulas and the Trueblood five-sign approach (Trueblood, 1994) in two samples of head-injured patients in rehabilitation, 33 of whom were tested twice (two months and 12 months postinjury), and 43 of whom were tested 4 times (at 2 months, 4 months, 8 months, and 12 months). All patients had sustained significant brain injury (loss of consciousness ≤ 24 hours = 27, coma of 1 to 7 days = 32, comatose > 1 week = 17). Specificity for the V-DS difference score was 70% at 2 months, but by 12 months had increased to 79% in the patients tested twice, and 86% in the patient tested four times. Similarly, at time 1, specificity for the DFS was 78% but rose to 88% at 12 months in the twice-tested group and 91% in the group tested four times. Interestingly, the five-sign approach showed an overall specificity of only 49% at 2 months but had risen to an average of 90% by 1 year. These data raise caution regarding the use of the effort indices in an acute head injury population due to excessive false-positive identifications but suggest that by 1 year postinjury, specificity is generally adequate.

Iverson and Tulsky (2003) report Digit Span data from the WAIS-III standardization sample (*n* = 2,450) and from six clinical groups, including TBI (*n* = 22), chronic alcohol abuse (*n* = 33), Korsakoff's syndrome (*n* = 12), left temporal lobectomy (*n* = 24), right temporal lobectomy (*n* = 16), and Alzheimer's disease (*n* = 38). The authors reported that a Digit Span scaled score of 4 or less occurred in less than 3% of the sample. A forward digit span of ≤ 4 occurred in ≤ 6% of individuals age > 54, while a backward span of ≤ 2 occurred in ≤ 6% of the entire sample. A V-DS difference of ≥ 5 was also rare and occurred in < 8% of the population; however, a difference score of > 2 occurred in approximately 21% of the sample, indicating that this cutoff is associated with an unacceptable false-positive rate.

The Digit Span scaled score, longest span forward and backward, and the V-DS difference did not significantly differ between the combined clinical group versus the normal group. In the clinical samples, a Digit Span scaled score below 6 was uncommon, occurring in only 8% of left temporal lobectomy patients, 5% of Alzheimer's patients, 5% of TBI patients, and in none of the other clinical groups. A cutoff score of ≤ 6 was associated with ≥ 90% specificity in all groups with the exception of the left temporal lobectomy group (12.5% false-positive rate). A forward digit span of ≤ 4 occurred in ≤ 8% of all clinical groups including Alzheimer patients (7.9%), and a backward span of ≤ 2 occurred in ≤ 8% of all clinical samples. A V-DS difference of ≥ 5 again was rare and occurred in ≤ 8% of the clinical comparison groups; however, a difference score of > 2 was relatively common, appearing in 14% of TBI, 24% of chronic alcohol abuse, 13% of right temporal lobectomy, and 11% of Alzheimer's patients. The authors recommend cutoffs of ≤ 5 for the ACSS, ≤ 4 for longest span forward (for persons under age 55), ≤ 2 for longest span backward, and ≤ 5 for V-DS difference.

Miller, Ryan, Carruthus, and Cluff (2004) examined the false positives rates for the V-DS scaled score difference in samples of alcohol abusers ($n = 30$), polysubstance abusers ($n = 43$), and TBI ($n = 27$). Patients were not in litigation or seeking compensation and were not suspected of malingering. None of the TBI or alcohol abuse patients were misclassified using the cutoff of greater than or equal to 6; 2% of the polysubstance abuse patients were misclassified.

SUMMARY AND CONCLUSIONS

The investigation of WAIS-R/WAIS-III scores as measures of effort has been a particularly prolific area of research; we tabulated a total of 38 studies, all but one dating from the 1990s and later. Simulators and real-world noncredible subjects generally perform comparably to brain-injured samples in overall IQ scores, although patterns of subtest performance differ between credible and noncredible groups as reflected in evidence of the effectiveness of DFS incorporating WAIS-R/WAIS-III subtests in identifying individuals with suspect effort. Studies have shown that Digit Span performance in particular, either in isolation or as contrasted with Vocabulary score, is particularly sensitive to noncredible performance.

However, of concern, sensitivity rates frequently appear to be substantially higher in simulating subjects, indicating that sensitivity values derived from simulation-only studies may be overestimates when applied to clinical settings. For example, Mittenberg et al. (2001) observed that approximately twice as many simulators as probable malingerers were detected with the discriminant function and Vocabulary minus Digit Span (72% and 56% vs. 44% and 25%, respectively). Greve et al. (2003) also observed modest hit rates in their probable malingerer sample; with discriminant function cut-scores sets to 89% specificity, sensitivity in their probable malingerer group was only 50%, and that Vocabulary minus Digit Span was only 14%. While sensitivity of < 40% has been reported in real-world suspect-effort patients for Digit Span ACSS ≤ 4 (Babikian et al., 2006; Heinly et al., 2005), Iverson and Franzen (1994, 1996) documented sensitivity rates of 75% to 90–95% using this cutoff in simulators. Likewise, Strauss et al. (2002), in examining RDS scores, observed 95% sensitivity in simulators using a cut-score of < 7, while others have found only a 39–45% identification rate in real-world non-credible samples (Babikian et al., 2006; Heinly et al., 2005). Evidence suggests that the amount of time malingerers have to prepare for feigning is a factor in the blatancy of their attempts at fabrication; Shum et al. (2004) noted that sensitivity rates were lower for digits forward < 6 in simulators given a week to prepare as compared to those allowed 10 minutes (74% vs. 62%). Real-world malingerers have months and even years to research and prepare for neuropsychological exams, and this likely explains the lower sensitivity rates found in this population.

RDS cutoff of ≤ 7 has been used in several real-world suspect-effort studies, with sensitivity rates ranging from 50% to 87% (Babikian et al., 2006; Etherton et al., 2005; Greiffenstein et al., 1994; Greiffenstein, Gola, & Baker, 1995; Heinly et al., 2005; Larrabee, 2003; Mathias et al., 2002; weighted average of 68%), but specificity may be unacceptable in moderate to severe TBI (57% to 94%; Etherton et al., 2005; Greiffenstein et al. 1994; Greiffenstein et al., 1995; Heinly et al., 2005; Larrabee, 2003; weighted mean of 81%), in a general neuropsychological clinic sample (76%; Babikian et al., 2006), and in patients with stroke (56%; Heinly et al., 2005); this cutoff may only have acceptable specificity in nonlitigating mild TBI patients (89% to 96%; Greiffenstein et al., 1995; Meyers & Volbrecht, 1998). Lowering the cutoff to ≤ 6 decreases sensitivity to between 38% and 57% (Babikian et al., 2006; Duncan & Ausborn, 2002; Heinly et al., 2005; Mathias et al., 2002; weighted average of 45%), but specificity is 88% or higher with the exception of stroke patients (70%; Heinly et al., 2005).

A Digit Span ACSS cutoff of ≤ 4 has been uniformly associated with specificity > 90% (Babikian et al., 2006; Heinly et al., 2005; Iverson & Franzen, 1994, 1996; Iverson & Tulsky, 2003), but sensitivity is low (19% to 32%; Babikian et al., 2006; Heinly et al., 2005). Raising the cutoff to ≤ 5 still limits false-positive identifications to ≤ 10% (Axelrod et al., 2006; Babikian et al., 2006; Etherton et al., 2006) with the exception of stroke patients (14% false-positive identifications; Heinly et al., 2005), but sensitivity increases to 36% to 47% (Axelrod et al., 2006; Babikian et al., 2006; Etherton, Bianchini, Greve, et al., 2006; Heinly et al., 2005).

Time scores for forward digit span, with sensitivities ranging from 37% to 50% (Babikian et al., 2006), may be particularly effective in identifying those noncredible individuals who use a test-taking strategy of slowed, but not necessarily inaccurate, performance.

A Vocabulary minus Digit Span ACSS cutoff > 2 is associated with good sensitivity (72%; Millis et al., 1998) but unacceptable specificity; 21% of the standardization sample of the WAIS-III exceeded this cutoff (Iverson & Tulsky, 2003) as well as 26% of college students (Demakis, 2004). Raising the cutoff to ≥ 5 only results in a ≤ 8% false-positive rate in the WAIS-III standardization sample and in patients with chronic alcohol abuse, Korsakoff's syndrome, left temporal lobectomy, right temporal lobectomy, and Alzheimer's disease (Iverson & Tulsky, 2003), although specificity rates are somewhat lower (79–86%) in primarily moderate to severe, nonacute TBI (Axelrod & Rawlings, 1999; Greve et al., 2003), with acute moderate/severe TBI patients showing an even greater false-positive rate (30%; Axelrod & Rawlings, 1999). The sensitivity of this index is greater in those noncredible subjects with higher IQ scores (Full Scale IQ > 85 = 50% sensitivity; Full Scale IQ ≤ 85 = 5% sensitivity), although this is difficult to interpret given that overall IQ scores are likely suppressed during efforts to feign. Perhaps these data indicate that individuals feigning less globally (hence the higher IQ scores) are more likely to show larger discrepancies between V-DS (i.e., they are only suppressing Digit Span performance); individuals adopting a feigning strategy of diffuse lowering of scores will be less likely to show differences between scores V-DS scores because they are suppressing both equally.

Data show that acute pain does not lower Digit Span (Etherton et al., 2005; Etherton, Bianchini, Greve, et al., 2006) or Symbol Search (Etherton, Bianchini, Heinly, et al., 2006); however, WAIS-III PSI and Digit Symbol are slightly lowered in response to laboratory-induced pain. As discussed by Salazar, Lu, Wen, and Boone (Chapter 18, this volume), Digit Span performance is impacted by cultural and linguistic factors, requiring some adjustment of cutoffs in some ethnic minorities and in patients who speak English as a second language.

The few studies examining a discriminant function employing all WAIS-R or WAIS-III subtests have documented comparable specificity values, although sensitivity rates have varied widely, making estimation of true levels of sensitivity problematic. Millis et al. (1998), using a cutoff ≥ .10536, reported sensitivity of 88% with specificity above 90% in moderate/severe TBI patients; however, Greve et al. (2003), using a cutoff of > 0, reported specificity of 83% with sensitivity of only 53%; raising the cutoff to .212 increased specificity to 89% while retaining sensitivity of 50%.

The WAIS-III WMI has been investigated as an effort index (Etherton, Bianchini, Greve, et al., 2006) but does not show any superiority over the Digit Span alone in a chronic pain/malingering sample, although interestingly in this study, Arithmetic was as sensitive as the Digit Span (47% hit rate). Other studies examining simulators and TBI patients have not found the Arithmetic subtest to be sensitive to the presence of simulation, raising the possibility that its sensitivity may be fairly specific to individuals feigning cognitive complaints in the context of alleged chronic pain, a hypothesis deserving of future research. The WAIS-III PSI has also been studied as an effort indicator by the same group (Etherton, Bianchini, Heinly, et al., 2006), but one of its subscales (Digit Symbol) actually performed better (detecting 50% of malingerers as compared to 28% for the full index at comparable specificity levels). A few other scattered reports have suggested that Digit Symbol (Etherton, Bianchini, Greve, et al., 2006; Inman & Berry, 2002; Trueblood, 1994; Youngjohn et al., 1995) and Picture Completion (Trueblood, 1994) may be suppressed in noncredible samples, but more data are needed in order to use these subtests clinically as effort indicators. Some investigators have recommended examination of qualitative indicators (e.g., two or more errors on WAIS-R Picture Completion items 1 through 5) or absurd responses (e.g., shapes of ball described a triangle), but these observations require replication. Also, in our experience, drawing of Digit Symbol codes upside down is pathognomonic for malingering, albeit this is very rare.

Finally, some intriguing data suggest that the discrepancy between premorbid and obtained IQs may be useful in identifying fabrication of lowered IQ level (Demakis et al., 2001; Trueblood, 1994), particularly given that IQ is not lowered in mild brain injury (Dikmen, Machamer, Winn, & Temkin, 1995).

Indicators derived from the WAIS are an efficient method of determining effort in that the test is typically administered in comprehensive neuropsychological assessments. Current recommended practice is to administer several effort tests interspersed through a test battery, but before various indicators can be used as independent measures of effort, it must be determined to what extent they are intercorrelated; highly correlated measures provide redundant information (Rosenfeld, Sands, & van Gorp, 2000). A recent study examining the correlations between eight separate effort indicators (Digit Span ACSS, Rey 15-Item Test, Rey Dot Counting Test, Rey Word Recognition Test, Rey Auditory Verbal Learning Test recognition trial, Rey–Osterrieth Complex Figure Test effort equation, Warrington Recognition Memory Test–Words, and b Test), showed that Digit Span was only modestly correlated with the other tests, with the exception of the Dot Counting Test (54% shared variance), suggesting that Digit Span generally provides nonredundant effort information (Nelson et al., 2003).

In conclusion, the various effort indices derived from the WAIS-R/WAIS-III appear to have relatively comparable sensitivity (approximately 50%) when cutoffs are set to acceptable specificity levels (i.e., ≥ 90%). Thus, performance exceeding cutoffs can be used to "rule in" noncredible performance; however, normal performance cannot be used to "rule out" malingering, given that approximately 50% of noncredible patients pass the indicators.

REFERENCES

Atkins v. Virginia, 536 U.S. 304 (2002).

Axelrod, B. N., Fichtenberg, N. L., Millis, S. R., & Wertheimer, J. C. (2006). Detecting incomplete effort with Digit Span from the Wechsler Adult Intelligence Scale–Third edition. *The Clinical Neuropsychologist, 20,* 513–523.

Axelrod, B. N., & Rawlings, D. B. (1999). Clinical utility of incomplete effort WAIS-R formulas: A longitudinal examination of individuals with traumatic brain injuries. *Journal of Forensic Neuropsychology, 1*(2), 15–27.

Babikian, T., Boone, K. B., Lu, P., & Arnold, G. (2006). Sensitivity and specificity of various Digit Span scores in the detection of suspect effort. *The Clinical Neuropsychologist, 20*(1), 145–159.

Bernard, L. C., McGrath, M. J., & Houston, W. (1993). Discriminating between simulated malingering and closed head injury on the Wechsler Memory Scale–Revised. *Archives of Clinical Neuropsychology, 8*(6), 539–551.

Butters, N., & Cermak, L. (1980). *Alcoholic Korsakoff's syndrome: An information processing approach.* San Diego: Academic Press.

Capruso, D. X., & Levin, H. S. (1992). Cognitive impairment following closed head injury. *Neurologic Clinics, 10*(4), 879–893.

Demakis, G. J. (2004). Application of clinically-derived malingering cutoffs on the California Verbal Learning Test and the Wechsler Adult Intelligence Test–Revised to an analog malingering study. *Applied Neuropsychology, 11*(4), 222–228.

Demakis, G. J., Sweet, J. J., Sawyer, T. P., Moulthrop, M., Nies, K., & Clingerman, S. (2001). Discrepancy between predicted and obtained WAIS-R IQ scores discriminates between traumatic brain injury and insufficient effort. *Psychological Assessment, 13*(2), 240–248.

Dikmen, S., Machamer, J. E., Winn, H. R., & Temkin, N. (1995). Neuropsychological outcome at 1-year posthead injury. *Neuropsychology, 9,* 80–90.

Duncan, S. A., & Ausborn, D. L. (2002). The use of reliable digits to detect malingering in a criminal forensic pretrial population. *Assessment, 9*(1), 56–61.

Etherton, J. L., Bianchini, K. J., Ciota, M. A., & Greve, K. (2005). Reliable Digit Span is unaffected by laboratory-induced pain: Implications for clinical use. *Assessment, 12,* 101–106.

Etherton, J. L., Bianchini, K. J., Greve, K. W., & Heinly, M. T. (2006). Sensitivity and specificity of reliable digit span in malingered pain-related disability. *Assessment, 12*(2), 130–136.

Etherton, J. L., Bianchini, K. J., Heinly, M. T., & Greve, K. W. (2006). Pain, malingering, and performance on the WAIS-III Processing Speed Index. *Journal of Clinical and Experimental Neuropsychology, 28,* 1218–1237.

Greiffenstein, M. F., Baker, R., & Gola, T. (1994). Validation of malingered amnesia measures with a large clinical sample. *Psychological Assessment 6*(3), 218–224.

Greiffenstein, M. F., Gola, T., & Baker, W. J. (1995). MMPI-2 validity scales versus domain specific measures in detection of factitious traumatic brain injury. *The Clinical Neuropsychologist, 9*(3), 230–240.

Greve, K. W., Bianchini, K. J., Mathias, C. W., Houston, R. J., & Crouch, J. A. (2003). Detecting malingered performance on the Wechsler Adult Intelligence Scale. Validation of Mittenberg's approach in traumatic brain injury. *Archives of Clinical Neuropsychology, 18*(3), 245–260.

Heaton, R. K., Smith, H. H., Jr., Lehman, R. A., & Vogt, A. T. (1978). Prospects for faking believable deficits on neuropsychological testing. *Journal of Consulting and Clinical Psychology, 46*(5), 892–900.

Heinly, M. T., Greve, K. W., Bianchini, K. J., Love, J. M., & Brennan, A. (2005). WAIS Digit Span-based indicators of malingered neurocognitive dysfunction. *Assessment, 12*, 429–444.

Hiscock, M., & Hiscock, C. K. (1989). Refining the forced-choice method for detection of malingering. *Journal of Clinical and Experimental Neuropsychiatry, 11*, 967–974.

Inman, T. H., & Berry, D. T. R. (2002). Cross-validation of indicators of malingering: A comparison of nine neuropsychological tests, four tests of malingering, and behavioral observations. *Archives of Clinical Neuropsychology, 17*, 1–23.

Iverson, G. L., & Franzen, M. D. (1994). The Recognition Memory Test, Digit Span, and Knox Cube Test as markers of malingered memory impairment. *Assessment 1*(4), 323–334.

Iverson, G. L., & Franzen, M. D. (1996). Using multiple objective memory procedures to detect simulated malingering. *Journal of Clinical and Experimental Neuropsychology, 18*(1), 38–51.

Iverson, G. L., & Tulsky, D. S. (2003). Detecting malingering on the WAIS-III. Unusual Digit Span performance patterns in the normal population and in clinical groups. *Archives of Clinical Neuropsychology, 18*(1), 1–9.

Johnson, J. L., Bellah, C. G., Dodge, T., Kelley, W., & Livingston, M. M. (1998). Effect of warning on feigned malingering on the WAIS-R in college samples. *Perceptual and Motor Skills, 87*(1), 152–154.

Johnstone, L., & Cooke, D. J. (2003). Feigned intellectual deficits on the Wechsler Adult Intelligence Scale-Revised. *British Journal of Clinical Psychology, 42*(Pt. 3), 303–318.

Klimczak, N. J., Donovick, P. J., & Burright, R. (1997). The malingering of multiple sclerosis and mild traumatic brain injury. *Brain Injury, 11*(5), 343–352.

Langeluddecke, P. M., & Lucas, S. K. (2003). Wechsler Adult Intelligence Scale—Third edition findings in relation to severity of brain injury in litigants. *Clinical Neuropsychology, 17*(2), 273–284.

Larrabee, G. J. (2003). Detection of malingering using atypical performance patterns on standard neuropsychological tests. *Clinical Neuropsychology, 17*(3), 410–425.

Mathias, C. W., Greve, K. W., Bianchini, K. J., Houston, R. J., & Crouch, J. A. (2002). Detecting malingered neurocognitive dysfunction using the reliable digit span in traumatic brain injury. *Assessment, 9*(3), 301–308.

Meyers, J. E., & Volbrecht, M. (1998). Validation of reliable digits for detection of malingering. *Assessment, 5*(3), 303–307.

Meyers, J. E., & Volbrecht, M. (2003). A validation of multiple malingering detection methods in a large clinical sample. *Archives of Clinical Neuropsychology, 18*(3), 261–276.

Miller, L. J., Ryan, J. J., Carruthers, C. A., & Cluff, R. B. (2004). Brief screening indexes for malingering: A confirmation of Vocabulary minus Digit Span from the WAIS-III and the Rarely Missed Index from the WMS-III. *Clinical Neuropsychology, 18*(2), 327–333.

Millis, S. R., Ross, S. R., & Ricker, J. H. (1998). Detection of incomplete effort on the Wechsler Adult Intelligence Scale-Revised: A cross-validation. *Journal of Clinical and Experimental Neuropsychology, 20*(2), 167–173.

Mittenberg, W., Patton, C., Canyock, E. M., & Condit, D. C. (2002). Base rates of malingering and symptom exaggeration. *Journal of Clinical and Experimental Neuropsychology, 24*(8), 1094–1102.

Mittenberg, W., Theroux, S., Aguila-Puentes, G., Bianchini, K., Greve, K., & Rayls, K. (2001). Identification of malingered head injury on the Wechsler Adult Intelligence Scale–3rd edition. *Clinical Neuropsychology, 15*(4), 440–445.

Mittenberg, W., Theroux-Fichera, S., Zielinski, R. E., & Heilbronner, R. L. (1995). Identification of malingered head injury on the Wechsler Adult Intelligence Scale–Revised. *Professional Psychology: Research and Practice, 26*(5), 491–498.

Nelson, N. W., Boone, K., Dueck, A., Wagener, L., Lu, P., & Grills, C. (2003). Relationships between eight measures of suspect effort. *Clinical Neuropsychology, 17*(2), 263–272.

Rawling, P., & Brooks, N. (1990). Simulation index: A method for detecting factitious errors on the WAIS-R and WMS. *Neuropsychology, 4*, 223–238.

Rogers, R., & Cavanaugh, J. L. (1983). "Nothing but the truth" . . . A reexamination of malingering. *Journal of Psychiatry and Law, 11*, 443–459.

Rosenfeld, B., Sands, S. A., & van Gorp, W. G. (2000). Have we forgotten the base rate problem? Methodological issues in the detection of distortion. *Archives of Clinical Neuropsychology, 15*, 349–359.

Shallice, T., & Warrington, E. K. (1977). Auditory-verbal short-term memory impairment and conduction aphasia. *Brain and Language, 4*(4), 479–491.

Sherman, D. S., Boone, K. B., Lu, P., & Razani, J. (2002). Re-examination of a Rey auditory verbal learning test/Rey complex figure discriminant function to detect suspect effort. *Clinical Neuropsychology, 16*(3), 242–250.

Shum, D. H., O'Gorman, J. G., & Alpar, A. (2004). Effects of incentive and preparation time on performance and classification accuracy of standard and malingering-specific memory tests. *Archives of Clinical Neuropsychology, 19*(6), 817–823.

Slick, D. J., Sherman, E. M., & Iverson, G. L. (1999). Diagnostic criteria for malingered neurocognitive dysfunction: Proposed standards for clinical practice and research. *Clinical Neuropsychology, 13*(4), 545–561.

Sterne, D. M. (1969). The Benton, Porteus and WAIS digit span tests with normal and brain-injured subjects. *Journal of Clinical Psychology, 25*(2), 173–177.

Strauss, E., Slick, D. J., Levy-Bencheton, J., Hunter, M., MacDonald, S. W., & Hultsch, D. F. (2002). Intraindividual variability as an indicator of malingering in head injury. *Archives of Clinical Neuropsychology, 17*(5), 423–444.

Suhr, J., Tranel, D., Wefel, J., & Barrash, J. (1997). Memory performance after head injury: Contributions of malingering, litigation status, psychological factors, and medication use. *Journal of Clinical and Experimental Neuropsychology, 19*(4), 500–514.

Sweet, J. J., King, J. H., Malina, A. C., Bergman, M. A., & Simmons, A. (2002). Documenting the prominence of forensic neuropsychology at national meetings and in relevant professional journals from 1990 to 2000. *Clinical Neuropsychology, 16*(4), 481–494.

Trueblood, W. (1994). Qualitative and quantitative characteristics of malingered and other invalid WAIS-R and clinical memory data. *Journal of Clinical and Experimental Neuropsychology, 16*(4), 597–607.

Trueblood, W., & Binder, L. M. (1997). Psychologists' accuracy in identifying neuropsychological test protocols of clinical malingerers. *Archives of Clinical Neuropsychology, 12*(1), 13–27.

Trueblood, W., & Schmidt, M. (1993). Malingering and other validity considerations in the neuropsychological evaluation of mild head injury. *Journal of Clinical and Experimental Neuropsychology, 15*(4), 578–590.

Wechsler, D. (1981). *Wechsler Adult Intelligence Scale–Revised.* San Antonio, TX: The Psychological Corporation.

Wecksler, D. (1997). *Wechsler Adult Intelligence Scale* (3rd ed.). San Antonio, TX: The Psychological Corporation.

Youngjohn, J. R., Burrows, L., & Erdal, K. (1995). Brain damage or compensation neurosis: The controversial post-concussive syndrome. *The Clinical Neuropsychologist, 9*, 112–123.

CHAPTER 7

Use of Standard Memory Tests to Detect Suspect Effort

Po H. Lu
Steven A. Rogers
Kyle Brauer Boone

Increased awareness of the prevalence of malingering of cognitive symptoms has prompted neuropsychologists to formulate strategies for the identification of feigned or exaggerated symptoms and suboptimal effort. Clinicians unanimously agree that one cannot rely on a single approach or instrument in detecting suspect effort. Instead, strong emphasis is placed on a multidimensional approach that integrates multiple sources of information including both psychometric and behavioral indices. The most commonly used approach is the inclusion of instruments specifically designed to discreetly assess motivation and effort in the testing procedures. Standard neuropsychological tests do not have built-in validity indices to detect exaggeration or defensive response bias, such as that found in the Minnesota Multiphasic Personality Inventory–2 (MMPI-2; Butcher, Dahlstrom, Graham, Tellegen, & Kaemmer, 1989). However, numerous commonly used cognitive tests have been found to be sensitive in detecting suboptimal effort because, similar to the rationale for specialized effort tests, they also capitalize on faulty knowledge held by the general public regarding the effects of brain injury. Therefore, examination of atypical performance on common neuropsychological measures can be particularly fruitful in providing clinically efficacious and practical means of identifying individuals exhibiting insufficient effort. The majority of standard neuropsychological tests are vulnerable to faking; therefore, it is vitally important to understand how suboptimal effort can affect performance on these measures and produce a set of classification functions to discriminate between feigned and sincere efforts.

Memory impairment is the most frequently reported complaint in patients presenting for neuropsychological assessment (Brandt, 1988), and it is the type of cognitive disability most likely to be feigned (Williams, 1998). A major component of a comprehensive neuropsychological evaluation involves the assessment of memory functioning, usually involving immediate and delayed recall of both verbal and visual material. There are known patterns of organic memory dysfunction (Delis, 1991; Trueblood, 1994), but malingerers frequently lack sufficient knowledge to mimic the symptoms of a true memory disorder and are likely to "overportray" the severity of impairment or produce improbable assessment outcomes that are inconsistent from those achieved by cooperative brain-injured patients (Gouvier, Prestholdt, & Warner, 1988). For example, naïve malingerers might not realize that recognition memory is easier than free recall, or that autobiographical memory, such as knowledge of one's name, age, date of birth, telephone number, and so on, remain relatively preserved even in amnesic patients (Wiggins & Brandt, 1988).

In this chapter, we review the effectiveness of five commonly used traditional measures of memory functioning, the Rey Auditory Verbal Learning Test, Rey–Osterrieth Complex Figure Test, California Verbal Learning Test, Warrington Recognition Memory Test, and Wechsler Memory Scale, in detecting suspect effort. We focus on those studies that have the most clinical utility, namely, investigations of real-world noncredible subjects as compared to credible brain injured patients. New cross-sectional data are presented for two of the effort indicators (Rey–Osterrieth Effort Equation, Rey Auditory Verbal Learning Test/Rey–Osterrieth discriminant function).

REY AUDITORY VERBAL LEARNING TEST

The Rey Auditory Verbal Learning Test (RAVLT) measures learning and short-term memory for a word list. The standard administration involves five successive presentations of 15 words; after each presentation, examinees are asked to recall as many words as they can. An interference trial involving a list of 15 different words is then administered, followed by postinterference recall of the original word list. A delayed-recall trial is administered after 20–30 minutes followed by a recognition trial, the format of which can vary widely. One format involves identifying target words embedded in a story format while another format employs a 30-word list with the original words interspersed among 15 foils.

Several studies have appeared regarding the effectiveness of the RAVLT for detecting noncredible performance. These investigations have consistently shown that when compared to credible brain-injured patients, individuals feigning cognitive impairment suppress performance on the recognition trial (Bernard, 1990; Binder, Kelly, Villanueva, & Winslow, 2003; Binder, Villanueva, Howieson, & Moore, 1993; Boone, Lu, & Wen, 2005; Chouinard & Rouleau, 1997; Greiffenstein, Baker, & Gola, 1994; Greiffenstein, Gola, & Baker, 1995; Haines & Norris, 2001; Inman & Berry, 2002; Meyers, Morrison, & Miller, 2001), with some evidence showing a higher rate of failure in recognizing words recalled at least three times on the learning trials (Suhr, Tranel, Wefel, & Barrash, 1997). However, findings regarding whether credible and noncredible subjects differ on remaining RAVLT variables have been inconsistent, with some authors reporting that individuals simulating memory impairment suppress performance on learning trials (Bernard, 1990; Greiffenstein et al., 1994; Greiffenstein, Baker, & Gola, 1996; Haines & Norris, 2001; Inman & Berry, 2002; Powell, Gfeller, Oliveri, Stanton, & Hendricks, 2004; Suhr et al., 1997) and free recall after either a distractor or an extended delay (Bernard, 1990; Binder et al., 2003; Greiffenstein et al., 1994; Inman & Berry, 2002; Powell et al., 2004; Suhr et al., 1997), fail to display a primacy effect (Bernard, 1991; Haines & Norris, 2001; Powell et al., 2004; Suhr et al., 1997; Suhr, 2002), and commit more false-positive errors on the recognition trial (Suhr et al., 1997), although others have failed to replicate these findings (Binder et al., 1993; Chouinard & Rouleau, 1997; Greiffenstein et al., 1994; Inman & Berry, 2002). The discrepancy in findings across investigations may be at least partially due to the use of simulators (volunteers instructed to fake) in some studies, rather than real-world noncredible patients.

A few of the aforementioned studies have examined classification accuracy in real-world noncredible samples for the recognition score, typically the most sensitive in discriminating between credible and noncredible performances. Binder et al. (1993) investigated recognition performance in 75 patients with mild traumatic brain injury (TBI) seeking compensation and 80 patients with brain dysfunction without incentive and found that a cutoff score of < 6 resulted in a sensitivity of 27% but with 95% specificity. A subset of the mild TBI patients was able to be assigned to either high ($n = 17$) or low motivation ($n = 24$) subgroups based on Portland Digit Recognition Test (PDRT) performance; the low-motivation group obtained significantly lower recognition scores than either the high-motivation or brain-damage-no-incentive ($n = 68$) groups; the latter two groups did not differ. Again using a cutoff of < 6, in a more recent study, Binder et al. (2003) reported 38% sensitivity in identifying 34 mild TBI litigants with poor motivation (failed PDRT) while maintaining high specificity in 22 mild head injury litigants with good motivation (passed PDRT) and 60 non-compensation-seeking moderate/severe TBI patients (95% and 92%, respectively).

Boone et al. (2005) suspected that failure to correctly recognize words presented first on the list might signal suspect effort because these words would in fact be the most strongly encoded. They found that double-weighting of correct recognition from the first five words of the list (primacy recognition) increased test sensitivity over that associated with the standard recognition score. A cutoff of ≤ 12 for recognition minus false positives plus number of words recognized from the first five words was associated with 74% sensitivity in 61 noncredible patients (determined by presence of motive to feign, failure on at least two other effort indicators, and at least one behavioral criteria), while misclassifying 10% of 88 credible neuropsychology clinic patients with no motive to feign. In contrast, the standard recognition score (cutoff ≤ 9) detected 67% of noncredible subjects at comparable specificity, while total words learned across the five learning trials was associated with only 43% sensitivity (cutoff ≤ 30).

In conclusion, RAVLT scores, particularly involving the recognition trial, appear to be an effective method for identifying noncredible performance, although more studies on real-world noncredible samples are needed. In addition, as discussed by Salazar, Lu, Wen, and Boone (Chapter 18, this volume), cutoffs may require adjustment for cultural factors.

REY–OSTERRIETH COMPLEX FIGURE TEST

André Rey (1941) originally devised the Rey–Osterrieth Complex Figure Test (ROCFT) to assess visual–perceptual organization and short-term retention of visual material in brain-damaged patients, and it still remains one of the most widely used measures of visual–spatial construction and visual memory. Administration of the test involves the presentation of a complex two-dimensional geometric design that the examinee must first copy and then recall after a varying interval of delay, ranging from immediately after exposure to 3 minutes to 30 minutes. The quality of performance is based on the accuracy and placement of the essential elements in the design.

Several studies on the detection of malingering using standard neuropsychological tests have examined the delayed-recall component of the ROCFT in capturing suspect effort (Bernard, 1990; Bernard, Houston, & Natoli, 1993; Chouinard & Rouleau, 1997; Demakis, 1999; Klimczak, Donovick, & Burright, 1997; Suhr et al., 1997; Lu, Boone, Cozolino, & Mitchell, 2003), a few of which have included real-world noncredible samples. Suhr et al. (1997) reported that a group of 31 compensation-seeking patients who sustained a mild head injury and were suspected of malingering (based on failed performance on a forced-choice measure [< 75% correct], improbable outcome, and/or improbable symptoms) performed significantly worse on ROCFT recall than 30 compensation-seeking mild TBI patients who did not meet criteria for suspected malingering, but not worse than 20 non-compensation-seeking mild to moderate TBI, 15 severe TBI, 30 depressed, and 29 somatization patients. Chouinard and Rouleau (1997) found that their dissimulation group (34 suspected malingerers and volunteer simulators) actually performed better than a clinical group (n = 39) comprising patients with amnesia, frontal lobe pathology, and moderate memory impairment on immediate-recall scores. These studies suggest that the ROCFT recall in isolation may lack discriminative power in separating noncredible subjects from all but mild TBI patients (who in fact show no chronic cognitive sequelae).

The introduction of a recognition trial for the ROCFT (Meyers & Meyers, 1995) raised the possibility of increasing the effectiveness of the measure in detecting suspect effort. The four-page recognition trial response sheets contain 12 individual designs from the original figure interspersed with 12 distractor items that are not part of the figure. After delayed recall, patients are asked to circle the designs that were part of the larger figure that they copied. Meyers and Volbrecht (1999) evaluated ROCFT performance in litigating (n = 35) versus nonlitigating (n = 48) mild head injury patients (less than 5 minutes of loss of consciousness) and 10 "malingerers" (based on litigating status and failure on effort measures) versus 25 simulators. All the malingerers and 80% of the simulators produced either an "Attention" memory error pattern (MEP), defined as equally impaired scores on immediate, delayed, and recognition trials, or a "Storage" MEP, operationalized as recognition scores worse than immediate or delayed trials (Meyers & Volbrecht, 1998). None of the nonlitigation subjects produced these patterns of errors.

However, Lu et al. (2003), using a different administration format (recognition trial immediately following 3-minute recall), found much lower sensitivity rates for the MEPs than those observed by Meyers and Volbrecht (1999) (26% for Attention MEP at ≥ 95% specificity; 50% for Storage MEP at 52% to 65% specificity). Lu et al. (2003) developed an alternative formula which incorporated the copy and recognition scores of the ROCFT while penalizing the endorsement of atypical foils on the recognition trial:

$$\text{E-score} = \text{copy score} + [(\text{true positive recognition} - \text{atypical recognition errors}) \times 3]$$

(Atypical recognition errors = #1, #4, #6, #10, #11, #16, #18, and #21.)

This combination score was validated on 58 patients with suspect effort (who were involved in litigation or seeking to obtain or maintain disability benefits, scored below cutoff on at least two of six tests designed to assess effort, and met at least one behavioral criterion for noncredible symptomatology) and 70 neuropsychology clinic patients with no motive to feign who were further classified into verbal memory impaired (< 9th percentile performance on the Wechsler Memory Scale–Revised/Wechsler Memory Scale–III [WMS-R/WMS-III] Logical Memory II or RAVLT delayed recall; n = 23), visual memory impaired (based on < 9th percentile performance on WMS-R/WMS-III Visual Reproduction II; n = 17) or nonmemory impaired (≥ 9th percentile on Logical Memory II, Visual Reproduction II, RAVLT delayed recall; $n = 30$). A cut-score of ≤ 45 correctly classified 74.1% of the suspect-effort participants while achieving specificity rates of 96% for verbal memory impaired, 88% for visual memory impaired, and 97% for non-memory impaired. Thus, these data suggested that this ROCFT effort equation is an effective effort indicator even in individuals with actual visual memory impairment.

Cross-Validation Data

Since the original publication, we have collected additional data on 53 noncredible patients and 35 clinic comparison patients who met the same inclusion and exclusion criteria as in the initial study (with the exception that an overall b Test E-score of ≥ 90 was employed rather cutoffs for four separate b Test scores). Table 7.1 shows descriptive statistics for age, education, and gender distribution for the two study groups. The clinic comparison patients had significantly more years of education, and the suspect-effort group had a higher proportion of men while the clinic comparison group was overrepresented by women.

Statistical examination (Kolmogorov–Smirnov test of normality) of the combination score revealed that it was normally distributed within each group. Age was not significantly related to test performance in either the suspect-effort group or the clinical comparison group; however, educational level was significantly correlated with test performance in the suspect-effort group (Pearson $r = .350$, $p = .01$), although the amount of test score variance accounted for by education was relatively small (12%). Within each group, no significant difference in test performance between men and women was observed.

Analysis of covariance with education as a covariate showed that the suspect-effort group obtained significantly worse scores compared to the clinic comparison patients (Table 7.1). Examination of specificity and sensitivity values, as reproduced in Table 7.2, showed that use of the previously

TABLE 7.1. Comparisons of Demographic Characteristics and the ROCFT Combination Score between Suspect Effort and Credible Clinic Patients

	Suspect effort ($n = 53$)	Clinic patients ($n = 35$)	Statistical tests	p-value
	Mean (SD)	Mean (SD)		
Age, years	40.2 (12.1)	44.6 (15.6)	$t = -1.50$	.14
Education, years	12.2 (2.7)	13.4 (2.5)	$t = -2.13$	.04
Gender, male/female	34/19	14/21	$\chi^2 = 4.96$	.03
Combination score	39.8 (17.1)	59.0 (12.5)	$F = 26.48$	.0001

TABLE 7.2. Classification Accuracy for ROCFT Combination Scores

Cutoff scores	Suspect effort Sensitivity ($n = 53$)	Clinic patients Specificity ($n = 35$)
≤ 43	56.6	91.4
≤ 44	62.3	91.4
≤ 45	64.2	88.6
≤ 46	66.0	88.6
≤ 47	67.9	85.7

published cutoff of less than or equal to 45 was associated with a specificity of 88.6%, which reflects a relatively small drop from the overall specificity of 94% obtained in the original study. However, sensitivity declined by approximately 15%; 64.2% of noncredible subjects were correctly identified in the cross-validation sample as compared to the 74.1% in the original study.

Thus, some loss in classification accuracy was found on cross-validation, although the ROCFT combination score was still associated with at least moderate sensitivity. Given that it is commonly included in neuropsychological exams (and thus the data are readily available with no additional administration time), and measures an aspect of cognitive function not often examined with regard to effort (e.g., visuoconstructional abilities), this equation would appear to be a valuable addition to cognitive effort measures. However, as discussed by Salazar, Lu, Wen, and Boone (Chapter 18, this volume), adjustment in cutoffs for cultural factors may be warranted.

RAVLT/ROCFT DISCRIMINANT FUNCTION

Bernard, Houston, and Natoli (1993) developed a discriminant function using the trial 1 and recognition score from the RAVLT and a 30-minute recall score from the Taylor (1959) figure. This discriminant function correctly classified 75% simulators ($n = 31$) and 100% of controls ($n = 26$). However, Sherman, Boone, Lu, and Razani (2002), substituting the ROCFT in place of the Taylor figure, found the formula to have poor discriminant ability, particularly regarding false-positive identifications. Specifically, they examined the function in a sample of 34 litigating/disability-seeking patients who also scored below cutoffs on at least two independent effort measures and met at least one behavioral criterion (e.g., implausible self-reported symptoms such as cannot see through glass); 34 neuropsychology clinic patients with documented cerebral insult including severe head trauma, stroke, and brain tumor/cyst and no motive to feign (i.e., not in litigation or attempting to obtain disability compensation); and 33 control subjects, and while they documented excellent sensitivity (97%), specificity was low (33% for patients, 61% for controls).

However, they were able to identify an alternative discriminant function which effectively separated the groups:

$$D = (.006 \times \text{RAVLT Trial 1}) - (.062 \times \text{ROCFT delay})$$
$$+ (.354 \times \text{RAVLT recognition}) - 2.508$$

A cutoff of $\leq -.40$ yielded a sensitivity of 71% while maintaining specificity at $\geq 91\%$ for brain injury patients and 100% for controls with 85% overall classification accuracy.

Cross-Validation Data

Since the original publication, we have collected additional data on 125 civil litigation/disability-seeking suspect-effort patients who met the same inclusion criteria as in the original study (with the exception that an overall b Test E-score of ≥ 90 was employed rather than cutoffs for four separate b Test scores), and 72 heterogeneous neuropsychology clinic comparison patients with no motive to feign, and who did not meet criteria for dementia or obtain a Full Scale IQ < 70. Table 7.3 shows descriptive statistics for age, education, and gender distribution for the two study groups. The clinic comparison patients averaged significantly more years of education, and the suspect-effort group had a higher proportion of men while the clinic comparison group was overrepresented by women.

Statistical examination (Kolmogorov–Smirnov test of normality) of the discriminant function revealed that it was not normally distributed within the clinical comparison group, necessitating use of nonparametric statistics. Age was not significantly related to test performance in either the suspect-effort group or the clinical comparison group, and education was not significantly correlated with test performance in the clinic group; however, a significant negative association between education and discriminant function was

TABLE 7.3. Comparisons of Demographic Characteristics and the RAVLT–ROCFT Discriminant Function between Suspect-Effort and Credible Clinic Patients

	Suspect effort ($n = 72$)	Clinic patients ($n = 125$)		
	Mean (SD)	Mean (SD)	Statistical tests	p-value
Age, years	41.6 (12.8)	43.4 (14.4)	$t = -0.90$	.37
Education, years	12.2 (2.2)	13.2 (2.8)	$t = -2.81$	.04
Gender, male/female	57/34	50/61	$\chi^2 = 6.21$	.01
Discriminant function	-0.63 (1.12)	1.01 (0.87)	$U = 1186.50$	.0001

TABLE 7.4. Classification Accuracy for RAVLT–ROCFT Disciminant Function Scores

Test and cutoff scores discriminant function	Suspect effort Sensitivity $n = 72$	Clinic patients Specificity $n = 125$
≤ 0.0	72.2	88.8
≤ –.10	66.7	91.2
≤ –.40	61.1	92.0

present in the suspect effort group (Spearman rho = –.367, p = .0001), although the amount of test score variance accounted for by education was relatively small (< 14%). Within each group, no significant difference in test performance between men and women was observed.

Due to the modest amount of test score variance accounted for by demographic variables, no attempt was made to adjust group comparisons for demographic variables. Mann–Whitney U test showed that the suspect effort patients performed significantly worse than the clinic comparison patients (Table 7.3).

Examination of specificity and sensitivity values, as reproduced in Table 7.4, revealed that use of the previously published cutoff of ≤ –.40 was associated with a specificity of 92.0%, which is essentially unchanged from the specificity of 91% obtained in the original study. However, sensitivity declined to 61.1%, as compared to the 71% documented previously. Adjustment of the cutoff score to ≤ –.10 improves the sensitivity to approximately 67% while maintaining specificity at 91%. In conclusion, available cross-validation data continue to demonstrate the efficacy of the ROCFT–RAVLT discriminant function in detection of suspect effort. However, as noted by Salazar, Lu, Wen, and Boone (Chapter 18, this volume), some adjustment in cutoffs for differing ethnic groups may enhance test effectiveness.

CALIFORNIA VERBAL LEARNING TEST

The California Verbal Learning Test (CVLT; Delis, Kramer, Kaplan, & Ober, 1987), a test of learning and short-term memory capacities, is very similar in format to the RAVLT, except that it contains 16 words and the words belong to one of four different semantic categories. It also contains two additional recall trials involving category cuing, and a recognition trial in a "yes/no" format.

Several simulation studies have investigated the utility of the CVLT in identifying noncredible performance (Coleman, Rapport, Millis, Ricker, & Farchione, 1998; Demakis, 1999; Klimczak et al., 1997).

Although these studies suggest that the CVLT has promise as a measure of effort, information regarding how simulators perform relative to controls is of limited clinical utility. Fortunately, several studies have also examined CVLT performance in real-world samples. Trueblood and Schmidt (1993), drawing subjects from a compensation-seeking mild TBI sample, found eight malingerers (based on significantly below-chance performance on a forced-choice measure) to score significantly below their eight demographically matched controls on CVLT recency, while the questionable validity patients (based on improbable test performance, e.g., grip strength = zero) scored significantly below their eight controls on CVLT total words learned across the five trials. Further, half of the questionable validity patients and 62% of the malingerers recognized fewer than 13 items. Subsequently, Trueblood (1994) observed 12 malingering and 10 questionable validity compensation-seeking mild TBI patients to perform significantly worse than matched patient controls on CVLT total and recognition, and the questionable validity subjects also scored more poorly on semantic clustering; groups did not differ in intrusions, recall consistency, or primacy effect. Recognition hits < 13 was associated with 75% sensitivity in the malingerers and 60% sensitivity in the questionable validity patients at ≥ 90% specificity. Total words learned across the five trials < 48 also resulted in 75% sensitivity at 91% specificity in malingerers, and 70% sensitivity at 100% specificity in questionable validity patients. Presence of one or more of these indicators was associated with 89% to 90% sensitivity at ≥ 90% specificity.

Millis, Putnam, Adams, and Ricker (1995) examined CVLT scores in 23 mild TBI patients actively pursuing personal injury or workers' compensation litigation and who scored at or below chance on the Warrington Recognition Memory Test as compared to 23 moderate/severe TBI patients with no incentive to feign and who obtained Warrington Recognition Memory Test scores > 25. The mild head injury patients achieved significantly lower CVLT total scores, recognition discriminability, recognition hits, and long-delayed cued recall. A linear discriminant analysis correctly classified 91% of the sample (91% sensitivity; 91% specificity). Recognition discriminability and recognition hits were also highly effective individually in separating groups; recognition discriminability was associated with sensitivity of 96% and specificity of 91%, while recognition hits yielded sensitivity of 83% at 96% specificity (specific cut-scores can be obtained from the first author).

Sweet et al. (2000) obtained CVLT data on 42 moderate to severe TBI patients (13 of whom were litigating), 21 compensation-seeking malingerers identified by independent criteria (Rey 15-Item Test, Multi-Digit Memory Test, Warrington Recognition Memory Test, Category Test algorithm), 25 malingering simulators provided with information regarding head injury sequelae, and 21 controls. Subjects were collapsed into credible and non-credible groups for the purpose of applying the Millis et al. (1995) discriminant function. Overall classification accuracy was lower than reported by Millis et al. (1995) (i.e., 79% vs. 91%); sensitivity was 74% but specificity was only 83%. However, adding recognition hits to the discriminant function improved classification to 85% (78% sensitivity, 91% specificity). Using the Millis et al. (1995) cutoffs for total words learned, long-delayed cued recall, recognition hits, and recognition discriminability, specificity in the TBI group was 83%, 83%, 90%, and 86%, respectively, while sensitivity in the real-world malingering group was 52%, 48%, 48%, and 57%, respectively. Using the Trueblood and Schmidt (1993; Trueblood, 1994) cutoff for recognition hits, sensitivity was 71% and specificity was 83%. Examination of intrusions and recognitions hits compared to long-delayed free recall were less effective in discriminating groups than the original discriminant function variables and recognition hits.

Slick, Iverson, and Green (2000) analyzed CVLT data from 193 compensation-seeking patients with TBI (131 negligible or mild, 62 moderate to severe). Sensitivity values for the negligible–mild TBI group ranged from 11% to 12%; a score below cutoffs for any of the variables occurred in 18% of the sample. Specificity values in the moderate/severe brain injury group, using the Millis et al. (1995) cutoffs for total words learned, long-delayed cued recall, recognition hits, and recognition discriminability, were 82%, 82%, 88%, and 91%, respectively; a score below cutoffs for any of the foregoing variables occurred in 31% of the sample. The authors raise concerns that CVLT effort indices may have higher than acceptable rates of false positive identifications. CVLT scores were unrelated to age and only weakly associated with education, although gender may have impacted performance; more men than women scored below cutoffs. Ashendorf, O'Bryant, and McCaffrey (2003) also found CVLT indices to be unrelated to age but failed to detect a relationship with gender.

Baker, Donders, and Thompson (2000) investigated specificity for the Millis et al. (1995) CVLT discriminant function and the Millis and Putnam (1997) CVLT logistic regression in a TBI sample with no motive to feign (60 mild, 35 moderate, and 39 severe). The discriminant function was associated with a false-positive rate of only 7.5%, although the logistic regression resulted in misclassification of 18.7% of the sample, particularly individuals with lower levels of education. Presence of prior psychiatric or substance abuse history, injury severity, and age were unrelated to false-positive identifications.

Curtis, Greve, Bianchini, and Brennan (2006) examined CVLT performance in patients with TBI with no incentive to feign ($n = 29$), incentive but no failed effort indicators ($n = 71$), suspect (incentive and any evidence of suspect effort; $n = 120$), and per Slick et al. (1999) criteria, definite ($n = 15$) and probable ($n = 40$) malingered neurocognitive dysfunction. The authors compared the efficacy of CVLT total correct recall (trials 1–5), recognition hits, discriminability, long-delayed cued recall scores, the Millis et al. (1995)

discriminant function, a logistic regression formula developed by Millis and Putnam (1997), and six logistic regression models developed by Millis and Volinsky (2001). The probable and definite malingerers significantly differed from the three other groups on all variables; the probable and definite malingering groups did not differ from each other except for models 1 through 4, the average of models 1 through 4, and the linear shrinkage model, with the definite group performing worse. To examine sensitivity, the probable and definite malingering groups were combined, and to estab- lish specificity, the no-incentive and incentive-only groups were combined. The most sensitive scores were recognition hits and the linear shrinkage model. Using a cutoff of ≤ 11 for recognition hits, specificity in mild or mod- erate/severe TBI was ≥ 90% with sensitivity at 60%; however, specificity val- ues were unacceptably low for comparison no-incentive patients with stroke (n = 183; 70%), memory disorder (n = 75; 64%), psychiatric disorder (n = 24; 79%), and brain tumor (n = 20; 75%). For the linear shrinkage model score of 0, sensitivity was slightly higher (66%) with comparable specific- ity in the no-malingered-neurocognitive-dysfunction TBI group; however, specificity was lower in the non-TBI groups (cerebral vascular accident; CVA = 62%, memory disorder = 52%; psychiatric disorder = 67%; and tumor (65%).

In 2000 the CVLT-II was published; it contains a new word list and includes a forced-choice recognition trial administered 10 minutes after the yes/no recognition trial. Extending effort research to the CVLT-II, Bauer, Yantz, Ryan, Warden, and McCaffrey (2005) imported the Millis et al. (1995) discriminant function and examined long-delayed forced-choice recognition hits in patients with postacute mild to moderate TBI (presence of incentive unreported), 29 of whom were identified as noncredible on the Word Memory Test, and 91 determined to have adequate effort. Delayed recognition hits, long-delayed forced-choice recognition hits, and long-delayed recognition discriminability differentiated the two groups, while immediate total recall and long-delayed cued recall did not uniquely contribute. The full model employing all five predictors correctly classified 75.8% of the sample, and, while specificity was high (95.6%), sensitivity was low (13.8%).

Root, Robbins, Chang, and van Gorp (2006) examined CVLT-II forced- choice recognition (including separate analyses of abstract and concrete items) and two types of critical item analysis (CIA; recognition [comparison of items recognized in yes/no format with items recognized in the forced- choice trial], and recall [comparison of items recalled with items recognized in forced-choice format]) in their investigation of effort in two groups of patients with mixed neuropsychiatric diagnoses and with incentive to feign: 27 individuals who passed the TOMM and/or VIP and 25 who failed these measures. Using a cutoff for forced-choice recognition of 14, sensitivity was 44% (93% specificity), although sensitivity was higher for concrete items in isolation (cutoff = 7; 56% sensitivity, 89% specificity). CIA sensitivity rates were substantially lower: 24% for CIA recall (cutoff = 2; 96% specificity) and 16% for recognition (cutoff = 2; 100% specificity).

In conclusion, the available literature suggests that the CVLT has some utility for detection of suspect effort, particularly in patients alleging symptoms in the context of mild TBI. However, specificity values appear to be problematic in patients with moderate to severe TBI, stroke, psychiatric conditions, memory disorder, and brain tumor, and in patients with lower levels of education. Research on the use of the CVLT as an effort indicator has been on the forefront of employing discriminant function analysis and logistic regression to test scores, a practice which will no doubt gain popularity in the quest to limit the effects of coaching on effort test performance. Consistent with research on the RAVLT, CVLT scores involving recognition data appear to be the most sensitive, although total words recalled across the five learning trials also discriminated between groups in several studies. However, some sensitivity values may have been inflated due to the practice in some studies of limiting the noncredible samples to those who were blatantly feigning symptoms (e.g., significantly below chance on forced-choice testing), while sensitivity in other studies was artificially lowered due to using litigation status as the sole criterion for group membership (not all litigants are malingering) or by using litigants deemed to be credible as the comparison group (effort indicators do not detect all noncredible subjects, therefore some noncredible subjects would be included in the credible group); true sensitivity values appear to range between 50% and 60%. Lack of consistent word recall across learning trials (Demakis, 1999) and semantic clustering (Trueblood, 1994) may be associated with feigning, observations which may serve to boost sensitivity if incorporated into existing CVLT effort algorithms. Research is particularly limited for the CVLT-II, although examination of the concrete items on the forced-choice recognition trial appears to show the most promise.

WARRINGTON RECOGNITION MEMORY TEST

The Warrington Recognition Memory Test (WRMT; Warrington, 1984) was designed to measure verbal (Words) and nonverbal (Faces) memory abilities. In the Words task, the patient is shown a series of 50 words and asked to rate subjective pleasantness of the words. The patient is then given a page with 50 pairs of words and instructed to choose, for each word pair, which word was previously shown from the earlier presentation of 50 words. Similarly, the WRMT–Faces is a test used to assess learning and recognition memory for nonverbal/visual material. The patient is shown 50 faces, comprised of black-and-white photographs of mostly Caucasian men, then presented with pairs of faces and asked to identify which one was previously shown. It should be noted that the Faces subtest is not nearly as sensitive to feigned symptoms as Words (Iverson & Franzen, 1994; 1998; Millis, 1992); therefore, this review focuses only on Words.

Even though the WRMT was not originally designed to detect malingered memory impairment, research has shown that the test, due to its forced-choice format, is well suited for detection of nonoptimal performance and feigned memory impairment.

Millis (1992) conducted the first study using the WRMT–Words to detect exaggerated memory impairment. Ten subjects with reported mild TBI who were pursuing financial compensation performed significantly worse than a group of 20 subjects who had documented moderate and severe TBIs and were not pursuing financial compensation. A cutoff score of 31 correctly classified 70% of the compensation-seeking patients with mild TBI with 90% specificity. A cutoff score of 29 only captured 50% of the patients with mild TBI but did not result in any false-positive identification.

In a subsequent study (Millis & Putnam, 1994), subjects with documented moderate to severe brain trauma ($n = 32$; litigation status unknown) were compared to compensation-seeking ($n = 19$) or noncompensation-seeking and/or returned to work ($n = 12$) subjects with mild head injury. The compensation-seeking group with mild TBI performed significantly worse than the two other groups, while the employed group with mild TBI scored highest; 29% of the compensation-seeking group with mild TBI scored < 25, in contrast to only 6% of the patients with moderate/severe TBI and none of the returned-to-work subjects with mild TBI.

Several other studies have examined WMRT–Words performance in simulators instructed to feign performance as compared to controls, patients with TBI, and neuropsychological clinic patients with and without memory impairment (i.e., ≤ 10th percentile on WMS-R Logical Memory I and II or Visual Reproduction I and II (Cato, Brewster, Ryan, & Giuliano, 2002; Iverson & Franzen, 1994, 1998; Suhr & Gunstad, 2000; Wogar, van den Broak, Bradshaw, & Szabadi, 1998). Warned simulators average 4 points higher than naïve simulators (Suhr & Gunstad, 2000). Iverson and Franzen (1994) reported that cutoffs of < 33 and < 40 were associated with 100% and 90% specificity, respectively, in patients with TBI (80% severe), and they subsequently described 100% specificity in nonlitigating memory impaired or nonmemory impaired hospital referrals for neuropsychological testing with a cutoff of < 38 (Iverson & Franzen, 1998); a cutoff of < 40 was associated with 90% specificity in the memory-impaired subjects and 100% specificity in those who were non-memory impaired.

In conclusion, the available literature suggests that the WRMT, specifically the Words section, shows discrimination of both litigating and simulating samples from actual brain-impaired subjects and controls. However, to date, no studies have appeared in which WRMT–Words data were examined in a real-world noncredible population as determined by failed performance on independent effort indicators. Accurate sensitivity data cannot be obtained through use of litigant pools because not all litigants are in fact malingering; sensitivity values will be an underestimate of true hit rate. Despite this limitation, the meager data on WMRT–Words sensitivity reveals high values although sample sizes have been small. As noted by Victor and Boone (Chapter 14, this volume), the WRMT–Words may be particularly effective in the differential between actual versus feigned mental retardation in that individuals with mentally retarded IQ scores typically perform well on this task. Further, WRMT–Words performance does not appear to be negatively impacted by English-as-a-second-language status or ethnicity (Salazar, Lu, Wen, and Boone, Chapter 18, this volume) or psychiatric disorder (depression or psychosis; Goldberg, Back-Madruga, and Boone, Chapter 13, this volume). Adding to its attractiveness, the WRMT–Words is typically briefer to administer than other forced-choice tasks (a single presentation and recognition trial and the latter is contained on a single page, eliminating page-turning time).

WECHSLER MEMORY SCALE

The Wechsler Memory Scale–Revised and the third edition (WMS-R and WMS-III, respectively; Wechsler, 1987, 1997) are the most often used measure of verbal and visual memory among neuropsychologists (Rabin, Barr, & Burton, 2005). Accordingly, the importance of identifying effective and efficient methods of screening for malingering on the WMS-R or WMS-III cannot be overstated. The WMS is composed of multiple subtests that contribute to various index scores; hence, numerous scores can be derived from the WMS. Several investigations have examined the efficacy of the WMS-R in detecting feigning of cognitive symptoms in simulating samples (Bernard, 1990; Bernard, Houston, & Natoli, 1993; Bernard, McGrath, & Houston, 1993; Johnson & Lesniak-Karpiak, 1997; Mittenberg, Azrin, Millsaps, & Heilbronner, 1993), and in real-world samples as summarized below.

Suchy and Sweet (2000) examined use of the WMS-R Information/Orientation subtest (unchanged in the WMS-III) in 50 benefit-seeking patients (40 of whom were reporting TBI); 12% obtained scores below all those of a clinical normative sample ($n = 312$), and an additional 24% achieved scores comparable to the lower 2% of this comparison sample.

Other researchers have examined the scores on Logical Memory and Visual Reproduction subtests with equivocal results. Greiffenstein et al. (1994) failed to find a significant group difference among probable malingering postconcussive patients (based on impaired cognitive scores and improbable outcomes; $n = 43$), credible postconcussive patients ($n = 30$), and patients with moderate/severe TBI ($n = 33$; some in litigation) but subsequently reported significant differences in performance on these scores between probable malingering (based on presence of impaired scores on cognitive testing and improbable outcomes) postconcussive patients involved in litigation ($n = 90$) and patients with severe TBI ($n = 60$; some in litigation), with the former group performing significantly worse (Greiffenstein et al., 1996). However, van Gorp et al. (1999), studying 20 probable malingerers (based on improbable symptom history, improbable outcome, and at least one failure on an independent effort indicator) and 61 nonmalingerers (although some may have had incentive to feign), found the former to significantly underperform on Visual Reproduction II but not on Visual Reproduction I or Logical Memory subtests. Binder et al. (2003) observed poor-motivation (failed PDRT) litigants with mild TBI ($n = 34$) to significantly underperform on Logical Memory I in comparison to noncompensation-seeking TBI patients with moderate/severe ($n = 60$), but good-motivation (passed PDRT) litigants with mild TBI ($n = 22$) did not perform significantly differ from either group. On Logical Memory II, the good-motivation group performed better than the poor-motivation group but not superior to the patients with moderate/severe brain-injury.

Iverson and Franzen (1996), employing the Logical Memory subtest and a forced-choice supplement, documented significantly poorer performance in 20 college students and 20 patients with various psychiatric disorders instructed to feign compared to performance under standard instructions and to that of neuropsychology patients with memory deficits. A cutoff of < 6 for Logical Memory I was associated with 100% specificity but only 18% sensitivity; raising the cutoff to < 14 led to 5% false-positive identifications and sensitivity of 60%. A cutscore of < 18 for the forced-choice adaptation had 100% specificity and 85% sensitivity. Subsequently, Martin, Franzen, and Orey (1998) used students and professionals familiar with the Logical Memory and Visual Reproduction subtests to rate the probability of selection for each intraitem choice for the Iverson and Franzen (1996) Logical Memory recognition trial and a Visual Reproduction recognition paradigm developed by Edith Kaplan. The averaged values were then assigned to the item selections of 15 college student controls, 15 college student simulators, 30 patients with moderate to severe TBI (litigation status unknown), and 7 litigating patients with mild TBI with questionable motivation based on below-cutoff performance on independent effort measures (21-Item Test, 16-Item Test) or severely impaired performance on standard memory tests. Controls outperformed all groups on Logical Memory and Visual Reproduction I and II scores as well as the summed probability value scores; patients with TBI performed significantly better than the two malingering groups, which did not differ from each other. Discriminant function analysis (malingering groups collapsed, and controls and TBI groups collapsed) employing a total recognition score and the summed probability value score revealed that only the latter entered the final discriminant function. Using a summed probability value score cutoff of ≤ 14, specificity in the TBI group was 93%, while sensitivity in the questionable malingering patients was 57%. Further, some multiple-choice selections were not endorsed by the TBI group but were chosen by malingering groups, which the authors suggest may also be independently useful in identifying poor effort.

Denney (1999) also developed a 50-item WMS-R Logical Memory forced choice task, and documented that 158 college students unfamiliar with the stories performed at chance on the measure (mean of 27.6 ± 3.93; range = 19 to 39). He illustrates the clinical use of this recognition trial in two case examples.

Various discriminant functions employing several WMS-R subtests have been examined in simulators (Bernard, 1990; Bernard, Houston, & Natoli, 1993; Bernard, McGrath, & Houston, 1993; Mittenberg et al., 1993), although findings have yet to be replicated in real-world noncredible samples.

Various studies have reported specificity data for a subtraction algorithm. Iverson, Slick, and Franzen (2000) found attention/concentration index scores substantially below general memory scores (> 25 points) in approximately 5% of a non-compensation-seeking inpatient substance abuse population (n = 332). Iverson and Slick (2001) documented only a 6.5% to 9.0% false-positive rate in 1,986 patients with acute TBI. Similarly, Slick, Hinkin, van Gorp, and Satz (2001) observed a false-positive rate of only 7% in non-compensation-seeking HIV-positive individuals (n = 55); however, the false-positive rate was elevated to 18% in patients with above-average general memory index scores. Hilsabeck et al. (2003), in studying 200 nonlitigants in nine diagnostic categories (TBI, brain tumor, stroke/vascular, Alzheimer's disease, epilepsy, depression/anxiety, medical problems, and no diagnosis), noted 92% specificity for the general memory index minus attention/ concentration index difference score cutoff of 25. Only 6.5% of the sample was misclassified as noncredible using a discriminant function employing all WMS-R subtests, although misclassification rates higher than 10% were found for stroke (24%) and patients with medical problems (11%).

With the introduction of the WMS-III in 1997, many of the findings in the aforementioned studies are not translatable to the current version due to significant differences in structure and format of the subtests. However, the inclusion of a recognition component in the WMS-III makes it ideal for applying a forced-choice paradigm in detecting suspect effort. Langeluddecke and Lucas (2003) studied 25 probable malingering (based on failed WRMT performance) litigants with mild TBI, 50 nonmalingering (passed the WRMT) litigants with mild TBI, and 50 litigants with severe

TBI who scored above chance on the WRMT (≥ 30). The authors reported significantly poorer performance in the malingering group for all of the subtests and indexes with Auditory Recognition Delay (ARD) Index yielding the greatest discrimination. Cutoff scores of < 43 on ARD and < 18 on word-list recognition resulted in excellent sensitivity (80% or higher) with specificity above 91%. The authors conclude that the ARD raw score, comprising the summation of scores on Logical Memory Delayed Recognition and Verbal Paired Associates Delayed Recognition, appears to be an extremely effective method of screening for inadequate effort. Despite significant group differences, classification rates for other WMS-III subtest and index scores, particularly visual recognition memory tests, were generally disappointing.

Lange, Iverson, Sullivan, and Anderson (2006) observed significantly lowered scores on the WMS-III Auditory Immediate Index, Immediate Memory Index, Auditory Delayed Index, General Memory Index (GMI), and Working Memory Index (WMI) in 145 litigants (19 with poor effort based on failed test of Memory Malingering or WRMT performance). Discriminant function analysis revealed the GMI to be the only predictor retained in the equation (89.5% sensitivity; 81.0% specificity). The WMI was subtracted from each of the other four indexes to create four memory–WMI discrepancy scores; groups were found to significantly differ on all four difference scores but classification rates were poor (58% to 68% sensitivity; 60% to 64% specificity).

Killgore and DellaPietra (2000) identified six items from the WMS-III Logical Memory recognition trial endorsed correctly at above-chance levels (i.e., 70–80%) by normal subjects naïve to story content (#12, #16, #18, #22, #24, #29); the weighted combination of these items was used to create a Rarely Missed Index (RMI). A cutoff score of 136 correctly classified 97% of 36 stimulators with no false-positive misidentifications among 51 heterogeneous neuropsychological clinic patients (litigation status unknown). In a discriminant function employing both the RMI and the total Logical Memory Delayed Recognition (LMDR) score, only RMI was retained in the equation, indicating that inclusion of LMDR score data did not enhance discrimination of groups over that of RMI alone. However, a subsequent study of the RMI in brain-injury litigants showed only 25% sensitivity in 20 suspected malingerers (based on poor performance on the Test of Memory Malingering or WRMT) and 41% sensitivity in 12 "borderline" malingerers (passed effort tests but cognitive test results were judged not to be reflective of actual functioning based on behavioral observations), although specificity in 126 litigants with good effort and 78 nonlitigant patients was high (91–95%) (Lange, Sullivan, & Anderson, 2005). In this study, noncredible groups scored significantly below credible groups on Logical Memory I and II. High specificity for the RMI was also confirmed by Miller, Ryan, Carruthers, and

Cluff (2004) in nonlitigating alcohol abusers (97%), substance abusers (95%), and head-injured patients (mild to severe; 93%).

Other individual WMS-III subtests have been investigated in terms of their utility in identifying suspect effort in simulators, such as the Faces subtest (Glassmire et al., 2003).

In conclusion, several studies have examined use of Wechsler Memory Scales, although most have employed the WMS-R rather than the newer version, the WMS-III, which is now more commonly used in clinical practice. Regarding the WMS-III, data have been contradictory regarding whether the ADI or the GMI is more sensitive to poor effort; both have high sensitivity (80% to 90%) and moderate to high specificity (81% to > 91%). Individual subtests, such as Logical Memory, Faces, Information/Orientation, and Word List recognition, may show promise for identifying noncredible performance, although preliminary data suggest that sensitivity is lower, with the possible exception of Word List recognition, than that found for index scores. In addition to reporting the results of group comparisons on individual subtests and index scores, several investigations have also employed novel approaches, such as discriminant functions, subtraction equations, tabulation of rarely missed items, and forced-choice supplements with individual items rated for plausibility and differentially weighted in summary scores, which have the possibility of enhancing test sensitivity.

CONCLUSION

The majority of patients presenting for neuropsychological evaluation report complaints of memory difficulties regardless of whether the pathology is neurological, psychiatric, physical, metabolic, or substance induced. It is therefore not surprising that memory impairment is the cognitive disability most likely to be feigned, necessitating the assessment of the veracity of memory complaint. The most popular strategy for assessing effort and motivation remains the administration of specialized measures, but the inclusion of several of these measures, particular those involving forced-choice recognition, can substantially lengthen test battery administration time. Given that the clinician is faced with the task of conducting a thorough neuropsychological evaluation under limited time constraints, a preferable alternative is to find patterns of performance that discriminate suspect effort and feigned or exaggerated deficits from true cognitive dysfunction with instruments that are already administered routinely as part of a standardized test battery. We reviewed numerous studies that have investigated the effectiveness of five commonly administered tests of memory functioning in detecting feigned or exaggerated memory impairment and found that in general, various variables can be extracted from the tests which demonstrate promise in discriminating noncredible effort from cooperative patients.

REFERENCES

Ashendorf, L., O'Bryant, S. E., & McCaffrey, R. J. (2003). Specificity of malingering detection strategies in older adults using the CVLT and WCST. *The Clinical Neuropsychologist*, *17*, 255–262.

Baker, R., Donders, J., & Thompson, E. (2000). Assessment of incomplete effort with the California Verbal Learning Test. *Applied Neuropsychology*, *7*, 111–114.

Bauer, L., Yantz, C. L., Ryan, L. M., Warden, D. L., & McCaffrey, R. J. (2005). An examination of the California Verbal Learning Test II to detect incomplete effort in a traumatic brain-injury sample. *Applied Neuropsychology*, *12*, 202–207.

Bernard, L. C. (1990). Prospects for faking believable memory deficits on neuropsychological tests and the use of incentives in simulation research. *Journal of Clinical and Experimental Neuropsychology*, *12*, 715–728.

Bernard, L. C. (1991). The detection of faked deficits on the Rey Auditory Verbal Learning Test: The effect of serial position. *Archives of Clinical Neuropsychology*, *6*, 81–88.

Bernard, L. C., Houston, W., & Natoli, L. (1993). Malingering on neuropsychological memory tests: Potential objective indicators. *Journal of Clinical Psychology*, *49*, 45–53.

Bernard, L. C., McGrath, M. J., & Houston, W. (1993). Discriminating between simulated malingering and closed head injury on the Wechsler Memory Scale—Revised. *Archives of Clinical Neuropsychology*, *8*, 539–551.

Binder, L. M., Kelly, M. P., Villanueva, M. R., & Winslow, M. M. (2003). Motivation and neuropsychological test performance following mild head injury. *Journal of Clinical and Experimental Neuropsychology*, *25*, 420–430.

Binder, L. M., Villanueva, M. R., Howieson, D., & Moore, R. T. (1993). The Rey AVLT Recognition Memory Task measures motivational impairment after mild head trauma. *Archives of Clinical Neuropsychology*, *8*, 137–147.

Boone, J. B., Lu, P., & Wen, J. (2005). Comparison of various RAVLT scores in the detection of noncredible memory performance. *Archives of Clinical Neuropsychology*, *20*, 310–319.

Brandt, J. (1988). Malingered amnesia. In R. Rogers (Ed.), *Clinical assessment of malingering and deception* (pp. 65–83). New York: Guilford Press.

Butcher, J. N., Dahlstrom, W. G., Graham, J. R., Tellegen, A., & Kaemmer, B. (1989). *Manual for administration and scoring MMPI-2*. Minneapolis: University of Minnesota Press.

Cato, M. A., Brewster, J., Ryan, T., & Giuliano, A. J. (2002). Coaching and the ability to simulate mild traumatic brain injury symptoms. *The Clinical Neuropsychologist*, *16*, 524–535.

Chouinard, M. J., & Rouleau, I. (1997). The 48-Pictures Test: A two-alternative forced-choice recognition test for the detection of malingering. *Journal of the International Neuropsychological Society*, *3*, 545–552.

Coleman, R. D., Rapport, L. J., Millis, S. R., Ricker, J. H., & Farchione, T. J. (1998). Effects of coaching on detection of malingering on the California Verbal Learning Test. *Journal of Clinical and Experimental Neuropsychology*, *20*, 201–210.

Curtis, K. L., Greve, K. W., Bianchini, K. J., & Brennan, A. (2006). California Verbal Learning Test indicators of malingered neurocognitive dysfunction. *Assessment*, *13*, 46–61.

Delis, D. C. (1991). Neuropsychological assessment in learning and memory. In F. Boller & J. Grafman (Eds.), *Handbook of neuropsychology* (Vol. 3, pp. 3–33). Amsterdam: Elsevier.

Delis, D. C., Kramer, H. H., Kaplan, E., & Ober, B. A. (1987). *California Verbal Learning Test*. San Antonio, TX: The Psychological Corporation.

Demakis, G. J. (1999). Serial malingering on verbal and nonverbal fluency and memory measures: An analog investigation. *Archives of Clinical Neuropsychology, 14*, 401–410.

Denney, R. L. (1999). A brief symptom validity testing procedure for Logical Memory of the Weschler Memory Scale–Revised which can demonstrate verbal memory in the face of claimed disability. *Journal of Forensic Neuropsychology, 1*, 5–26.

Glassmire, D. M., Bierley, R. A., Wisniewski, A. M., Greene, R. L., Kennedy, J. E., & Date, E. (2003). Using the WMS-III Faces subtest to detect malingered memory impairment. *Journal of Clinical and Experimental Neuropsychology, 25*, 465–481.

Gouvier, W. D., Prestholdt, P. H., & Warner, M. S. (1988). A survey of common misconceptions about head injury and recovery. *Archives of Clinical Neuropsychology, 3*, 331–343.

Greiffenstein, M. F., Baker, W. J., & Gola, T. (1994). Validation of malingered amnesia measures with a large clinical sample. *Psychological Assessment, 6*, 218–224.

Greiffenstein, M. F., Baker, W. J., & Gola, T. (1996). Comparison of multiple scoring methods for Rey's malingered amnesia measures. *Archives of Clinical Neuropsychology, 11*, 283–293.

Greiffenstein, M. F., Gola, T., & Baker, W. J. (1995). MMPI-2 validity scales versus domain specific measures in detection of factitious traumatic brain injury. *The Clinical Neuropsychologist, 9*, 230–240.

Haines, M. E., & Norris, M. P. (2001). Comparing student and patient simulated malingerers' performance on standard neuropsychological measures to detect feigned cognitive deficits. *The Clinical Neuropsychologist, 15*, 171–182.

Hilsabeck, R. C., Thompson, M. D., Irby, J. W., Adams, R. L., Scott, J. G., & Gouvier, W. D. (2003). Partial cross-validation of the Wechsler Memory Scale–Revised (WMS-R) General Memory–Attention/Concentration Malingering Index in a nonlitigating sample. *Archives of Clinical Neuropsychology, 18*, 71–79.

Inman, T. H., & Berry, D. T. R. (2002). Cross-validation of indicators of malingering: A comparison of nine neuropsychological tests, four tests of malingering, and behavioral observations. *Archives of Clinical Neuropsychology, 17*, 1–23.

Iverson, G. L., & Franzen, M. D. (1994). The Recognition Memory Test, Digit Span, and Knox Cube Test as markers of malingered memory impairment. *Assessment, 1*, 323–334.

Iverson, G. L., & Franzen, M. D. (1996). Using multiple objective memory procedures to detect simulated malingering. *Journal of Clinical and Experimental Neuropsychology, 18*, 38–51.

Iverson, G. L., & Franzen, M. D. (1998). Detecting malingered memory deficits with the Recognition Memory Test. *Brain Injury, 12*, 275–282.

Iverson, G. L., & Slick, D. J. (2001). Base rates of the WMS-R malingering index following traumatic brain injury. *American Journal of Forensic Psychology, 19*, 5–13.

Iverson, G. L., Slick, D. J., & Franzen, M. D. (2000). Evaluation of a WMS-R Malingering Index in a non-litigating clinical sample. *Journal of Clinical and Experimental Neuropsychology, 22*, 191–197.

Johnson, J. L., & Lesniak-Karpiak, K. (1997). The effect of warning on malingering on memory and motor tasks in college samples. *Archives of Clinical Neuropsychology, 12*, 231–238.

Killgore, W. D. S., & DellaPietra, L. (2000). Using the WMS-III to detect malingering: Empirical validation of the Rarely Missed Index (RMI). *Journal of Clinical and Experimental Neuropsychology, 22*, 761–771.

Klimczak, N. J., Donovick, P. J.,& Burright, R. (1997). The malingering of multiple sclerosis and mild traumatic brain injury. *Brain Injury, 11*, 343–352.

Lange, R. T., Iverson, G. L., Sullivan, K., & Anderson, D. (2006). Suppressed working memory on the WMS-III as a marker for poor effort. *Journal of Clinical and Experimental Neuropsychology, 28*, 294–305.

Lange, R. T., Sullivan, K., & Anderson, D. (2005). Ecological validity of the WMS-III Rarely Missed Index in personal injury litigation. *Journal of Clinical and Experimental Neuropsychology, 27*, 412–424.

Langeluddecke, P. M., & Lucas, S. K. (2003). Quantitative measures of memory malingering on the Wechsler Memory Scale–Third edition in mild head injury litigants. *Archives of Clinical Neuropsychology, 18*, 181–197.

Lu, P. H., Boone, K. B., Cozolino, L., & Mitchell, C. (2003). Effectiveness of the Rey–Osterrieth Complex Figure Test and the Meyers and Meyers recognition trial in the detection of suspect effort. *The Clinical Neuropsychologist, 17*, 426–440.

Martin, R.C., Franzen, M. D., & Orey, S. (1998). Magnitude of error as a strategy to detect feigned memory impairment. *The Clinical Neuropsychologist, 12*, 84–91.

Meyers, J. E., & Meyers, K. R. (1995). *Rey Complex Figure Test and Recognition Trial.* Odessa, FL: Psychological Assessment Resources.

Meyers, J. E., Morrison, A. L., & Miller, J.C. (2001). How low is too low, revisited: Sentence repetition and AVLT-Recognition in the detection of malingering. *Applied Neuropsychology, 8*, 234–241.

Meyers, J. E., & Volbrecht, M. (1998). Validation of memory error patterns on the Rey Complex Figure and Recognition Trial. *Applied Neuropsychology, 5*, 120–131.

Meyers, J. E., & Volbrecht, M. E. (1999). Detection of malingerers using the Rey Complex Figure and Recognition Trial. *Archives of Clinical Neuropsychology, 6*, 201–207.

Miller, L. J., Ryan, J. J., Carruthers, C. A., & Cluff, R. B. (2004). Brief screening indexes for malingering: A confirmation of Vocabulary minus Digit Span from the WAIS-III and the Rarely Missed Index from the WMS-III. *The Clinical Neuropsychologist, 18*, 327–333.

Millis, S. R. (1992). The Recognition Memory Test in the detection of malingered and exaggerated memory deficits. *The Clinical Neuropsychologist, 6*, 406–414.

Millis, S. R., & Putnam, S. H. (1994). The Recognition Memory Test in the assessment of memory impairment after financially compensable mild head injury: A replication. *Perceptual and Motor Skills, 79*, 384–386.

Millis, S. R., & Putnam, S. H. (1997, June). *The California Verbal Learning Test in the assessment of financially compensable mild head injury: Further development.* Paper presented at the meeting of the International Neuropsychological Society, Bergen, Norway.

Millis, S. R., Putnam S. H., Adams K. H., & Ricker, J. H. (1995). The California Verbal Learning Test in the detection of incomplete effort in neuropsychological testing. *Psychological Assessment, 7*, 463–471.

Millis, S. R., & Volinsky, C. T. (2001). Assessment of responses bias in mild head injury: Beyond malingering tests. *Journal of Clinical and Experimental Neuropsychology*, *23*, 809–828.

Mittenberg, W., Azrin, R., Millsaps, C., & Heilbronner, R. (1993). Identification of malingered head injury on the Wechsler Memory Scale–Revised. *Psychological Assessment*, *5*, 34–40.

Powell, M. R., Gfeller, J. D., Oliveri, M. V., Stanton, S., & Hendricks, B. (2004). The Rey AVLT serial position effect: A useful indicator of symptom exaggeration? *The Clinical Neuropsychologist*, *18*, 465–476.

Rabin, L. A., Barr, W. B., & Burton, L. A. (2005). Assessment practices of clinical neuropsychologists in the United States and Canada: A survey of INS, NAN, and APA Division 40 members. *Archives of Clinical Neuropsychology*, *20*, 33–65.

Root, J. C., Robbins, R. N., Chang, L., & van Gorp, W. (2006). Detection of inadequate effort on the California Verbal Learning Test (2nd ed.): Forced choice recognition and critical item analysis. *Journal of the International Neuropsychological Society*, *12*, 688–696.

Sherman, D. S., Boone, K. B., Lu, P., & Razani, J. (2002). Re-examination of a Rey Auditory Verbal Learning Test/Rey Complex Figure discriminant function to detect suboptimal effort. *The Clinical Neuropsychologist*, *16*, 242–250.

Slick, D. J., Hinkin, C. H., van Gorp, W. G., & Satz, P. (2001). Base rate of a WMS-R Malingering Index in a sample of non-compensation-seeking men infected with HIV-1. *Applied Neuropsychology*, *8*, 185–189.

Slick, D. J., Iverson, G. L., & Green, P. (2000). California Verbal Learning Test indicators of suboptimal performance in a sample of head-injury litigants. *Journal of Clinical and Experimental Neuropsychology*, *22*, 569–579.

Suchy, Y., & Sweet, J. J. (2000). Information/Orientation subtest of the Wechsler Memory Scale–Revised as an indicator of suspicion of insufficient effort. *The Clinical Neuropsychologist*, *14*, 56–66.

Suhr, J. A. (2002). Malingering, coaching, and the serial position effect. *Archives of Clinical Neuropsychology*, *17*, 69–77.

Suhr, J. A., & Gunstad, J. (2000). The effects of coaching on the sensitivity and specificity of malingering measures. *Archives of Clinical Neuropsychology*, *15*, 415–424.

Suhr, J., Tranel, D., Wefel, J., & Barrash, J. (1997). Memory performance after head injury: Contributions of malingering, litigation status, psychological factors, and medication use. *Journal of Clinical and Experimental Neuropsychology*, *19*, 500–514.

Sweet, J. J., Wolfe, P., Satlberger, E., Numan, B., Rosenfeld, J. P., Clingerman, S., et al. (2000). Further investigation of traumatic brain injury versus insufficient effort with the California Verbal Learning Test. *Archives of Clinical Neuropsychology*, *15*(2), 105–113.

Taylor, E. M. (1959). *Psychological appraisal of children with cerebral deficits*. Cambridge, MA: Harvard University Press.

Trueblood, W. (1994). Qualitative and quantitative characteristics of malingered and other invalid WAIS-R and clinical memory data. *Journal of Clinical and Experimental Neuropsychology*, *16*, 597–607.

Trueblood, W., & Schmidt, M. (1993). Malingering and other validity considerations in the neuropsychological evaluation of mild head injury. *Journal of Clinical and Experimental Neuropsychology*, *15*, 578–590.

van Gorp, W. G., Humphrey, L. A., Kalechstien, A. L., Brumm, V. L., McMullen, W. J., & Stoddard, M. A. (1999). How well do standard clinical neuropsychological tests identify malingering? A preliminary analysis. *Journal of Clinical and Experimental Neuropsychology, 21,* 245–250.

Warrington, E. K. (1984). *Recognition Memory Test: Manual.* Berkshire, UK: NFER-Nelson.

Wechsler, D. (1987). *Wechsler Memory Scale–Revised.* San Antonio, TX: The Psychological Corporation.

Wechsler, D. (1997). *Wechsler Memory Scale* (3rd ed.). San Antonio, TX: The Psychological Corporation.

Wiggins, E. C., & Brandt, J. (1988). The detection of simulated amnesia. *Law and Human Behavior, 12,* 57–58.

Williams, J. M. (1998). The malingering of memory disorder. In C. R. Reynolds (Ed.), *Detection of malingering during head injury litigation* (pp. 105–132). New York: Plenum Press.

Wogar, M. A., van den Broek, M. D., Bradshaw, C. M., & Szabadi, E. (1998). A new performance-curve method for the detection of simulated cognitive impairment. *British Journal of Clinical Psychology, 37,* 327–339.

CHAPTER 8

Validity Indicators
within Executive Function Measures

Use and Limits in Detection of Malingering

Jerry J. Sweet
Nathaniel W. Nelson

The detection of neuropsychological malingering has evolved in a relatively short span of time from an approach that initially was limited almost exclusively to impressionistic clinical judgment to one that involves multiple methods and multiple levels of decision making. Evidence of this transition appeared in less than 10 years (cf. Faust, Hart, Guilmette, & Arkes, 1988; Nies & Sweet, 1994) and at approximately 10 years was highly visible (cf. the large literature cited in Sweet, 1999). In fact, the growth of the relevant literature during the 1990s concerning insufficient effort (IE) and malingering was nothing short of impressive and continues to constitute a major portion of the clinical research published annually in the three major journals relied on by American clinical neuropsychologists (Sweet, King, Malina, Bergman, & Simmons, 2002).

There are at least two reasons why the use of multiple symptom validity indicators (i.e., cognitive effort indices derived from standard ability tests) should be used in addition to or in conjunction with symptom validity tests (i.e., cognitive effort measures). First, cognitive effort fluctuates throughout the course of any evaluation (e.g., it may be sufficient at time 1, mediocre at time 2, and clearly insufficient at time 3). In other words:

> Invalid responding or performance is not a dichotomous phenomenon. Examinees may vary their performances along a continuum from complete effort and honesty to a complete lack thereof. Similarly, effort and honesty may vary from one point in the evaluation to another. (Bush et al., 2005, p. 422)

As such, multiple cognitive effort assessments on multiple occasions during a single evaluation allow the examiner to develop an understanding of the chronology of an individual's effort at various points during testing. This fact is the fundamental reason that we should not assume that effort performance on initial symptom validity testing necessarily represents an individual's effort across an entire evaluation, and why we do not simply stop testing if we find IE early in, or perhaps at the outset of, the evaluation. Regarding the latter circumstance, discontinuance of an entire set of ability tests solely because of initial IE does a disservice to both the patient and the examiner; the patient is not afforded the opportunity to perform at capacity on standard ability tests, and the examiner remains ignorant of whether the patient might have provided useful information regarding cognitive ability independent of IE.

Second, in addition to tracking an individual's effort across time, it is generally assumed that multiple symptom validity tests, as well as symptom validity indicators derived from standard ability tests, yield nonredundant information regarding cognitive effort (Nelson et al., 2003). Administration of multiple effort measures increases the incremental validity of the examiner's conclusions regarding the patient's effort performances. In keeping with the spirit of the widely used "Slick criteria" (Slick, Sherman, & Iverson, 1999), which operationalize diagnostic conclusion of "malingering" as a probabilistic statement based on multiple measures and sources of information, inclusion of multiple effort measures and consideration of multiple embedded validity indicators ensure greater diagnostic confidence. Because it is not expedient to continually administer multiple symptom validity tests during the course of an already very lengthy test battery, tests with embedded symptom validity indicators allow the examiner to continually monitor for IE while concurrently assessing an individual's cognitive ability.

A subset of the literature pertaining to detection of IE and malingering using traditional tests of ability relates to measures of executive function. A succinct definition of executive function has been offered by Lezak, Howieson, and Loring (2004), who describe executive functions as "capacities that enable a person to engage successfully in independent, purposive, self-serving behavior" (p. 35). For the purposes of this chapter, we find it useful to consider the more detailed description offered by Ettlin and Kischka (1999) in operationalizing human prefrontal functions.

> They include high-level mental activities such as motor control and programming (suppression of reflexes and motor impulses, rapid switches in move-

ments, programming and performance of complex series of movements); mental control (flexibility in shifting, resistance to interference, e.g., the ability to reverse automatized series); personality and emotion (initiative, self-monitoring, control of aggressive and sexual impulses); and fluency, creativity, and planning. (p. 233)

Aside from the clinical task of identifying invalid responding that potentially signals malingering, clinical assessment of the domain of executive function is noteworthy for being among the most challenging tasks facing neuropsychologists (cf. Damasio & Anderson, 2003; Osmon, 1999, and more generally the excellent texts by Miller & Cummings, 1999, and Stuss & Knight, 2002). This chapter does not address in detail the well-known complex nature of evaluating executive function but instead focuses almost exclusively on the degree to which concepts (e.g., invalid responding, compromised effort, unrealistically poor performances, and nonneurological patterns of performance) related to detection of malingering can be measured and quantified using traditional tests that putatively assess executive functioning. Thus, the present chapter has the following goals: (1) summarize the extant literature on assessment of executive function relevant to malingering, and (2) provide recommendations for clinical application, emphasizing the limits of executive measures in this regard. The following commonly used putative measures of executive function are included in this review: Wisconsin Card Sorting Test, Category and Booklet Category Test, verbal and figural fluency tasks, Stroop Color–Word Test, and the Trailmaking Test (parts A and B).

LITERATURE REVIEW OF RELEVANT TESTS

Wisconsin Card Sorting Test

Bernard, McGrath, and Houston (1996) examined the utility of the Wisconsin Card Sorting Test (WCST) as an effort indicator in groups of simulating malingerers, controls, closed head-injured patients of undisclosed severity, and patients with mixed etiologies. The authors hypothesized that malingerers would display statistically contrasting patterns of fewer *categories completed* (an obvious indicator) obtained relative to the number of *perseverative responses* and/or *perseverative errors* (subtle indicators). A series of discriminant functions were conducted, comparing malingerers versus controls, malingerers versus head-injured patients, and malingerers versus the other patients. For malingerers versus controls, *categories completed* was the only WCST index to meet criteria for inclusion (in contrast to *total errors, perseverative responses, perseverative errors*, and *other responses*), suggesting that it was the only index to discriminate between groups (100% sensitivity, 92% specificity). For malingerers versus closed head injury patients, *categories com-*

pleted and *perseverative errors* entered into the analysis and yielded an overall classification of 86% sensitivity and 94% specificity. For malingerers versus other patients, *categories completed* and *perseverative responses* met inclusion criteria and yielded 58% sensitivity and 100% specificity. The authors interpreted these findings to support the pattern of performance hypothesis for subtle versus obvious effort indicators. The authors' expectation that the WCST *other responses* would be a subtle indicator of poor effort was not supported, perhaps because of the low frequencies of *other responses* across groups, which would preclude usefulness as a discriminative indicator. Bernard et al. (1996) also explored the validity of their discriminant function equations by discussing their use in eight real-world referrals identified on separate bases as likely malingerers, with six correctly identified by the WCST discriminant functions.

Donders (1999) examined the specificity of the Bernard et al. (1996) WCST malingering formula in 130 patients with mild, moderate, or severe traumatic head injury who had no external incentives for poor performance. Basically, the motivation for the study was that if Bernard's formula was to be of use, it should demonstrate a false-positive error rate of no greater than 10% in a genuine head-injured sample. The Bernard formula yielded a false-positive error rate of only 5% ($n = 7$). Three of these seven patients had a history of severe head injury, whereas the other four had mild head injuries complicated by posttraumatic stress disorder (PTSD) ($n = 2$) or severe pain ($n = 2$). Donders interpreted the 5% false-positive rate to be acceptable and more accurate than other existing malingering formulas. Donders speculated that the formula may produce more false-positive errors with increasing age.

Suhr and Boyer (1999) attempted to replicate and extend the findings of Bernard et al. (1996) in using the WCST to discriminate between groups of undergraduates (simulators and controls) and patients (probable malingerers and mild–moderate head-injured patients). In addition to the variables employed by Bernard et al., Suhr and Boyer included *failure to maintain set* (*FMS*) in their analyses as *FMS* errors are relatively rare in both normal and brain-injured cohorts. For this reason, they regarded the *FMS* as a potential "subtle" variable. All four groups were compared across *categories completed*, *errors*, *perseverative errors*, and *FMS*. As might be expected, the simulators and probable malingerers performed worse than the head-injured and normal groups. In attempts to predict groups using WCST variables, the authors found *categories completed* and *perseverative errors* to be very highly (negatively) correlated. They therefore used only *categories completed* and *FMS* to predict group classifications, with logistic regression resulting in 70.7% sensitivity (correctly identified simulators) and 87.1% specificity (correctly identified normal students). In the patient samples, the same predictors (*FMS*, *categories completed*) yielded 82.4% sensitivity (probable malingerers) and 93.3% specificity (motivated head-injured patients). Suhr and Boyer

(1999) concluded that their findings support the use of WCST as an indicator of possible feigned cognitive impairment. In the undergraduate sample, the malingerers completed half as many categories, while making twice as many *FMS* errors, a pattern that was similar in the patient groups. Because of the multicollinearity between *categories completed* and *perseverative errors*, and the usefulness of *FMS* in discriminating groups, the authors suggest that their findings did not completely replicate those of Bernard et al. Bernard et al. (1996) found *categories completed* to distinguish simulators and controls, while Suhr and Boyer (1999) found *categories completed* and *FMS* to significantly discriminate between groups.

Miller, Donders, and Suhr (2000) examined the utility of the Bernard and Suhr formulae in a sample of 90 patients with mild and severe traumatic brain injury (TBI), including 13 individuals who had shown insufficient effort on either the Warrington Recognition Memory Test (WRMT) or the Test of Memory Malingering (TOMM; Tombaugh, 1996). The Bernard formula identified three of the nonmalingerers as likely malingerers, and the Suhr and Boyer formula identified four of the nonmalingerers as likely malingerers (three of which were also identified by the Bernard formula). However, none of the individuals identified as malingering by the formulae were in litigation or showed insufficient effort on the WRMT or TOMM. Although having produced specificities of 96% (Bernard formula) and 95% (Suhr and Boyer formula), and a negative predictive accuracy of 86%, the formulae demonstrated 0% sensitivity and 0% positive predictive accuracies, which were "disappointing and concerning." The authors suggest that the latter findings may be related to the fact that Bernard developed the formulae using undergraduate simulators rather than real-life malingerers, though this argument would not explain the poor performance of the Suhr formula, as it was developed on the basis of actual patients. The low base rate in the Miller et al. (2000) study relative to the Suhr and Boyer (1999) study may also have influenced the results, as would variability of effort within the test battery. Miller et al. interpreted their findings as not supporting the application of existing malingering formulas for the WCST in clinical practice and cautioned against their use.

Greve and Bianchini (2002) examined the specificities of the Bernard and Suhr WCST malingering formulas in a number of normal (two college student) and clinical (substance abuse, severe TBI, cerebrovascular accident [CVA], and two mixed neurological) samples. The Bernard formula showed the following false-positive error rates: 2.3% (college student sample 1), 15.8% (college student sample 2), 20.5% (substance abuse), 41.7% (severe TBI), 12% (CVA), 7.8% (mixed neurological sample 1), and 13.3% (mixed neurological sample 2). The Suhr formula showed false-positive error rates of: 0% (normal college sample 1), 1.3% (normal college sample 2), 18.2% (substance abusers), 26.1% (severe TBI), 26.5% (CVA), 14.1% (mixed neurological sample 1), and 20.3% (mixed neurological sample 2). The Bernard and Suhr formulae were also applied by diagnostic category in two separate clinical samples to examine false-positive errors, with widely varying rates and sample sizes (Bernard: 0 – 42.9%; Suhr: 0 – 42.8%). The authors interpret these findings to represent an "unacceptably high" rate of false-positive errors (especially in severe TBI for the Bernard equation, and severe TBI, CVA, and mixed sample using the Suhr formula). Greve and Bianchini (2002) conclude that the Bernard equations may be useful in samples similar to those in which they were derived, but the Suhr equations "appear too inaccurate to produce a reliable index of malingering" (p. 51). They also suggest that the reason the equations did not perform better may be related to false assumptions about how honest clinical and dishonest malingering groups perform on the WCST (i.e., there are multiple approaches that a malingerer might choose). They state that "researchers must first empirically identify the various approaches to malingering on a given test and then apply DFA [discriminant function analysis] to derive equations which are sensitive to those specific strategies" (p. 53).

Greve, Bianchini, Mathias, Houston, and Crouch (2002) examined classification accuracies of four possible WCST malingering indicators (including the Bernard and Suhr formulas and two types of unique responses) in 89 patients with mild or moderate to severe TBI who were nonmalingering or malingering according to the Slick et al. (1999) criteria. The authors report sensitivities, specificities, and predictive accuracies according to various combinations of the Bernard, Suhr, and unique responses, stratified into controls, incentive only, probable malingering, and suspect malingering. *Unique responses* and the Bernard and Suhr formulae identified at least one-third of the probable malingerers with a false-positive rate of about 10%. The perfect match-missed marker (i.e., failure to match identical deck and stimulus cards) had perfect specificity but limited sensitivity (about 10%). The Suhr formula/unique responses were found sensitive to two different approaches to malingering on the WCST; in combination, they correctly identified two-thirds of the probable malingerers with a decline in specificity to as low as 40%. The Bernard formula shared "a substantial amount of variance with the Suhr formula and did not detect any malingerers that were not already detected using one of the other methods" (p. 189). Greve et al. (2002) suggest that their findings revealed three approaches to malingering used by the probable malingerers. First (as tapped by the Suhr formula and its dependence on *FMS*) is the strategy to "avoid too many consecutive correct responses." This was the most common strategy employed with half of the probable malingerers having shown this pattern. Second is the strategy to avoid matching to any of the three dimensions. Unique responses were uncommon, but > 1 *unique response* may be pathognomonic and highly specific. "It is rare indeed for a person to generate a unique response by missing a perfect match" (p. 189), and three of the probable malingerers did this. Third is a strategy that involves responding validly on the WCST, which was evident in a third of the probable malingering group. Individuals in this group may not have perceived the WCST to be measuring the cognitive domain they were attempting to feign or perhaps viewed it as not associated with TBI sequelae.

King, Sweet, Sherer, Curtiss, and Vanderploeg (2002) conducted three studies to further examine the utility of WCST indices in the detection of feigned cognitive impairment. Study 1 consisted of 33 patients with moderate to severe chronic TBI and 27 litigants with evidence of IE. IE litigants performed significantly worse across nearly all traditional WCST indices relative to the TBI group. Logistic regression resulted in an overall accuracy of 77% in discriminating the two groups. The Bernard and Suhr formulae yielded acceptable specificity (94% for Bernard, 88% for Suhr) but lower sensitivity (63% for Bernard, 59% for Suhr). The authors also introduced five new WCST variables as possible discriminators of IE, but results of multivariate analysis of variance and logistic regression did not support their usefulness. Study 2 examined WCST effort variables across the IE group and an acute moderate–severe TBI group. The only significant differences between the IE and acute TBI groups was observed for *categories completed, trials to first category,* and *FMS* (with the IE group performing worse on all three). The acute TBI group performed significantly worse relative to the chronic TBI group on all variables, except for *nonperseverative errors, FMS,* and the *other responses.* The Bernard et al. formula yielded a specificity of 73% in the acute TBI group. At a 90% probability of IE, 97% of the acute TBI group was accurately classified. The Suhr formula at the same 90% cutoff resulted in 75% of the acute TBI group being accurately classified. Study 3 included 130 Veterans Administration (VA) patients with mild to severe TBI who were less acute than the patients with TBI in Study 2. The IE group performed significantly worse than the VA sample on *all* 10 basic WCST variables. The VA group performed significantly better than the acute TBI group, except for *FMS.* No significant differences were observed between the VA and chronic TBI patients. The Bernard formula correctly classified 95% of the VA group. With a 90% cutoff, logistic regression resulted in 99% specificity for the VA group. The Suhr equation yielded 85% specificity. The authors conclude that the results of their three studies support the position that valid effort, but not necessarily insufficient effort, can be identified via WCST performances. King et al. suggest that the WCST can be useful in assessing test validity, in contrast to the positions of Miller et al. (2000) and Greve and Bianchini (2002). They conclude that their findings demonstrated "robust specificity with the logistic regression formula evaluated across our present samples; however, readers should note that we have not demonstrated robust sensitivity across forensic samples" (King et al., 2002, p. 520).

Ashendorf, O'Bryant, and McCaffrey (2003) examined the specificity of previously suggested WCST and California Verbal Learning Test (CVLT) malingering detection strategies in a sample of normal elders. For the

WCST, the authors employed formulas by Bernard et al. (1996) and Suhr and Boyer (1999). A conservative 90% likelihood of malingering cutoff was applied to the Suhr formulas, as was done in a study by Greve et al. (2002). Results suggested that two of the Bernard strategies were significantly related to age; none were related to gender. Specificities of the Bernard formulas ranged from 55.1%, 75.7%, and 91.4%, whereas the Suhr WCST formulas yielded specificities of 62.7% and 47.6%. Similarly, specificity rates for unique response cutoffs ranged from 47.6% (> 0), 72.4% (> 1), and 91.4% (> 5), whereas cutoffs for the WCST *perfect matches missed* resulted in 86.5% specificity (> 0) and 95.1% (> 1) specificity. Ashendorf et al. (2003) suggest that, the decline in WCST performance that accompanies increasing age significantly affects the Bernard and Suhr equations. With more impaired elderly individuals, Ashendorf et al. believe that the equations result in increasing false positive rates.

To summarize, research surrounding WCST cognitive effort indices has been mixed. Variables such as age and TBI severity may obscure the ability to identify invalid WCST performances. The most effective use of WCST in detecting insufficient cognitive effort entails the use of multivariate formulae rather than the use of any single WCST index. The clinician should be aware that most of the extant literature pertaining to WCST and detection of IE includes head-injured samples; conclusions regarding effort in samples demonstrating impaired WCST performances as a result of alternative conditions should be made with caution.

Category Test and Booklet Category Test

An extensive overview of the historical development within the Category Test and Booklet Category Test of validity indicators has been published by Sweet and King (2002). In this next section, we revisit some of this historical literature and extend the review of studies to the present.

Simmel and Counts (1957) appear to have been the first to note that subtests I and II of the Category Test are very easy from the objective standpoint of very few errors being made on this test by normal individuals or brain-damaged patients. This fact has been noted uniformly by subsequent researchers (e.g., Laatsch & Choca, 1991) and eventually influenced attempts to identify indicators of invalid responding and malingering on the Category Test and Booklet Category Test.

In one of the first American group studies of simulated cognitive impairment on neuropsychological measures, Heaton, Smith, Lehman, and Vogt (1978) observed performances of simulated malingerers and non-litigating head-trauma patients on a variety of common neuropsychological measures, including the Category Test. Interestingly, in light of the general tendency of malingerers to perform worse than genuine, well-motivated, neurological patients, the study by Heaton et al. found head-injured patients to have a significantly greater number of total errors on the Category Test than malingerers. A similar finding of better performance on the Category Test in terms of fewer errors was reported by Goebel (1983). *Such findings have not been reported in any subsequent study of the Category Test, either with malingerers or with simulators.* That is, in every subsequent study of the Category Test or Booklet Category Test, as is the case with nearly all investigations of performance on traditional tests by simulators or probable malingerers in real-world samples, worse performances have been reported in the samples of individuals whose effort is compromised.

The next published use of the Category Test pertaining to malingering was a seminal but unpublished study by Bolter, Picano, and Zych (1985), who were the first to employ a within-test validity indicator. This research identified a series of items within the Category Test that were rarely answered incorrectly by neurological patients and therefore were deemed relevant to determination of performance validity. In numerous subsequent studies, these items were referred to as either the "Bolter Index" or the "Bolter items."

Undoubtedly limited by small sample size (only eight malingerers and eight questionably invalid subjects), Trueblood and Schmidt (1993) did not find support for the "rare errors" suggested by Bolter et al. for the Category Test. Mean errors on subtest VII, however, were statistically higher in the malingering, but not in the "invalid" group, relative to controls, and 100% of patients with good effort were correctly classified. However, small sample sizes likely do not allow reasonable generalizations of findings from this study.

Tenhula and Sweet (1996) conducted two studies to evaluate five potential Booklet Category Test indicators in addition to the traditional error score representing total number of errors on the task. The five validity indicators were subtest I and II errors, subtest VII errors, Bolter items, newly identified "easy" items, and newly identified "difficult" items. In Study 1, the authors observed Booklet Category Test (BCT) performances in a group of 34 normals, 28 simulators, and 26 patients with mild to severe head injury. Study 2 consisted of a cross-validation of Study 1 and evaluated BCT performances in another group of 24 normal controls, 17 simulators, and 24 patients with mild to severe head injury. Procedures were identical in both studies. Discriminant function analyses (DFA) from the Study 1 sample resulted in hit rates from 68.2% (for "difficult" items) to 92.0% (using subtest VII), with 100% specificity in the DFA that used items from subtests I and II. Classifications were very similar in the Study 2 individuals, ranging from 64.6% (for the "difficult items") to 89.2% (for "easy" items). A double cross-validation (i.e., applying DFAs from Study 1 to individuals in Study 2 and vice versa) was conducted, which resulted in hit rates ranging from 80% (using the "difficult" items) to 96.9% (using subtest VII). In light of the similar findings across Studies 1 and 2, additional discriminant functions were conducted combining subjects from both studies. Hit rates ranged from

72.5% ("difficult" items) to 92.2% (combined errors on subtests I and II), with 100% specificity and 73.3% sensitivity for the latter. Based on these findings, optimal cutoff scores were developed for each of the indices, with the greatest overall hit rate being that of combined errors on subtests I and II (91.5%) with 98.1% specificity and 75.6% sensitivity.

Ellwanger, Tenhula, Rosenfeld, and Sweet (1999) conducted a simulation experiment that examined the utility of event-related potentials (ERPs) and the BCT in the detection of feigned cognitive impairment. ERP performances on the P3 Multi-Digit Memory Test (P3MDMT; an adaptation of a forced-choice digit recognition procedure to ERP instrumentation) were compared with BCT performance in a sample of 10 undergraduates simulating brain injury and 11 student controls. Overall BCT hit rates varied from 66.7% (Total number of errors) to 95.2% (combined errors on subtest I and II). Subsequent DFA yielded an overall correct classification rate of 76.2% using the Bolter items and 85.7% using traditional subtest scores. The P3MDMT intraindividual analysis resulted in an overall correct classification rate of 90.5% and 80% sensitivity. Based on a positive outcome for either the P3MDMT or use of subtests I and II on the BCT, all simulators were correctly classified. These results provided further support for the merits of the BCT in the detection of feigned cognitive impairment, especially when employed in concert with other forms of detection strategies (in this case ERP analysis).

DiCarlo, Gfeller, and Oliveri (2000) conducted a replication and extension study of the methods used by Tenhula and Sweet (1996). Specifically, DiCarlo et al. employed BCT cutoffs for combined subtest I and II errors, subtest VII errors, total errors, "easy" item errors, and number of criteria exceeded in a sample of 30 patients with TBI of undisclosed severity, 32 coached simulators, 30 uncoached simulators, and 30 controls. A unique aspect of the DiCarlo study was the inclusion of the coached or presumably more sophisticated simulation group, as previous research has suggested that informed simulators may possess the capacity to perform akin to genuinely impaired individuals. The authors hypothesized that coached simulators would commit significantly fewer errors than uncoached simulators on the Tenhula and Sweet indicators. Postexperimental questioning suggested that the coached simulators reported that they "missed only difficult items" more often and answered "at least half of the items correctly" more often than uncoached simulators. Nearly 97% of the coached simulators reported that they utilized suggested strategies. As predicted, both simulation groups produced more errors across indices relative to both the controls and TBI patients. Coached simulators were misclassified significantly more often than the uncoached simulators for all indices except for the subtest VII errors. This suggested that coached simulators were able to effectively employ test-taking strategies on four of the five malingering indicators. Although overall hit rates were quite impressive across each of the five indicators, a decision rule of > 1 error on subtests I and II was the most sensitive indicator of malingering, regardless of coaching strategy or presence of TBI (76% of all simulators correctly identified, 100% of controls and TBI patients correctly identified). The total number of BCT errors yielded the lowest overall classification rates. Based on these findings, the authors concluded that the Tenhula and Sweet (1996) cutoffs (especially using a decision rule of > 1 error on subtests I and II) were adequate indicators of symptom validity.

Williamson et al. (2003) compared results of the Word Memory Test (WMT; Green, Allen, & Astner, 1996) and results of a subset of the validity indicators of the BCT from Tenhula and Sweet (1996) in 244 patients with either mild head injury or moderate–severe TBI. When participants were assigned to good- and poor-effort groups according to the BCT total number of validity indicators, the poor-effort group was significantly older and less educated than the valid-effort group. The WMT and the BCT total combined errors on subtests I and II disagreed 27% of the time in the total sample and 20% of the time in the subset of patients with moderate–severe TBI. Further, substantial differences were observed between cognitive effort groups (as identified by either WMT or BCT indicators) on numerous tests of ability and personality functioning associated with valid or poor cognitive effort. One of the most important findings of this study is the lack of agreement demonstrated between poor performance on cognitive effort measures and two of the BCT validity indicators from Tenhula and Sweet (1996). In sum, the authors suggest that the Tenhula and Sweet (1996) criteria be employed cautiously, especially with moderate–severe TBI patients.

We have seen thus far two separate attempts to characterize "easy" or rarely missed items, those being Bolter et al. (1985) and Tenhula and Sweet (1996). A third attempt was made by Barrett and Putnam (1998), who identified 46 items rarely missed in a sample of patients with moderate to severe TBI, most of whom were litigating. Despite the very different initial sample used to identify the rarely missed items, the specific items chosen overlapped substantially with the prior studies. For example, the analysis by Barrett and Putnam identified all the items from subtest I and all but one item from subtest II. If one excludes all the items from the first two subtests from consideration, then the remaining Barrett and Putnam rarely missed items show overlap with 12 chosen by Bolter and 12 chosen by Tenhula and Sweet. Unfortunately, the effectiveness of the three item pools was not compared in this unpublished study.

Reitan and Wolfson (1997) demonstrated that litigants and nonlitigants differed significantly on the total error score of the Category Test. Noting that second administration of the Category Test in nonlitigants was associated with an improvement in the total error score, Reitan and Wolfson compared retest performance between litigants and nonlitigants. Nonlitigants *improved* on average, whereas litigants *worsened* on average. These results suggest that performance across time on the Category Test may be useful in identifying unexpected or unrealistic findings that may be invalid.

Forrest, Allen, and Goldstein (2004) conducted two studies to explore the effectiveness of previously suggested Category Test validity indicators in detection of feigned cognitive impairment. In Study 1, their sample consisted of 195 schizophrenic (SZ) patients, 177 patients with various forms of brain damage (BD; such as substance-related dementia, head trauma, vascular disorders, or demyelinating disorders), and 229 controls (with neither SZ nor BD). Category Test indices included errors on subtests I and II, errors on subtest VII, total errors, error rate proportions on subtests I–VI versus subtest VII, and error rate proportions on subtest V versus subtest VI. Results showed the expected patterns of performance, with the BD group making the most errors, followed by the SZ and control groups. Very few errors were observed on subtests I and II in any of the groups (mean I and II combined performances were 1.22 for the BD group, 1.02 for the SZ group, and .84 for the control group). All mean group performances were better on subtest VII than on subtests I through VI, and on subtest VI than on V. Differences from subtests I–VI minus VII were not significant between groups. The BD group showed less V to VI improvement relative to the other groups. As 27% of the sample did proportionately worse on subtest VII than on the average of the other subtests, the authors suggest that VII may not be as effective in detecting malingering as other indices. Ten percent of the sample did not do better on subtest VI than on subtest V. Consistent with the findings of others (Tenhula & Sweet, 1996; DiCarlo et al. 2000), on the basis of their first study, Forrest et al. (2004) suggest that subtests I and II may be the best indicator of malingering on the BCT.

The second study by Forrest et al. (2004) compared BCT performances across three groups: 25 undergraduate controls, 75 undergraduate simulators, and the 177 BD patients from Study 1 (the SZ and control groups for Study 1 were thought to be less relevant to the simulation of "structural brain damage"). Malingering simulators performed significantly worse on most Category indices than the two other groups, with errors on subtests I and II being the best discriminator between simulating and good effort groups. Stepwise DFA (with subtest I errors, total errors, and subtest II errors entered) resulted in an 83% classification accuracy (64% for the controls, 73% of malingerers, and 91% of BD patients). Further DFA between malingerers and BD participants resulted in 89% classification accuracy, with 76% of the simulator group and 95% of the BD group classified correctly. As with the first discriminant function, subtest I errors, total errors, and subtest II errors were entered to the exclusion of the other indices. Overall, the authors suggest that their results across both studies support the use of previously suggested BCT indices in detection of feigned cognitive impairment, especially use of subtests I and II. Unlike Sweet and King (2002), who had suggested caution in using such indices outside a TBI context, Forrest et al. suggest their findings provide support for use Category Test validity indicators in "heterogeneous neurological populations."

In summary, a variety of studies spanning several decades have documented BCT-embedded validity indicators, some of which appear to be more useful than others. Use of BCT "easy" items (subtests I, II, Bolter items, etc.), or those that are rarely missed by normal and brain-injured individuals, appears to be useful in detecting invalid performance, whereas the use of "difficult" items has not been supported. As with the WCST, it is prudent to consider multiple BCT validity indicators within the context of pure effort tests, demographics, other test results, and injury severity, before concluding that overall BCT performance is likely invalid.

Verbal and Visual Fluency

In an analogue study of 21 malingering simulators and 21 controls, Demakis (1999) observed between-group performances on a number of standard neuropsychological measures, including two common executive fluency measures (Controlled Oral Word Association, COWA; Ruff Figural Fluency Test, RFFT). Measures were administered twice, with a 3-week delay between administrations. Demakis found that while simulators' COWA and RFFT performances were significantly worse than those of controls, the malingerers showed almost the same rate of improvement on repeat testing as controls. For instance, whereas mean number of designs generated on the RFFT in the control group was 100.9 at time 1 and 117.7 on time 2 (16.5% improvement), the simulator group's mean number of generated designs was 63.2 on time 1 and 71.5 on time 2 (13.1% improvement). For COWA, the mean number of words generated in the control group was 37.8 at time 1 and 43.4 on time 2 (14.8% improvement), and the simulator group's mean number of words generated was 29.5 on time 1 and 30.2 on time 2 (only a 2.4% percent improvement). Demakis (1999) suggests that simulators "may assume that neurologically damaged patients do not improve with repeat testing and thus may attempt to perform as poorly on the second testing as they did on initial testing" (p. 408), which was evident on verbal testing but not on nonverbal testing. Interestingly, brain-injured patients have been shown to have a different, usually reduced, practice effect compared to normals (e.g., Wilson, Watson, Baddeley, Emslie, & Evans, 2000), suggesting the possibility that the simulators' adoption of this strategy could be difficult to distinguish from genuine injury. The Demakis (1999) study did not include a TBI comparison group and could not address this possibility.

van Gorp et al. (1999) examined a wide variety of standard neuropsychological ability measures, including a verbal fluency task, in a group of preidentified malingerers and nonmalingerers. No statistical differences were observed between groups, and the verbal fluency task did not contribute a significant proportion of variance in a discriminant function analysis.

Vickery et al. (2004) observed COWA and other test performances in head-injured and community volunteers. Groups were divided in four partitions, resulting in simulators who had experienced head injury versus honest controls and volunteer simulators who had not experienced head injury versus honest conditions. Simulators who had previously experienced head injury performed significantly worse than motivated head injury controls and significantly worse than non-head-injured simulators. Effort measures, such as the Letter Memory Test, were able to identify the simulators, but no data were provided regarding classification accuracy using the COWA results alone.

Backhaus, Fichtenberg, and Hanks (2004) examined a variety of neuropsychological test performances, including COWA, in three groups: clinical participants with mild TBI, clinical participants with moderate–severe TBI, and litigants who demonstrated IE on cognitive effort tests (i.e., WRMT [Warrington, 1984]; TOMM [Tombaugh, 1996]). Raw score ability performances were obtained at varying percentiles in the moderate–severe TBI group, and then mild TBI and IE performances were observed at these same percentiles. The IE group generated significantly ($p < .01$) fewer words than the mild TBI group (IE $M = 31.80$, $SD = 10.21$; mild TBI $M = 39.68$, $SD = 9.22$). Although the authors provide classification accuracy data based on percentiles derived from their own participants with moderate–severe TBI, the data provided are inadequate for guiding clinical practice. For example, by traditional clinical standards, the IE group mean performance was within a range most clinicians would consider to represent "normal limits." Differently, we are concerned that a cutoff based on the midpoint of moderate to severe TBI is a rarely used approach in the relevant IE and malingering literature (cf. Frederick, 2000, uses the midpoint of the range of documented *memory* impairment, such as recall ability to set an expectation regarding the easier task of recognition, and argues for the use of a *personal* floor effect) and precludes application to any litigant claiming other than a mild injury. Though many researchers have used moderate to severe TBI comparison groups to establish reasonable expectations for litigant performance, these studies nearly invariably select a cutoff that represents infrequently seen abnormal performance, perhaps representing 90–100% specificity, as a means of identifying IE (e.g., Millis, 1992, pp. 412–413).

In summary, in the few studies available, there are no data presently available on fluency tasks that would suggest that statistically significant mean score differences in simulators or malingerers and either controls or motivated patients are associated with classification of individual cases.

Stroop Color–Word Test

Lu, Boone, Jimenez, and Razani (2004) administered the Stroop Test (Comalli, Wapner, & Werner, 1962) to six patients with claims of complete loss of reading ability as a result of either limitations in education or a TBI.

The Stroop is a common executive measure that involves the ability to inhibit one's overlearned reading response. All six participants met the Slick et al. (1999) criteria for probable malingering of neurocognitive dysfunction based on numerous failures on cognitive effort measures. Although claiming to be unable to read, the participants nevertheless showed marked difficulty on the color-interference trial and frequently made reading errors (i.e., reading the name of presented words rather than the ink colors). This suggested that they were indeed inhibiting a reading response, contrary to their claims of being unable to read. The authors note that the ability to inhibit the reading response is an extremely difficult task relative to naming colors alone. Therefore, when an individual claims to have lost all reading ability but nevertheless shows a significant difficulty in inhibiting the reading response, it is clear that the individual has not lost the ability to read at all. For this reason, Lu et al. (2004) suggest that the Stroop Test may be "the most powerful and pathognomonic indicator" of feigned impairment in individuals claiming to have lost the ability to read. The authors note that their findings contrasted with those of Osimani, Alon, Berger, and Abarbanel (1997), who found an inverse Stroop effect in their simulator sample. However, their findings concurred with those of van Gorp et al. (1999), who observed the presence of a Stroop effect in a sample of probable malingerers and nonmalingerers. Lu et al. suggest that the former study's finding of an inverse Stroop effect may have been related to the fact that they did not include real-life malingerers.

van Gorp et al. (1999) examined Stroop color naming and interference performances in a group of independently identified malingerers (based in part on symptom validity testing) and nonmalingerers. Both of these indices were significantly worse in the malingering group, and both contributed a significant amount of variance in a subsequent discriminant function between groups. The authors suggest that malingerers may have difficulty accurately presenting themselves as impaired on timed tasks, such as the Stroop Test, in relation to difficulty gauging what substantiates impaired timed performance and the inability to time themselves. The very large Stroop Interference standard deviation in the malingering group (98.24) relative to the nonmalingering group (31.59) supports the notion that malingerers have difficulty gauging what constitutes an impaired performance. van Gorp et al. suggest that level of performance on the Stroop may help identify malingering.

Vickery et al. (2004) administered a variety of both cognitive effort measures and standard ability measures to groups of moderately to severely head-injured patients and demographically matched controls. None of the participants were seeking any form of compensation. Per the suggestions of others (e.g., Rogers, 1997), the authors employed a "four-group design" that consisted of patient status (patient vs. control) and instructional set (feigned symptoms vs. standard). Such a design maintains the internal validity inherent in simulation designs and at the same time increases external validity (generalizability) by using both normal and clinical groups. Among the standard ability measures administered was the Stroop Neuropsychological Screening Test (Trenerry, Crosson, DeBoe, & Leber, 1989). The head-injured simulating group performed worse than each of the other three groups on the Stroop. Across multiple ability measures, the authors found comparable main effects for both instruction set and patient status but did not find a significant interaction effect. The absence of an interaction effect suggests that, "whatever factors may contribute to ability to feign successfully, simply experiencing a genuine head injury does not appear to be one of them" (Vickery et al., 2004, p. 46). Nevertheless, there was a main effect for instruction set on the Stroop.

The Stroop Neuropsychological Screening Test (Trenerry et al., 1989) was among the 11 ability measures included in the aforementioned Backhaus et al. (2004) study. As with COWA, the IE group performed significantly worse ($p < .01$) in identifying colors on the interference page of the Stroop than the mild TBI group (IE $M = 61.25$, $SD = 28.30$; mild TBI $M = 104.39$, $SD = 11.71$).

As with the previous section on fluency tasks, there is currently no research evidence that the Stroop can be used to make individual classifications pertaining to malingering, despite some evidence that decreased motivation and effort reduces Stroop performance. The possible exception would be in a small subset of malingerers alleging total inability to read; in these subjects, the Stroop interference task may identify those who inadvertently engage in what they claim to be unable to do.

Trailmaking Test

Heaton et al. (1978) examined Trailmaking Test (TMT) performances in simulated malingerers and head-injured (severity unspecified) patients. No significant differences were observed between groups on TMT A time to completion or number of errors committed. The head-injured group took somewhat longer than the simulation group on TMT B time to completion, but this difference was not statistically significant. The head-injured group did demonstrate significantly more errors on TMT B (mean of 2.00) relative to the simulators (mean of .81).

Trueblood and Schmidt (1993) examined a wide variety of neuropsychological symptom validity indicators derived from standard ability tests in eight malingering and eight litigants showing questionable validity, including TMT B. The malingering group performed statistically less than chance on a modified version of the Hiscock and Hiscock (1989) forced-choice symptom validity test (SVT) procedure, and the invalid group showed intact SVT performance, with questionable performances on a range of standard ability tests (e.g., zero grip strength). Cognitive ability performances for the malingering and the invalid groups were compared with separate control groups that were matched by age, education, and gender. Mean completion time on TMT B was substantially longer in the malingering group (131.0s) relative to matched controls (77.4s), and statistically longer in the invalid group (158.9s) relative to matched controls (54.9s). The malingering group averaged .6 errors on TMT B compared to .5 errors in the matched control group, whereas the invalid group averaged 1.4 errors compared to 0 mean errors in the matched control group. Although the authors did not explicitly address the TMT findings in their discussion, their study provided initial support for the notion that the TMT may be relevant to the task of identifying insufficient cognitive effort.

van Gorp et al. (1999) administered an extended battery of standard neuropsychological measures to malingerers (based on a variety of *a priori* criteria, including substandard performances on cognitive effort tests) and nonmalingerers. Although malingerers demonstrated longer times to completion for both TMT A and B, only the TMT B minus A discrepancy score was statistically different between groups, with malingerers showing longer discrepancies. The significantly different mean discrepancy scores between groups could suggest that malingerers are unable to "calibrate" performances between TMT A and B in an appropriately believable manner. Further, the authors suggest that for timed tasks, such as the TMT and Stroop Test, malingerers may have difficulty successfully feigning impairment because they are (1) unaware of how slowly a genuinely impaired individual might perform, and (2) unable to track their own times while completing the tasks.

Ruffolo, Guilmette, and Willis (2000) examined TMT time to completion and error rates in five groups: controls, experimental simulators, and outpatients with mild head injury, moderate–severe head injury, or suspect-effort head injury. An omnibus effect was found across groups for both performance errors and time to completion, with the simulating group making more errors and taking longer to complete the TMT A than each of the other groups. For TMT B, the simulating group made significantly more errors than each of the other groups. However, the suspect effort head-injury group took longer to complete TMT B than the other groups, followed by the simulator group. The authors also found that the TMT B/A ratio was lower in the simulator group than in the mild and moderate–severe head-injured groups, but the ratio in the suspect effort head-injury group was comparable with the ratios of the head-injury groups. Overall, the authors suggest that four or more errors on either TMT A or B may suggest suspect effort, and observation of both error rates and completion times on the TMT "may be useful for neuropsychologists during assessments when malingering is possible or suspected" (Ruffolo et al., 2000, p. 229). Limitations of this study include having had only seven subjects in the suspect-effort head-injury group. Also, the authors did not report classification accuracies despite significant between-group differences for TMT A and B completion times, instead stating that "there was significant variability with completion times for both the TMT-A and TMT-B among the head-injured groups that precluded establishing a definite cut-off" (p. 228).

Haines and Norris (2001) included TMT A and B as part of an extended battery administered to five volunteer groups: normal control student (NCST), normal control VA (NCVA), mild traumatic brain-injured VA (MTBI), simulated malingerer student (SMST), and simulated malingerer VA (SMVA). An omnibus group difference was observed across groups, and post hoc analysis revealed that the SMVA group performed significantly worse than all the other groups on both Trails A and B, including the SMST group, suggesting that simulating groups are not necessarily comparable. The authors suggest that their findings may support the use of standard measures, such as the TMT, in detecting malingering.

Iverson, Lang, Green, and Franzen (2002) examined TMT error scores, ratio scores, and completion times in a large sample of patients with acute TBI (head injuries varying from uncomplicated mild, mild with skull fracture, complicated mild, to moderate–severe). These groups differed most significantly on TMT A and B completion times, though the B/A ratio was also statistically significant. The authors then reported cutoff scores for rarely observed performances (< 5%) in the overall TBI group on the TMT (> 63 seconds for TMT A; > 200 seconds for TMT B; < 1.49 for B/A ratio), and evaluated their utility as effort indicators in a large group of compensation-seeking head-injured individuals (classified as very mild injury, well-defined injury, and suspected malingering). The malingering group had demonstrated suboptimal performances on either the Computerized Assessment of Response Bias or WMT. TMT A and B completion times were significantly different across groups (with the malingering group performing significantly worse) for TMT A and B completion times, but in contrast to Ruffolo et al. (2000), no differences were observed for the TMT ratio. Positive predictive validities for both TMT A and B completion times were 100% in the very mild head-injury group (inclusive of genuine vs. suspect individuals) but were less impressive for the well-defined head-injury group. This finding suggested that TMT A and B completion time scores may be a good indicator of poor effort, but only when an individual has sustained a very mild head injury. Further, although specificity was very impressive across groups (ranging from 87% to 100%) for all three TMT indices, sensitivities were very poor across groups (ranging from 2.4% to 18.5%). Overall, in their words, "the results of this study do not support the use of the TMT as a reliable predictor of exaggerated deficits or poor effort during neuropsychological testing" (Iverson et al., 2002, p. 405).

O'Bryant, Hiscock, Fisher, and McCaffrey (2003) observed TMT performances of 27 MTBI litigants and 67 nonmalingering MTBI litigants. Because the TMT may be sensitive to brain injury *and* suboptimal effort, the authors hypothesized that it would demonstrate poor utility as an indicator of suspect effort. Litigants were classified as malingering based on suboptimal performances on the TOMM and/or the Rey 15-Item Memory Test. Malingerers demonstrated significantly slower performance times on both portion A and B relative to the nonmalingering group but did not show significantly greater numbers of errors on either test. Further, the B/A ratio was not statistically significant between groups. A DFA was also conducted on the TMT ratio score and the TMT A and B time combined. Results were significant for the ratio score but classified only 44.8% of the nonmalingerers and 63.0% of the malingerers correctly. DFA for the A and B times combined was also significant, with 85% of the nonmalingerers but only 63% of the malingerers classified correctly. Although the finding that malingerers performed more poorly on TMT A and B is consistent with the notion that malingerers perform more poorly on standard measures overall (e.g., van Gorp et al., 1999), additional levels of analysis led O'Bryant et al. (2003) to conclude that "none of the TMT variables adequately differentiated between TBI litigants suspected of malingering and those not suspected of malingering" (p. 73).

Backhaus et al. (2004) found their IE group to perform significantly worse ($p < .01$) on TMT B relative to the mild TBI group (IE $M = 144.28$, $SD = 94.51$; mild TBI $M = 72.12$, $SD = 35.41$). As with the COWA and Stroop results of Backhaus mentioned previously, we have serious concern about the cutoffs considered to be suggestive of suboptimal performance and possible malingering.

In summary, it seems clear that compromised effort results in slower performances on the TMT. However, TMT scores alone are not able to correctly classify a sufficient number of individual cases of possible malingerers to support its use as a reliable indicator of malingering.

PRACTICE RECOMMENDATIONS: USES AND LIMITS

In the foregoing review of relevant literature pertaining to the use of executive function measures to identify IE and the subset of individuals showing IE who are in fact malingering, there is a wide range of effectiveness. Given that the tests reviewed measure actual ability within a domain that is universally recognized to be difficult to assess, it does not seem at all surprising to find that the alternative use of these tests as possible indicators of malingering would also meet with limited success, and in some instances no success. At this stage of the development of the scientific literature pertaining to executive measures, we believe the following practice recommendations are prudent:

1. Do *not* rely on COWA, RFFT, and TMT as independent indicators of IE. Instead, when other better-validated indicators of effort and response validity have been failed, examine the results of these executive measures to determine whether the degree of impaired performance, if present, is realistic in light of the individual's relevant demographics (e.g., age and education) and given the alleged cause of the individual's condition. In this sense, limit consideration of these particular executive measures to identifying discrepancies from expected performance levels that would more likely represent IE than genuine injury. Note that even in this limited application, these specific measures do *not* offer useful information regarding possible conscious attempts to perform poorly in order to obtain an external reward. That is, they do not allow any statement with regard to ruling malingering in or out, even when insufficient effort is present. These comments also apply to the Stroop Test with the exception that it may have a unique role in documenting feigned inability to read.

2. With regard to the WCST, results of numerous independent investigations using various WCST-derived scores have produced mixed results related to effort and malingering. It is possible that age (Donders, 1999; Ashendorf et al., 2003) can affect diagnostic accuracy. In addition, although not affected by Glasgow Coma Scale or loss of consciousness, a modest significant effect of posttraumatic amnesia on WCST variables suggests that injury severity and acuity may affect the ability of the WCST to identify invalid responses (King et al., 2002). Nearly all the applications of the WCST to identifying invalid responses have been multivariate rather than application of simple cutoffs, which can be viewed as a strength in terms of being more difficult for examinees and claimants to undermine. The formulae that have been the most frequently researched are in fact somewhat similar in often identifying the same WCST variables of interest (*categories completed, FMS*), though on different samples and often with different weightings, which has resulted in a range of effectiveness (cf. King et al., 2002). It appears that WCST approaches to identifying response validity may be better at identifying a valid response set than one that is a result of IE.

At this point, we recommend that clinicians not rely exclusively on only one formulaic approach with regard to using the WCST to identify invalid responding. Instead, we compute the following formulae: Bernard et al. (1996), Suhr and Boyer (1999), and King et al. (2002). The results of these three approaches are considered collectively alongside numerous other validity indicators within traditional tests of ability, and, of course, in the context of stand-alone effort tests. This approach is in keeping with numerous cautionary statements to consider only the WCST among multiple measures of response validity and effort and to make decisions regarding effort and possible malingering within the context of the overall pattern of results (Bianchini et al., 2003; Larrabee, 2003), as well as to consider "the broader context of injury-related factors (e.g., initial severity indicators) and credibility/reasonableness of claimed injuries" (King et al., 2002, p. 520).

Finally, clinicians should note that the vast majority of WCST studies related to effort and malingering have been with head-injured participants. Though perhaps the results will generalize to other neurological samples, this should not be assumed. In almost any type of patient sample, significant worsening of scores on repeat evaluation is unexpected and much more likely to be caused by compromised effort, or in some instances a significant change in emotional functioning, than a previously acquired stable neurological condition.

3. As with the WCST, the Category Test and BCT research has been produced by different investigators across decades, but with some interesting uniformity. With the exception of the Williamson, Green, Allen, and Kohling (2003) study, investigators dating back to the 1950s (Simmel & Counts, 1957) have reported that some of the 208 items of the Category Test are so easy that normal individuals and brain-damaged individuals invariably do not make errors on these items. Different methodologies have produced varying subsets of items that are objectively "easy" or "rarely missed." Subtests I and II have consistently been reported to be so easy that genuine brain dysfunction produces very few errors across patients. As with the WCST, the application of various methods of identifying invalid response sets with the Category Test and BCT can be affected by variables such as age and education, and possibly very severe injury (Sweet & King, 2002). We recommend that multiple validity indicators of the Category Test and BCT be examined but exclude "difficult items" from consideration. We do not rely on the test's validity indicators when education is below the high school level or when the examinee is elderly or has suffered a very severe injury. In fact, we generally do not administer a BCT to such individuals. Also, when any individual fails only a single indicator, we typically do not conclude that the response set for the test is necessarily invalid. Consistent with our recommendations for the WCST, the Category Test and BCT validity indicators should be used in a broader context of the validity indicators of other tests, stand-alone effort tests, demographics, the overall picture of injury history, and postinjury course, as well as the consistency and reasonableness of symptom presentation as it pertains to the injury in question.

SUMMARY

Identifying the presence of insufficient effort and its effects on neuropsychological tests can at times be a very difficult undertaking. As alluded to earlier, if all that was needed was a single stand-alone effort test at the beginning of the test battery then the professional journals and national meetings of clinical neuropsychologists would not be so well stocked with relevant research and discussion of methods to determine response bias, response validity, effort, and malingering. In reality, clinicians who are active in forensic cases and therefore have evaluated numerous litigants and claimants know very well that effort and response validity can vary from one portion of an evaluation to another, and sometimes from one test to another in the same portion of the evaluation. Ideally, clinical researchers will develop effective validity indicators for every single neuropsychological test in common use. Even with such methodology, use of stand-alone effort measures will remain necessary for at least two reasons. First, we are not aware of any embedded index that has consistently demonstrated classification accuracies that are as impressive as those demonstrated by dedicated cognitive effort measures. Second, even when embedded measures have demonstrated excellent classification accuracies in identifying insufficient cognitive effort, we must continually consider the possibility that standard ability effort indices may also be sensitive to a variety of conditions (e.g., severe brain injury, profoundly severe dementia, and learning disability) or other variables (e.g., age and education) to which cognitive effort measures may not be sensitive. Validity indicators of executive function tests such as the WCST and BCT at times will not be consistent with results of pure effort tests, both because specificity and sensitivity may differ but also because the actual effort expended by an examinee can vary within an evaluation. In this regard, we agree with the conclusion of King et al. (2002) made in reference to the WCST and would generalize this conclusion to the BCT and all other traditional ability tests, namely, that "validity indicators within a specific test of ability likely have greater relative utility in determining the validity of that test's performances than the broader issue of malingering as an overall diagnostic conclusion" (p. 520). To us, this observation seems axiomatic. We believe clinicians offering opinions in forensic cases would do well to keep this in mind.

REFERENCES

Ashendorf, L., O'Bryant, S. E., & McCaffrey, R. J. (2003). Specificity of malingering detection strategies in older adults using the CVLT and WCST. *The Clinical Neuropsychologist, 17*, 255–262.

Backhaus, S. L., Fichtenberg, N. L., & Hanks, R. A. (2004). Detection of sub-optimal performance using a floor effect strategy in patients with traumatic brain injury. *The Clinical Neuropsychologist, 18*, 591–603.

Barrett, P., & Putnam, S. (1998). *Empirical data as an aide for assessing performance validity on the Halstead Category Test for mild head injury patients*. Paper presented at the annual meeting of the National Academy of Neuropsychology, Washington, DC.

Bernard, L., McGrath, M., & Houston, W. (1996). The differential effects of simulating malingering, closed head injury, and other CNS pathology on the Wisconsin Card Sorting Test: Support for the "pattern of performance" hypothesis. *Archives of Clinical Neuropsychology, 11*, 231–245.

Bianchini, K., Houston, R., Greve, K., Irvin, R., Black, F. W., Swift, D., et al. (2003). Malingered neurocognitive dysfunction in neurotoxic exposure: An application of the Slick criteria. *Journal of Occupational and Environmental Medicine, 45*, 1087–1099.

Bolter, J. F., Picano, J. J., & Zych, K. (1985). *Item error frequencies on the Halstead Category Test: An index of performance validity*. Paper presented at the annual meeting of the National Academy of Neuropsychology, Philadelphia.

Bush, S. S., Ruff, R. M., Tröster, A. I., Barth, J. T., Koffler, S. P, Pliskin, N. H., et al. (2005). Symptom validity assessment: Practice issues and medical necessity. NAN policy & planning committee. *Archives of Clinical Neuropsychology, 20*, 419–426.

Comalli, P. E., Jr., Wapner, S., & Werner, H. (1962). Interference effects of Stroop Color–Word Test in childhood, adulthood, and aging. *Journal of Genetic Psychology, 100*, 47–53.

Damasio, A. R., & Anderson, S. W., (2003). The frontal lobes. In K. Heilman & E. Valenstein (Eds.), *Clinical neuropsychology* (4th ed., pp. 404–446). New York: Oxford University Press.

Demakis, G. J. (1999). Serial malingering on verbal and nonverbal fluency and memory measures: An analogue investigation. *Archives of Clinical Neuropsychology, 14*, 401–410.

DiCarlo, M. A., Gfeller, J. D., & Oliveri, M. V. (2000). Effects of coaching on detecting feigned cognitive impairment with the Category Test. *Archives of Clinical Neuropsychology, 15*, 399–413.

Donders, J. (1999). Specificity of a malingering formula for the Wisconsin Card Sorting Test. *Journal of Forensic Neuropsychology, 1*, 35–54.

Ellwanger, J., Tenhula, W., Rosenfeld, J. P., & Sweet, J. (1999). Identifying simulators of cognitive deficit through combined use of neuropsychological test performance and event-related potentials (ERPs). *Journal of Clinical and Experimental Neuropsychology, 21*, 866–879.

Ettlin, T., & Kischka, U. (1999). Bedside frontal lobe testing: The "frontal lobe" score. In B. L. Miller & J. L. Cummings (Eds.), *The human frontal lobes: Functions and disorders* (pp. 233–246). New York: Guilford Press.

Faust, D. Hart, K. Guilmette, T. J., & Arkes, H. R. (1988). Neuropsychologists' capacity to detect adolescent malingerers. *Professional Psychology: Research and Practice, 19*, 508–515.

Frederick, R. I. (2000). A personal floor effect strategy to evaluate the validity of performance on memory tests. *Journal of Clinical and Experimental Neuropsychology, 22*, 720–730.

Forrest, T. , Allen, D., & Goldstein, G. (2004). Malingering indexes for the Halstead Category Test. *The Clinical Neuropsychologist, 18*, 334–347.

Goebel, R. (1983). Detection of faking of the Halstead–Reitan Neuropsychological Test Battery. *Journal of Clinical Psychology, 39*, 731–742.

Green, P., Allen, L. M., & Astner, K. (1996). *The Word Memory Test: A user's guide to the oral and computer-administered forms, U.S. Version 1.1*. Durham, NC: CogniSyst.

Greve, K., & Bianchini, K. (2002). Using the Wisconsin Card Sorting Test to detect malingering: An analysis of the specificity of two methods in nonmalingering normal and patient samples. *Journal of Clinical and Experimental Neuropsychology, 24*, 48–54.

Greve, K., Bianchini, K., Mathias, C., Houston, R., & Crouch, J. (2002). Detecting malingered performance with the Wisconsin Card Sorting Test: A preliminary investigation in traumatic brain injury. *The Clinical Neuropsychologist, 16*, 179–191.

Haines, M. E., & Norris, M. P. (2001). Comparing student and patient simulated malingerers' performance on standard neuropsychological measures to detect feigned cognitive deficits. *The Clinical Neuropsychologist, 15*, 171–182.

Heaton, R. K., Smith, Jr., H. H., Lehman, R. A. W., & Vogt, A. T. (1978). Prospects for faking believable deficits on neuropsychological testing. *Journal of Consulting and Clinical Psychology, 46*, 892–900.

Hiscock, M., & Hiscock, C. (1989). Refining the forced-choice method for the detection of malingering. *Journal of Clinical and Experimental Neuropsychology, 11*, 967–974.

Iverson, G. L., Lang, R. T., Green, P., & Franzen, M. D. (2002). Detecting exaggeration and malingering with the Trail Making Test. *The Clinical Neuropsychologist, 16*, 398–406.

King, J. H., Sweet, J. J., Sherer, M., Curtiss, G., & Vanderploeg, R. (2002). Validity indicators within the Wisconsin Card Sorting Test: Application of new and previously researched multivariate procedures in multiple traumatic brain injury samples. *The Clinical Neuropsychologist, 16*, 506–523.

Laatsch, L., & Choca, J. (1991). Understanding the Category Test by using item analysis. *Psychological Assessment: A Journal of Consulting and Clinical Psychology, 3*, 701–704.

Larrabee, G. (2003). Detection of malingering using atypical performance patterns on standard neuropsychological tests. *The Clinical Neuropsychologist, 17*, 410–425.

Lezak, M. D., Howieson, D. B., & Loring, D. W. (2004). *Neuropsychologcial assessment* (4th ed.). New York: Oxford University Press.

Lu, P., Boone, K. B., Jimenez, N., & Razani, J. (2004). Failure to inhibit the reading response on the Stroop Test: A pathognomonic indicator of suspect effort. *Journal of Clinical and Experimental Neuropsychology, 26*, 180–189.

Miller, A., Donders, J., & Suhr, J. (2000). Evaluation of malingering with the Wisconsin Card Sorting Test: A cross-validation. *Clinical Neuropsychological Assessment, 2*, 141–149.

Miller, B. L., & Cummings, J. L. (1999). *The human frontal lobes: Functions and disorders.* New York: Guilford Press.

Millis, S. R. (1992). The Recognition Memory Test in the detection of malingered and exaggerated memory deficits. *The Clinical Neuropsychologist, 6*, 406–414.

Nelson, N. W., Boone, K., Dueck, A., Wagener, L., Lu, P., & Grills, C. (2003). Relationships between eight measures of suspect effort. *The Clinical Neuropsychologist, 17*, 263–272.

Nies, K., & Sweet, J. (1994). Neuropsychological assessment and malingering: A critical review of past and present strategies. *Archives of Clinical Neuropsychology, 9*, 501–552.

O'Bryant, S., Hilsabeck, R., Fisher, J., & McCaffrey, R. (2003). Utility of the Trail

Making Test in the assessment of malingering in a sample of mild traumatic brain injury. *The Clinical Neuropsychologist, 17*, 69–74.

Osimani, A., Alon, A., Berger, A., & Abarbanel, J. M. (1997). Use of the Stroop phenomenon as a diagnostic tool for malingering. *Journal of Neurology, Neurosurgery and Psychiatry, 62*, 617–621.

Osmon, D. C. (1999). Complexities in the evaluation of executive functions. In J. Sweet (Ed.), *Forensic neuropsychology: Fundamentals and practice* (pp. 185–226). Lisse, Netherlands: Swets & Zeitlinger.

Reitan, R. M., & Wolfson, D. (1997). Consistency of neuropsychological test scores of head-injured subjects involved in litigation compared with head-injured subjects not involved in litigation: Development of the Retest Consistency Index. *The Clinical Neuropsychologist, 11*, 69–76.

Rogers, R. (1997). Researching dissimulation. In R. Rogers (Ed.), *Clinical assessment of malingering and deception* (2nd ed., pp. 398–426). New York: Guilford Press.

Ruffolo, L. F., Guilmette, T. J., & Willis, W. G. (2000). Comparison of time and error rates on the Trail Making Test among patients with head injuries, experimental malingerers, patients with suspect effort on testing, and normal controls. *The Clinical Neuropsychologist, 14*, 223–230.

Simmel, M. S., & Counts, S. (1957). Some stable determinants of perception, thinking, and learning: A study based on the analysis of a single test. *Genetic Psychology Monographs, 56*, 3–157.

Slick, D. J., Sherman, E. M. S., & Iverson, G. L. (1999). Diagnostic criteria for malingered neurocognitive dysfunction: Proposed standards for clinical practice and research. *The Clinical Neuropsychologist, 13*, 545–561.

Stuss, D. T., & Knight, R. T. (2002). *Principles of frontal lobe function*. New York: Oxford University Press.

Suhr, J., & Boyer, D. (1999). Use of the Wisconsin Card Sorting Test in the detection of malingering in student simulator and patient samples. *Journal of Clinical and Experimental Neuropsychology, 21*, 701–708.

Sweet, J. (1999). Malingering: Differential diagnosis. In J. Sweet (Ed.), *Forensic neuropsychology: Fundamentals and practice* (pp. 255–285). Lisse, Netherlands: Swets & Zeitlinger.

Sweet, J. J., & King, J. H. (2002). Category Test validity indicators: Overview and practice recommendations. *Journal of Forensic Neuropsychology, 3*, 241–274.

Sweet, J., King, J., Malina, A., Bergman, M., & Simmons, A. (2002). Documenting the prominence of forensic neuropsychology at national meetings and in relevant professional journals from 1990–2000. *The Clinical Neuropsychologist, 16*, 481–494.

Tenhula, W., & Sweet, J. (1996). Double cross-validation of the Booklet Category Test in detecting malingered traumatic brain injury. *The Clinical Neuropsychologist, 10*, 104–116.

Tombaugh, T. N. (1996). *Test of Memory Malingering*. Toronto, Ontario, Canada: MultiHealth Systems.

Trenerry, M. R., Crosson, B., DeBoe, J., & Leber, W. R. (1989). *The Stroop Neuropsychological Screening Test*. Odessa, FL: Psychological Assessment Resources.

Trueblood, W., & Schmidt, M. (1993). Malingering and other validity considerations in the neuropsychological evaluation of mild head injury. *Journal of Clinical and Experimental Neuropsychology, 15*, 578–590.

van Gorp, W. G., Humphrey, L. A., Kalechstein, A., Brumm, V. L., McMullen, W. J., Stoddard, M., et al. (1999). How well do standard clinical neuropsychological tests identify malingering? A preliminary analysis. *Journal of Clinical and Experimental Neuropsychology, 21,* 245–250.

Vickery, C., Berry, D. T. R., Dearth, C., Vagnini, V., Baser, R., Cragar, D., et al. (2004). Head injury and the ability to feign neuropsychological deficits. *Archives of ClinicalNeuropsychology, 19,* 37–48.

Warrington, E. K. (1984). *Recognition memory test manual.* Berkshire, UK: NFER-Nelson.

Williamson, D. J., Green, P., Allen, L., & Rohling, M. (2003). Evaluating effort with the Word Memory Test and Category Test—Or not: Inconsistencies in compensation-seeking sample. *Journal of Forensic Neuropsychology, 3,* 19–44.

Wilson, B. A., Watson, P. C., Baddeley, A. D., Emslie, H., & Evans, J. J. (2000). Improvement or simply practice? The effects of twenty repeated assessments on people with and without brain injury. *Journal of the International Neuropsychological Society, 6,* 469–479.

CHAPTER 9

Use of Motor and Sensory Tests as Measures of Effort

Ginger Arnold
Kyle Brauer Boone

Individuals feigning brain injury are often under the misconception that any type of brain injury inevitably causes impairments in motor speed/coordination/strength and sensation. However, literature shows that such skills are relatively insensitive to cerebral dysfunction (e.g., grip strength; Haaland, Temkin, Randahl, & Dikmen, 1994). Thus, if actual brain-injured patients perform relatively well, and noncredible patients underperform on motor and sensory tests, such measures have the potential to be particularly effective effort measures. Although some attempts have been made to develop effort profiles and cutoff scores for motor and sensory tests, these measures have received much less attention than effort indices from other neuropsychological tests.

This chapter reviews the literature concerning detection of suboptimal effort on Grooved Pegboard, Finger Tapping, Grip Strength, Jamar Grip, Hand Movements subtest from the Kaufman Assessment Battery for Children, the Static Steadiness test, Tactile Finger Recognition, Finger Tip Number Writing, Seashore Rhythm Test, and Speech Sounds Perception Test. Data tables for each study can be found in Appendix 9.1 at the end of the chapter. We discuss recommendations for the clinical use of these tests in detecting noncredible performance and make suggestions for future research on this topic.

MOTOR TASKS

Grooved Pegboard

Johnson and Lesniak-Karpiak (1997) examined Grooved Pegboard perfor-mance in 87 undergraduates with no history of concussion or peripheral injury to hands or arms randomly assigned to three groups: (1) simulators without warning, (2) simulators with warning (i.e., that simulated perfor-mance could be detected), and (3) controls. The unwarned simulators were significantly slower than controls with both hands; the warned simulators scored intermediate to both groups and did not significantly differ from either. The dominant hand was consistently faster than the nondominant hand in all groups, and group differences were more pronounced for the dominant hand.

In a similar study, Rapport, Farchione, Coleman, and Axelrod (1998) recruited 92 college undergraduates who were excluded if they had suffered a loss of consciousness or significant neurological event, had a peripheral motor disturbance, had a Full Scale IQ lower than one standard deviation below the mean, or used medication that might alter cognition. In contrast to the Johnson and Lesniak-Karpiak (1997) study, Rapport et al. (1998) observed that controls significantly outperformed both naïve and coached malingerers (the latter were provided with description of deficits associated with mild brain injury and with cues regarding how to avoid detection), and that the naïve malingerers scored significantly worse than the coached sub-jects. Examination of mean scores suggests that the malingering groups par-ticularly underperformed with the dominant hand.

Inman and Berry (2002) examined Grooved Pegboard performance in 92 undergraduates divided into four groups: (1) those with a history of mild head injury who were asked to exaggerate their deficits on neuropsychologi-cal testing, (2) those with a history of head injury who were asked to put forth their best effort, (3) a group of noninjured analog malingerers, and (4) a group of noninjured controls. Injured participants were excluded if they were seeking compensation for their injury at the time of testing, if their injury had occurred more than 5 years prior to the study, and if they had been diagnosed with a severe mental illness, such as major depression or schizophrenia. Students were excluded from the "normal" group if they had suffered a blow to the head that resulted in a loss of consciousness, or if they had been diagnosed with a severe mental illness. Non-head-injured students were matched to the head-injured groups on age, gender, years of education, and race. Simulators were compensated and were cautioned not to be too blatant in their feigning to avoid detection. Results indicated that the simu-lating groups were significantly slower than the honest groups with both hands, but differences were more pronounced for the dominant hand.

Thus, these studies indicate that simulators, at least unwarned and uncoached simulators, may score significantly below controls and postconcussive patients not in litigation on Grooved Pegboard, with a greater effect noted with the dominant hand. However, knowledge as to how simulators perform relative to controls and mild brain-injured patients (who by weeks or months postaccident have returned to cognitive baseline) is of limited value; what is needed is information regarding how malingerers score compared to patients with significant brain injury, an issue addressed by the following three studies.

Heaton, Smith, Lehman, and Vogt (1978) compared 16 volunteer malingerers with 16 nonlitigating moderate to severe head trauma patients who had no peripheral injury to upper extremities. Malingerers were told to imagine that they were in litigation and that test results would influence the amount of the financial settlement, and they were encouraged to feign "the most severe disabilities they could, without making it obvious to the examiner that they were faking" (p. 894). Malingerers were informed that they would be paid $25 with an extra $5 if they feigned convincingly; however, all were paid $30. No significant difference was observed between the malingerers and patients in Grooved Pegboard time; however, examination of mean scores suggests that the head-injured group performed more poorly than the simulating group, although the large variability in performance in the head-injured group appears to have precluded detection of group differences.

Binder and Willis (1991) reported Grooved Pegboard performance in mild head injury litigants evaluated approximately 2 years postinjury, all of whom had normal brain imaging (when available) and no focal neurological abnormalities at any time after injury. The sample was divided into good- and poor-effort subgroups based on performance on the Portland Digit Recognition Test (PDRT); the low-effort group ($n = 10$) had scores of ≤ 15 correct on the 36 difficult items or ≤ 30 on total score, while the high-effort group ($n = 19$) achieved scores of ≥ 23 on the hard items. The low-effort group performed significantly poorer on Grooved Pegboard than the good-effort group but also had significantly less education. It is unclear whether this impacted test performance independent of effort.

Greiffenstein, Baker, and Gola (1996) compared the Grooved Pegboard performance of 40 moderate to severe brain-injury clients Glasgow Coma Scale ([GCS] ≤ 12; litigation status not reported) with that of 131 litigating postconcussion syndrome patients. All brain injury patients showed unambiguous motor abnormalities on neurological examination including unilateral or bilateral weakness, hyperactive tendon reflexes indicative of spasticity, upgoing plantars, endpoint ataxia during finger-to-nose testing, and dysdiadochokinesia. Patients with dense hemiplegia were excluded. All postconcussive subjects had injuries resulting in < 1 hour of posttraumatic amnesia, remained in the hospital less than 24 hours postinjury, underwent cognitive remediation in outpatient centers with no effect or worsening of symptoms, claimed three or more persistent cognitive or emotional symptoms lasting more than 1 year, reported disability in at least one social role (work, school, or homemaking), and had normal physical and neurological exams throughout the treatment course. All postconcussive subjects also obtained at least one motor skill T score ≤ 40 determined from age/gender/education-specific norms (Heaton, Grant, & Mathews, 1991).

Prior to group comparisons, groups were divided by gender. For both men and women, no significant differences in Grooved Pegboard completion times for either the dominant or nondominant hand were found between postconcussive and moderate/severe brain injury groups, although this appears to be due to extreme variability in Grooved Pegboard performance in the brain injury sample, especially for the nondominant hand. In fact, examination of mean scores for brain injury and postconcussive females reveals that, on average, the less injured group was performing more poorly with the dominant hand than the more severely injured group, a nonsensical finding and one that indicates that postconcussive group was not performing with adequate effort. However, these findings are specific to that subset of moderate-to-severe head-injured patients with documented motor dysfunction and postconcussive patients who obtain at least one lowered motor test score.

van Gorp et al. (1999) examined archival data on mild-to-moderate head injury patients, 20 of whom were suspected of malingering, and 61 of whom were judged to be credible. Subjects were assigned to the suspected malingering group if they met any of these criteria: (1) improbable symptoms, such as claiming severe memory disturbance following an accident in which there was no loss of consciousness; (2) total disability in work or a major social role after 1 year from a mild closed-head injury in which loss of consciousness was less than 1 hour; (3) claims of remote or autobiographical memory loss; and (4) at least one failure on a cognitive effort test (Rey 15-Word Memory Test < 5, Rey 15-Item Memory Test < 9, or a forced-choice digit recognition test). The litigation status of subjects was not reported, but it was noted that all patients "may have been motivated to malinger their performance" (van Gorp et al., 1999, p. 246). No subject had preexisting or concomitant neurological disorder (e.g., seizures, hematoma, and stroke), learning disability, substance abuse infection, or uncontrolled or labile hypertension. Groups did not significantly differ in Grooved Pegboard performance, although this appeared to be an artifact of wide variability in scores; on average, the suspected malingerers required 20 seconds more to complete the task with the dominant hand. Of interest, the suspected malingerers showed a much smaller difference score (dominant hand minus nondominant hand), than nonmalingerers, suggesting that malingerers particularly suppressed dominant hand performance.

In summary, the available studies show significantly lowered Grooved Pegboard performance in simulators versus controls and nonlitigating postconcussive patients, and between "poor effort" versus "good effort" postconcussive litigants. However, no significant differences have been observed in Grooved Pegboard scores between simulators or real-world suspect-effort individuals and patients with moderate-to-severe brain injury. However, examination of mean scores showed that, in most reports, the noncredible subjects were taking longer to complete the task than head-injured patients. The lack of significant group differences between moderate/severe brain injury patients and noncredible subjects appears in some cases to be an artifact of reduced power due to small sample size, possible incomplete exclusion of malingerers from the credible groups (e.g., litigation status was not reported), and/or large variability in performance in the groups. Some of this variability may have been due to failure in some reports to stratify groups by gender; data suggest that women may have higher scores than men on Grooved Pegboard (Polubinski & Melamed, 1986), and if groups do not have comparable gender distribution, the effect of effort on Grooved Pegboard performance will be obscured. In addition, none of the studies provide data on sensitivity and specificity values for particular cutoff scores. Failure to detect group differences could occur when data are not normally distributed and parametric statistical analyses are employed. However, the frequency distribution data used to determine sensitivity/specificity are less impacted by outliers. Thus, it is conceivable that Grooved Pegboard cutoffs may be at least moderately sensitive to suspect effort at acceptable specificity values (i.e., $\geq$ 90%) despite no significant differences in group means.

At the current time, Grooved Pegboard does not appear appropriate for use as an effort indicator due to lack of evidence that suspect-effort individuals score differently than patients with significant brain injury. However, Grooved Pegboard may in fact have potential as a measure of effort. This can only be determined by future studies that control for the effect of gender and examine sensitivity and specificity of specific cutoff scores in addition to comparisons of group means, with specificity values specifically provided for homogenous patient groups. In addition, a consistent finding was that dominant hand performance was more suppressed in poor effort groups than was nondominant hand performance, indicating that future studies on Grooved Pegboard as an effort measure should focus on this performance parameter.

Finger Tapping Test

Over the past two decades the Finger Tapping test has yielded mixed results in studies of its sensitivity to detecting noncredible performance. However, the most recent data appears to confirm its usefulness in differentiating malingerers from credible patients.

In the study by Heaton et al. (1978; study described previously), simulating malingerers scored significantly worse on the Finger Tapping test than moderate-to-severe head-injured patients. Finger Tapping test data were also obtained on college student controls, naïve malingerers, and coached malingerers in the Rapport et al. (1998) study described earlier. The control group performed significantly better with both hands than coached and naive malingerers whose tapping scores were statistically equivalent.

Vickery et al. (2004) investigated finger-tapping performance in 46 head-injured and 46 normal volunteers randomly assigned to credible or feigning groups. The head injury group generally had moderate to severe head injuries as reflected in a mean admitting GCS of 8.6 and loss of consciousness > 1 hour (mean of 13.8 days; SD = 40.1). Eighty-five percent had positive neuroimaging and 34% required neurosurgical intervention. The sample averaged 41.3 days of posttraumatic amnesia (SD = 47.9). None were compensation seeking for their injury, and none had a significant history of substance abuse. They averaged 61.7 months postinjury (SD = 40.5). Community volunteers were matched to the head injury groups on demographic characteristics and had no history of significant neurological, psychiatric, substance abuse, or head injury with loss of consciousness. Those in the malingering groups were read a scenario indicating that they were being tested to determine their readiness to return to work and to document disability. They were told to avoid obvious feigning and detection and then given a coaching sheet that included commonly experienced head injury symptoms and tips for avoiding detection. All subjects were informed they would receive $75 when they completed the testing; those in the malingering groups were told they would receive an extra $20 if they were successfully undetected. The head-injured patients performed significantly worse than volunteers, and those instructed to feign scored significantly lower than those instructed to perform with their best effort. Results showed that head-injured patients were not better able to successfully feign neuropsychological deficits than noninjured individuals.

However, inconsistent findings have been noted in studies comparing real-world malingerers against patients with brain injury. Trueblood and Schmidt (1993) examined outpatients who were in litigation or seeking disability compensation, almost all of whom met criteria for mild head injury (i.e., loss of consciousness < 20 minutes, posttraumatic amnesia < 24 hours, "no neurological evidence of structural damage," and a GCS score of 13–15). Testing was completed an average of 14.8 months postinjury. Patients were divided into four groups: (1) malingering (n = 8); (2) questionable validity (n = 8); (3) credible patients (n = 8) matched to malingerers by age (within 6 years), gender, and education (within 2 years); and (4) credible patients (n = 8) matched to questionable validity patients by age (within 9 years), gender, and education (within 3 years). Patients who performed significantly below chance on a symptom validity test (SVT) were placed in the malingering group. Those placed in the questionable validity group scored at or above chance on the SVT but had at least one highly improbable result on neuropsychological tests (i.e., a score of 0 on Grip Strength or two or more face imperceptions on face–hand stimulation). No significant differences in finger-tapping performance were observed across groups, although this is likely an artifact of reduced power given that performance in the non-credible groups was consistently 80% of that of the patient controls.

In the Greiffenstein et al. (1996) study, also described earlier, no significant differences in dominant and nondominant hand performance were observed between moderate/severe brain injury with motor abnormalities and atypical outcome postconcussive patients in gender-segregated analyses, although the postconcussive subjects obtained mean scores below the moderate/severe brain injury subjects on dominant hand performance (but scored higher on the nondominant hand).

Similar results were observed in a study by Binder, Kelly, Villanueva, and Winslow (2003), who investigated three groups of litigating patients: 34 patients with mild head injury with demonstrated poor effort as determined by performance on the PDRT, and two groups of patients (22 mild head injury and 60 moderate to severe brain injury) who showed good effort by scoring ≥ the second percentile on the PDRT. Mild head injury patients had posttraumatic amnesia ≤ 6 hours, a GCS (when available) of ≥ 13 at hospital admission, and CT (computed tomography) and MRI (magnetic resonance imaging) scans (when available) that did not indicate skull fracture or intracranial lesions. Moderate-to-severe head injury patients had posttraumatic amnesia > 24 hours, admitting acute hospital GCS ≤ 12, or CT scan positive for skull fracture or intracranial lesion. No significant group differences in Finger Tapping scores for dominant and nondominant hands were observed, although the poor motivation group did obtain average T scores below those of both other groups, particularly in the dominant hand.

In contrast, Binder and Willis (1991; study summarized previously) observed poor-effort postconcussive litigants to score significantly lower on a summed Finger Tapping score than good-effort mild head injury litigants, although the former group also had significantly less education.

More recently, Larrabee (2003) observed credible head injury patients to outperform definite and probable malingerers on the Finger Tapping test. Patients in the definite malingered neurocognitive dysfunction (MND) group were 24 personal injury litigants without objective medical evidence of brain injury or damage (normal labs and imaging) and who had a worse than chance performance on the PDRT. He compared them to 27 moderate to severe closed-head-injury patients (moderate was defined as GCS of 9–12 or 13–15 with CT or MRI abnormalities; severe was defined by GCS of 8 or less). Some of these were in litigation, although they did not significantly differ in test performance from head injury patients not in litigation. Effort test data were available on 10 of these subjects and was consistent with trauma severity. He found that a combined Finger Tapping score (sum of the average for dominant and nondominant hands) cutoff of < 63 correctly identified 40% of malingerers and 93.5% of moderate-to-severe head injury patients. No head injury patient scored < 39 and only one scored < 62 while

12% of MND patients scored < 39. He then compared the definite MND patients to 17 probable MND patients who were in litigation, failed at least two SVTs, and had no psychiatric, neurological, or developmental factors that could account for invalid test performance. As can be seen in Appendix 9.1, the latter group actually obtained a summed Finger Tapping score lower than the definite malingering subjects, as well as below that of the head injury group and two other clinical, nonlitigating groups: one with neurological disorders ($n = 13$) and one with psychiatric disorders ($n = 14$).

Backhaus, Fichtenberg, and Hanks (2004) examined Finger Tapping performance in a mild traumatic brain injury group ($n = 25$), a moderate-to-severe traumatic brain injury group ($n = 70$), and a poor-effort group ($n = 25$). The moderate-to-severe traumatic brain injury comparison group consisted of patients who had medically documented brain injuries, were determined by a rehab team to have functional losses and in need of treatment for cognitive deficits, had a GCS below 13 upon admission to the emergency room, and had positive neuroimaging (when available). Twenty-seven of these patients were in litigation, but their test performance was not statistically different from that of the nonlitigating patients, and none were deemed noncredible by a multidisciplinary treatment team. The mild traumatic brain injury group had experienced loss of consciousness and/or a period of post-traumatic confusion and/or had positive neuroimaging (when available). Patients were excluded from the group if they had GCS < 13, their neurocognitive profile was inconsistent with head trauma history, they were involved in litigation, or they were over age 60. The poor-effort patients were seeking compensation for their injuries, had histories of mild head trauma as reflected by GCS score of = 15, no history of loss of consciousness > 30 minutes or posttraumatic confusion > 1 hour, and no abnormalities on neuroimaging. All met Slick, Sherman, and Iverson (1999) criteria for probable or definite malingered performance.

Percentiles which corresponded to the 10th, 25th, 50th, and 90th percentiles in the moderate/severe traumatic brain injury group were calculated. Dominant hand cutoffs of 43.6 and 37.7 corresponded to 50th and 25th percentiles, respectively, for the moderate/severe brain injury group and were associated with 84% and 100% specificity, respectively, in the mild traumatic brain injury group with sensitivity in the poor effort group at 48% and 32%, respectively. For the nondominant hand, cutoffs of 38.9 and 32.9 corresponded to 87.5% and 100% specificity, respectively, in the mild traumatic brain injury patients, with 56% and 28% sensitivity in the poor-effort litigants, respectively.

Arnold et al. (2005) compared Finger Tapping scores of 77 noncredible patients with heterogeneous presenting diagnoses against those of credible patients in six diagnostic groups: moderate to severe closed head injury (loss of consciousness ≥ 12 hours and/or posttraumatic amnesia ≥ 24 hours; $n = 24$), dementia ($n = 31$), low IQ (FSIQ ≤ 70; $n = 18$), psychosis ($n = 27$), depression (n = 42), and healthy older controls (n = 18). Patients in the noncredible group were in litigation or attempting to secure disability compensation and failed at least two cognitive effort indices as well as at least one behavioral criterion (e.g., pattern of neuropsychological test scores not consistent with medical or psychiatric condition). In contrast, none of the credible patients were involved in litigation or were attempting to obtain disability compensation, and they did not meet the aforementioned criteria for noncredible presentation. Patients were excluded from the study if they had obvious motor problems (i.e., tremor, dystonia, severe coordination problems, paralysis, or a recent hand or arm injury from which they had not fully recovered).

Men were found to tap faster than women, requiring that groups be divided by gender. Noncredible male and female patients tapped significantly slower than their comparison group counterparts. Dominant hand score proved to be more sensitive to noncredible performance than other scores (nondominant, sum of both hands, difference between dominant and nondominant), especially for women. Sensitivity, specificity, and positive and negative predictive values were calculated for various dominant hand cutscores and are presented in Appendix 9.1. With specificity set at 90% for the comparison groups combined, a dominant-hand cutoff score of ≤ 35 for men yielded 50% sensitivity, while a score of ≤ 28 yielded 61% sensitivity for women. Of interest, sensitivity values were lower in the subgroup of noncredible subjects who were claiming symptoms secondary to traumatic brain injury (i.e., 50% for women, 41% for men), suggesting, as the studies by the Binder et al. (2003) and Greiffenstein et al. (1996) predicted, that the Finger Tapping test is less effective in the detection of noncredible traumatic brain injury subjects, particularly men, than in the identification of suspecteffort patients with other presenting diagnoses. Specificity values for specific cutoff scores varied significantly across the comparison groups, indicating that cutoffs should be adjusted for the particular differential diagnosis (see Appendix 9.1).

The variability in findings from the real-world studies examining Finger Tapping performance as a measure of effort may be at least partly related to possible failure to completely exclude noncredible subjects from credible groups in some studies. For example, Greiffenstein et al. (1996) did not report the litigation status of their moderate/severe head-injured sample, and head injury controls in the Trueblood and Schmidt (1993) and Binder et al. (2003) studies were in litigation. Further, in the latter two studies, the criteria for assigning subjects to the malingering versus credible groups was based on either performance on a single effort indicator or gross failure on psychometric measures (significantly below chance on forced-choice measure, zero performance on motor testing), which is generally only observed in rather blatant, unsophisticated malingerers (Binder & Willis, 1991). Thus, it is possible in these studies that a significant number of individuals who were feigning were included in the credible group. In contrast, Arnold et al.

(2005) and Backhaus et al. (2004) either excluded litigants from the credible comparison group or ensured that the subset of litigants performed comparably to nonlitigating head injury controls, and Larrabee (2003) noted that the SVT results that were available on his head-injured control sample were consistent with injury severity.

Thus, in conclusion, the available data does suggest that the Finger Tapping test has utility for the discrimination of suspect effort. Sensitivity averages between 40% and 50% (at adequate specificity levels) in head injury samples but may actually be higher in samples feigning symptoms in the context of conditions other than head injury. However, the Greiffenstein et al. (1996) data suggest caution in using Finger Tapping as measure of effort in head injury populations with documented motor abnormalities; mean Finger Tapping scores in their moderate/severe head-injured sample were lower than averages reported in other studies employing moderate/severe head-injured patients (cf. Binder et al., 2003; Heaton et al., 1978; Larrabee, 2003). As with Grooved Pegboard, dominant hand performance appears to be more sensitive to suspect effort than nondominant or summed performance. The Arnold et al. (2005) data suggest that gender and presenting diagnosis should be considered when selecting cutoff scores. While age effects have been reported for tapping performance (cf. Mitrushina, Boone, Razani, & D'Elia, 2005), older normal samples in the Arnold et al. (2005) study did not obtain lowered specificity values, indicating that no adjustment for age is required in using tapping as a measure of effort.

Grip Strength

Rapport et al. (1998), in a study described earlier, compared Grip Strength performance in three college student groups: (1) controls, (2) naïve malingerers, and (3) coached malingerers. The control group performed significantly better with both hands than coached and naive malingerers whose mean grip strength scores were statistically equivalent.

Grip strength performance has also been found to differ between noncredible subjects and credible brain-injured populations. For example, in the Heaton et al. (1978) study, described earlier, simulators were observed to score significantly poorer than moderate-to-severe brain injury patients.

Similarly, Greiffenstein et al. (1996), in a study described previously, found that moderate/severe brain injury patients with motor abnormalities outperformed atypical outcome postconcussive patients on both dominant and nondominant hands in separate gender analyses, with a greater difference noted for the dominant hand; the postconcussive groups performed comparably to patients with partial flaccid paralysis.

In a more recent study of litigating patients, Greiffenstein and Baker (2006) investigated Miller and Cartlidge's (1972) inverse dose–response assertion that the more minor the compensable injury, the greater the likelihood of deficit simulation. Late postconcussive syndrome claimants (n = 607) were alleging disability of > 1 year. The moderate-to-severe brain-injured group (n = 159) consisted of patients with GCS $\leq$ 12 at hospital admission, inpatient stays of 1 week or more, and at least one acute focal neurological finding either on radiographic scanning or during admission physical. Substantial gender effects were present necessitating gender-specific group comparisons. The postconcussive syndrome patients obtained significantly lower grip strength scores than the moderate/severe head injury patients, and higher admitting or field GCS scores correlated with a lower mean grip strength. Cutoff scores were established for "possible" (defined as performance $\leq$ moderate to severe head injury reference group mean) and "probable" (defined as performance $\leq$ minus 1 SD of the moderate-to-severe reference group mean) noncredible performance.

In contrast to the foregoing studies, the Inman and Berry (2002) study (described earlier) found no difference for either dominant or nondominant hand Grip Strength performance between groups of undergraduates (1) with a history of mild head injury asked to exaggerate deficits, (2) with a history of head injury asked to perform their best, (3) without a history of head trauma asked to feign injury, and (4) without a history of head trauma asked to put forth their best effort. However, this may have been an artifact of small sample size; for example, head injury malingerers averaged a dominant hand T score 7 points below that of head injury controls (although only a 4-point difference was observed in nondominant hand performance).

In conclusion, most studies to date have demonstrated that noncredible patients and simulating malingerers routinely underperform as compared to credible patients on grip strength. In fact, some studies have suggested that grip strength may be the most effective motor test for detecting noncredible performance (Greiffenstein et al., 1996; Greiffenstein & Baker, 2006; Heaton et al., 1978; Rapport et al., 1998). However, while significant group differences have typically been obtained, no data on sensitivity/specificity values have been published, thus limiting the clinical application of this measure in differentiating between actual versus feigned performance. A prominent gender effect is present, indicating that future attempts to develop cut-scores should segregate data by gender.

Jamar Grip

A number of studies have been published on detecting feigned hand injuries with the Jamar hydraulic hand dynamometer used by occupational therapists and physical therapists. Some investigations have shown that simulators perform worse than credible patients and that their scores across handle position trials show a flatter bell curve than those of credible patients (Niebuhr & Marion, 1987, 1990; Stokes, Landrieu, Domangue, & Kunen, 1995). However, other data have indicated that subjects can approximate reduced degrees of strength (e.g., 30% effort or 50% effort) with fairly good accuracy (Niebuhr & Marion, 1990), which predicts that malingerers may well be able to reproduce reduced strength in a credible manner. In addition, the effectiveness of these methods of detecting submaximal performance has not been demonstrated across all studies, and the general consensus is that more accurate methods of determining noncredible performance must be developed (Ashford, Nagelburg, & Adkins, 1996; Lechner, Bradbury, & Bradley, 1998; Robinson & Dannecker, 2004; Shechtman, Gutierrez, & Kokendofer, 2005). The interested reader is referred to publications by De Smet and Londers (2003), Dvir (1999), Hoffmaster, Lech, and Niebuhr (1993), Niebuhr and Marion (1987, 1990), Niebuhr, Marion, and Hasson (1993), Schapmire et al. (2002), Smith, Nelson, Sadoff, and Sadoff (1989), and Tredgett and Davis (2000).

Motor Function Patterns

Attempts have been made to detect suspect effort through abnormal patterns in performance across motor tasks. Haaland et al. (1994) reported normal grip strength but relatively poor Finger Tapping in traumatic brain injury 1 year after injury, which indicated that complex motor skills are more affected by severe brain trauma than are simpler skills. As outlined by Greiffenstein et al. (1996), grip strength only requires contraction of flexor muscle groups with inhibition of extensor groups, while Grooved Pegboard involves integration of visual and tactile feedback with rapid, sequenced excitatory and inhibitory motor signals. Finger Tapping is of intermediate complexity, requiring speeded motor movements without a sequencing component and minimal visual and tactile inputs.

Greiffenstein et al. (1996; study described earlier) investigated performance on Grip Strength, Finger Tapping, and Grooved Pegboard for moderate-to-severe brain injury patients with motor abnormalities as compared to atypical outcome postconcussive syndrome patients. The moderate/severe brain injury group produced a motor dysfunction pattern consistent with impairment on more complex tasks and sparing of performance on simpler tasks (Grooved Pegboard < Finger Tapping < Grip Strength), while the postconcussive syndrome patients tended to produce the opposite pattern (Grooved Pegboard > Finger Tapping > Grip Strength). The authors conclude that a pattern incongruent with the hierarchical structure of motor control systems is suggestive of noncredible performance.

Rapport et al. (1998; study described previously) examined whether the Greiffenstein et al. (1996) findings of the noncongruent motor profile in postconcussive syndrome patients were robust to coaching of malingered test performance in three groups of college students: (1) control, (2) naïve malingerer, and (3) coached malingerer. Group comparisons demonstrated that performance was comparable across the three tests in the control group.

In contrast to the findings of Greiffenstein et al. (1996), in the naïve malingerer group, grip strength and finger tapping performances were equivalent and significantly better than Grooved Pegboard scores. Coached malingerers showed no difference between Grip Strength and Finger Tapping, but tapping was worse than Grooved Pegboard.

The sensitivities of the Greiffenstein et al. (1996) nonphysiological performance patterns (i.e., Grip Strength < Finger Tapping; Finger Tapping < Grooved Pegboard; Grip Strength < Grooved Pegboard) as indices of malingering proved to be poor. One or more of these rare signs were present in 89.7% of the control group although none exhibited the full pattern; 62.1% had a lower score on Grip Strength than on Finger Tapping, 41.4% scored better on Grooved Pegboard than Finger Tapping, and 51.7% performed worse on Grip Strength than Grooved Pegboard. Sensitivity of the Grip Strength < Finger Tapping < Grooved Pegboard profile for detecting naïve malingerers was only 6.5% for the complete pattern and 39% for two or more rare signs. In contrast and surprisingly, 25% of coached malingerers displayed the complete profile and 62.5% demonstrated two or more rare signs. Malingerers with lower IQs showed more rare indices than did malingerers with higher IQs (an all the more noteworthy finding given the likely restricted range of IQ in a college sample), which suggested that this pattern might be reflective of an unsophisticated approach to feigning.

The discrepancy in findings across the Greiffenstein et al. (1996) and Rapport et al. (1998) studies is puzzling and may be related to demographic and other differences in the samples employed in the two studies, and/or the limitations of analog malingering research versus use of real-world noncredible samples.

Although both the Greiffenstein et al. (1996) and Rapport et al. (1998) studies had comparable percentages of females in the noncredible groups (57% to 59%), the Greiffenstein et al. (1996) postconcussive samples were in their late 30s and averaged less than 12 years of education, while the Rapport et al. (1998) college student simulators were in their mid-20s and averaged 14.5 years of education. It is possible that unskilled and blue-collar occupational groups, which likely constituted the Greiffenstein et al. (1996) sample, are required to engage in lifting and pulling as a prominent part of their jobs, and therefore grip strength would be a particularly salient skill on which they might focus their efforts to feign disability. In contrast, for young, well-educated samples whose current and anticipated future jobs do not involve hand strength, feigning attempts would be less likely to focus on Grip Strength measures. However, for these individuals, finger speed (for typing) might be viewed as more critical in the job market, hence the somewhat lowered scores in tapping and peg placement (at least in the coached malingerers). These findings raise the intriguing possibility that feigning attempts are shaped by what the malingerer views as important job skills, and feigning strategies on neuropsychological testing may somewhat differ across occupational groups (e.g., white-collar/professionals vs. unskilled/blue-collar). Alternatively, Rapport et al. (1998) suggested the Greiffenstein et al. (1996) noncredible motor profile may be related to an unsophisticated approach to malingering associated with lowered IQ.

Further, the Greiffenstein et al. (1996) postconcussive sample was selected based on lowered performance on at least one motor task and thus may not be representative of the larger persistent postconcussive population. The data on Finger Tapping performance in isolation suggests that sensitivity in head-injured samples hovers slightly below 50%, indicating that approximately half of noncredible head injury patients are not significantly underperforming on that motor task. Further, the Arnold et al. (2005) study showed that noncredible Finger Tapping performance was somewhat less common in a noncredible head injury population than in individuals feigning symptoms in the context of other alleged conditions. Thus, while poor motor performance may be common in postconcussive litigants, it is not ubiquitous. It is possible that the nonphysiological motor profile identified by Greiffenstein et al. (1996) is only present in the subset of persistent postconcussive patients who incorporate motor dysfunction as a part of their feigned presentation.

Currently, the available data on motor pattern analysis to detect suboptimal effort is contradictory and corroboration is required before the technique can be used clinically. In addition, given the gender differences in motor task performance (i.e., women > men on Grooved Pegboard, men > women on Grip Strength and Finger Tapping), there are likely to be gender differences in motor profile performance in both brain-injured and malingering populations. Combined data across male and female samples may produce profiles that are not representative of either gender. Finally, future research should examine whether motor patterns differ as a function of socioeconomic status and/or IQ.

Hand Movements Subtest
from the Kaufman Assessment Battery for Children

One study (Bowen & Littell, 1997) focused on the Hand Movements subtest of the Kaufman Assessment Battery for Children (KABC; Kaufman & Kaufman, 1983) as a measure of effort in adults. The authors compared 21 patients involved in a lawsuit or filing for workers' compensation with 25 non-compensation-seeking patients and previously published data on normal healthy adults (n = 80; Barry & Riley, 1987). Nonlitigants had diagnoses of early-onset cerebrovascular disorder, arteriovenous malformation, aneurysm, traumatic brain injury, neoplastic disease, and hydrocephalus; all had brain lesions verified by brain imaging. Most compensation-seeking patients reported mild concussions without positive imaging studies, although two had sustained severe brain injury, two had moderate brain injuries, three claimed mental stress, and two presented with chronic fatigue syndrome. Overall, compensation-seeking patients performed worse than nonlitigants, who performed worse than healthy adults. The mean for the compensation-seeking group was equivalent to that of children between the ages of 4 years, 10 months through 4 years, 11 months. In contrast, the non-compensation-seeking patient mean score was within the normal range. Approximately 90% of the patient group obtained a score of ≥ 10, while only 34% of the litigation group scored at this level. Thus, sensitivity for this cutoff is 66%.

In conclusion, these data suggest that this hand-sequence task appears to have promise in the detection of suspect effort, although given the small sample size, the findings require replication. Further, although no relationship to gender was observed in the current study, normative data have revealed a modest gender effect (Barry & Riley, 1987), which should be considered in future studies. Also, age effects have been observed in normal samples; whether age adjustments to cutoffs are necessary requires investigation.

Static Steadiness Test

Heaton et al. (1978; described earlier) found no significant difference in performance between simulating and moderate–severe brain injury groups on the Static Steadiness Test, included in the Klove–Matthews Motor Steadiness Battery. However, this appears to have been an artifact of marked variability in performance, particularly in the head-injured group. To date, there has been no further empirical investigation of the use of the Static Steadiness test in detection of suspect effort.

SENSORY TASKS

Tactile Finger Recognition (Finger Agnosia) and Finger Tip Number Writing

Heaton et al. (1978; study described earlier) documented that volunteer malingerers made significantly more errors than nonlitigating patients with moderate to severe brain injury on the finger agnosia test but did not significantly differ on number of errors on the Finger Tip Number Writing task.

Subsequently, Binder and Willis (1991; study described earlier) found that poor-effort postconcussive litigants committed more errors on a combined finger agnosia/Finger Tip Number Writing score than good-effort litigants with mild brain injury, although groups also differed in educational level. Similarly, Trueblood and Schmidt (1993; study described previously), observed significantly more errors on the finger agnosia task between malingerers and head injury controls and on both the finger agnosia and Finger

Tip Number Writing tasks between questionable validity patients and their head injury controls. Employing a cutoff score of > 3 errors for both hands on the finger agnosia task, sensitivity was 50% in malingerers and 75% in questionable validity patients, with 94% specificity in mild injury controls. Similarly, a cutoff of > 5 total errors on the Finger Tip Number Writing task was associated with 62% sensitivity in both noncredible groups with a false-positive identification rate of 6%.

Youngjohn, Burrows, and Erdal (1995) obtained neuropsychological test data on 55 persistent postconcussive syndrome subjects attempting to secure financial compensation for their injuries, nearly half of whom showed noncredible performance on effort indicators (PDRT, Dot Counting Test). These authors reported that while few errors were committed on the sensory–perceptual section of the neuropsychological evaluation, those that that did occur were present on Finger Tip Number Writing (right-hand mean = 3.63 ± 3.77, left-hand mean = 2.54 ± 3.10) and Tactile Finger Recognition (right-hand mean = 1.70 ± 2.52; left-hand mean = 1.43 ± 2.71).

Binder et al. (2003; study previously described) observed that poorly motivated patients with head injury made significantly more errors with both the right and left hands on Tactile Finger Recognition (finger agnosia) and Finger Tip Number Writing than good-motivation groups with mild and moderate–severe head injury. In fact, effect sizes were larger for Tactile Finger Recognition (1.94 for the right hand and 1.39 for the left hand) and Finger Tip Number Writing (1.10 for the right hand and .77 for the left hand) than those for all other tests in a comprehensive neuropsychological test battery (e.g., the next largest effect size was the Rey Auditory Verbal Learning Test [RAVLT] recognition, $d = .90$).

For Tactile Finger Recognition, use of a cutoff which corresponded to < 10th percentile (> 4 errors combined for both hands) in the moderate–severe brain injury group resulted in identification of 56% of noncredible patients. The false-positive identification rate was only 7% in the good-motivation individuals with moderate to severe head injury, but the false-positive rate in the good-motivation group with mild head injury was inexplicably more than double (i.e., 18%). The finding that the group with mild head injury made more errors than the group with moderate–severe injury is nonsensical and suggests that some noncredible patients were inadvertently included in the credible group with mild head injury.

For Finger Tip Number Writing, use of a cutoff closest to ≤ 10th percentile (> 17 errors with both hands) in the good-motivation group with moderate–severe injury, yielded sensitivity of only 18%; although specificity was 95% in the group with moderate–severe head injury and 100% in the group with mild head injury. However, it is likely that the cutoff could be lowered, while still retaining false-positive identifications ≤ 10%, with a concomitant rise in sensitivity.

In conclusion, the available studies suggest that both Tactile Finger Recognition and Finger Tip Number Writing may have hit rates for identification of suspect effort of ≥ 50% at acceptable specificity (i.e., ≥ 90%), but that Tactile Finger Recognition (finger agnosia) may be the more effective of the two measures. These tasks have been underutilized in research and clinical practice, despite the surprising finding that effect sizes in comparisons of credible and noncredible groups may be larger than those for more commonly used effort indices (e.g., RAVLT recognition). Recommended cut-scores for finger agnosia were similar across studies (> 3 vs. > 4), although Finger Tip Number Writing cutoffs have varied from > 5 to > 17, indicating that further research is needed to identify the most effective cutoffs.

Seashore Rhythm Test

Heaton et al. (1978; study described earlier) found no significant difference in the Seashore Rhythm Test performance between volunteer simulators and nonlitigating patients with moderate to severe head trauma.

In contrast, Trueblood and Schmidt (1993; study summarized earlier) observed that malingerers and questionable validity patients performed significantly worse than credible patients on this test. A cutoff score of ≥ 8 errors was associated with 63% sensitivity in malingerers and 50% sensitivity in questionable validity patients at 100% specificity (no false positives).

Similarly, Inman and Berry (2002; described previously) found that undergraduates with and without a history of minor head injury instructed to malinger made significantly more errors than subjects with and without a history of minor head injury who were asked to perform with their best effort. Use of Trueblood and Schmidt's (1993) cutting score resulted in a specificity of 98%, although sensitivity was only 27%.

More recently, Ross et al. (2006) examined SRT performance in 46 compensation-seeking patients with mild to very mild head injuries (post-traumatic amnesia [PTA] < 60 minutes) who were judged to be probable malingerers based on poor performance on the Warrington Recognition Memory Test (< 33 on Words or Faces, and < 41 on the remaining subtest), a WAIS-R discriminant function of > .1011, and a raw score of > 20 on the MMPI-2 Fake Bad Scale (FBS). Data were also obtained on a comparison group of 49 non-compensation-seeking patients with head injuries (62.2% mild to very mild [PTA < 60 minutes]; 32.7% moderate [PTA 1 to 24 hours], and 8.1% severe [PTA > 1 day]); 7 obtained FBS scores ≥ 21, and 5 obtained WAIS-R discriminant functions of > .1011. The probable malingerer group had less education (12.0 vs. 13.4 years); however, education was not a significant predictor of SRT performance. A cutoff of ≥ 8 errors was associated with 76.1% sensitivity, but with specificity of only 73.5%; raising the cutoff to ≥ 10 errors achieved acceptable specificity (92%), but sensitivity dropped to 59%.

In conclusion, data have been generally supportive of the effectiveness of the Seashore Rhythm Test in the identification of noncredible performance; however, recommended cut scores and associated sensitivity and specificity rates have not been consistent across investigations. While earlier studies, which employed simulators or were limited by small ns have recommended a cut score of ≥ 8 errors, the most recent data, obtained in a large real-world noncredible sample, suggest that the cut score must be raised to ≥ 10 to maintain adequate specificity, although this cut score only identifies slightly more than half of noncredible subjects.

Speech Sounds Perception Test

Heaton et al. (1978; summarized previously) reported that malingerers made significantly more errors on the Speech Sound Perception Test than patients with moderate to severe brain injury.

Trueblood and Schmidt (1993; described earlier) were able to establish a cutoff score for Speech Sounds Perception (errors > 17) that correctly identified seven malingerers (87% sensitivity) and three questionable validity patients (38% sensitivity), while yielding only one false positive (94% specificity).

Ross et al. (2006; described previously) observed that the optimal Speech Sounds Perception Test score to maintain false positive identification $\leq 10\%$ was ≥ 13 errors (70% sensitivity), which is probably more reliable than the cut score of > 17 recommended by Trueblood and Schmidt (1993) due to the larger sample sizes in the former study. Thus, the Speech Sounds Perception Test may have utility in the detection of suboptimal performance although additional corroborating studies are required. Further, the confounding effect of poor reading ability on test performance as it impacts specificity requires careful assessment.

CONCLUSIONS AND RECOMMENDATIONS

Motor and sensory tasks are generally brief and are already incorporated in many neuropsychological examinations, thus making them attractive options as effort indicators. Further, they are better suited to capture feigned symptoms involving motor and sensory function than other types of effort indicators, most of which test for fabricated memory impairment. Unfortunately, while data on comparisons of credible and noncredible groups have been consistently reported, cut-scores and accompanying sensitivity and specificity information, required for clinical use of the tests, are less frequently available. Current information suggests that sensitivity may only be moderate, and thus the tests are primarily useful in "ruling in" rather than "ruling out" noncredible performance. That is, a positive finding is a strong indicator of poor effort, but a passed performance does not preclude the presence of suboptimal performance. The Finger Tapping test has garnered the most research attention, but some studies suggest that grip strength, hand-sequence tasks, Tactile Finger Recognition (finger agnosia), Seashore Rhythm Test, and Speech Sounds Perception Test may be as or more effective in identifying suspect performance and are deserving of additional investigation. Gender effects are prominent on motor tasks, necessitating the use of separate gender-based cut-scores, and there are also some suggestions that socioeconomic status, IQ, and educational and/or occupational level may influence feigning strategies and should be considered in future research on these tasks.

Most studies have only examined the impact of actual versus feigned head injury on test performance, and there is evidence that these data may underestimate the effectiveness of these measures as effort tools in patients with suspect effort with claimed brain injury from other than traumatic head injury causes. Head injury malingerers may particularly focus on verbal memory measures to showcase their deficits (Nitch, Boone, Wen, Arnold, & Warner-Chacon, 2006), while patients feigning symptoms associated with other claimed causes may be more inclined to fake motor (Arnold et al., 2005) or sensory (Greve, Bianchini, & Ameduri, 2003) impairment, necessitating that validation studies include alleged etiologies other than traumatic brain injury. As shown in the Arnold et al. (2005) study, cut-scores vary as a function of clinical comparison group, and data are needed on effort indicators for various discrete diagnostic categories, such as epilepsy, stroke, chronic pain, depression, psychosis, Alzheimer's disease, and mental retardation, in addition to head injury.

Use of discrete patterns of performance across several motor tasks has met with limited success. Analyses incorporating multiple motor and/or sensory tasks could examine for patterns of performance in a more detailed manner and would shed light on whether some motor tests should be weighted more heavily than others in the identification of suspect effort. Further, Rapport et al. (1998) recommended examining consistency of motor performance across repeated administrations on the assumption that malingerers are less able to replicate consistent scores across successive evaluations; empirical verification of this hypothesis is needed.

Modifications in test administration could have the potential of enhancing effectiveness of motor/and sensory tasks as effort indicators. For example, there is evidence that tapping in the right hand is suppressed (while left hand tapping is facilitated) when subjects complete verbal tasks (anagram solution and verbal memory) due to increased demands on left-hemisphere function (Fearing, Browning, Corey, & Foundas, 2001; Yeary, Patton, & Kee, 2002), or when standing on the right or left foot only as compared to sitting or standing on both feet (Gabbard & Hart, 2002). In contrast, left hand tapping is lowered when subjects complete concurrent manual rotation or block design arrangement tasks due to recruitment of the right hemisphere in the spatial tasks (Hellige & Longstreth, 1981; Yeary et al., 2002). Individuals feigning motor impairment are not likely to be aware of these phenomena, and may perform atypically when presented with these task paradigms. In addition, available data suggest that variations in lighting and noise do not impact motor test performance (Harrison & Pauly, 1990), which may not be appreciated by individuals feigning motor impairment; as a result, non-credible subjects may demonstrate unexpected findings on motor exam when subjected to changes in light and noise levels. Finally, examination of qualitative aspects of test performance may be a useful adjunct to quantitative scores; for example, on Finger Tapping, some noncredible patients exhibit nonorganic "fast/slow" tapping patterns.

In conclusion, the empirical study of motor and sensory tasks as measures of effort is in its infancy, but evidence suggests that these measures may have a unique role as effort indicators during neuropsychological assessment.

REFERENCES

Arnold, G., Boone, K. B., Lu, P., Dean, A., Wen, J., Nitch, S., et al. (2005). Sensitivity and specificity of Finger Tapping Test scores for the detection of suspect effort. *Journal of Clinical and Experimental Neuropsychology*, *19*, 105–120.

Ashford, R. F., Nagelburg, S., & Adkins, R. (1996). Sensitivity of the Jamar Dynamometer in detecting submaximal grip effort. *Journal of Hand Surgery*, *21*, 402–405.

Backhaus, S. L., Fichtenberg, N. L., & Hanks, R. A. (2004). Detection of sub-optimal performance using a floor effect strategy in patients with traumatic brain injury. *The Clinical Neuropsychologist*, *18*, 591–603.

Barry, P., & Riley, J. (1987). Adult norms for the Kaufman Hand Movements Test and single-subject design for acute brain injury rehabilitation. *Journal of Clinical and Experimental Neuropsychology*, *9*, 449–455.

Binder, L. M., Kelly, M. P., Villanueva, M. R., & Winslow, M. M. (2003). Motivation and neuropsychological test performance following mild head injury. *Journal of Clinical and Experimental Neuropsychology*, *25*, 420–230.

Binder, L. M., & Willis, S. C. (1991). Assessment of motivation after financially compensable minor head trauma. *Psychological Assessment: A Journal of Consulting and Clinical Psychology*, *3*, 175–181.

Bowen, M., & Littell, C. (1997). Discriminating adult normals, patients, and claimants with a pediatric test: A brief report. *The Clinical Neuropsychologist*, *11*, 433–435.

De Smet, L., & Londers, J. (2003). Repeated grip strength at one month interval and detection of voluntary submaximal effort. *Acta Orthopedica Belgica*, *69*, 142–144.

Dvir, Z. (1999). Coefficient of variation in maximal and feigned static and dynamic grip efforts. *American Journal of Physical Medicine and Rehabilitation*, *78*, 216–221.

Fearing, M. K., Browning, C. A., Corey, D. M., & Foundas, A. L. (2001). Dual-task performance in right- and left-handed adults: A finger-tapping and foot-tapping study. *Perceptual and Motor Skills*, *92*, 323–334.

Gabbard, C., & Hart, S. (2002). Effects of standing and sitting on finger-tapping speed in healthy adults. *Journal of Orthopaedic and Sports Physical Therapy*, *32*, 525–529.

Greiffenstein, M. F., & Baker, W. J. (2006). Miller was (mostly) right: Head injury severity inversely related to simulation. *Legal and Criminal Psychology*, *11*, 131–145.

Greiffenstein, M. F., Baker, W. J., & Gola, T. (1996). Motor dysfunction profiles in traumatic brain injury and postconcussion syndrome. *Journal of the International Neuropsychology Society*, *2*, 477–485.

Greve, K. W., Bianchini, K. J., & Ameduri, C. J. (2003). Use of a forced choice test of tactile discrimination in the evaluation of functional sensory loss: A report of 3 cases. *Archives of Physical Medicine and Rehabilitation*, *84*, 1233–1236.

Haaland, K. Y., Temkin, N., Randahl, G., & Dikmen, S. (1994). Recovery of simple motor skills after head injury. *Journal of Clinical and Experimental Neuropsychology*, *16*, 448–456.

Harrison, D. W., & Pauly, R. S. (1990). Manual dexterity, strength, fatigue, and perseveration: An initial test of asymmetry in cerebral activation. *Perceptual and Motor Skills*, *70*, 739–744.

Heaton, R. K., Grant, I., & Matthews, C. G. (1991). *Comprehensive norms for an expanded Halstead-Reitan Battery: Demographic corrections, research findings, and clinical applications.* Odessa, FL: Psychological Assessment Resources.

Heaton, R. K., Smith, H. H., Lehman, A. W., & Vogt, A. T. (1978). Prospects for faking believable deficits on neuropsychological testing. *Journal of Consulting and Clinical Psychology*, *46*, 892–900.

Hellige, J. B., & Longstreth, L. E. (1981). Effects of concurrent hemisphere-specific activity on unimanual tapping rate. *Neuropsychologia*, *19*, 395–405.

Hoffmaster, E., Lech, R., & Niebuhr, B. R. (1993). *Journal of Medicine*, *35*, 788–794.

Inman, T. H., & Berry, D. T. R. (2002). Cross-validation of indicators of malingering. A comparison of nine neuropsychological tests, four tests of malingering, and behavioral observations. *Archives of Clinical Neuropsychology*, *17*, 1–23.

Johnson, J. L., & Lesniak-Karpiak, K. (1997). The effect of warning on malingering on memory and motor tasks in college samples. *Archives of Clinical Neuropsychology*, *12*, 231–238.

Kaufman, A., & Kaufman, N. (1983). *Kaufman Assessment Battery for Children: Administration and scoring manual.* Circle Pines, MN: American Guidance Service.

Klove, H. (1963). Clinical neuropsychology. In F. M. Forster (Ed.), *The medical clinics of North America.* New York: Saunders.

Larrabee, G. J. (2003). Detection of malingering using atypical performance patterns on standard neuropsychological tests. *The Clinical Neuropsychologist*, *17*, 410–425.

Lechner, D. E., Bradbury, S. F., & Bradley, L. A. (1998). Detecting sincerity of effort: A summary of methods and approaches. *Physical Therapy*, *78*, 867–888.

Mathews, C. G., & Klove, H. (1964). *Instruction manual for the Adult Neuropsychology Test Battery.* Madison: University of Wisconsin Medical School.

Miller, H., & Cartlidge, N. (1972). Simulation and malingering after injuries to the brain and spinal cord. *Lancet, 1*, 580–585.

Mitrushina, M., Boone, K. B., Razani, J., & D'ELia, L. F. (2005). *Handbook of normative data for neuropsychological assessment* (2nd ed.). New York: Oxford University Press.

Neibuhr, B. R., & Marion, R. (1987). Detecting sincerity of effort when measuring grip strength. *American Journal of Physical Medicine, 66*, 16–24.

Niebuhr, B. R., & Marion, R. (1990). Voluntary control of submaximal grip strength. *American Journal of Physical Medicine and Rehabilitation, 69*, 96–101.

Niebuhr, B. R., Marion, R., & Hasson, S. M. (1993). Electromyographic analysis of effort in grip strength assessment. *Electromyographic Clinical Neurophysiology, 33*, 149–156.

Nitch, S., Boone, K. B., Wen, J., Arnold, G., & Warner-Chacon, K. (2006). The utility of the Rey Word Recognition in the detection of suspect. *The Clinical Neuropsychologist, 20*, 873–887.

Polubinski, J. P., & Melamed, L. E. (1986). Examination of the sex difference on the Symbol Digit Substitution Test. *Perception and Motor Skills, 62*, 975–982.

Rapport, L. J., Farchione, T. J., Coleman, R. D., & Axelrod, B. N. (1998). Effects of coaching on malingered motor function profiles. *Journal of Clinical and Experimental Neuropsychology, 20*, 89–97.

Reitan, R. M. (1955). Certain differential effects of left and right cerebral lesions in human adults. *Journal of Comparative and Physiological Psychology, 48*, 474–477.

Robinson, M. E., & Dannecker, E. A. (2004). Critical issues in the use of muscle testing for the determination of sincerity of effort. *Clinical Journal of Pain, 20*, 392–398.

Ross, S. R., Putnam, S. H., Millis, S. R., Adams, K. M., & Krukowski, R. (2006). Detecting insufficient effort using the Seashore Rhythm and Speech Sounds Perception Tests in head injury. *The Clinical Neuropsychologist, 20*, 798–815.

Schapmire, D., St. James, J. D., Townsend, R., Stewart, T., Delheimer, S., & Focht, D. (2002). Simultaneous bilateral testing: Validation of a new protocol to detect insincere effort during grip and pinch strength testing. *Journal of Hand Therapy, 15*, 242–250.

Schectman, O., Gutierrez, Z., & Kokendofer, E. (2005). Analysis of the statistical methods used to detect submaximal effort with the five-rung grip strength test. *Journal of Hand Therapy, 18*, 10–18.

Slick, D., Sherman, E., & Iverson, G. (1999). Diagnostic criteria for malingered neurocognitive dysfunction: Proposed standards for clinical practice and research. *The Clinical Neuropsychologist, 13*, 545–561.

Smith, G. A., Nelson, R. C., Sadoff, S. J., & Sadoff, A. M. (1989). Assessing Sincerity of effort in maximal grip strength tests. *American Journal of Physical Medicine and Rehabilitation, 68*, 73–80.

Stokes, H. M., Landrieu, K. W., Domangue, B., & Kunen, S. (1995). Identification of low-effort patients through dynamometry. *Journal of Hand Surgery, 20*, 1047–1056.

Tredgett, M. W., & Davis, T. R. (2000). Rapid repeat testing of grip strength for detection of faked hand weakness. *Journal of Hand Surgery, 25*, 372–375.

Trueblood, W., & Schmidt, M. (1993). Malingering and other validity considerations in the neuropsychological evaluation of mild head injury. *Journal of Clinical and Experimental Neuropsychology, 15,* 578–590.

van Gorp, W. G., Humphrey, L., Kalechstein, A., Brumm, V., McMullen, W. J., Stoddard, M., et al. (1999). How well do standard clinical neuropsychological tests identify malingering? A preliminary analysis. *Journal of Clinical and Experimental Neuropsychology, 21,* 245–250.

Vickery, C. D., Berry, D. T. R., Dearth, C. S., Vagini, V. L., Baser, R. E., Cragar, D. E., et al. (2004). Head injury and the ability to feign neuropsychological deficits. *Archives of Clinical Neuropsychology, 19,* 37–48.

Yeary, S. A., Patton, J. N., & Kee, D. W. (2002). Asymmetries in finger-tapping interference produced by mental versus manual rotation of Shepard and Metzler type objects. *Brain and Cognition, 50,* 324–334.

Youngjohn, J. R., Burrows, L., & Erdal, K. (1995). Brain damage or compensation neurosis? The controversial post-concussive syndrome. *The Clinical Neuropsychologist, 9,* 112–123.

APPENDIX 9.1. DATA TABLES

Arnold et al. (2005)

Sensitivity and Specificity Values for Dominant-Hand Women's Finger Tapping Scores

	Sensitivity		Specificity						
	Total noncredible	Noncredible head injured	Total credible	Head injured	Depressed	Psychotic	Mentally retarded	Dementia	Older adults
n	33	12	77	7	21	17	8	16	8
≤ 15	18	17	99	100	100	100	100	94	100
≤ 28	**61**	**50**	**92**	**100**	**95**	**88**	**87**	**75**	**100**
≤ 32	70	67	86	100	95	88	87	62	100
≤ 35	73	67	79	86	95	65	87	66	100
≤ 38	76	67	65	57	90	53	87	25	87

Note. Finger Tapping scores were the average number of taps for three 10-second trials.

Sensitivity and Specificity Values for Dominant-Hand Men's Finger Tapping Scores

	Sensitivity		Specificity						
	Total noncredible	Noncredible head injured	Total credible	Head injured	Depressed	Psychotic	Mentally retarded	Dementia	Older adults
n	44	22	81	16	21	10	9	15	10
≤ 21	21	18	99	100	100	100	100	93	100
≤ 33	43	32	94	94	100	100	89	87	100
≤ 35	**50**	**41**	**90**	**87**	**95**	**90**	**78**	**87**	**100**
≤ 38	55	46	86	87	95	90	78	80	100
≤ 40	57	46	81	81	86	90	56	80	100

Note. Finger Tapping scores were the average number of taps for three 10-second trials.

Positive Predictive Values (PPV) and Negative Predictive Values (NPV) for Dominant-Hand Finger Tapping Test Score for Different Base Rates

	15% base rate		30% base rate		50% base rate	
Cutoff	PPV %	NPV %	PPV %	NPV %	PPV %	NPV %
Women						
≤ 15	75	87	86	74	91	55
≤ 28	63	93	80	85	87	70
≤ 32	48	94	68	87	83	73
≤ 35	39	94	60	87	78	85
≤ 38	28	94	48	86	69	73
Men						
≤ 21	80	88	89	74	93	55
≤ 33	53	90	76	79	87	62
≤ 35	50	91	68	80	84	64
≤ 38	45	91	67	82	83	65
≤ 40	35	92	58	82	77	67

Backhaus, Fichtenberg, and Hanks (2004)

	Poor-effort litigants ($n = 25$)		Mild TBI ($n = 25$)		
	M	SD	M	SD	p
Age	39.20	10.94	34.72	10.73	<.150
Education	12.56	1.76	13.08	2.61	<.414
Months postinjury	27.76	34.34	5.64	6.34	<.004
Finger Tapping— dominant hand	40.72	11.58	50.25	5.84	<.01
Finger Tapping— nondominant hand	36.78	10.29	45.03	4.56	<.01

Note. Finger Tapping scores calculated based on Reitan (1955).

Raw Scores for the 10th, 25th, 50th, 75th, and 90th Percentiles in a Brain Injury Rehabilitation Database of the Moderate to Severe Postacute Cases

	n	10th	25th	50th	75th
Tapping—dominant hand	67	29.6	37.7	43.6	48.8
Tapping—nondominant hand	68	23.5	32.9	38.9	43.2

Sensitivity, Specificity, Positive Predictive Power, Negative Predictive Power, and Overall Correct Classification for Finger Tapping Test for Moderate to Severe Brain-Injured Patients

	Sensitivity	Specificity	PPV	NPP	Overall correct
Tapping—dominant hand					
<50th	48	84	75	62	66
<25th	32	100	100	60	66
<10th	16	100	100	54	58
Tapping—nondominant hand					
<50th	56	88	82	66	71
<25th	28	100	100	58	64
<10th	16	100	100	54	58

Note. All in percentages.

Binder, Kelly, Villanueva, and Winslow (2003)

	Mild head injury, poor motivation (n = 34)		Mild head injury, good motivation (n = 22)		Moderate to severe head injury (n = 60)		
	M	SD	M	SD	M	SD	p
Age	40.97	10.94	39.64	12.33	30.77	10.15	>.07
Education	11.29	2.30	12.59	2.48	12.22	2.22	<.05[a]
Gender	18 women, 13 men		18 women, 14 men		17 women, 12 men		
Tapping–dominant hand	41.47	12.29	48.10	9.75	44.62	9.49	>.05
Tapping–nondominant hand	38.88	12.56	42.86	8.53	41.91	8.96	>.05

Note. The Finger Tapping Test was administered in three 10-second trials for both the dominant and nondominant hands, and the average number of taps per trial was converted into age, gender, and education-adjusted T-scores (Heaton et al., 1991).
[a] Moderate to severe head injury group was younger than both mild head injury groups.

Binder and Willis (1991)

	Mild head injury, poor effort (n = 10)		Mild head injury, good effort (n = 19)		
	M	SD	M	SD	p
Age	41.50	7.58	37.79	11.36	
Education	9.90	3.54	13.37	2.11	.001
Finger Tapping	71.89	16.54	88.44	11.84	.003
Grooved Pegboard	192.67	48.39	141.59	24.51	.001
Tactile Finger Recognition and Finger Tip Number Writing	18.13	7.43	3.61	3.47	.001

Note. Finger Tapping score is the sum of the average performance of both hands (three trials per hand). Grooved Pegboard (device not specified) is the time for each hand summed. Errors for Tactile Finger Recognition and Finger Tip Number Writing were summed.

Bowen and Little (1997)

	Litigant-claimants (n = 21)		Patients (n = 25)		Normals (n = 80)		
	M	SD	M	SD	M	SD	p
Kaufman Assessment Battery for Children—Hand Movements subtest	8.0	4.90	13.08	3.60	15.4	3.17	<.006

Note. Demographic data are limited: The only data available for the Normal group were an age range from 20 to 50. There was no difference between the patient and litigant-claimant groups for age (M = 38.4) or education (M = 14.1). Gender distribution was relatively even across groups except for a trend for more females in the litigant-claimant group.

Greiffenstein, Baker, and Gola (1996)

	PCS[a] females (n = 78)		PCS[a] males (n = 53)		TBI[b] females (n = 10)		TBI[b] males (n = 30)	
	M	SD	M	SD	M	SD	M	SD
Age	38.92	11.97	37.00	8.80	32.40	11.02	35.65	12.59
Education	11.40	1.47	11.33	1.68	11.18	1.25	11.12	1.24
Glasgow Coma Scale	15.00	0.00	15.00	0.00	9.09	3.08	8.72	2.69
Hospital Days	0.06	0.25	0.04	0.03	49.27	41.60	71.88	80.67
Tapping— dominant hand	33.32	13.23	36.86	14.09	34.09	14.19	39.40	12.07
Tapping— nondominant hand	31.95	12.17	36.58	12.50	28.55	16.40	34.35	12.23
Pegboard—dominant hand	86.04	11.36	101.35	46.40	77.27	31.15	132.23	95.53
Pegboard— nondominant hand	95.62	47.74	107.46	47.32	113.90	101.90	155.60	157.07
Grip—dominant hand	14.47	8.67	31.47	15.02	21.20	8.66	41.37	12.86
Grip—nondominant hand	13.91	7.82	30.80	15.09	15.70	10.23	38.26	13.37

Note. Finger Tapping was measured with the Halstead Finger Oscillation test with mean number of taps in the best three trials. Grip strength was measured in kilograms with the Smedley Dynamometer. Scores for both measures were converted to age, education, and gender-adjusted T-scores according to Heaton et al. (1991) norms. Dominant and nondominant T-scores were summed and divided by 2 to obtain the average for each task. The LaFayette Grooved Pegboard was used. Scores are recorded as seconds to completion.
[a] PCS, Postconcussive syndrome.
[b] TBI, traumatic brain injury.

Greiffenstein and Baker (2006)

	1991–1999 cohort PCS[a] (n = 300)		Moderate– severe TBI[b] (n = 91)		2000–2004 cohort PCS[a] (n = 307)		Moderate– severe TBI[b] (n = 61)	
	M	SD	M	SD	M	SD	M	SD
Age	35.89	11.80	33.14	12.50	42.70	12.20	38.02	15.40
Education	12.90	3.40	11.36	1.40	11.40	2.30	11.96	1.90
Gender	159 women, 141 men		24 women, 67 men		141 women, 166 men		18 women, 43 men	
Grip— dominant hand	29.64	15.10	37.43	12.30	29.50	14.30	36.90	12.60

Note. Grip strength was measured in kilograms with the Smedley Dynamometer. Scores were the average of four trials (two for each hand).
[a] PCS, postconcussive syndrome.
[b] TBI, traumatic brain injury.

Grip Strength Means, Standard Deviations, and Cutoff Scores Divided by Gender under Two Certainty Levels (Possible and Probable)

	1991–1999 moderate–severe TBI cohort				2000–2004 moderate–severe TBI cohort			
	M	SD	Possible	Probable	M	SD	Possible	Probable
Grip–females	26.44	10.50	< 26 kg	≤ 16 kg	25.63	10.00	< 25 kg	≤ 16 kg
Grip–males	41.37	10.30	< 41 kg	≤ 31 kg	40.03	10.00	< 40 kg	≤ 29 kg

Note. Grip strength was measured in kilograms with the Smedley Dynamometer. Scores were the average of four trials (two for each hand).

Heaton, Smith, Lehman, and Vogt (1978)

	Malingerers (n = 16)		Head injured (n = 16)		
	M	SD	M	SD	p
Age	24.4	7.5	26.7	6.5	>.05
Education	12.9	2.4	11.9	1.6	>.05
Gender	5 women, 11 men		3 women, 13 men		
Tapping Score	63.1	17.1	80.2	21.4	<.05
Pegboard Score	3.9	.9	6.3	7.3	>.05
Grip Strength	45.8	20.8	76.4	30.5	<.01
Seashore Rhythm (correct)	21.40	4.50	23.80	4.10	>.05
Speech Sounds (errors)	23.80	12.60	10.60	7.30	<.001
Finger Agnosia (errors)	7.20	5.60	3.50	3.70	<.05
Hole-Type Steadiness					
Steadiness	10.10	11.60	26.50	39.30	>.05
Hits	75.30	60.30	99.10	84.00	>.05

Note. Finger Tapping score is the sum of the mean score for each hand for 20-second trials. Grooved Pegboard (instrument unspecified) score is recorded as time in seconds per peg. Grip strength (specific instrument used not indicated) score is the sum of both hands in kg. Finger agnosia errors are summed for both sides of the body.

Inman and Berry (2002)

	Head-injured malingering (n = 21)		Noninjured malingering (n = 23)		Head-injured controls (n = 24)		Noninjured controls (n = 24)		
	M	SD	M	SD	M	SD	M	SD	p
Age	18.67	.91	18.91	1.27	18.67	1.69	18.42	.88	>.05
Education	12.48	.98	12.83	1.19	12.25	.61	12.21	.51	>.05
Gender	10 women, 11 men		16 women, 7 men		14 women, 10 men		16 women, 8 men		
Pegboard–dominant hand	38.24	11.90	32.17	12.95	43.67	9.87	45.33	11.30	<.01

(continued)

Inman and Berry (2002) *(continued)*

	Head-injured malingering (n = 21)		Noninjured malingering (n = 23)		Head-injured controls (n = 24)		Noninjured controls (n = 24)		
	M	SD	M	SD	M	SD	M	SD	p
Pegboard–nondominant hand	40.05	9.10	34.91	10.00	42.04	8.59	45.13	10.89	<.01
Grip–dominant hand	41.24	8.60	41.65	8.10	48.71	9.09	42.49	6.31	>.05
Grip–nondominant hand	43.29	6.62	42.30	9.36	47.50	8.70	44.04	5.79	>.05
Seashore Rhythm–T-score	40.91	10.94	43.83	14.49	53.00	9.83	54.75	12.39	<.01
Seashore Rhythm–(errors)	6.62	4.65	5.39	4.75	2.63	2.12	2.63	2.63	<.01

Note. Grooved Pegboard (instrument unspecified) scores were transformed to T-scores using Heaton et al. (1991) norms. Grip strength (instrument unspecified) scores were converted to age, education, and gender-corrected normative T-scores from the Heaton norms (Heaton et al., 1991).

Johnson and Lesniak-Karpiak (1997)

	Unwarned simulators (n = 8)		Warned simulators (n = 8)		Controls (n = 8)		
	M	SD	M	SD	M	SD	p
Age	19.80	.90	19.60	1.02	19.4	1.02	
IQ	107.17	9.62	107.97	8.11	107.6	28.78	
Pegboard–dominant hand	78.59	32.49	71.10	16.18	60.69	6.79	<.008
Pegboard–nondominant hand	82.38	32.52	76.59	19.27	66.03	8.43	<.021

Note. Grooved Pegboard (Klove, 1963) scores indicated in seconds taken to complete task.

Larrabee (2003)

	Definite MND[a] (n = 24)		Moderate to severe CHI (n = 27)		
	M	SD	M	SD	p
Age	39.33	11.78	34.80	16.78	<.28
Education	12.54	2.25	12.56	2.56	<.98
Gender	12 women, 12 men		13 women, 14 men		
Months posttrauma	32.70	13.00	44.50	85.00	<.48
Finger Tapping Score	70.97	26.72	83.43	10.48	

Note. Finger Tapping score is dominant plus nondominant hand raw score.
[a] MND, malingered neurocognitive dysfunction.

	Definite MND[a] (n = 24)		Probable MND (n = 17)		Neurological (n = 13)		Psychiatric (n = 14)		
	M	SD	M	SD	M	SD	M	SD	p
Age	39.33	11.78	43.06	11.39	49.92	13.16	45.29	12.21	<.32
Education	12.54	2.25	11.26	1.44	14.42	2.75	14.57	1.99	<.05
Gender	12 women, 12 men		5 women, 12 men		5 women, 8 men		8 women, 6 men		
Finger Tapping Score	70.97	26.72	66.86	30.27	90.31	11.94	89.39	10.70	

Note. Finger Tapping score is dominant plus nondominant hand raw score.
[a] MND, malingered neurocognitive dysfunction.

Rapport, Farchione, Coleman, and Axelrod (1998)

	Naïve malingerers (n = 31)		Coached malingerers (n = 32)		Controls (n = 29)		
	M	SD	M	SD	M	SD	p
Age	24.10	6.70	24.50	5.90	23.40	6.40	> .15
Education	14.40	1.10	14.50	.90	14.60	1.20	> .15
Gender	18 women, 13 men		18 women, 14 men		17 women, 12 men		
NAART IQ	100.60	6.20	101.00	5.30	103.60	7.90	> .15
Tapping—dominant hand	29.68	18.82	29.59	15.47	50.41	10.16	
Tapping—nondominant hand	30.35	19.55	28.78	15.85	48.59	9.02	
Grip—dominant hand	30.61	16.93	32.59	11.97	46.86	8.66	
Grip—nondominant hand	31.45	18.29	32.22	12.60	46.52	9.30	
Pegboard—dominant hand	26.35	18.88	34.66	16.74	50.83	10.13	
Pegboard—nondominant hand	27.06	15.65	35.12	15.22	47.07	8.58	

Note. Finger Tapping scores represented mean number of taps in five consecutive trials within 5 points. Grip strength scores reflected kg of pressure on Smedley dynamometer. Lafayette Grooved Pegboard scores were measured as time in seconds taken to complete task. Data are reported as adjusted T-scores using the normative data from Heaton et al. (1991).

Ross et al. (2006)

	Probable malingerers (n = 46)		Head injury group (n = 49)	
	M	SD	M	SD
Age	40.2	12.0	37.5	14.1
Education	12.0	2.4	13.4	2.7
Gender	50% male		59% male	
Ethnicity	63% white		78% white	

(continued)

Ross et al. (2006) *(continued)*

	Probable malingerers (*n* = 46)	Head injury group (*n* = 49)
Seashore Rhythm Test		
Cut score ≥ 8 errors	76% sensitivity	74% specificity
Cut score ≥ 10 errors	59% sensitivity	92% specificity
Speech Sounds Perception		
Cut score ≥ 10 errors	72% sensitivity	76% specificity
Cut score ≥ 13 errors	70% sensitivity	90% specificity

Trueblood and Schmidt (1993)

	Malingering (*n* = 8)		Patient control (*n* = 8)		Invalid (*n* = 8)		Patient control (*n* = 8)		
	M	Range	*M*	Range	*M*	Range	*M*	Range	*p*
Age	37.4	20–54	37.4	19–58	36.0	23–52	37.9	23–56	> .05
Education	12.0	10–15	11.6	8–14	12.5	9–17	12.1	10–14	> .05
Gender	4 women, 4 men		4 women, 4 men		7 women, 1 man		7 women, 1 man		
Tapping	73.0	38–102	91.5	65–112	72.0	22–103	88.8	72–103	
Seashore Rhythm (errors)	11.00	0–17	4.90	3–8*	8.40	3–15	3.30	0–8*	
Speech Sounds (errors)	20.50	5–30	6.60	3–16*	14.60	4–43	5.60	1–20	
Finger Tip Number Writing (errors)	6.80	1–15	2.30	0–8*	10.10	2–25	4.00	0–2*	
Finger Agnosia (errors)	2.60	0–9	.60	0–3	7.3	0–17	1.40	0–5*	

*Note. Finger Tapping is recorded as number of taps for both hands.
p < .05.

van Gorp et al. (1999)

	Suspected malingerers (n = 20)		Nonmalingerers (n = 61)		
	M	SD	M	SD	p
Age	40.50	11.51	35.35	12.96	.14
Education	12.70	3.30	13.53	4.27	.26
Pegboard—dominant hand	89.56	26.80	69.42	11.29	>.1
Pegboard—nondominant hand	92.72	31.49	79.31	21.68	>.1

Note. The Grooved Pegboard (Matthews & Klove, 1964) scores are not clearly defined.

Vickery et al. (2004)

	Head-injured malingerers (n = 23)		Community volunteer malingerers (n = 23)		Head-injured controls (n = 23)		Community volunteer controls (n = 23)		p	
	M	SD	M	SD	M	SD	M	SD	IS[a]	HS[b]
Age	29.9	11.3	32.5	10.5	34.1	14.8	38.7	14.0	.178	
Education	12.9	2.1	12.7	2.0	12.5	2.0	12.7	2.3	.921	
Tapping—dominant hand	30.3	15.8	37.2	13.2	38.5	11.3	47.2	10.0	.001	.006

Note. Finger Tapping scores recorded as T-scores.
[a] IS, instruction set status.
[b] HIS, head injury status.

CHAPTER 10

The MMPI-2 Fake Bad Scale in Detection of Noncredible Brain Injury Claims

Manfred F. Greiffenstein
David Fox
Paul R. Lees-Haley

Neuropsychologists conducting examinations in medicolegal circumstances typically evaluate for misrepresentation of cognitive status. Prospects for obtaining monetary compensation and powerful social benefits (sympathy, work release, lowered expectations) may provide strong incentives to exaggerate or fabricate cognitive deficits. But many persons reporting cognitive dysfunction resulting from compensable causes (traffic crashes, slip and falls, occupational injury, toxic exposures) may additionally report changes in physical health, personality, or emotional reactivity (Butcher & Miller, 1999; Sbordone & Liter, 1995). As a result, neuropsychologists must provide additional objective assessment of malingered and/or exaggerated emotional disorders in addition to evaluating for feigned cognitive defect.

This chapter focuses on techniques developed from the Minnesota Multiphasic Personality Inventory that are useful for detecting misrepresented personality and somatic change in a neuropsychological context. Over a decade of research has shown the Fake Bad Scale (FBS; Lees-Haley, English, & Glenn, 1991) to be sensitive to both feigned brain injury and promotion of nonpsychotic emotional syndromes. The purpose of this chapter is to:

- Review the history of MMPI/MMPI-2 validity scales in forensic contexts.
- Describe the conceptual and empirical deficiencies of the tradi-

tional MMPI-2 validity scales in settings where secondary gain is present.
- Summarize the development, psychometric properties, validity, and diagnostic efficiency of the FBS.
- Recommend best practices in using FBS and MMPI-F-family in forensic neuropsychological settings.

HISTORICAL BACKDROP

From the inception of standardized measures, psychologists recognized that personality tests were vulnerable to misrepresentation and deception. Lore has it that in the 1920s, Hermann Rorschach selected inkblots to make deception difficult. It was hypothesized that projective testing makes feigning more effortful and risky because "right" and "wrong" answers are not obvious. The advent of multiple-choice personality tests with face-valid items made it easier for even naïve respondents to discriminate abnormal from normal answers. The most commonly used of these tests is the Minnesota Multiphasic Personality Inventory (MMPI), updated in 1989 to the Minnesota Multiphasic Personality Inventory-2 (MMPI–2; Butcher, Dahlstrom, Tellegen, & Kaemmer, 1989; Butcher et al., 2001). Because of the ease with which a person could produce an abnormal MMPI profile not accurately reflective of his or her actual psychological condition, validity scales for detection of negative response bias (exaggeration of symptoms) and positive response bias (minimization of symptoms) were added at or soon after development of the MMPI.

The basic validity scales embedded in the MMPI are the Lie (L), Infrequency (F), and Correction (K) scales. The 64-item F scale was developed by selecting deviant responses endorsed by < 10% of the standardization sample, although empirically the base rate was < 5% for most items (Dahlstrom, Welsh, & Dahlstrom, 1975). The 15-item L scale was rationally developed "to identify deliberate or intentional efforts to evade answering the test frankly and honestly" (Dahlstrom, Welsh, & Dahlstrom, 1972, p. 108). The K scale was later developed to improve discrimination of normal from abnormal profiles in cases in which mentally ill persons hid psychopathology (Dahlstrom et al., 1972). The derivative Gough Dissimulation Index (F–K) was proposed in 1947. When the MMPI was restandardized into the MMPI-2, additional validity scales were developed, including the Fb ("Backpage" F) scale consisting of items rarely endorsed in the second half of the test, and the Infrequency–Psychopathology scale (Fp; Arbisi & Ben-Porath, 1995). The Fp items were selected for a frequency of < 20% in psychiatric inpatients as Fp was intended to address exaggeration in otherwise genuine psychiatric patients, although they did not distinguish between plausible and implausible clinical histories, a theme that is developed in later sections. Along with the F scale, the Fb, and the

Fp are based on the premise that frequent endorsement of infrequent items is suggestive of symptom exaggeration, or "faking bad." The F, Fb, Fp, and F–K scales are collectively termed the MMPI-2 "F-family."

There is a surprising dearth of research on the F-family's validity in *natural* samples. Inspection of the classic *MMPI Handbooks* (Dahlstrom et al., 1972, 1975) revealed all F-family studies relied on *simulation* (analog) designs, meaning undergraduates or community volunteers were asked to feign disorders or personality styles. Berry et al. (1995) summarized the construct validity of the F-family in detection of distortion but compiled only studies examining MMPI validity patterns in coached volunteers. Lim and Butcher (1996) recognized the limitations of simulation studies and concluded: "Particularly we recommend more studies of faking be constructed in real-world settings or non-analogue studies to examine further the generalizability of findings" (p. 24). Despite recognition of a 60-year dearth of applied (nonanalog) studies on the F-family, research with real-world forensic samples by MMPI-2 advocates has been almost nonexistent, with the exception of those studying the FBS. The next section describes the empirical and conceptual deficiencies of the F-family in more detail.

LIMITATIONS OF THE F-FAMILY

The F-family is based on the theoretical assumption that overendorsement of unusual symptoms is a sign of malingering. This position implies all malingering is alike. Although the MMPI-2 is the most frequently used psychometric scale in neuropsychological forensic settings (Lees-Haley, Smith, Williams, & Dunn, 1996), there is little scientific basis for assuming the F-family can detect any form of feigned psychological abnormality or simulated neuropsychological impairments as they present in noncriminal settings. Greiffenstein, Gola, and Baker (1995) first drew attention to this issue, observing probable neurocognitive malingering but unremarkable F-family scores in persons with remote head injury. There is no doubt that extremely elevated F-family scores "rule in" profile invalidity. The problem with the F-family is unproven sensitivity and the related concept of negative predictive power, meaning no proven ability to rule out all forms of exaggeration or feigned mental disorders in personal injury settings.

Content Validity

General

Lanyon and Almer (2001) argue that measurement of self-serving misrepresentations requires psychometrics tailored to the nature of the misrepresentation. Empirical studies show that F-family contains items tailored to a clinical setting where overreporting of *psychotic* presentations would predominate. Steadily increasing F scale elevations are accompanied by higher elevations on scales 6 and 8 but decreasing elevations on scales 1, 2, 3, 4, 7, and 9 (Hathaway & Meehl, 1951). Hence, F elevations are associated with a picture of paranoid schizophrenia. It follows then that situations in which misrepresentations do not involve pretending psychosis where denial of psychopathology is rare, the F-family may lack content validity.

Somatic and Nonpsychotic Exaggeration

Content validity means the degree to which a test measures all the facets of a clinical phenomenon. The F-family is designed to capture feigned severe psychopathology but has little content reflective of somatic misrepresentation. Larrabee (1998) points out that the F-scale shares only one item in common with scales 1 (Hypochondriasis; Hs) and 3 (Hysteria; Hy). F shows a modest correlation with Hs (.41–.46) and a negligible one with Hy (.07–.10) in the normative sample, per the administration manual. Keller and Butcher's (1991) book on the MMPI-2 and chronic pain shows low scores on the F scale despite drawing almost all cases from the workers' compensation system. The appendices to Keller and Butcher (1991) allow scoring of the FBS. The mean FBS score for chronic pain patients was 22.4 versus 13.8 for the normal sample.

Misrepresentation of emotional distress other than psychosis is another domain the F-family was not tailored for and does not capture. This is a crucial weakness because spurious complaints in litigated brain injury settings rarely simulate a psychosis. Personal injury plaintiffs feigning mental illness do not "act crazy" but just try to show major distress, heightened emotionality, or high reactivity to stressful events. One study (Greiffenstein et al., 1995) showed the F scale to be less sensitive to noncredible brain injury claims than content-valid effort measures. Later, Greiffenstein, Baker, Gola, Donders, and Miller (2002) documented the F and F-K scales to be insensitive to illogical head injury histories, while Greiffenstein, Baker, Axelrod, Peck, and Gervais (2004) found the entire F-family unable to differentiate patently spurious from genuine posttraumatic stress disorder (PTSD). Rogers, Sewell, Martin, and Vitacco (2003) observed much larger group effects when simulators were asked to fake psychosis than when they were asked to fake neurotic variants.

Role-Play Validation and Generalization

A limitation of the F-family is validation based on role-play simulation using undergraduates (Lim & Butcher, 1996). Referring again to both *Handbooks*, all studies of F-family validity from 1945 to 1975 rely on role-play simulation. This methodology grossly inflates validity coefficients or group differences.

The basic formula for role-play simulation is to instruct naïve undergraduates or community volunteers to feign psychopathology, model ideal mental health, or imagine a specific personality. In the first scenario (i.e., feigning mental illness), predictably, students and volunteers typically produce *extreme* F-family elevations that represent crude stereotypes of mental illness and malingering. Rogers et al. (2003) conducted a meta-analysis of MMPI/MMPI-2 validity scales and reported huge group effects when relying on undergraduate simulators feigning mental illness (Cohen's effect size = 4.0). In contrast, litigants with psychiatric histories score less than one-half standard deviation above nonlitigating patients (Cohen's effect size = 0.4). Rothke et al. (2000) showed that Social Security Disability applicants, a population at risk for exaggeration, produced much lower Fp scores than undergraduates simulating various disorders. Clearly, undergraduates distort responses differently than actual compensation seekers. A fair conclusion is that role play has limited generalization to real-world samples.

THE FAKE BAD SCALE

In light of the F-family's limitations, there were some earlier attempts to develop alternative validity scales focused more on the spectrum of nonpsychotic presentations. Gough (1954) believed that item endorsement would be different between those people pretending to be "experiencing a psychoneurotic reaction" and those who actually were. He developed the Dissimulation Scale (Ds) on which scores represented "the product of the stereotypic views that normal subjects have about psychoneurotic patients" (Dahlstrom et al., 1972, p. 151). It was later revised by Gough into the Ds-r and remains scorable on the MMPI-2. Later, Butcher and Harlow (1987) argued that scales 1 (Hypochondriasis) and 3 (Hysteria) were most predictive of malingering in industrial injury, because of content reflective of medically unexplained somatic complaints. Working in Gough's tradition of investigating nonpsychotic misrepresentation, the present third author (Lees-Haley) developed a scale that would measure the kind of symptom overreporting specific to the medicolegal context.

Item Pool Development

Lees-Haley et al. (1991) voiced concern with the MMPI-2 F-family's value in the types of response distortion seen during personal injury litigation. Based on experience with compensation seekers claiming psychological and/or neuropsychological damages, Lees-Haley observed that litigants with implausible-sounding case histories produced unremarkable MMPI-2 F-family scores, an observation shared by others (e.g., Butcher & Miller, 1999). Instead, plaintiffs misrepresenting psychological symptoms voiced marked distress, functional impairment, and great *suffering* blamed on the legal cause of action. Lees-Haley et al. (1991) hypothesized that the MMPI F-family may not detect the type of response distortion common in psychological damages claims. The authors set out to create a new MMPI-2-derived scale designed to capture the exaggerated suffering of some litigants.

The litigation-related items were selected on an empirical basis much like the MMPI clinical scales, using a mixed-group validation design. Lees-Haley et al. (1991) gave the MMPI-2 to medical outpatients asked to simulate mental illness (role-play simulation strategy), personal injury litigants classified as malingering distress, and litigants with genuine-appearing symptom histories (known-groups strategy). The resulting frequency counts resulted in 43 items with higher endorsements in the role-play simulation and probable malingering groups. The authors then conducted a post hoc, rational analysis of the chosen items. They concluded that the items reflected a dual strategy of (1) exaggerating postinjury emotional distress but also (2) underreporting or minimizing preincident personality problems. More concretely, such litigants put effort into appearing honest and psychologically normal except for the influence of the alleged incident. They downplay the presence or severity of preexisting psychopathology and hide antisocial or other behavior that would discredit them while overemphasizing disability within the limits of plausibility. Hence, there are elements of both "faking bad" and "faking good" in spurious presentations during *civil* medicolegal presentations. Such presentations are not contradictory but goal oriented: These dual tactics may leave a global impression that the plaintiff was ideally well adjusted in the past but is now very distressed. The authors termed this new 43-item set the "Fake Bad Scale" (see Appendix 10.1 for scoring key).

Normative Data and Psychometric Properties

Greene (2000) reported means and central dispersions for the FBS based on the entire MMPI-2 normative sample. Males endorsed a mean of 11.7 items ($SD = 3.81$) and females averaged 13.76 ($SD = 4.14$). Using z-scores of +1.5 SDs and +2 SDs to calculate FBS cutoffs representing the 93rd and 98th percentiles by gender results in the following scores:

Males FBS scores	Females FBS scores
1.5 SD = 17	1.5 SD = 20
2.0 SD = 19	2.0 SD = 22

These results provide evidence that elevated scores on the FBS are rare among community residing persons not claiming mental health disorders.

FBS has been found to be normally distributed in the normative sample (males skewness = 0.52, kurtosis = 0.56; females skewness = 0.57, kurtosis =

TABLE 10.1. Normative Characteristics of the Fake Bad Scale

Author	n	Skewness	Kurtosis
Lees-Haley[a]	213 medicolegal	−.105	−.485
Greenberg & Lees-Haley[a]	269 medicolegal	−.094	−.453
Lees-Haley[a]	650 medicolegal	−.04	−.223
Fox	873 medicolegal	−.096	−.46
Fox	149 psychiatric outpatients	.268	−.778
Millis	23 severe TBI	2.11	5.76

[a] These samples share some data and are not fully independent.

0.96; Greene, personal communication, 2005); in personal injury claimants (Males skewness = .015, kurtosis = −.496; Females skewness = .087, kurtosis = .024; Lees-Haley, personal communication, July 2005); and in a sample of patients with severe traumatic brain injury (TBI) (skewness = 0.52, kurtosis = −0.32; Ross, personal communication, April 15, 2005). Table 10.1 reproduces additional data on FBS score distribution. These distribution features suggest that the FBS represents a normally distributed variable amenable to statistical analysis and probability estimation. This is unlike the F, Fb, and Fp, which are not normally distributed in medicolegal samples (Fox, 2005).

Use of the FBS with the 370-Item MMPI-2 and with Incomplete Data

To extend its usefulness to the MMPI-2 short form, Fox examined 707 protocols from several contexts (medical legal, psychiatric, and nonmental health referrals) to establish empirically derived coefficients for predicting full FBS scores when only the 370-Item form MMPI-2 is administered. Full and partial FBS scores based on the 370-Item form (FBS-S) were extracted from complete protocols. Regression analyses using the FBS-S score and demographic variables were used to predict full FBS scores. Demographics were found to be noncontributory. Fox found that the full FBS score can be accurately prorated from the FBS-S (those items appearing in the 370-Item form of the MMPI-2). There is a modest advantage in using the empirically derived coefficient rather than a rationally derived estimate, although both are adequate. Fox provided coefficients and a table for prorating FBS-S scores.

Nelson, Parsons, Grote, Smith, and Sisung (2006) noted that "clinicians may not always have access to True FBS (T-FBS) scores, such as when True-False answer sheets are unavailable or published research studies do not report FBS raw scores" (p. 1) and performed a cross-validation of Larrabee's (2003a) linear regression formula that provides estimated FBS (E-FBS) scores derived from weighted validity and clinical T-scores. They concluded that E-

FBS scores correlated very highly with T-FBS scores, particularly for women. They further concluded that "When matching to T-FBS "high" and "low" scores, the E-FBS scores demonstrated the highest hit rate (92.5%) through use of Lees-Haley's (1992) revised cutoffs for men and women. These same cutoffs resulted in excellent overall specificity for both the T-FBS scores (92.5%) and E-FBS scores (90.6%)" (p. 1). They stated, "The authors conclude that the E-FBS represents an adequate estimate of T-FBS scores in the current epilepsy sample. Use of E-FBS scores may be especially useful when clinicians conduct the MMPI-2 short form, which does not include all of the 43 FBS items but does include enough items to compute each of the validity and clinical T-Scores. Future studies should examine E-FBS sensitivity in compensation-seekers with incomplete effort" (p. 1).

Reliability

Reliability of psychological scales is typically conceptualized as having two characteristics: internal consistency (i.e., do the items of the scale measure a single construct?) and temporal stability. Because scales such as the FBS measure a particular time-limited behavior (symptom exaggeration) rather than a persisting psychological trait, temporal stability is probably not a meaningful measure.

Even internal consistency may be difficult to measure because Lees-Haley designed the scale to have multiple factors. In fact, analysis of internal consistency has shown there to be several factors in the scale. In heretofore unpublished data, Fox (2005) examined each item of the FBS for a sample consisting of 873 individuals in workers' compensation, personal injury, or disability claim cases. A factor analysis yielded a figure of .88 for these data on the Kaiser–Meyer–Olkin and Bartlett's tests, which suggests that there is a meaningful factor structure to the scale. Most of the variance was accounted for by five factors.

Sensitivity

Sensitivity is an important characteristic of all psychological scales. Sensitivity is defined as a scale's ability to detect conditions or traits known to be present. If the FBS measures increased reporting of symptoms in excess of injury characteristics, the FBS should be elevated in criterion groups at risk for symptom misrepresentation. Groups in civil litigation alleging persistent emotional and neuropsychological symptoms are at higher risk for overreporting of symptoms. The existence of a compensable injury or a lawsuit does not automatically mean exaggeration is present but findings of malingering prevalence rates in the 40% range (e.g., Mittenberg, Patton, Canyock, & Condit, 2002) make litigation groups the ideal natural group to study.

Numerous studies examined FBS sensitivity to misrepresented brain injury. Millis, Putnam, and Adams (1995) were the first to investigate FBS validity patterns in a pseudoneurological population and reported higher FBS scores in litigants with remote mild trauma versus patients with moderate–severe closed head injury (CHI). Martens, Donders, and Millis (2001) examined 100 consecutive head injury patients using gender-specific FBS criteria; they found individuals pursuing litigation were five times more likely to have positive FBS scores than nonlitigants. Other studies relied on a known-groups paradigm to form criterion groups (Greiffenstein, Baker, & Gola, 1994; Rogers, 1997). Putnam, Millis, and Adams (1998) reported an FBS cutoff score of 22 resulted in a 93% correct classification of persons selected for poor scores on simple two-choice memory tests. Greiffenstein et al. (2002) reported acceptable diagnostic efficiency in discriminating (1) illogical versus logical symptom evolution and (2) litigation versus non-litigating status in 277 participants with mixed head injury and financial features. Ross, Millis, Krukowski, Putnam, and Adams (2004) used the Warrington Recognition Memory Test to bifurcate head injury groups and reported a combined hit rate of 92% in discriminating 59 probable malingerers alleging mild CHI, from 59 nonlitigating patients with moderate–severe CHI. Bianchini et al. (2003), using the Slick, Sherman, and Iverson (1999) criteria for identifying malingering, found elevated FBS scores in four persons with suspicious toxic exposure claims. Larrabee's (2003d) cross-validation study used atypical patterns on genuine neuropsychological tests as his operational criterion and found the FBS was the most sensitive test of five different validity indicators, which included reliable digit span (Greiffenstein et al., 1994), with a reported combined hit rate of 83.6%. This was comparable to the optimal cutoff score of > 21 Larrabee reported in an earlier study of malingered neurocognitive dysfunction (Larrabee, 2003a). Larrabee (2003c) settled on an FBS score of 22 showing good sensitivity and specificity in discriminating litigants with definite malingered neurocognitive dysfunction. In a study of pain questionnaires as potential tools for detecting exaggerated pain, Larrabee (2003c) concluded that until further cross-validation is available, pain questionnaires should be used in conjunction with other evidence of symptom exaggeration and poor effort, including measures such as the FBS, Portland Digit Recognition Test, and Word Memory Test.

Detection of spurious emotional injury claims is another branch of FBS research. Two studies used known-groups designs. Lees-Haley (1992) used rational grounds to divide a heterogeneous sample of 119 litigants into believable and spurious claimants. A cutoff of > 23 for men and > 25 for women correctly classified 75% of male and 74% of female spurious PTSD claimants and 96% of male and 92% of female controls. Greiffenstein et al. (2004) compared the FBS with the F-family in the detection of implausible PTSD claims. The implausible group showed a FBS mean of 27 versus 20 in a recent (but still compensable) PTSD group; the severe but litigating PTSD group scored intermediate. Differential prevalence studies generally show mean FBS scores at or above 20. In a study of a sample of 492 personal injury plaintiffs, the mean FBS score for plaintiffs was 20.8 (Lees-Haley, 1997). Using a differential design, Posthuma and Harper (1998) studied 95 personal injury litigants, reporting FBS means of 22 (SD = 6.7) for both males and females, higher than in groups not seeking compensation. Interestingly, child custody litigants scored low on the FBS, tentatively suggesting that the adversarial process per se is not a factor in the FBS. Tsushima and Tsushima (2001) compared 120 patients involved in personal injury litigation to 251 nonlitigants and found a litigation related FBS mean of 21 (SD = 7) versus means less than 18 for the other groups. Martinez, Mittenberg, Gass, and Quintar (2005) used discriminant function analysis to predict forensic status in a heterogeneous sample of disability seekers and genuine patients. The FBS was overall superior to the F-family and a raw score of ≥ 22 represented specificity of 0.90.

A smaller number of studies examined FBS sensitivity using simulation (analog) designs. Diagnosis specific criteria were made available to volunteers asked to feign various disorders, and results indicated that inmates asked to feign insanity produced a mean FBS of 22 (SD = 6) (Iverson, Henrichs, Barton, & Allen 2002); genuine psychiatric patients asked to exaggerate their psychopathology underperformed on FBS relative to the F scale (Rogers, Sewell, & Ustad, 1995); community volunteers feigning brain injury produced significantly higher FBS scores (mean = 25) versus honest responders (Dearth et al., 2005); and college students misrepresenting PTSD performed poorly on the FBS (Elhai, Gold, Sellers, & Dorfman, 2001). Cramer (1995) showed simulators produced higher FBS scores when asked to feign anxiety symptoms than when asked to feign psychosis. Interestingly, the simulators produced extreme scores on the F-family with both the neurotic and psychotic scripts. A tentative generalization from simulation studies is that the FBS better captures feigned neurological and neurotic status but the F-family captures misrepresentation of the severest psychopathology.

Specificity

Specificity refers to a scale's ability to rule out conditions or traits known to be absent. In the context of validity testing, a good scale should identify persons known for making genuine self-report ("not faking"). Specificity is closely related to positive predictive power, which means the probability of detecting a target symptom given a score predicting that symptom. Starting with the MMPI-2 standardization sample, Greene (1997) reported 1,167 males produced a mean FBS score of 11.7 (SD = 3.8), while 1,376 females averaged an FBS of 13.76 (SD = 4). Specificity calculations relative to the original cut score of 20 results in .984 for males and .956 for females. The remainder of this section summarizes FBS performance in psychological examinees not reported as seeking compensation for their distress. Two approaches are next reviewed: studies reporting grouped data and those providing actuarial data. The latter are more conducive to calculating specificity.

Table 10.2 summarizes a number of studies reporting central dispersion statistics for the FBS in examinees without any obvious incentive to exaggerate. Lees-Haley et al. (1991) estimated mean FBS scores for the 540 psychiatric inpatients described in the MMPI-2 manual. The mean score was 19.1 for women and 16.9 for men; standard deviations could not be calculated because of the grouped data. Posthuma and Harper (1998) gave the MMPI-2 to child custody litigants. They reported a mean FBS of 15.5 (SD = 3.5) in female child custody litigants and a mean of 13.5 (SD = 3.1) in male custody litigants. Tsushima and Tsushima (2001) documented an FBS mean of 17 (SD = 6) among 208 psychology clinic referrals and 11 (SD = 3) in 43 persons undergoing preemployment screenings; females scored slightly higher in both cases. Meyers, Millis, and Volkert (2002) found an FBS mean of 18 (SD = 6) in a nonlitigating sample of 100 chronic pain patients with serious neurological illnesses. Table 10.1 summarizes mean and central dispersion data for many studies. The table shows the highest mean FBS scores were achieved by the 48 persons seen shortly after life-threatening workplace stressors but before litigation (Greiffenstein et al., 2004). Hence, *potential* compensability may be associated with higher FBS scores in otherwise nonlitigating groups. Two generalizations can be made. First, females score higher on the FBS by roughly two items. Second, a sizable minority of females with psychiatric histories score above 20, assuming normal kurtosis. As a practical matter, the latter finding will have relatively little effect on most forensic neuropsychologists because the majority of plaintiffs deny having a history of psychiatric outpatient treatment and the overwhelming majority denies any history of inpatient psychiatric treatment.

Numerous studies reported actuarial FBS data in groups presenting for psychological testing but not seeking compensation. Tsushima and Tsushima's (2001) large sample of psychology clinic patients showed 15% of females and 7% of males scored above 24. Iverson et al. (2002) performed a specificity-only study examining FBS scores in mixed groups of male non-litigants. The original cutoff score of > 20 misclassified 30% of seriously ill outpatients awaiting organ transplants and 24% of inpatient substance abusers but only 4% of inmates. However, cut-scores of > 26 kept false-positive errors below 10% (specificity > 90%). Miller and Donders (2001) found FBS scores > 23 in only 4% of persons with moderate severe brain injury seen clinically 1 year postinjury. In an unpublished study, Fox (2005) reported no job applicant (N = 69) scored above 20 and only 9% of 80 criminal probationers scored > 23. Woltersdorf (2005) gave the FBS to a large sample of patients with unequivocal neurological disease and found none that exceeded a raw score of 20. Meyers et al. (2002) observed that no nonlitigating

TABLE 10.2. Fake Bad Scale Performances in Groups Rated as Genuine on a Priori Basis

First author (year)	Group	n	Mean score	SD
Greene (1997)	MMPI-2 normative sample–males	1,138	11.7	3.8
Greene (1997)	MMPI-2 normative sample–females	1,462	13.8	4.1
Iverson (2002)	Federal prison inmates (males)	25	9.8	4.1
Fox (2005)	Probationers	80	15.51	5.64
Fox (2005)	Job applicants	69	13.52	2.97
	Medical patients			
Millis (1995)	Moderate–severe traumatic brain injury	20	16.1	4.9
Iverson (2002)	Medical outpatients–transplant candidates–males	20	15.3	7.6
Millis (1999)	Severe TBI	23	15.09	5.51
	Psychiatric patients			
Lees-Haley (1991)	MMPI-2 psychiatric sample–estimated, males	–	16.9	–
Lees-Haley (1991)	MMPI-2 psychiatric sample (females)	–	19.1	–
	Patients with chronic psychiatric problems	42	22.1	5.8
Iverson (2002)	Male veterans–inpatient substance abuse unit	25	15.6	6.4
	Child custody litigants			
Posthuma (1998)	No alleged abuse–males	–	13.8	3.0
Posthuma (1998)	No alleged abuse–females	–	13.8	3.0
Posthuma (1998)	Alleged physical abuse–males	–	13.6	3.1
Posthuma (1998)	Alleged physical abuse–females	–	15.1	3.6
Posthuma (1998)	Alleged sexual abuse–males	–	13.5	3.1
Posthuma (1998)	Alleged sexual abuse–females	–	16.0	3.5
	Personal injury			
Greiffenstein (2004)	Presumed credible work-stress claimants[a]	48	20.1	2.3
Fox (2005)	Litigants rated as credible on a priori basis	21	19.1	5.5

[a] Mostly workplace robberies; took place in compensable context but seen early.

chronic pain patient scored higher than 29 on the FBS, and Ross et al. (2004) documented that no CHI subject scored over 26. Martens et al. (2001) found 22% of mixed CHI patients to score above gender-specific FBS cutoffs of 23 and 25. The ratio of positive to absent psychiatric histories was 2:1 in patients with FBS above cutoffs but 1:5 in those below cutoffs; in addition, scores above cutoffs were more common in females. Larrabee (2003a) further reported a combined error rate of 16% associated with FBS of 22 or higher, superior to base rate prediction alone with malingering prevalence of > 16% and < 84% (Gouvier, 1999). Per Ross et al., who obtained a lower combined error rate of .10, an FBS cut-score of 22 or more will be effective when the base rate of malingering is > 10% and < 90% (Gouvier, 1999). However, preaccident psychiatric history as a moderator was not examined.

Table 10.3 presents a summary of FBS specificity data. Only studies involving patients without external incentive were included, although unspoken incentives can never be ruled out. The data of Butcher, Arbisi, Atlis, and McNulty (2003) are not included for lack of extra-test data necessary to

TABLE 10.3. Summary of FBS Frequency and Specificity Data for Clinical Groups with Known Nonlegal Status

First author (year)	Group	n	FBS cut score ≤ 20	≤ 22	≤ 25	≤ 28	≤ 29
Miller (2001)	Severe TBI	28	25	25	27	27	28
Tsushima (2001)	Psychiatric patient female	111	89	100	105	108	109
Tsushima (2001)	Psychiatric patient male	97	65	76	87	94	96
Iverson (2002)	Medical Ill males	20	14	15	16	19	20
Iverson (2002)	Substance abusers, male	25	19	21	23	25	25
Iverson (2002)	Inmates, males	50	48	50	50	50	50
Meyers (2002)	Moderate–severe CHI	59	50	54	56	59	59
Larrabee (2003b)	CHI	29	23	25	27	29	29
Ross (2004)	Clinical TBI	41	36	37	39	41	41
Greiffenstein (2005)	Nontraumatic brain diseases	29	17	24	27	29	29
Greve (2006)	Nontraumatic brain diseases	132	107	121	128	132	132
Greve (2006)	Moderate–severe CHI, no incentive	18	14	14	16	18	18
Fox (2005)	Probationers (criminal)	80	64	69	73	79	80
Fox (2005)	Job applicants	69	68	69	69	69	69
Barr (2005)	Inpatient epilepsy unit	51	35	42	46	49	51
Woltersdorf (2005)	Mixed neurology	150	150	150	150	150	150
Martinez (2005)	Acute head trauma	63	52	58	60	63	63
	Cumulative total	1,052	876	950	999	1,040	1,049
	Specificity		.833	.903	.950	.988	.997

gauge believability, as recommended by Butcher and Williams (1992). Table 10.3 shows that specificity is 83% for scores above Lees-Haley et al.'s (1991) original cut-score of 20, probably an unacceptable level of false-positives. False-positive errors drop to < 10% at FBS ≥ 23 and become negligible at above 25. At 30 and above, false-positive errors are < 1%. Hence, an FBS score > 29 is associated with near perfect confidence in finding symptom magnification.

Some generalizations about FBS specificity are now warranted. First, an FBS score ≥ 23 provides increasing evidence of symptom exaggeration, because of its association with a 10% false-positive rate; many researchers use an a priori specificity of 0.9. Second, females as a group tend to score an average of 2 points higher on the FBS than males, irrespective of clinical status. Third, Iverson et al.'s (2002) and Meyer et al.'s (2002) data suggest that persons with severe but *objectively manifested* physiological distress (drug withdrawal, severe illnesses) will score relatively high on the FBS, requiring upward adjustment of the FBS cut-score. Fourth, scores above the original cutoff of 20 are associated with psychiatric treatment histories in females. Finally, scores of 30+ never or rarely produce false-positive errors. Put differently, the positive predictive power of the FBS > 29 is virtually 100%.

Construct Validity

Construct validity is defined as the degree to which an operational measure captures an underlying concept. Two methods are generally relied on: *convergent validity* or the degree to which your measure correlates with measures capturing the same construct, and *discriminant validity*, the degree to which your measure departs from tests measuring a different concept. Correlational analyses and factor analysis are the preferred means of investigating construct validity.

Studies that compare the FBS with F-family patterns address discriminant validity. A recurring theme of this chapter is that the two scales capture different forms of pseudoabnormalities, and to this extent groups with subjective medical disability should score higher on the FBS than on the F-family. In comparison to the FBS, studies utilizing natural groups (as opposed to paid simulators) consistently show the F-family's insensitivity to misrepresented brain injury in persons without radiological or electrophysiological abnormalities (Eyler, Diehl, & Kirkhart, 2000; Greiffenstein et al., 1995; Larrabee, 1997, 1998, 2003a, 2003b; Ross et al., 2004); persons with implausible PTSD (Greiffenstein et al., 2004; Lees-Haley, 1992); litigated distress (Posthuma & Harper, 1998; Tsushima & Tsushima, 2001); and medically unexplained pain (Larrabee, 1998). In the only study using a mixed-group validation design to examine MMPI-2 validity scales in a personal injury context, Crawford, Greene, and Dupart (2006) asked undergraduates to feign depression blamed on industrial accidents. They assigned dimensional values representing the base rate for malingering to genuine depressed inpatients and the student simulators. They reported only FBS generated acceptable true and false-positive rates. A nice summary of findings can be found in a recent meta-analysis by Nelson, Sweet and Demakis (2006). These authors performed a meta-analysis of the FBS in which they examined the weighted mean effect sizes of commonly used MMPI-2 validity scales. They found that the FBS had the largest grand effect size (.96) in a comparison of FBS, L, F, K, Fb, Fp, F-K, O-S, Ds2, and Dsr2. They concluded that "the FBS performs as well as, if not superior to, other validity scales in discriminating overreporting and comparison groups" and "the preponderance of the present literature supports the scale's use within forensic settings" (Nelson et al., 2006, p. 39).

Natural samples of persons seeking compensation for unexplained medical symptoms outside neurology are of special interest. The FBS is used as a measure of bodily oriented exaggeration, so the FBS should be elevated in such populations relative to the F-family. Staudenmeyer and Phillips (2007) administered the MMPI-2 to 70 litigants reporting subjective organ failure blamed on low toxic exposure, a claim the authors termed "idiopathic environmental intolerance" (IEI). The IEI group's mean FBS T-score was above 70, but F and Fp were close to the MMPI-2 standardization group mean. Binder, Storzbach, and Salinsky (2006) consecutively evaluated 14 persons claiming multiple chemical sensitivities (MCS) as the basis for subjective disability. The mean FBS score for the MCS group was 27, compared to 17 for genuine seizure patients and 20 for nonepileptic seizure patients.

Studies relevant to convergent validity are those showing significant correlations between the FBS and validity scales sensitive to malingered cognitive deficit. Greiffenstein et al. (2002) reported a negative correlation between FBS and finger tapping (high FBS scorers tap more slowly), evidence the FBS captures exaggerated physical deterioration. Slick, Hopp, Strauss, and Spellacy (1996) found that FBS scores were correlated both with response time scores and number of items correct on the Victoria Symptom Validity Test (VSVT) for both easy and hard items. Eyler et al. (2000) reported that FBS showed an association with atypical cognitive score patterns (e.g., Digit Span below Vocabulary) and somatic exaggeration scales of the MMPI-2 but not with the F-family. In contrast, others have observed modest correlations between FBS and F-family scales (Butcher et al., 2003; Greiffenstein et al., 2002).

Another approach is to include the FBS in factor analyses of various well-established validity scales, such as the F-family. Fox and Lees-Haley recently examined the factor structure of the validity scales of the MMPI-2 in 650 medicolegal cases. Using a principal components analysis, 73% of the variance was accounted for by three components. The first component (exaggeration) was composed of the F-family of scales and the FBS. The second component (defensiveness) consisted of the FBS and scales L and K. The final component (unreliability) loaded with Trust Response Inconsistency (TRIN) and Variable Response Inconsistency (VRIN). Subsequent analysis supported this factor structure in subgroups composed of individuals who were employed, not employed, or with verified brain injury. Those without brain injury showed only two factors—exaggeration and defensiveness. This pattern is similar to that previously reported by Fox, Gerson and Lees-Haley (1995). These findings imply that the FBS does measure symptom over-reporting as well as other techniques of "impression management."

Greiffenstein, Baker, and Gola (1996) made the first tentative statement of FBS construct validity, concluding that it predominantly measured exaggerated physical disability. This was later supported by Ross et al. (2004). Greiffenstein et al. (2002) later termed the FBS a "hybrid" scale quantifying overreporting of nonpsychotic symptoms from multiple domains. Butcher et al. (2003) published data showing FBS correlated highest with Health Concerns and significantly with most other Content scales *except* for Bizarre Mentation, consistent with diffuse overreporting of nonpsychotic symptoms. Hence, the FBS appears to quantify the nonspecific symptom reporting of litigants producing diffusely elevated MMPI-2 profiles despite acceptable F scales that Butcher and Miller (1999) address. Greiffenstein (2005) has unpublished data bearing on this issue. Based on Butcher and Miller's (1999) notion of using the MMPI-2 to determine whether physical or psychological symptoms are consistent with a claimed disability in a personal injury evaluation, the first author defined exaggerated disability as multisystem complaints in gross excess of initial injury characteristics. If the FBS is a measure of exaggerated disability, a good test of this hypothesis is to examine FBS elevations as a function of initial injury severity. Using the Glasgow Coma Scale (GCS) as an operational measure of initial injury severity, Greiffenstein analyzed unpublished FBS, F, and Fb data on 481 late postconcussion claimants from his patient database. This sample was more than 2 years post-head injury, mostly minor, and all were seen for either disability recertification or litigation related examinations. Figure 10.1 shows a clear inverse dose–response relationship between FBS scores and initial injury severity. The more minor the injury, the higher mean FBS, and the more severe the injury (GCS < 9), the lower the score. In contrast, the F and Fb scales showed no significant association with severity in this large sample of disability applicants. Tests of linearity with a one-way analysis of variance (ANOVA) showed a significant association (F (1,478) = 64, p < .0001). Neither F nor Fb showed significant linearity (p = .10 and .08, respectively). Multiple regression analysis showed R = –.34 for FBS, compared to –.07 and –.08 for the other validity scales.

Criticisms of the FBS

There are two published papers critical of the FBS by Bury and Bagby (2002) and Butcher et al. (2003). These papers are presently in wide circulation among trial lawyers and introduced during cross-examination. In view of the

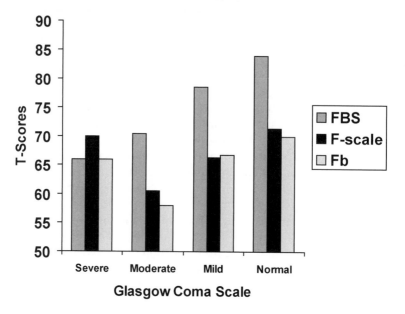

FIGURE 10.1. Dose–response relationship between severity of initial head injury and MMPI-2 validity scales in patients with persistent disability claims.

adversarial context in which these publications can be misused, it is important to take a scholarly approach to these papers, addressing valid points as well as challenging the obvious weaknesses.

In brief review, Bury and Bagby (2002) examined F-family and FBS validity in the differentiation of coached from what they termed "bona fide" PTSD claimants. Their PTSD group consisted of industrial workers seeking disability status years after workplace stressors; the coached group consisted of undergraduate simulators offered token prize money to fake PTSD under four training levels. Logistic regressions analyses indicated Fp and F produced high hit rates. Bury and Bagby (2002) were critical of the FBS, concluding that it produced high false positives and could not detect simulation by undergraduates. In their specificity-only study, Butcher et al. (2003) used a differential prevalence design to examine FBS endorsement rates in various settings. They conducted item, correlational, and frequency analyses on over 19,000 archived MMPI-2 profiles from inpatient psychiatric, general medical, chronic pain, litigation, and correctional settings. Their findings included alpha coefficients > .80 within the personal injury group; FBS scores ≥ 25 in 24% of females with "chronic pain"; and FBS > 25 in 20% of female psychiatric inpatients. Despite a clear gender-by-setting interaction, Butcher et al. (2003) interpreted these data to support *blanket dismissal* of the FBS ("It is recommended that the FBS not be used in clinical settings nor should it be used during disability evaluations to determine malingering," p. 473). The authors further warned of "grave consequences" for users of the FBS, and accused the FBS of bias against females, without mentioning that different norms have been used for males and females throughout the history of the MMPI and MMPI-2.

Many methodological and inferential problems of these two studies do not support the blanket conclusions offered. Issues common to both studies are (1) absence of external criterion for plausibility of self-report (see Butcher & Williams, 1992) and (2) picking samples historically associated with secondary gain. Bury and Bagby (2002) chose as "genuine" a large group of workers seeking compensation for persistent subjective disability long after vaguely described workplace stressors. Interestingly, Bury and Bagby (2002) reported a mean FBS of 27 in this group, but Greiffenstein et al. (2004) also found a mean of 27 in their indisputably implausible PTSD group. Hence, the Bury and Bagby (2002) PTSD group likely contained many persons misrepresenting their mental health in the service of compensatory ends. Similarly, Butcher et al. (2003) relied on an outpatient "chronic pain" group, a population known for secondary gain features such as narcotic access, dependency-seeking tactics, and compensation. For example, Keller and Butcher's (1991) study of MMPI-2 profiles in chronic pain patients was based on "many patients in the Workers' Compensation system" (p. 74). It should not be surprising that Butcher and colleagues found patients scoring above critical FBS thresholds. A reasonable alternate conclusion is that both studies were biased against the FBS by treating samples historically associated with secondary gain as "genuine."

There are other difficulties specific to each study. Published challenges to Butcher et al.'s (2003) paper note many issues including partisan literature review ignoring supportive studies (Lees-Haley & Fox, 2004); mischaracterization of the FBS and its proper use (Greve & Bianchini, 2004); mischaracterization of the Greiffenstein et al. (2002) findings; misinterpretation of the alpha coefficient (Larrabee, 2003c); assumption that the F scale is a "gold standard" (Greiffenstein et al., 2004); uncritical acceptance of MMPI-2 profiles without contextual details (Larrabee, 2003c; Greiffenstein et al., 2004); and reliance on a differential prevalence design (Greiffenstein et al., 2004). One cannot calculate false-positive rates in the absence of extra-test data, a known weakness of the differential prevalence design (Rogers, 1997). Interpreting the MMPI-2 in isolation from extra-test data is contrary to previous methodological recommendations. For example, in their text *Essentials of MMPI-2 and MMPI-A Interpretation*, Butcher and Williams (1992) write: "Basic demographic and setting characteristics are important considerations because they set the stage for test interpretation by which to judge the client's MMPI-2. *One can gauge the believability of a personality study by considering the individual's performance in light of the background factors*" (p. 186, emphasis added). Butcher and Williams (1992) go on to mention a court setting as a contextual factor to gauge the plausibility of a profile. In addition, Butcher and Miller (1999) describe the features of malingered MMPI-2 profiles with F-family scores < 100-T seen in personal injury litigation. They note that litigants exaggerating postaccident adjustment problems showed "no selective responding" and many clinical scales > 70-T.

In summary, the only reasonable criticism supported by Butcher et al.'s (2003) paper is a finding previously established in the FBS literature: Females with past psychiatric histories score higher on the FBS than other clinical groups. Otherwise, the data of Bury and Bagby (2002) and Butcher et al. (2003) actually *support* use of the FBS. The lack of FBS/F overlap bolsters the discriminant validity of the FBS, while the high alpha coefficient in the litigation group and high FBS endorsement rates in chronic pain patients upholds the convergent validity of the FBS. Butcher et al.'s (2003) blanket dismissal of the FBS is unsupportable and inconsistent with Butcher's published advice for considering nonspecific symptom overreporting as grounds for suspicion (Butcher & Miller, 1999) and incorporating extra-test factors such as legal status and historical plausibility (Butcher & Williams, 1992). In fact, we argue that the FBS quantifies Butcher and Miller's (1999) view that nonselective symptom endorsement is a means of detecting litigation related exaggeration when the F scale is not extremely elevated.

Recommendations for Current Use of the FBS

The FBS appears to be a valid measure of exaggerated disability and physiological suffering, most of all in the context of litigated minor head injury. We want to leave the reader with a set of best practice guidelines based on our critical reading of the published studies to date. We recommend the following:

• *Joint use.* Use the FBS and MMPI-2 F-family jointly. They work in complementary fashion to detect multiple forms of misrepresentation. The F scale detects feigned severe psychopathology and the FBS inflated emotional and somatic suffering. The MMPI-2 F-family is more useful in criminal settings and the FBS in civil settings.

• *General FBS threshold.* An FBS score ≥ 23 justifies concerns about symptom validity. The risk of false positives declines as scores increase in the 20s. Final conclusions depend on score magnitude and moderator variables.

• *Gender and history as moderators.* Consider cutting scores of 29 and above in females with preinjury psychiatric histories. Keep in mind persons with mental illness can still exaggerate disability in the service of regressive ends.

• *Injury severity as moderator.* In cases with historical or radiological evidence negative for cerebral dysfunction, relatively lower FBS scores (23–24) are grounds for suspecting exaggeration. With severe brain injury with residual neurological signs (such as anosmia), adjust cut-score to 26 and up.

- *Medical history as a moderator variable.* In cases of serious, active medical disease, especially diseases with complex and multiple symptom complaints, interpret FBS scores with caution or rely on scores of 30+. Consult with a medical colleague if unsure of disease status.

- *General prohibitions.* Never use the FBS alone; combine FBS score with behavior observations and other validity test indicators; avoid the original 1991 cut-score of 20 because of false positives; as of this writing, too little is known about FBS in criminal settings for use in insanity pleas (the F scale remains particularly useful in criminal settings); a positive FBS score does not automatically rule out the coexistence of genuine problems, but it does indicate magnification of problems in such cases.

- Scores of 30 and above have a 99–100% probability (Bayes "posterior probability") of indicating promotion of suffering across all settings. FBS scores in this range provide the greatest confidence irrespective of gender, medical, or psychiatric context.

- *Ideal for neuropsychologists.* The FBS is highly recommended for use in forensic neuropsychology contexts, where somatic dysfunction and emotional complaints are evaluated in conjunction with neurocognitive issues.

- *Can be prorated from the MMPI-2 short form.* Fox (2004) demonstrated that a reasonable estimate of the full FBS can be made when only the first 370 items are administered.

CONCLUDING COMMENTS

An extensive review of the literature demonstrates that neuropsychologists conducting forensic (civil) evaluations have a reasonable scientific basis for using the FBS. The strengths of the FBS include validation in diverse clinical and litigated samples; consistent demonstrations of sensitivity to symptom implausibility and disability seeking; proven association with malingered cognitive deficit; discriminant validity illustrated by superiority over the MMPI-2 F-family in natural groups; acceptable specificity dependent on cut-score; large samples; and convergent validity demonstrated by correlations with measures of nonpsychotic malingering. Overall, the FBS is a good measure of exaggerated disability irrespective of whether comorbid genuine problems are present or not. A recognized weakness is higher FBS scores in females with psychiatric histories, a problem easily remedied by increasing the cut-score, as is usual and customary with other MMPI-2 scales and neuropsychological measures. An important maxim is that *persons with genuine psychopathology can still voluntarily exaggerate disability to serve regressive ends or unknown external benefits.* We are not the first and will not be the last to offer that maxim. Keller and Butcher (1991), in their analysis of MMPI-2 profiles produced by patients from the workers' compensation system, concluded: "Secondary gain is probably a more complicated concept among these [chronic pain] patients than simply whether or not financial reinforcement is available" (p. 92).

The forensic neuropsychologist should be prepared to both justify use of the FBS and defend it against admissibility challenges. Much has been made of the "threat of *Daubert*" as a bar to admission of psychological tests (*Daubert v. Merrill-Dow Pharmaceuticals*, 1993). We believe the threat is over-blown and despite over a decade of post-*Daubert* jurisprudence, validity measures and other psychological tests are commonly used in the courtroom (Greiffenstein & Cohen, 2005). The *Daubert* decision makes the trial judge the gatekeeper of scientific evidence and requires the court to examine scientific evidence for indicia of validity and relevance. Although there is no legal requirement that the *Daubert* indicia be applied like an exhaustive checklist, the FBS satisfies many of the known conditions for legal admission. The FBS has a known error rate, has generated and continues to generate testable hypotheses, has been published in a diverse array of peer-reviewed journals, and is accepted by well-published forensic specialists. In a survey of neuropsychologists' assessment of effort and malingering, Sharland (2005) found that the FBS is the third most frequently used measure of effort in neuropsychological evaluations.

ACKNOWLEDGMENTS

We wish to thank William Barr, Scott Millis, William Tsushima, Mitchell Woltersdorf, and Wiley Mittenberg for providing additional data from their studies. Roger Greene provided a prepublication draft of a book chapter containing many useful analytical concepts and literature, and his colleague Eric Crawford provided a preprint of an FBS paper.

REFERENCES

Arbisi, P. A., & Ben-Porath, Y. S. (1995). An MMPI-2 infrequent response scale for use with psychopathological populations: The Infrequency Psychopathology scale, F(p). *Psychological Assessment, 7*, 424–431.

Barr, W. B. (2005, December). *Rates of invalid MMPI-2 responding in patients with epileptic and nonepileptic seizures.* Poster session presented at the American Epilepsy Society annual meeting, Washington, DC.

Berry, D., Wetter, M., Baer, R., Youngjohn, J., Gass, C., Lamb, D., et al. (1995). Overreporting of closed head injury symptoms on the MMPI-2. *Psychological Assessment, 7*, 517–523.

Bianchini, K. J., Houston, R. J., Greve, K. W., Irvin, T. R., Black, F. W., Swift, D. A., et al. (2003). Malingered neurocognitive dysfunction in neurotoxic exposure: An application of the Slick criteria. *Journal of Occupational and Environmental Medicine, 45*, 1087–1099.

Binder, L. M., Storzbach, D., & Salinsky, M. C. (2006). MMPI-2 profiles of persons with multiple chemical sensitivity. *The Clinical Neuropsychologist, 20*, 848–857.

Bury, A. S., & Bagby, R. M. (2002). The detection of feigned uncoached and coached posttraumatic stress disorder with the MMPI-2 in a sample of workplace accident victims. *Psychological Assessment, 14*, 472–484.

Butcher, J. N., Arbisi, P. A., Atlis, M. M., & McNulty, J. L. (2003). The construct validity of the Lees-Haley Fake Bad Scale: Does this scale measure somatic malingering and feigned emotional distress? *Archives of Clinical Neuropsychology, 18*, 473–485.

Butcher, J. N., Dahlstrom, W. G., Graham, J. R., Tellegen, A., & Kaemmer, B. (1989). *MMPI-2 manual for administration and scoring.* Minneapolis: University of Minnesota Press.

Butcher, J. N., Graham, J. R., Ben-Porath, Y. S., Tellegen, A., Dahlstrom, W. G., & Kaemmer, B. (2001). *MMPI-2: Manual for administration, scoring and interpretation. Revised Edition.* Minneapolis: University of Minnesota Press.

Butcher, J. N., & Harlow, T. C. (1987). Personality assessment in personal injury cases. In I. B. Weiner & A. K. Hess (Eds.), *Handbook of forensic psychology* (pp. 128–154). Oxford, UK: Wiley.

Butcher, J. N., & Miller, K. B. (1999). Personality assessment in personal injury litigation. In A. K. Hess & I. B. Weiner (Eds.), *Handbook of forensic psychology* (2nd ed., pp. 104–126). New York: Wiley.

Butcher, J. N., & Williams, B. L. (1992). *Essentials of MMPI-2 and MMPI-A interpretation* Minneapolis: University of Minnesota Press.

Cramer, K. M. (1995). The effects of description clarity and disorder type on MMPI-2 fake-bad validity indices. *Journal of Clinical Psychology, 51*, 831–840.

Crawford, E. F., Greene, R. L., & Dupart, T. (2006). MMPI-2 assessment of malingered emotional distress related to a workplace injury: A mixed group validation. *Journal of Personality Assessment, 86*, 217–221.

Dahlstrom, W. G., Welsh, G., & Dahlstrom, L. (1972). *An MMPI handbook: Vol. I. Clinical interpretation.* Minneapolis: University of Minnesota Press.

Dahlstrom, W. G., Welsh, G., & Dahlstrom, L. (1975). *An MMPI handbook: Vol. II. Research applications.* Minneapolis: University of Minnesota Press.

Daubert v. Merrell-Dow Pharmaceuticals, 509 U.S. 579 (1993).

Dearth, C. S., Berry, D. T. R., Vickery, C. D., Vagnini, V. L., Baser, R. E., Orey, S. A., et al. (2005). Detection of feigned head injury symptoms on the MMPI-2 in head injured patients and community controls. *Archives of Clinical Neuropsychology, 20*, 95–110.

Elhai, J. D., Gold, S. N., Sellers, A. H., & Dorfman, W. I. (2001). The detection of malingered posttraumatic stress disorder with MMPI-2 Fake bad indices. *Assessment, 8*, 221–236.

Eyler, V. A., Diehl, K. W., & Kirkhart, M. (2000). Validation of the Lees-Haley Fake Bad Scale for the MMPI-2 to detect somatic malingering among personal injury litigants. *Archives of Clinical Neuropsychology, 15*, 835–835.

Fox, D. D. (2004, November). *Prorating the Fake Bad Scale of the MMPI-2: Empirically derived equations*. Poster presented at the annual meeting of the National Academy of Neuropsychology, Seattle, WA.

Fox, D. D. (2005). *Distributional characteristics and factor analysis of MMPI-2 F-family and Fake Bad Scale*. Unpublished raw data.

Fox, D. D., Gerson, A., & Lees-Haley, P. R. (1995). Interrelationship of MMPI-2 validity scales in personal injury claims. *Journal of Clinical Psychology, 51*, 42–47.

Gough, H. G. (1954). Some common misconceptions about neuroticism. *Journal of Consulting Psychology, 18*, 287–292.

Gouvier, W. D. (1999). Base rates and clinical decision making in neuropsychology. In J. J. Sweet (Ed.), *Forensic neuropsychology. Fundamentals and practice* (pp. 27–37). Lisse, The Netherlands: Swets & Zeitlinger.

Greene, R. L. (1997). Assessment of malingering and defensiveness on multiscale inventories. In R. Rogers (Ed.), *Clinical assessment of malingering and deception* (2nd ed., pp. 169–207). New York: Guilford Press.

Greene, R. L. (2000). *MMPI-2/MMPI: An interpretive manual* (2nd ed.). Needham Heights, MA: Allyn & Bacon.

Greiffenstein, M. F. (2005). *Inverse trauma-response relationships in the MMPI-2 F-family and Lees-Haley Fake Bad Scale*. Unpublished raw data.

Greiffenstein, M. F., Baker, W. J., Axelrod, B., Peck, T. A., & Gervais, R. (2004). The Fake Bad Scale and MMPI-2 F-Family in detection of implausible psychological trauma claims. *The Clinical Neuropsychologist, 18*, 573–590.

Greiffenstein, M. F., Baker, W. J., & Gola, T. (1994). Validation of malingered amnesia measures with a large clinical sample. *Psychological Assessment, 6*, 218–224.

Greiffenstein, M. F., Baker, W. J., & Gola, T. (1996). What kind of faking does the *Fake Bad Scale* measure? *American Psychology–Law Society Newsletter*, APA Convention Issue.

Greiffenstein, M. F., Baker, W. J., Gola, T., Donders, J., & Miller, L. J. (2002). The FBS in atypical and severe closed head injury litigants. *Journal of Clinical Psychology, 58*, 1591–1600.

Greiffenstein, M. F., & Cohen, L. (2005). Neuropsychology and the law: Principles of productive attorney-neuropsychologist relations. In G. J. Larrabee (Ed.), *Forensic neuropsychology* (pp. 29–91). New York: Oxford University Press.

Greiffenstein, M. F., Gola, T., & Baker, W. J. (1995). The MMPI-2 validity scales versus domain specific measures in the detection of factitious brain injury. *The Clinical Neuropsychologist, 9*, 230–240.

Greve, K. W., & Bianchini, K. J. (2004). Response to Butcher et al., The construct validity of the Lees-Haley Fake Bad Scale [Letter to the editor]. *Archives of Clinical Neuropsychology, 19*, 337–339.

Greve, K. W., Bianchini, K. J., Love, J. M., Brennan, A., & Heinley, M. T. (2006). Sensitivity and specificity of the MMPI-2 validity indicators to malingered neurocognitive dysfunction in traumatic brain injury. *The Clinical Neuropsychologist, 20*, 491–512.

Hathaway, S. R., & Meehl, P. E. (1951). *An atlas for clinical use of the MMPI*. Minneapolis: University of Minnesota Press.

Iverson, G. L., Henrichs, T. F., Barton, E. A., & Allen, S. (2002). Specificity of the MMPI-2 Fake Bad Scale as a marker for personal injury malingering. *Psychological Reports, 90*, 131–136.

Keller, L. S., & Butcher, J. N. (1991). *Assessment of chronic pain with the MMPI-2.* Minneapolis: University of Minnesota Press.

Lanyon, R. I., & Almer, E. R. (2001). Multimodal assessment of self-serving misrepresentation during personal injury evaluation. *American Journal of Forensic Psychology, 19*(3), 5.

Larrabee, G. J. (1997). Neuropsychological outcome, post concussion symptoms, and forensic considerations in mild closed head trauma. *Seminars in Clinical Neuropsychiatry, 2,* 196–206.

Larrabee, G. J. (1998). Somatic malingering on the MMPI and MMPI-2 in personal injury litigants. *The Clinical Neuropsychologist, 12,* 179–188.

Larrabee, G. J. (2003a). Detection of symptom exaggeration with the MMPI-2 in litigants with malingered neurocognitive dysfunction. *The Clinical Neuropsychologist, 17,* 54–68.

Larrabee, G. J. (2003b). Exaggerated MMPI-2 symptom report in personal injury litigants with malingered neurocognitive deficit. *Archives of Clinical Neuropsychology, 18,* 673–686.

Larrabee, G. J. (2003c). Exaggerated pain report in litigants with malingered neurocognitive dysfunction. *The Clinical Neuropsychologist, 17,* 395–401.

Larrabee, G. J. (2003d). Detection of malingering using atypical performance patterns on standard neuropsychological tests. *The Clinical Neuropsychologist, 17,* 410–425.

Lees-Haley P. R. (1992). Efficacy of MMPI-2 validity scales and MCMI-II modifier scales for detecting spurious PTSD claims: F, F-K, Fake Bad Scale, ego strength, subtle-obvious subscales, DIS, and DEB. *Journal of Clinical Psychology, 48,* 681–689.

Lees-Haley, P. R. (1997). MMPI-2 base rates for 492 personal injury plaintiffs: Implications and challenges for forensic assessment. *Journal of Clinical Psychology, 53,* 745–755.

Lees-Haley, P. R., English, L. T., & Glenn, W. J. (1991). A Fake Bad Scale on the MMPI-2 for personal injury claimants. *Psychological Reports, 68,* 203–210.

Lees-Haley, P. R., & Fox, D. D. (2004). Commentary on Butcher, Arbisi, Atlis, and McNulty (2003) on the Fake Bad Scale. *Archives of Clinical Neuropsychology, 19,* 333–336.

Lees-Haley, P. R., Smith, H. H., Williams, C. W., & Dunn, J. T. (1996). Forensic neuropsychological test usage: An empirical survey. *Archives of Clinical Neuropsychology, 11*(1), 45–51.

Lim, J., & Butcher, J. N. (1996). Detection of faking on the MMPI-2: Differentiation among faking bad, denial, and claiming extreme virtue. *Journal of Personality Assessment, 67,* 1–25.

Martens, M., Donders, J., & Millis, S. R. (2001). Evaluation of invalid response sets after traumatic head injury. *Journal of Forensic Neuropsychology, 2,* 1–18.

Martinez, G., Mittenberg, W., Gass, C. S., & Quintar, B. (2005, October). *Validation of the MMPI-2 FBS scale in clinical malingerers and nonlitigating patients.* Poster session presented at the annual meeting of the National Academy of Neuropsychology, Tampa, FL.

Meyers, J. E., Millis, S. R., & Volkert, K. (2002). A validity index for the MMPI-2. *Archives of Clinical Neuropsychology, 17,* 157–169.

Miller, L. J., & Donders, J. (2001). Subjective symptomatology after traumatic head injury. *Brain Injury, 15*, 297–304.

Millis, S. R., Putnam, S. H., & Adams, K. M. (1995, March 19). *Neuropsychological malingering and the MMPI-2: Old and new indicators*. Paper presented at the 30th Annual Symposium on Recent Developments in the Use of the MMPI, MMPI-2 and MMPI-A, St Petersburg Beach, FL.

Mittenberg, W., Patton, C., Canyock, E. M., & Condit, D. C. (2002). Base rates of malingering and symptom exaggeration. *Journal of Clinical and Experimental Neuropsychology, 24*, 1094–1102.

Nelson, N. W., Parsons, T. D., Grote, C. L., Smith, C. A., & Sisung, J. R. (2006). The MMPI-2 Fake Bad Scale: Concordance and specificity of true and estimated scores. *Journal of Clinical and Experimental Neuropsychology, 28*(1), 1–12.

Nelson, N. W., Sweet, J. J., & Demakis, G. J. (2006). Meta-Analysis of the MMPI-2 Fake Bad Scale: Utility in forensic practice. *The Clinical Neuropsychologist, 20*(1), 39–58.

Posthuma, A. B., & Harper, J. F. (1998). Comparison of MMPI-2 responses of child custody and personal injury litigants. *Professional Psychology: Research and Practice, 29*, 437–443.

Putnam, S. H., Millis, S. R., & Adams, K. M. (1998, August). Consideration of impression management in the neuropsychological examination with the MMPI-2. Paper presented at the annual meeting of the American Psychological Association, San Francisco.

Rogers, R. (1997). Introduction. In R. Rogers (Ed.), *Clinical assessment of malingering and deception* (pp. 1–19). New York: Guilford Press.

Rogers, R., Sewell, K. W., Martin, M. A., & Vitacco, M. J. (2003). Detection of feigned mental disorders: A meta-analysis of the MMPI-2 and malingering. *Assessment, 10*, 160–177.

Rogers, R., Sewell, K. W., & Ustad, L. L. (1995). Feigning among chronic outpatients on the MMPI-2: A systematic examination of fake-bad indicators. *Assessment, 2*, 81–89.

Ross, S. R., Millis, S. R., Krukowski, R. A., Putnam, S. H., & Adams, K. M. (2004). Detecting probable malingering on the MMPI-2: An examination of the Fake bad Scale in mild head injury. *Journal of Clinical and Experimental Neuropsychology, 26*, 115–124.

Rothke, S. E., Friedman, A. F., Jaffe, A. M., Greene, R. L., Wetter, M. W., Cole, P. et al. (2000). Normative data for the F(p) Scale of the MMPI-2: Implications for clinical and forensic assessment of malingering. *Psychological Assessment, 12*, 335–340.

Sbordone, R. J., & Liter, J. C. (1995). Mild traumatic brain injury does not produce post-traumatic stress disorder. *Brain Injury, 9*, 405–412.

Sharland, M. J. (2005, November 14). *A survey of neuropsychologists' beliefs and practices with respect to the assessment of effort*. Poster presented at the annual meeting of the National Academy of Neuropsychology, Session C, Tampa, FL.

Slick, D. J., Hopp, G., Strauss, E., & Spellacy, F. J. (1996). Victoria Symptom Validity Test: Efficiency for detecting feigned memory impairment and relationship to neuropsychological tests and MMPI-2 validity scales. *Journal of Clinical and Experimental Neuropsychology, 18*, 911–922.

Slick, D. J., Sherman, E. M., & Iverson, G. L. (1999). Diagnostic criteria for malingered neurocognitive dysfunction: Proposed standards for clinical practice and research. *The Clinical Neuropsychologist, 13*, 545–561.

Staudenmayer, H., & Phillips, S. (2007). MMPI-2 validity, clinical, and content scales and the Fake Bad Scale for personal injury litigants claiming idiopathic environmental intolerance. *Journal of Psychosomatic Research, 62*, 61–72.

Tsushima, W. T., & Tsushima, V. G. (2001). Comparison of the Fake Bad Scale and other MMPI-2 validity scales with personal injury litigants. *Assessment, 8*(2), 205–212.

Woltersdorf, M. A. (2005, October). *FBS in clinical and forensic practice sample in Midwest.* Poster session presented at annual meeting of the National Academy of Neuropsychology, Tampa, FL.

APPENDIX 10.1. FBS ANSWER KEY

Following are the MMPI-2 items and scored direction of answering for the Fake Bad Scale (FBS):

- Add 1 point if marked True: 11, 18, 28, 30, 31, 39, 40, 44, 59, 111, 252, 274, 325, 339, 464, 469, 505, 506
- Add 1 point if marked False: 12, 41, 57, 58, 81, 110, 117, 152, 164, 176, 224, 227, 248, 249, 250, 255, 264, 284, 362, 373, 374, 419, 433, 496, 561

PART III

COGNITIVE EFFORT TESTING IN VARIOUS CLINICAL POPULATIONS

CHAPTER 11

Malingering Mild Traumatic Brain Injury

Behavioral Approaches Used by Both
Malingering Actors and Probable Malingerers

John E. Meyers

The assessment of motivation/symptom validity is an important consideration in modern-day neuropsychological assessment. As an example, Green, Rohling, Lees-Haley, and Allen (2001) found that motivation accounted for a larger amount of variance than did severe brain injury. To attempt to reference the hundreds of articles published on malingering and malingering assessment would be tedious and unnecessary. In short, the assessment of motivation/symptom validity has become the standard of practice in neuropsychology, and many different methods are used.

In neuropsychological practice, a group of neuropsychological tests are generally given as part of an assessment. Russel (1998) points out that a battery of tests must be validated. The discussion here centers on the use of a well-validated battery of tests. The Meyers Neuropsychological Battery (MNB) is a well-researched and published neuropsychological battery (Meyers & Rohling, 2004; Rohling, Meyers, & Millis, 2003; Volbrecht, Meyers, & Kaster-Bundgaard, 2000). Norms for the MNB are based on more than 1,700 subjects and covers the age ranges of 6 to 90+ years (Meyers, 2004). The MNB consists of 16 commonly used neuropsychological tests that generate 34 variables which are used to compare with a database of over 3,000 subjects. The battery showed a test–retest reliability of $r = .86$, and comparing normal, depressed, and chronic pain patients with mild traumatic brain injury showed a sensitivity of 90% and a specificity of 98.9% with an overall correct classification rate of 96.1%.

The MNB has nine internal motivation/validity items, which are explained in detail in several publications (e.g., Meyers & Volbrecht, 2003; Meyers, Morrison, & Miller, 2001; Meyers & Diep, 2000; Meyers & Volbrecht, 1999; Meyers, Galinsky, & Volbrecht, 1999; Meyers & Volbrecht, 1998a, 1998b) (see also Table 11.1). In summary, the internal validity checks consist of nine individual methods, each with a cutoff level that produced a 0 false-positive rate, and when combined with all methods, 0 false-positive rate of failure of no more than one of the nine specific motivation/validity items is used (Meyers & Volbrecht, 2003). Using this method, failure on two or more of the specific motivation/validity items would result in a failure on the validity check. This same criteria (two or more failures) was presented by Slick, Sherman, and Iverson (1999). Both the research on the nine internal validity checks and the criteria presented by Slick et al. (1999) independently of each other conclude that probable malingering should be considered when failure on two or more of the internal validity checks are achieved. Persons for whom these internal validity items are probably not appropriate are detailed by Meyers and Volbrecht (2003). Specifically, persons for whom the nine validity items are not appropriate include those who are not testable or who are institutionalized.

There are a number of good symptom validity tests that can be added to a battery of neuropsychological tests (e.g., see Chapter 4, this volume). The one concern I have regarding an "added test of malingering" is that a person simply could be told to "do good" on the computer test, and then the individual would be free to purposefully perform poorly on the battery of tests and still pass the symptom validity tests. But with internal validity items, the motivational component on the tests can be assessed as the battery of tests

TABLE 11.1. The Nine Internal Validity Items for the MNB

Internal validity item	Raw
Forced Choice	≤10
Judgment of Line Orientation	≤12
Sentence Repetition	≤9
Token Test	≤150
Reliable Digits	≤6
AVLT Recognition	≤9
Dichotic Listening	≤9
Memory Error Pattern	≤3
Finger Tapping Difference	≥10

Note. 0 false-positive rate cutoff score).

are given. Failure on one of the internal validity items suggests variability in motivation, but failure on two or more indicates motivation that is too variable or purposefully poor performance. Based on previous publications the following nine internal validity checks are used in this study.

These nine items use a variety of methods. The forced-choice (FC) task uses a score that would be at or below random responding. That is, even if a person had not previously heard any of the words used, a random response would still produce a score of 10. The cutoff scores on Judgment of Line Orientation (JOL), Sentence Repetition (SR), and Rey Auditory Verbal Learning Test (AVLT) Recognition (AVLT REC) are based on performance that would be improbably low for subjects with 30 days or more of loss of consciousness (LOC), based on a 0 false-positive rate. Reliable Digit Span (RDS) and the Dichotic Listening Both Ears score are based on a 0 false-positive rate for persons with less than 7 days of LOC. The Token Test (TT) uses a process of the harder items first then giving the easier items, as most tests start out with the easiest items and progresses to harder. The score is set with a 0 false-positive rate for persons who had less than 14 days of LOC.

The Memory Error Pattern (MEP) uses a configuration relationship between scores on the Rey Complex Figure Test (RCFT) (Meyers & Meyers, 1995a, 1995b). An Attention Pattern is usually found in persons who are at Rancho Level 4–5. An Encoding pattern is generally found in persons who are at Rancho 5–6, and a Storage Pattern is generally found in persons at Rancho 6. A Retrieval or Normal MEP may be found at Rancho Level 7–8. Therefore, a person who is able to live independently would not be expected to achieve an Attention (1), Encoding (2), or Storage (3) MEP.

The Finger Tapping method uses a comparison of performance on tests that also use the index finger with the performance on the dominant hand Finger Tapping mean score. This of course assumes that the dominant-hand index finger is present and that the patients used their dominant hand to perform the tasks that calculate the expected performance. The formula used is:

{[Difference score = (ROCFT Copy Raw Score × .185) + (Digit Symbol Scale Score × .491) + (Block Design Scale Score × .361)] + 31.34)} – Average Dominant Hand Finger Tapping

If the actual performance is 10 or more points below the expected performance, impaired motivation to do well is suggested.

There have been several previous studies identifying patterns of performance indicative of poor effort (Millis, 1992; Millis, Putnam, Adams, & Richer, 1995) as well as atypical patterns of problem solving (Suhr & Boyer, 1999) and finger tapping performance (Heaton, Smith, Lehman, & Vogt, 1978; Mittenberg, Rotholc, Russell, & Heilbronner, 1996; Larrabee, 2003). Poor performance on RDS (Greiffenstein, Baker, & Gola, 1994, Meyers &

Volbrecht, 1998a, 1998b) has also been found, and improbable relationships between scores (Mittenberg, Theroux-Fichera, Zielinski, & Heilbronner, 1995) have been investigated. Regression equations have also been used to identify poorly motivated performance (Suhr & Boyer, 1999; Heaton, Chelune, Talley, Kay, & Curtiss, 1993). The MNB validity items use similar approaches as published by other authors.

BEHAVIORAL MALINGERING

This study was undertaken to provide information on how persons who choose to purposefully perform poorly on neuropsychological tests go about performing poorly. A sample of 20 participants (Group 1) who were normal community-dwelling individuals with no history of significant injury were asked to take the MNB as if they were trying to present themselves as having an acquired serious brain injury (i.e., from a motor vehicle accident) but not to get caught "faking." None of these persons had any "specific" training in brain injury, six had CPR training, and two had first aid training through the Boy Scouts. Table 11.2 provides a description of the demographic make up of this group.

Prior to taking the battery of tests, the subjects were interviewed and asked to describe what their approach to "malingering" on the tests would be. Then, following the administration of the MNB, they were asked to describe their approach to "malingering" and any differences or additional methods they had used or would use. In summary, they reported:

"I would think about how I would look like, if I had a brain injury (think about and plan what I would say to the doctor)."
"I would find information about brain injury (lawyer, Internet, library, ask someone)."
"I would make up a story (symptoms) and stick to it. I would say it is getting worse."
"I would try to make it look like I had trouble concentrating (paying attention, got confused easily)."

TABLE 11.2. Group 1 (Normal Community-Dwelling Individuals Asked to "Malinger")

Demographics	Range
Age	18–44 years
Education	11–19 years
Gender	13 female, 7 male
Ethnicity	1 African American, 2 Asian, 16 Caucasian, 1 Hispanic

"I would pretend the testing was too hard."
"If I got tired of the testing, I would just get mad and walk out."
"I would forget easily and complain about my memory."
"I would say I
- had headaches."
- had memory problems (forget family members, personal information, and short term memory problems)."
- had trouble concentrating."
- had dizziness."
- had a hard time figuring things out."
- got mad easily."
- was frustrated, depressed."
"I would say I can't work anymore."
"I would try to make you think I am an honest person by telling you I am a good person (lay minister, Sunday school teacher, volunteer)."

Following the MNB they were interviewed again and asked about any additional strategy during the testing or additional things they would do and what tests were the easiest to "malinger on":

"I did not try to malinger on all the tests, I only picked the ones that I thought I could fake on, and not get caught (could malinger on any test, just get them wrong)."
"I would tell my lawyer that the testing was too hard."
"I would tell my lawyer that I was too tired (anxious, scared) to do good on the testing, or that the testing was unfair in some form."

Next the participants were asked which tests they thought were easiest to "malinger on." First, they were asked to describe the testing task in their own words and then were shown the test materials to identify which tests they meant:

"Repeating things [Digit Span, SR]."
"The instruction following [TT]."
"The one with the earphones [dichotic listening] that I had to pay attention to."
"Tests that I had to remember anything on [FC, AVLT, RCFT]."
"The one where you had to look at the lines or draw [JOL, RCFT]."
"The one with the pictures I had to name [Boston Naming]."
"The one with the '1,2,3,4' numbers [Category]."
"The figuring-out ones [Arithmetic, Block Design, Information]."
"Be slow at doing things [Finger Tapping, anything with time limit]."
"Anything you could just say 'I don't know' to. Don't get them all wrong, sometimes just get some wrong."

Then the participants were asked to tell how they "malingered" on the tests.

Sentence Repetition and Digit Span
"Slow repeating, substitute words/numbers, say a few words/numbers
    then pause then give rest of the sentence or digits incorrectly, try to
    look confused or forgetful and complain about memory."

Token Test
"Say sentence out loud, then do it wrong. Pick up wrong token."

Dichotic Listening
"Alternate responses from one ear to the other. Do a few on one ear
    then the other and back. Not respond to one ear. Mix up words."

Memory Tests
"Just say 'I don't know.' Act confused, insert made up words/designs.
    Leave out things. Forget things from past and also short term."

JOL
"Pick one number off (near correct response), just get them wrong."

Boston Naming
"Just say 'I don't know' or give wrong name."

Category
"Just keep naming wrong numbers. Keep doing same number until it
    came to that number being correct then give a different number. Try
    not to get too many right in a row."

Arithmetic, Information
"Just keep saying I don't know, give up easy, pretend to be confused."

Block Design
"Get the blocks right except for one block, reverse the blocks. Go fast at
    the beginning then keep turning the blocks until the time runs out.
    Just keep turning the blocks till the time ran out."

Timed Tasks
"Start out ok then go slow."

The descriptions of the tests represent the nature of the tasks as perceived by the participants, which in turn determined how easily the participants felt the tasks would be to malinger. For example, it was not the repeating of digits but the task of repeating "things" that was described.

These results are similar to those reported by Iverson (1995), who indicated behaviors that were identified as "malingering" behaviors. These
behaviors were developed by asking undergraduates, community volunteers,
psychiatric inpatients, and federal inmates what they would do to "malinger"

on a neuropsychological assessment. Iverson (1995) described strategies that would be used: to act confused, stick to one's story, pretend memory problems, go blank, space off, get frustrated or upset, respond slowly with hesitations, research memory loss, pretend testing was too hard, and be forgetful.

It is interesting to note that in the Iverson (1995) study, persons reported researching about how to present as having a brain injury. During the current study, again persons reported researching about brain injury and specifically cited talking to their lawyer and using the Internet as the most common source of information on how to fake a brain injury. These findings are similar to those reported by Youngjohn (1995) and Youngjohn, Lees-Haley, and Binder (1999) that attorneys are a source of information on how to "fake" an injury. Wetter and Corrigan (1995) reported that almost 50% of the attorneys felt that clients referred for psychological testing should be coached on the validity scales on the tests. Results from this study appear to be consistent with previously published information.

The next analysis was to identify how those behaviors that have been identified would appear on a neuropsychological battery. An analysis of the failure rates on each of the internal validity checks on the MNB were examined. A pool of 105 consecutive litigating referrals were then collected. The pool of subjects was divided by the individual's performance on the validity items. Persons who failed on one item were classified as Group 2, those who failed on two or more were classified as Group 3, and those who failed on no validity items were classified as Group 4. All subjects in Groups 2, 3, and 4 were involved in litigation. Litigation was due to complaints of traumatic brain injury (i.e., motor vehicle accident).

Comparing the three groups (2–4) using a chi square showed no difference in handedness, gender, or ethnicity ($p > .05$). Using an analysis of variance (ANOVA) there was no difference in age, education, months since injury, LOC (not all were reporting LOC, but all who did were reporting less than 1 hour of LOC), posttraumatic amnesia, and Full Scale IQ ($p > .05$) Barona, Reynolds, & Chastain, 1984). The overall test battery mean (OTBM) was significantly different between the groups ($p = < .001$). A Scheffe post hoc test shows Group 3 is significantly different from Groups 2 and 4 but Groups 2 and 4 were not different from each other although Group 2 did have a slightly lower OTBM than Group 4.

From these data it is clear that those who are attempting to present themselves as more impaired than they are tried to perform below their expected level of performance. As can be seen in Table 11.3, the two groups that performed at least adequately (Groups 2 and 4) showed OTBMs that were not significantly different from each other. The OTBM for the Malingering Actors group (1) was 29. The Group 3 (failed two or more validity items) participants showed an OTBM that was more than a standard deviation below the other two groups (2 and 4), although the three groups did not differ significantly on important demographic variables.

TABLE 11.3. Demographics for Groups

Group		Age	Education	Loss of consciousness	Posttraumatic amnesia	Months since injury	Overall test battery mean
Group 2	Mean	38.5	11.8	.04	.6	44.5	42.2
	SD	14.3	3.1	.2	3.1	91.2	6.9
Group 3	Mean	44.8	12.1	.4	1.3	52.8	34.7
	SD	10.5	3.1	2.1	6.3	55.9	6.5
Group 4	Mean	39.9	12.3	.1	.6	36.6	45.6
	SD	13.7	2.3	.5	2.2	85.1	4.6

These data show a very well known effect: that those who exhibit poor motivation perform more poorly than those who exhibit adequate motivation. This has been reported in other studies (e.g., Green, Rohling, Lees-Haley, & Allen, 2001).

Examining the failures on the validity items shows that the actors demonstrated more failures in general compared to the actual patient groups but that the pattern of failures was similar. The failures were not due to demographic differences between the groups but to motivational differences. The most common failures on validity items in order are AVLT, RDS, Dichotic Listening, Finger Tapping, SR, TT, MEP, JOL, and FC.

Previously published estimated "malingering" rates have been variable depending on the methods used. In a summary of 11 studies, Larrabee (2003) found 548/1363 subjects (40%) identified with motivated performance deficits suggestive of malingering. In this current dataset only 21.9% would have been identified as having impaired motivation to do well on the testing. If one considers the variable motivation group (Group 2) and the impaired motivation group (Group 3) then the overall identified rate of impaired motivation was 44%, which is very similar to that reported by Larrabee (2003). It may be that the method used (failure on two or more of the individual validity items) may be somewhat conservative. Given that the cutoff scores for each method were set at a 0 false-positive rate and the failure on two or more of these methods when combined was also set at a 0 false-positive rate, it is easy to see that this method is more conservative than most. As Table 11.4 indicates, Groups 1, 2, and 3 show failures on the validity items.

The two internal validity checks that showed the highest failure rate in the variable motivated group (Group 2) were RDS and Finger Tapping. These two internal validity tasks are probably more sensitive to motivation perhaps because on "their face," they appear to be difficult tasks. Therefore, these two tests may be able to pick up more subtle variability in motivation.

TABLE 11.4. Failure Rates on Individual Validity Tests

Frequency of failure on internal validity items	Group 1 Actors ($n = 20$)	Group 2 Failed 1 ($n = 24$)	Group 3 Failed 2+ ($n = 23$)	Group 4 Failed 0 ($n = 58$)
Sentence Repetition	13(65%)	1(4%)	7(30%)	0
Token Test	12(60%)	0(0%)	5(21%)	0
FC	12(60%)	0(0%)	1(4%)	0
Memory Error Pattern	12(60%)	2(8%)	5(21%)	0
Dichotic Listening Both	10(50%)	2(8%)	9(39%)	0
Judgment of Line Orientation	10(50%)	0(0%)	5(21%)	0
AVLT Recognition	10(50%)	2(8%)	13(56%)	0
Reliable Digits	10(50%)	7(29%)	10(43%)	0
Finger Tapping	8(40%)	10(41%)	8(34%)	0

Clearly, those in the impaired motivation group (Group 3) often failed these two internal validity checks as well. Adherence to the failure on two or more items is also accentuated by these findings. Variable motivation until it is sufficient to produce two failures would not be sufficient to invalidate the battery of neuropsychological testing. But some specific areas of test results may be unusable for interpretation. If an internal validity check such as AVLT Recognition is failed (and no other validity checks are failed) one might simply report that the performance on memory items was too variable for reliable interpretation. If only RDS is failed, one may conclude that performance on working memory and attention tasks was too variable to be reliably interpreted. Similarly, performance on Finger Tapping might suggest that performance in tasks of speed that involve the hands was too inconsistent/variable to be reliably interpreted. This is clearly another benefit of internal validity checks. From Table 11.5 it can also be observed that memory is probably the most common cognitive deficit that is malingered.

Based on the behaviors that were reported by the Malingering Actors (Group 1), behavioral descriptions were gathered for each of the 105 subjects by a master's-level testing technician. This technician was blind to the purpose to the data gathering and was asked only to indicate the behaviors observed during the assessment. The behaviors were then tabulated. Table 11.5 includes a summary of the reported behavior.

A chi square comparing each of the 12 observed behaviors with the three groups (2–4) showed that only behaviors 2, 3, 8, 11, 12, and 13 were different between the groups ($p < .05$). The reported symptoms of headache, memory problems, difficulty concentrating, and so forth were not different between the groups ($p > .05$). Those differences that were significant were also obvious differences such as complaining that the testing was too hard, walking out on the testing, getting angry during the testing, spending time trying to convince the evaluator of one's sincerity, and complaining about

TABLE 11.5. Behavioral Observations During and after Testing

	Groups		
	2	3	4
1. Reported being confused or asked for clarification	24 (100%)	22 (95%)	53 (91%)
2. Stated that the testing was too hard*	5 (20%)	7 (30%)	4 (6%)
3. Walked out before completing the testing*	0 (0%)	2 (8%)	0 (0%)
4. Reported memory problems	24 (100%)	23 (100%)	57 (98%)
5. Reported headaches	7 (29%)	8 (34%)	27 (46%)
6. Reported trouble concentrating	24 (100%)	23 (100%)	58 (100%)
7. Reported dizziness/head foggy/trouble focusing	17 (70%)	16 (69%)	43 (74%)
8. Got visibly angry during testing*	0 (0%)	4 (17%)	0 (0%)
9. Reported being depressed/sad/frustrated	20 (83%)	21 (91%)	47 (81%)
10. Reported had trouble working	24 (100%)	22 (95%)	57 (98%)
11. Claimed to forget biographical data (names, ages of children, etc.)*	0 (0%)	1 (4%)	0 (0%)
12. Invoked deity/personal virtue (one person reported he was a lay minister, did lots of community service, and so should be believed; one brought "Sunday school" lesson to "work on during breaks")*	0 (0%)	2 (8%)	0 (0%)
13. Following testing reported to lawyer that the testing was too hard/unfair (not all depositions have been done; therefore, these numbers may be higher)*	0 (0%)	6 (26%)	0 (0%)

*Groups significantly different $p < .05$.

the testing to one's lawyer. These data clearly support the need for use of symptom validity tests given that there are no clear differences between the complaints of well-motivated and not well-motivated subjects. Using patient complaints or behavior (with a few obvious exceptions) to distinguish between well motivated (to do best on the testing) and motivated to do poorly on the testing would be unreliable. Specific validity items must be included as part of the assessment.

From an anecdotal perspective those who failed the validity check showed more "don't know" responses on memory items (visual and verbal). On SR a common approach was to give the first part of the sentence correctly, then to pause and then to give a partial correct answer. Those with adequate motivation generally gave the sentence (even if incorrect) as one phrase without a pause. An example, if the sentence was "The boy stood on the shore looking at the ships" (not a real test item). Those who failed the validity check might say, "The boy stood on the shore (pause) seeing a boat." On Dichotic Listening, those who failed this validity item often showed an alternating pattern, that is, some correct on one ear then some correct on the other ear and alternating every few items, although a single ear suppression was also found. Nearly correct responses, such as consistently off one number on JOL or one incorrect on Block Design was also noted. On the Category Test, a common approach was to keep giving the same number then, when that number would be correct, to give a different number. These are not the only approaches used but were common.

These data indicate that those who are attempting to present themselves as being more impaired than they actually are often tend to be organized in their approach (i.e., near-correct responses). Also, "malingering" is not done on all tests. Instead, selected items may be "malingered on." It is clear that validity of performance needs to be assessed across the assessment battery (i.e., internal validity checks) not just "special add-in tests." This is not to suggest that add-in tests are not useful, but internal validity items should be considered too.

HOW WELL WERE THE "MALINGERERS" ABLE TO SIMULATE A BRAIN INJURY?

The next part of this study was to identify how well persons could simulate a brain injury. To do this, seven groups of subjects were selected from a database of more than 3,000 subjects collected from consecutive referrals between 1997 and 2004. Six brain injury groups (Groups 5–10) and one probable malingering group (Group 11) were selected. All brain-injured subjects were personally treated by the author in either an inpatient or an outpatient setting. All subjects in Groups 5–9 had documented LOC as identified by third-party witness (i.e., nursing notes, emergency room physician, ambulance personnel, and witnesses at the scene). The sixth group consisted of persons with identified bifrontal injury on MRI (magnetic resonance imaging). Regardless of LOC, the persons in Group 10 were not part of the Groups 5–9. All subjects in groups 5–10 passed the validity check by failing no more than one of the internal individual validity items. None of these subjects were in litigation at the time of the assessment (except Group 11). The seventh group (Probable Malingerers, Group 11) consisted of litigants claiming brain injury who failed the internal validity check by failing two or more of the individual validity checks and met Slick et al. (1999) criteria for Probable Malingerers. These data were previously published in several studies (Meyers & Volbrecht, 2003; Rohling et al., 2003; and some additional subjects collected since those studies were published).

The group data from the malingering actors (Group 1) was compared to Groups 5–11 in the following way. A correlation was performed between the Malingering Actors (Group 1) and the seven test groups. A configuration match was derived by first calculating the OTBM for each group. Then, examining each individual test score on the MNB, if the score was above the OTBM (for the individual group), a "+" is scored. If the score was below the OTBM then a "–" was scored. If the score equaled the OTBM then a "0" was scored. That is, each group's scores were compared with that group's OTBM. The Configuration Match is the percent agreement between the groups for the "+, –, and 0" values. This method creates a measure of agreement in the "direction" of the scores, that is, going up or down in the same place (i.e., on a graph). (See Table 11.6.)

As can be seen from these data, the profile of the malingering actors (Group 1) was most similar to the Probable Malingerers (Group 11), and the pattern that the Malingering Actors showed was most similar to frontal lobe

TABLE 11.6. Group Descriptive Data and Results Comparing the Correlation and Configuration Scores between the Malingering Actors (Group 1) and the TBI Groups (5–11)

Group by LOC (n)	Mean age	Mean education	Months postinjury	Correlation	Configuration	Overall test battery mean
5. < 5 minutes (27)	32	12	16	.49	.56	46
6. Up to 1 hour (22)	34	13	13	.53	.59	45
7. 1–24 hours (40)	32	13	8	.61	.59	41
8. 1–7 days (56)	25	11	20	.60	.68	39
9. 8–90 days (72)	31	12	84	.58	.65	33
10. Bifrontal (12)	61	14	1	.62	.68	37
11. Probable malingerers (94)	41	11	30	.86	.82	32

brain injury patients (Group 10). The correlation between the Malingering Actors and the bifrontal group was .86, suggesting a strong relationship. This clearly shows the similarity of the Malingering Actors and the Probable Malingerers. The correlation between the Probable Malingerers and the bifrontal group was .79 and the Configuration Match was .85. These findings suggest that those who are attempting to present themselves as more impaired (i.e., poor motivation to do well on the testing) show a pattern of scores that is most similar to patients with bifrontal injuries. The correlation between the Probable Malingerers (Group 11) and Groups 5–10 were .67, .71, .83, .76, .80, and .85, respectively. These data show that Malingering Actors (Group 1) and Probable Malingerers (Group 11) show a pattern of performance that is similar to patients with bifrontal injuries (at about 1 month postinjury). These correlations also show that when persons are attempting to perform poorly (Groups 1 and 11) they are likely to show a pattern of scores that suggest moderate to severe traumatic brain injury. That is, that the level of impaired performance is greatly out of proportion to the level of LOC. (See Figure 11.1.)

A study published by Rohling et al. (2003) used the Dikmen dataset (Dikmen, Machamer, Winn, & Temkin; 1995) and the MNB (Midwest) database showed that performance on the Halstead–Reitan Neuropsychological Battery (HRNB) and the MNB were very similar in there sensitivity to brain injury. The combined database was used to generate the expected level of performance based on LOC. Figure 11.1 shows that with a particular level of LOC there is a level of OTBM that would be expected. As an example, an OTBM score of 32 would not be expected until a LOC of 28 days or more. Therefore, a person who performs at a level expected for individuals who have a much longer LOC than reported would be out of proportion to what is expected. The mean score of the Probable Malingerers was 32 and the Malingering Actors was 29; these scores are consistent with the average performance of persons with about a month of LOC. Figure 11.1 presents the slope of expected performance based on LOC. As you can see, both those that were Malingering Actors and Probable Malingerers had an unrealistically low performance as indicated on the OTBM.

DO BRAIN INJURIES GET WORSE OVER TIME?

One of the approaches to malingering discussed by the Malingering Actors (Group 1) was to report that their cognitive difficulties were getting worse over time. With this in mind, the database of over 3,000 subjects was searched using the criteria of traumatic brain injury (TBI), 18 years of age or older, nonlitigating, passed all the validity checks, tested more than 1 year postinjury, and given the full MNB. Using these criteria, the OTBM was

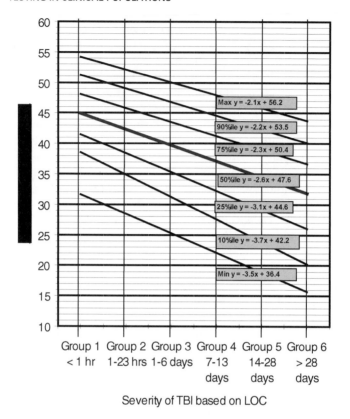

Severity of TBI based on LOC

FIGURE 11.1. Level of expected OTBM by length of loss of consciousness (LOC). From Rohling, Meyers, and Millis (2003). Copyright 2003 by Taylor & Francis. www.psypress.com/journals.asp. Reprinted by permission.

examined for those who had multiple evaluations. Table 11.7 show the demographics of the individuals in the group. Also included are the length of LOC and self-reported posttraumatic amnesia (PTA) or confusion.

Examining Table 11.8, we can see that the consistency of performance across performance for individuals with adequate motivation did not show a significant decline over time. The greatest decline for any individual was 2.5 T-score points for one individual who was also later diagnosed not only with a TBI but also multiple sclerosis (MS). For other persons who did not have any intervening injury or neurological disease the greatest drop was 1.5 T-score points. In a previous study the MNB showed a .86 test–retest reliability score (Meyers & Rohling, 2004).

Given these findings, it would not be expected that there would be a decline in cognitive functioning; this of course assumes similar batteries of tests having been given with similar norms. It was found that over time

TABLE 11.7. Demographic Description of Multiple Test Subjects

Subject no.	Age	Education	Gender	Handedness	Ethnicity	Days LOC	Days PTA
1	29	9	M	R	Caucasian	25	55
2	20	12	F	R	Caucasian	28	30
3	66	12	F	R	Caucasian	Minutes	Minutes
4	45	18	F	R	Caucasian	2	2
5	19	12	F	R	Caucasian	8	30
6	26	15	F	R	Caucasian	8	14
7	43	16	F	R	Caucasian	Minutes	45
8	53	12	F	R	Caucasian	21	33
9	41	12	M	R	African American	1	1
10	42	14	M	R	Caucasian	14	30
11	28	11	M	R	Caucasian	30	300
12	48	12	M	R	Caucasian	8	8
13	20	12	F	L	Caucasian	28	95

Note. LOC, loss of consciousness (as identified in medical records); PTA, posttraumatic amnesia or confusion, reported by patient as the length of time his or her confusion lasted; M, male; F, female.

TABLE 11.8. Overall Test Battery Means for Multiple Test Subjects

Subject no.		Testing 1	Testing 2	Testing 3	Testing 4	Testing 5	Testing 6
1	OTBM (M)	38.10(96)	44.97(110)				
2	OTBM (M)	38.65(14)	41.32(24)				
3	OTBM (M)	43.94(13)	43.26(24)				
4[a]	OTBM (M)	48.73(25)	46.25(85)				
5	OTBM (M)	29.82(13)	32.50(54)				
6	OTBM (M)	44.79(63)	44.56(67)				
7	OTBM (M)	51.59(32)	55.24(36)	53.65(54)			
8	OTBM (M)	29.44(113)	31.29(134)				
9	OTBM (M)	51.35(19)	49.88(28)				
10	OTBM (M)	30.88(21)	31.35(45)	32.30(70)			
11	OTBM (M)	24.29(42)	26.15(61)				
12	OTBM (M)	39.76(23)	38.38(60)				
13	OTBM (M)	26.24(12)	26.62(21)	30.74(26)	30.09(33)	29.85(39)	33.10(68)

Note. OTBM, overall test battery mean, T score; (M), months postinjury at the time of the testing. The largest drop in scores between testing was 1.59 T score points (without additional injury). Therefore, a decline of 5 points in the OTBM would be inconsistent with traumatic brain injury.
[a] This patient was later diagnosed with MS in addition to TBI. Drop from first testing to second testing was 2.48 T score points.

scores would be the same or show improvement, unless some other intervening neurological event was present. Therefore, a decline in function of 5 T-score points or more could be an indication of reduced motivation to perform well (this of course assumes no intervening neurological disease). Subject 3 had not had medication for possible seizure disorder at any time. Subjects 2, 9, and 12 had antiseizure medications in the past but only briefly. Subject 4 was on antiseizure medications and medication for MS (added after first testing). Subjects 1, 5, 6, and 11 were on seizure medications at the time of the first assessment and the medications had been stopped prior to the second assessment. For the rest of the subjects no changes in medications were reported between the different times of the assessments. All had been treated with selective serotonin reuptake inhibitors, currently or after their injury at some point. Medication changes may have had some effect on test scores, but no clear pattern was observed. Subject 13 was assessed as part of a study of effects of hyperbaric oxygen (HBO) treatment. She had a series of treatments between the third assessment and the fourth. The fifth assessment was after treatment sets. Assessment six was a follow-up to the HBO treatment.

The persons selected for this experiment were all at least 1 year postinjury when assessed and so would be expected to be fairly stable in their recovery. It was observed that some persons did show improved scores, suggesting that continued cognitive improvement past a year may be expected. The approach presented by the Malingering Actors to "do worse" as time goes on appears to be an important sign to examine for declining motivation.

CONCLUSION

From the data presented, it was found that it was easy for nonsophisticated persons with no specific training in brain injury to report symptoms of brain injury; likewise, it was easy to do poorly on neuropsychological testing and have those test results appear like a moderate to severe traumatic injury. The time postinjury, the length of LOC, and PTA, along with demographic variables, were not related to performance on the internal validity items. Not all tests are malingered equally. The nature of the task and the person's feelings that he or she can malinger on that task without being "caught" determine which tasks are malingered. Persons with no specific training in brain injury are able to "fake" a pattern of scores that looks like a brain injury. However, "faked" performance is much below the expected level of performance compared to the LOC.

Behavioral observations showed that the "approach" to malingering described by the Malingering Actors and the behaviors of Probable Malingerers (using the Slick et al., 1999, criteria) were similar. Cognitive com plaints presented by those who do and those who do not pass the validity checks are similar; therefore, reliance on "reported" symptoms to assess for validity is inappropriate, specific validity checks are needed. Unsophisticated persons with no background in brain injury report the types of cognitive and behavioral complaints commonly associated with brain injury. In short, it is easy to fake cognitive impairment or brain injury.

Six of the 20 persons in the Malingering Actor group reported they would use their lawyer as a source of information on how to "malinger" on the neuropsychological tests. It is interesting that attorneys were felt to be a source of information on how to "malinger." The implications of this are similar to that reported by Youngjohn (1995) and Youngjohn et al. (1999) that attorneys are or are perceived as a source of information on how to "fake" an injury.

The most common pattern of performance by persons attempting to present themselves as brain injured was a "frontal pattern." These Malingering Actors were able to present with a "moderate to severe injury." The implications of this are clear—that performance on a battery of tests that is disproportionately low compared to the expected level of performance is a characteristic of those who have poor motivation to perform well. Performance that declines between assessments with similar batteries of tests and no additional neurological injury could also be suspect. The data presented show that TBI patients generally score similarly on serial testing when a similar battery of tests is given. It would not be expected that there would be a change of 5 points or more on the OTBM as change is generally less than 2 T-points unless additional injury occurs between the two assessments.

These results underscore the need for validity testing as part of a neuropsychological assessment. Internal validity items should be used to assess motivation for all assessments, especially those in a medical/legal setting. Failure on two or more validity checks suggest that the data are not reliable to determine brain injury or cognitive impairment. However, the data would be usable as an assessment of poor motivation to perform well. Failure on only one validity check may only invalidate a portion of the assessment and thus should be interpreted as "variable motivation," not "impaired motivation."

The information presented in this chapter addresses the behavioral methods people employ when attempting to malinger or to present themselves as more impaired than they actually are. People that have no training in brain injury are able to present themselves as impaired on cognitive tasks. They are also able to present symptoms of brain injury and describe how they would present those symptoms during a neuropsychological evaluation. The most common pattern of neuropsychological deficits presented by untrained individuals who have been asked to malinger and by probable malingerers is a "frontal pattern."

The complaint that brain injury "gets worse" as time goes on was also examined, and it is clear, with serial testing, that the overall test battery performance remains consistent unless there is some type of intervening injury. A traumatic brain injury of itself does not get "worse as time goes on."

The data presented underscore the need for validity checks contained within the neuropsychological assessment. The validity checks should address multiple avenues or approaches that may be used by individuals who are presenting themselves as more impaired than they actually are. It is clear from the information presented in this chapter that not everyone uses the same approach to malingering, but there are some commonalities, including the attempt to present oneself as honest and believable, but still significantly impaired. When caught in their malingering attempts, the malingering actors often report to their lawyer that they were nervous or anxious, or they make an excuse as to why the testing was "invalid." This is also the behavior noted in probable malingerers. The behavioral reports of the malingering actors and the behavioral observations of the probable malingerers were similar, giving insight into the behavioral aspects of the process of malingering.

REFERENCES

Barona, A., Reynolds, C. R., & Chastain, R. (1984). A demographically based index of premorbid intelligence for the WAIS-R. *Journal of Consulting and Clinical Psychology, 52*, 885–887.

Dikmen, S. S., Machamer, J. E., Winn, H. R., & Temkin, N. R. (1995). Neuropsychological outcome at 1-year post head injury. *Neuropsychology, 9*, 80–90.

Green, P., Rohling, M. L., Lees-Haley, P. R., & Allen, L. M. (2001). Effort has a greater effect on test scores than severe brain injury in compensation claimants. *Brain Injury, 15*(12), 1045–1060.

Greiffenstein, M. F., Baker, W. J., & Gola, T. (1994). Validation of malingered amnesia measures with a large clinical sample. *Psychological Assessment, 6*, 218–224.

Heaton, R. K., Chelune, G. J., Talley, J. L., Kay, C. G., & Curtiss, G. (1993). *Wisconsin Card Sorting Test manual. Revised and expanded.* Odessa, FL: Psychological Assessment Resources.

Heaton, R. K., Smith, H. H., Jr., Lehman, R. A., & Vogt, A. J. (1978). Prospects for faking believable deficits on neuropsychological testing. *Journal of Consulting and Clinical Psychology, 46*, 892–900.

Iverson, G. (1995). Qualitative aspects of malingering memory deficits. *Brain Injury, 9*(1), 35–40.

Larrabee, G. J. (2003). Detection of malingering using atypical performance patterns on standard neuropsychological tests. *The Clinical Neuropsychologist, 17*(3), 410–425.

Meyers, J. E. (2004). Meyers Neuropsychological Battery (MNB). Computer Software. Meyers Neuropsychological Services. Available at: www.meyersneuropsychological.com.

Meyers, J. E., & Diep, A. (2000). Assessment of malingering in chronic pain patients using neuropsychological tests. *Applied Neuropsychology, 7,* 133–139.

Meyers, J. E., Galinsky, A., & Volbrecht, M. (1999). Malingering and mild brain injury: How low is too low. *Applied Neuropsychology, 6,* 208–216.

Meyers, J. E., & Meyers, K. R. (1995a). *Rey Complex Figure Test and Recognition Trial: Professional manual.* Odessa, FL: Psychological Assessment Resource.

Meyers, J. E., & Meyers, K. R. (1995b). The Rey Complex Figure and Recognition Trial under four different administration procedures. *The Clinical Neuropsychologist, 9,* 65–67.

Meyers, J. E., Morrison, A. L., & Miller, J. C. (2001). How low is too low, revisited: Sentence Repetition and AVLT-Recognition in the detection of malingering. *Applied Neuropsychology, 8*(4), 234–241.

Meyers, J. E., & Rohling, M. L. (2004). Validation of the Meyers Short Battery on Mild TBI patients. *Archives of Clinical Neuropsychology, 19,* 637–651.

Meyers, J. E., & Volbrecht, M. (1998a). Validation of memory error patterns on the Rey Complex Figure and Recognition Trial. *Applied Neuropsychology, 5,* 120–131.

Meyers, J. E., & Volbrecht, M. (1998b). Validation of reliable digits for detection of malingering. *Assessment, 5,* 301–305.

Meyers, J. E., & Volbrecht, M. (1999). Detection of malingerers using the Rey Complex Figure and Recognition Trial. *Applied Neuropsychology, 6*(4), 201–207.

Meyers, J. E., & Volbrecht, M. E. (2003). A validation of multiple malingering detection methods in a large clinical sample. *Archives of Clinical Neuropsychology, 18*(3), 261–276.

Millis, S. R. (1992). The Recognition Memory Test in the detection of malingered and exaggerated memory deficits. *The Clinical Neuropsychologist, 6,* 406–414.

Millis, S. R., Putnam, S. H., Adams, K. M., & Ricker, J. H. (1995). The California Verbal Learning Test in the detection of incomplete effort in neuropsychological evaluation. *Psychological Assessment, 7,* 463–471.

Mittenberg, W., Rotholc, A., Russell, E., & Heilbronner, R. (1996). Identification of malingered head injury on the Halstead–Reitan Battery. *Archives of Clinical Neuropsychology, 11,* 271–281.

Mittenberg, W., Theroux-Fichera, S., Zielinski, R. E., & Heilbronner, R. Z. (1995). Identification of malingered head injury on the Wechsler Adult Intelligence Scale–Revised. *Professional Psychology: Research and Practice, 26,* 491–498.

Rohling, M. L., Meyers, J. E., & Millis, S. R. (2003). Neuropsychological impairment following traumatic brain injury: A dose–response analysis. *The Clinical Neuropsychologist, 17,* 289–302.

Russel, E. W. (1998). In defense of the Halstead–Reitan Battery: A critique of Lezak's review. *Archives of Clinical Neuropsychology, 13,* 365–381.

Slick, D. J., Sherman, E. M. S., & Iverson, G. L. (1999). Diagnostic criteria for malingered neurocognitive dysfunction: Proposed standards for clinical practice and research. *The Clinical Neuropsychologist, 13,* 545–561.

Suhr, J. A., & Boyer, D. (1999). Use of the Wisconsin Card Sorting test in the detection of malingering in student simulator and patient samples. *Journal of Clinical and Experimental Neuropsychology, 21,* 701–708.

Volbrecht, M., Meyers, J. E., & Kaster-Bundgaard, J. (2000). Neuropsychological outcome of head injury using a short battery. *Archives of Clinical Neuropsychology, 15,* 251–265.

Wetter, M., & Corrigan, S. (1995). Providing information to clients about psychological tests: A survey of attorneys' and law students' attitudes. *Professional Psychology: Research and Practice, 26,* 474–477.

Youngjohn, J. R. (1995). Confirmed attorney coaching prior to neuropsychological evaluation. *Assessment, 2,* 279–283.

Youngjohn, J. R., Lees-Haley, P. R., & Binder, L. M. (1999). Comment: Warning malingerers produces more sophisticated malingering. *Archives of Clinical Neuropsychology, 14,* 511–515.

CHAPTER 12

Including Measures of Effort in Neuropsychological Assessment of Pain- and Fatigue-Related Medical Disorders

Clinical and Research Implications

Julie Suhr
Brad Spickard

Over the last two decades, research has clearly demonstrated the need to address effort as a factor contributing to neuropsychological test results in mild traumatic brain injury, in both the clinical and research setting. However, the use of effort measures in other disorders in which there are cognitive complaints is still in its infancy. In several medical disorders characterized by pain, fatigue, or other subjectively judged physical symptoms, cognitive complaints are extremely common and are often cited as major factors in disability associated with these conditions (Bennett, 1996; Iverson & McCracken, 1997; Schnurr & MacDonald, 1995). Furthermore, many clinicians and researchers believe findings of poor neuropsychological performance are evidence for brain dysfunction and thus brain-based etiology for these medical disorders (e.g., Arnold et al., 2002; Bell, Primeau, Sweet, & Lofland, 1999; Crombez, Eccleston, Baeyens, Van Houdenhove & Van Den Broeck, 1999; Jamison, Sbrocco, & Paris, 1988; Landro, Stiles, & Sletvold, 1997; Lawrie, MacHale, Cavanagh, O'Carroll, & Goodwin, 2000).

Although poor effort is a variable often overlooked in neuropsychological studies of chronic pain- and fatigue-related disorders, malingering is perceived to be relatively common in such disorders. For example, Mittenberg, Patton, Canyock, and Condit (2002) surveyed American Board of Clinical Neuropsychology members in active practice, asking them to estimate rates of cognitive malingering in personal injury, disability, criminal, and medical litigation cases. The base rates for malingering averaged around 30% for patients seeking compensation or actively involved in litigation, regardless of clinical setting. By diagnostic group, surveyed psychologists estimated a 39% malingering rate in patients with fibromyalgia and a 34% malingering rate in patients with other pain/somatoform disorders. Estimated base rates for malingering were much lower for patients not seeking compensation or involved in litigation, averaging 7 to 12%.

Objective test data support the impression of clinicians with regard to poor effort in pain and other medical disorders, particularly in the context of disability claims. For example, Gervais, Rohling, Green, and Ford (2004) examined rates of failure on three common instruments for assessing poor effort (the Word Memory Test, the Computerized Assessment of Response Bias, and the Test of Memory Malingering) in an archive of patient data from referrals related to workers' compensation, disability, or personal injury claims. The majority of the sample consisted of musculoskeletal pain patients with orthopedic injuries (66%), another 9% had diagnoses of fibromyalgia/chronic fatigue syndrome, approximately 5% reported chronic pain associated with repetitive strain, and around 10% of the sample consisted of non-pain-related diagnoses (anxiety, posttraumatic stress disorder, depression). Of note, none of the participants had head-injury-associated claims, yet cognitive complaints (as assessed by the Memory Complaints Inventory) were extremely common, with 84% of claimants indicating that pain symptoms interfered with their memory and 80% indicating that memory problems interfered with their ability to work. Although the three tests were not equally sensitive to invalid performance, a significant percentage of the group of individuals seeking disability for their pain/fatigue failed at least one effort test (e.g., 43% failure on the Word Memory Test).

These data suggest that a large number of patients with pain and fatigue syndromes exaggerate or malinger their cognitive impairments, yet very little is done to address this concern in either the clinical or research arena. Ignoring a factor that could account for a significant amount of the variance in cognitive performance in an individual patient's cognitive profile increases the likelihood of a clinician making diagnostic errors and/or suggesting consequences that are unfounded (such as cognitive-related disability). In the research setting, ignoring a factor that could account for a significant amount of the variance in cognitive performance in studies of patients with such disorders may lead to misunderstanding of the true relation of cognitive impairment (and, by extension, brain dysfunction) to those disorders. In this chapter, we demonstrate the importance of considering poor effort in both clinical and research-based neuropsychological assessment of medical conditions, using fibromyalgia, chronic fatigue syndrome, multiple chemical sensitivity, and non-head-injury-associated chronic pain as illustrative conditions.

FIBROMYALGIA

Fibromyalgia is a systemic condition characterized by complaints of generalized pain and multiple tender points, with numerous other associated symptoms, including fatigue, stiffness, and cognitive complaints. Fibromyalgia is a significant cause of long-term disability (Gordon, 1999; White & Harth, 1999). Although not part of the diagnostic criteria, cognitive complaints are frequently seen in patients diagnosed with fibromyalgia (Glass & Park, 2001; Grace, Nielson, Hopkins, & Berg, 1999; Komaroff & Goldenberg, 1989; Wolfe, Ross, Anderson, Russell, & Hebert, 1995). However, evidence for cognitive impairment in fibromyalgia is inconsistent; for any study finding impairment in a particular neuropsychological construct or with a specific neuropsychological measure, one can find another study that did not find impairment in that construct or with that measure.

Various explanations for the presence of cognitive impairment in fibromyalgia have been suggested by investigators, including psychological correlates of the illness such as depression (Ahles, Khan, Yunus, Spiegel, & Masi, 1991; Grace et al., 1999; Kaplan, Meadows, Vincent, Logigian, & Steere, 1992; Wallace, 1997), sleep difficulties (Cote & Moldofsky, 1997), neuroendocrine abnormalities leading to hypocortisolism (Sephton et al., 2003), cerebral dysfunction (Johansson et al., 1995; Landro et al., 1997; Mountz et al., 1995), and attentional distraction from pain (Grisart, Van der Linden, & Masquelier, 2002). However, no consistent evidence has emerged to clearly implicate any of these hypothesized causes. In fact, some researchers have found evidence inconsistent with their own hypotheses. For example, Sephton et al. (2003) speculated that higher cortisol levels in patients with fibromyalgia would be associated with worse memory performance, but the opposite was demonstrated in their study. Cote and Moldofsky (1997) expected to find a diurnal variation in cognitive performance based on hypothesized sleep irregularities in fibromyalgia but instead found consistently impaired cognitive performance across time. Grisart et al. (2002) applied the cognitive attention model of pain to fibromyalgia, hypothesizing that patients with fibromyalgia would show worse attention, given their more generalized pain, than patients with other chronic pain disorders and healthy controls but actually found enhanced attention performance in fibromyalgia relative to these groups.

Why are neuropsychological results in fibromyalgia so inconsistent and sometimes opposite of prediction? Above and beyond the usual methodological concerns when comparing studies (sample size, selection of control groups, sensitivity of cognitive measures used, etc.), we speculate that lack of control for poor effort can account for some of the discrepancies. Table 12.1 presents a list of neuropsychological studies in fibromyalgia, illustrating the samples used and whether or not effort measures were included in the battery. It is clear that few published studies of cognitive impairment in fibromyalgia controlled for poor effort in their data. In fact, there is little acknowledgement of the need to consider the effort as an important variable in this population; of the studies that do not include effort measures, only Dick, Eccleston, and Crombez (2002) even suggest the need to use such measures in future studies.

The lack of control for poor effort in existing studies on neuropsychological outcome in fibromyalgia is all the more notable in the face of data suggesting a high rate of failure on effort tests in this disorder. For example, Gervais et al. (2001) found that 24% of a sample of patients with fibromyalgia already on or actively applying for disability scored below very conservative cutoffs on the Cognitive Assessment of Response Bias (CARB), 30% of them scored below conservative cutoffs for the Word Memory Test

TABLE 12.1. Review of Neuropsychological Studies of Fibromyalgia

Authors (year)	Source of fibromyalgia sample	Litigation/ disability status	Control for effort?
Kaplan et al. (1992)	Patients referred for cognitive testing due to complaints.	Unknown	No
Landro et al. (1997); Sletvold et al. (1995)	Patients recruited from fibromyalgia association (same sample both studies).	Unknown	No
Cote & Moldofsky (1997)	Patients from clinic sample.	Unknown	No
Grace et al. (1999)	Patients in multidisciplinary treatment program.	Unknown	No
Park et al. (2001)	Patients currently in treatment.	Unknown	No
Dick et al. (2002)	Patients seeking treatment.	Unknown	No
Grisart et al. (2002)	Two samples of patients recruited from pain treatment centers.	Unknown	No
Suhr (2003)	Patients recruited after completing research-based treatment.	Unknown	Yes
Sephton et al. (2003)	Patients participating in stress reduction study.	31% disabled	No
de Gier et al. (2003)	Patients recruited from fibromyalgia association.	38% employed	No

(WMT), and 35% scored below cutoffs on one or both of these tests. By comparison, in the group of patients with fibromyalgia who were not on disability or applying for disability, none scored below cutoffs on the CARB and 4% scored below cutoffs on the WMT. Furthermore, in the control group of patients with rheumatoid arthritis, no patients scored below the cutoff on either measure.

Another fibromyalgia study that included an effort measure was Suhr (2003). Participants were patients with fibromyalgia (meeting standard diagnostic criteria and diagnosed by a rheumatologist) who had completed participation in a large treatment study. Patients with fibromyalgia were compared to a group of individuals with various chronic pain disorders (osteoarthritis, chronic headache, low back pain, rheumatoid arthritis) who had also completed participation in a research-based treatment project, and to a healthy age-matched control group. As a part of the neuropsychological test battery, the Auditory Verbal Learning Test was administered and a version of the Exaggeration Index for the Auditory Verbal Learning Test—Expanded was calculated (EIAVLT-X; Barrash, Suhr, & Manzel, 2004; Suhr, Gunstad, Greub, & Barrash, 2004). EIAVLT-X scores demonstrated that 5 of 28 participants with fibromyalgia and 5 of 27 participants with other chronic pain diagnoses failed the EIAVLT-X, while none of the control group participants failed. After excluding individuals who failed the effort test, there was no difference in cognitive performance among any of the groups, although patients with fibromyalgia still self-reported more depression, pain, fatigue, and cognitive complaints.

What do such findings suggest for existing fibromyalgia research? The Suhr (2003) and Gervais et al. (2001) studies both used samples directly recruited for a neuropsychological research project after completion of a treatment research project. Yet they were clinical samples, and in Gervais's sample, a high percentage of participants were either on disability or actively seeking it at the time of their neuropsychological evaluation. Such findings suggest that individuals recruited specifically for research after completing treatment protocols still fail effort tests, and Gervais's findings also suggest that failure on effort measures is strongly tied to disability status. Of the studies summarized in Table 12.1, five recruited participants from clinic referrals who were actively in treatment, while three more recruited individuals from a fibromyalgia association. Litigation/disability status was unreported for all studies, with the exception of Sephton et al. (2003), who noted that 31% of the sample were totally disabled, despite having physical symptom scores milder on average than other samples they had studied, and de Gier, Peters, and Vlaeyen (2003), who indicated that 38% of the sample were employed. We suggest that, given data on the percentage of patients with fibromyalgia who fail effort tests, a significant proportion of the samples tested may have invalidly low cognitive scores, driving down the overall mean for the fibromyalgia patient group. Then, when this inaccurate group average is compared to control samples, the results suggest an overall poorer performance in the group with fibromyalgia as a whole.

A few studies describe their neuropsychological findings in enough detail to support this speculation. For example, Grace et al. (1999) indicated that 23.3% of their group of fibromyalgia patients scored 2 standard deviations or more below the mean of at least one neuropsychological measure administered in their battery, leading them to conclude that a subgroup of their sample of fibromyalgia patients was "at risk for having clinically significant impairment." It may be that the vast majority of this subgroup gave poor effort on the cognitive tests, creating an invalidly lowered overall mean for the group as a whole. Gervais et al. (2001) conducted follow-up analyses that lend further support to this hypothesis. When their group of fibromyalgia patients on disability was divided into those who passed the WMT effort subtests versus those who did not, those who failed scored significantly lower on all WMT subtests than those who passed; in fact their scores on memory-related subtests of the WMT fell 1 to 1.6 standard deviations below means relative to samples of patients with severe traumatic brain injury or documented memory impairment. Thus, those who failed the effort subtests also looked extremely impaired on the memory measures.

To further illustrate this point, we reanalyzed data from Suhr (2003), examining specifically the excluded participants who had performed abnormally on the effort test. Analysis of the 10 individuals who failed revealed that they performed significantly worse than controls on the Digit Symbol subtest of the Wechsler Adult Intelligence Scale–III (WAIS-III) and Trail-making Test B. As described earlier, when the noncredible subjects were removed from the samples, no differences in cognitive performance were found between patients and controls. However, when the participants who failed effort tests were returned to their claimed diagnostic groups and the data were reanalyzed, the group of individuals with fibromyalgia performed significantly worse than controls on the Auditory Verbal Learning Test, Digit Symbol and Arithmetic subtests of the WAIS-III, and Trailmaking Test B; in addition, both pain groups performed significantly worse than controls on Controlled Oral Word Association. Thus, leaving individuals with invalid performance in the overall sample would have dramatically changed the results of the study and its implications for neuropsychological impairment in fibromyalgia.

CHRONIC FATIGUE SYNDROME

Another medically unexplained disorder that has received a great deal of recent neuropsychological attention is chronic fatigue syndrome. Chronic fatigue syndrome is characterized by the experience of debilitating fatigue with no clear somatic explanation. Chronic fatigue syndrome can also be accompanied by multiple pain symptoms, and cognitive complaints are very common (Michiels, Cluydts, Fischler, & Hoffman, 1996; Vercoulen et al., 1998). As in fibromyalgia, neuropsychological findings in chronic fatigue syndrome do not demonstrate a consistent pattern of cognitive impairment; many of the most recent studies in this area, as described below, acknowledge this difficulty in their literature reviews. Some studies have also taken note of the high variability in test scores observed in their samples, emphasizing that it would be inappropriate to generalize the average cognitive scores to all patients with chronic fatigue syndrome, if only a subgroup of patients is impaired (Michiels et al., 1996; Vercoulen et al., 1998). However, reasons for severe impairment in a subgroup of patients are not often considered. Table 12.2 summarizes recent neuropsychological findings with regard to sample source, litigation/disability status, and the role of effort tests in the research battery. It is clear that these studies as a whole do not control for poor effort, nor do the authors of these studies consider poor effort as a potential explanatory factor when interpreting their study results, even when results are inconsistent with known patterns of central nervous system dysfunction, hypotheses regarding the etiology of the cognitive impairment, or with existing neuropsychological literature.

As in fibromyalgia, few neuropsychological studies have included effort measures in studies of chronic fatigue. In one (Busichio, Tiersky, DeLuca, & Natelson, 2004) of the 141 patients with chronic fatigue syndrome in the sample, only 34 were administered an effort test (the Test of Memory Malingering, or TOMM). Of the 34 who did complete the TOMM, none failed. This failure rate seems unusual given other findings in the literature, but concerns have been raised about the sensitivity of the TOMM to poor effort (Gervais, Green, & Allen, 1999; Gervais et al., 2004; Green, Berendt, Mandel, & Allen, 2000). Also, the disability status of the patients who participated in Busichio et al. (2004) study was not reported. Other investigations that have specifically examined performance on effort tests in individuals with chronic fatigue syndrome have found high failure rates. For example, van der Werf, Prins, Jongen, van der Meer and Bleijenberg (2000) found a 30% failure rate on a forced-choice effort task in a sample of patients with chronic fatigue syndrome who were participating in longitudinal fatigue and treatment studies; 13% of a control group of patients with multiple sclerosis also failed the forced-choice effort test. Notably, a high percentage of patients with chronic fatigue syndrome who failed the forced-choice effort test also scored in the clinically significantly impaired range on a symbol digit task. In a second study, van der Werf, de Vree, van der Meer, and Bleijenberg (2002) found a 23% failure rate in their sample of individuals with chronic fatigue syndrome, using the same forced-choice effort measure as in their 2000 study. On the other hand, Binder, Storzbach, Campbell, Rohlman, and Anger (2001) did not find failures on a computerized forced-

TABLE 12.2. Review of Recent Neuropsychological Studies of Chronic Fatigue Syndrome

Authors (year)	Source of chronic fatigue syndrome sample	Litigation/disability status	Control for effort?
Grafman et al. (1993)	Patients participating in National Institutes of Health research.	Unknown	No
Joyce et al. (1996)	Individuals meeting chronic fatigue syndrome diagnostic criteria in final stage of prospective community-based study of viral infection.	Most not seeking treatment for chronic fatigue syndrome at time of study	No
Marcel et al. (1996)	Unknown.	Described as homebound/bedridden/ unable to work full time	No
Michiels et al. (1996)	Patients from larger research project.	74.3% unable to work	No
Christodoulou et al. (1998)	Patients referred by self or physician for testing.	Unknown	No
Michiels et al. (1998)	Patients recruited from a fatigue clinic, 95% complained of cognitive impairment.	Average patient described as unable to carry out normal activity/do active work	No
Michiels et al. (1999)	Patients recruited from clinic.	Unknown	No
Johnson et al. (1998)	Patients recruited for free medical workup and referral to chronic fatigue syndrome center.	Unknown	No
Vercoulen et al. (1998)	Patients from existing database (referrals for testing).	Unknown	No
Lawrie et al. (2000)	Patients recruited from self-help group and clinic.	Unknown	No

Study	Description		
van der Werf et al. (2000)	Patients in ongoing research project.	Unknown	Yes
Dobbs et al. (2001)	Patients in treatment.	Unknown	No
Ross et al. (2001)	Patients who had been in prior chronic fatigue syndrome studies.	Unknown	No
Short et al. (2002)	Patients recruited through their physicians.	Unknown	No
Morriss et al. (2002)	Consecutive attenders at an outpatient clinic for chronic fatigue syndrome.	Unknown	No
Arnold et al. (2002)	Patients with chronic fatigue syndrome versus healthy controls.	Unknown	No
van der Werf (2002)	Unknown.	Unknown	Yes
Tiersky et al. (2003)	Unknown.	Unknown	No
de Lange et al. (2004)	Unknown.	Unknown	No
DeLuca et al. (2004)	Patients referred by self or physician for study.	Unknown	No
Busichio et al. (2004)	Unknown.	Unknown	Partial[a]
Mahurin et al. (2004)	Volunteer twin registry, selected twins discordant for chronic fatigue syndrome.	Unknown	No

[a] Thirty-four of 141 patients with chronic fatigue syndrome, given TOMM, all "passed" (no data provided).

267

choice effort task in their sample of Persian Gulf War veterans with chronic fatigue syndrome.

Many researchers have speculated about the neurophysiological causes for neuropsychological impairment in chronic fatigue syndrome, though in many cases results have been inconsistent with their hypotheses (e.g., Lawrie et al., 2000; Morriss, Robson, & Deakin, 2002; Arnold et al., 2002). Lawrie and colleagues (Lawrie, MacHale, Power, & Goodwin, 1997; Lawrie et al., 2000) have suggested that the reason for neuropsychological test failure in chronic fatigue syndrome is a "failure in effort mobilization." They argue that higher-order motor and cognitive processing requires more brain "effort," and impairment in higher-order working memory or motor/executive skills in chronic fatigue syndrome thus lead to cognitive compromise. However, such an explanation would not account for the subgroup of patients with chronic fatigue syndrome who fail tests that *appear to* require cognitive effort but in fact are easy even for cognitively compromised individuals—effort tests. We suggest that it is the *perception* of required effort that is at issue, and thus the explanation for neuropsychological findings in a subset of individuals with chronic fatigue syndrome is a psychological, not a neurological, one. However, such a speculation cannot be fully assessed without consistent use of effort measures in this and related populations.

MULTIPLE CHEMICAL SENSITIVITY

Evidence suggests that there is a large overlap in the physical and cognitive symptoms and even medical findings among individuals diagnosed with various medically unexplained physical disorders (Aaron & Buchwald, 2001). For example, patients diagnosed with chronic fatigue syndrome and fibromyalgia report sensitivities to various substances at similar rates to individuals diagnosed with multiple chemical sensitivity (Fiedler, Kipen, DeLuca, Kelly-McNeil, & Natelson, 1996; Labarge & McCaffrey, 2000), and patients with multiple chemical sensitivity are often also diagnosed with chronic fatigue syndrome or fibromyalgia (Bell, Baldwin, & Schwartz, 1998; Sparks, 2000).

There are few published neuropsychological studies of individuals diagnosed with multiple chemical sensitivity; in a 2000 review of the literature, Labarge and McCaffrey found little evidence of a consistent cognitive profile for individuals with this diagnosis, and they strongly recommended that future studies include effort measures in order to address concerns about the role of poor effort in explaining the inconsistent findings in the literature. Such a recommendation is extremely important, given the high rate of disability, workman's compensation, and major changes to lifestyle that accompany this diagnosis. Yet when we searched for more recent articles addressing neuropsychological impairment in this disorder, we found few published studies, none of which addressed the issue of poor effort with an effort measure.

In a fascinating report, Smith and Sullivan (2003) examined the neuropsychological performance of 36 individuals diagnosed with chronic fatigue syndrome who had been referred to an allergy specialist for testing due to complaints of chemical sensitivity. About 75% of the sample had specific neuropsychological complaints, and most were seeking compensation (such as disability). A standard allergen exposure protocol was administered. Substances to which each person reported a reaction were then further examined using a double-blind exposure paradigm. Individuals were tested before and 1 hour postexposure to either the reactive agent or a placebo (randomly administered on 2 separate exposure days). The testing battery included memory, attention, motor speed, coordination, and visuospatial measures. Each patient was also asked to predict whether they received the reactive agent. There was a general trend toward worse neuropsychological performance postexposure, regardless of whether the reactive agent or the placebo was the substance used. Interestingly, the patients' *beliefs* about what they had been exposed to were the strongest predictor of neuropsychological test performance, particularly in psychomotor processing speed and memory ability. Although this study did not measure effort per se, the findings were consistent with a psychological rather than a physiological explanation for their findings, and supportive of our hypothesis that at least some minority of patients with similar medical concerns have invalidly low neuropsychological performance on tests, a hypothesis that cannot be fully tested without consistent inclusion of effort measures in neuropsychological research.

CHRONIC PAIN

Cognitive complaints are among the most frequently reported complaints for individuals with chronic head/neck pain (Nicholson & Martelli, 2004) and are also frequent in other types of chronic pain, particularly among patients involved in litigation or other secondary gain associated with their pain symptoms (Iverson, King, Scott, & Adams, 2001). The vast majority of literature on chronic pain and neuropsychological functioning is from posttraumatic pain associated with head injury or whiplash. There are fewer studies of non-head injury associated chronic pain and its cognitive effects (e.g., low back pain, nontraumatic headache, and rheumatoid arthritis). It is clear from examining this literature that poor effort is an explanatory variable not considered in these studies, despite recommendations for the use of effort measures in clinical practice with pain patients (Martelli, Zasler, Bender, & Nicholson, 2004). For example, Bell et al. (1999) explored whether neuropsychological impairment was present in migraine populations, based on existing migraine research findings that suggested evidence of persistent and subtle brain dysfunction secondary to cranial neurovascular dysfunction. They studied 20 patients with migraine (most with aura), 20 patients with chronic pain (mostly back, more than 50% actively seeking disability compensation), and 20 patients with mild traumatic brain injuries (50% seeking compensation, some with headaches). Interestingly, although all the patients with traumatic brain injury were screened for poor effort with the Multi-Digit Memory Test, leading to exclusion of three participants, this test was not used in either of the other two groups. This study demonstrates that there is recognition of the need to control for poor effort in mild traumatic brain injury but minimal recognition of a need to consider this factor in other clinical populations.

Lack of effort assessment in chronic pain research is highlighted in a review article by Hart, Marelli, and Zasler (2000) that examined the effect of chronic pain on neuropsychological functioning. Participants in the studies reviewed did not have a history of traumatic brain injury, and some of the research studies included individuals involved in litigation. Neuropsychological impairment was found in patients with chronic pain disorders in several studies reviewed by the authors, suggesting significant chronic pain-associated impairment in attentional capacity, processing speed, and psychomotor speed. However, of the 23 studies reviewed, only one study, conducted by Schmand et al. (1998), tested for poor effort. Hart et al. (2000) included this study in their review because the patients had chronic whiplash injuries without concurrent traumatic brain injury and without loss of consciousness at the time of injury; all were seen on average 2 years since injury and many were being seen as part of litigation. Of 108 patients in the study, 43 scored below cutoffs on the forced-choice effort measure, and these individuals performed as poorly on the neuropsychological battery as did patients with a history of severe head injury. Patients who passed the forced-choice test did not perform as well on neuropsychological tests as normal controls but did perform significantly better than patients who did not pass the forced-choice test. Excluding the Schmand et al. (1998) study, studies demonstrating neuropsychological impairment as a result of chronic pain that were reviewed by Hart et al. (2000) did not take into account the effects of poor effort on their results, and we have been unsuccessful in locating more recent nontraumatic pain studies that have addressed this significant limitation.

Although more recent chronic pain studies have made attempts to improve research controls (recruiting participants who are not just treatment seekers, controlling for headache state, conducting repeated measures within subject designs), often disability and litigation rates are not reported. Without addressing disability and litigation rates, and without inclusion of measures of poor effort, it is largely unknown what effect poor effort has on results of these studies. For example, studies that find a significant drop in cognitive functioning during migraine relative to premigraine state conclude that this reflects temporary brain dysfunction. We argue that rather than pointing to brain dysfunction as the sole cause of lower test scores, poor effort may play a role in an individual's performance on neuropsychological tests during times of migraine and recovery.

As with fibromyalgia and chronic fatigue syndrome, there is evidence for the need to assess for effort in other non-head-injury-related chronic pain disorders. For example, Meyers and Diep (2000) assessed effort in 108 chronic pain patients, 55 of whom were seeking disability for symptoms associated with their pain, including cognitive complaints. Participants were assessed for poor effort using cutoffs on standard neuropsychological tests obtained from existing effort studies. Twenty-nine percent of the litigation group failed two or more of six neuropsychological indicators of poor effort, versus none within the nonlitigation group. More recently, Meyers and Volbrecht (2003) studied a large sample of individuals with various diagnoses, including two subgroups of individuals reporting chronic pain attributed to many etiologies (but no head injury history), and found that 26% of the group currently in litigation related to chronic pain failed two or more tests validated in previous studies as indices of poor effort. In contrast, none of the group of patients with chronic pain but not involved in litigation failed two or more effort tests. Their results further emphasize the importance of considering secondary gain as a factor. The Gervais et al. (2004) study described briefly above provides further support for this issue. They studied a large sample of referrals to a private practice for neuropsychological assessment, described in more detail earlier. Some of the referrals were for workman's compensation/disability/personal injury claims, and others were vocational assessment referrals (patients who might receive extended benefits to pay for vocational training if cognitive competencies were demonstrated with evaluation). All referrals had been administered the WMT, the CARB, and the TOMM, as part of an extensive neuropsychological research battery. In the disability-associated referrals, 43% failed the WMT, 25% failed the CARB, and 17% failed the TOMM. Among those referred for vocational assessment, 12% failed the WMT, 4% failed the CARB, and 1% failed the TOMM. Those who failed the TOMM virtually always failed one of the other effort measures and also had the lowest neuropsychological scores in the sample, suggesting that performance on the neuropsychological measures was related to poor effort and not reflective of cognitive dysfunction.

IMPLICATIONS

The evidence reviewed previously suggests that it is necessary to consider the role poor effort plays in neuropsychological assessment of individuals with pain- and fatigue-related medical conditions, particularly when the clinical evaluation occurs in the context of a clear secondary gain. Furthermore, it is necessary to assess for this variable in neuropsychological studies of these conditions, in order to account for a variable that may explain the inconsistencies in existing research. However, it is also clear that not all individuals with such disorders fail effort tasks. Thus, it would be erroneous to conclude that *all* individuals with these disorders have poor effort, based on the data presented; in fact, studies using effort measures suggest that the majority of individuals with these diagnoses do not have poor effort.

Even in individuals who perform poorly on effort tests, it cannot always be concluded that the failure is due to deliberate and conscious attempts to deceive (i.e., malingering). Other possible nonneurological contributions can and should be considered. For example, Boone and Lu (1999) found that persons with 1-3/3-1 MMPI (Minnesota Multiphasic Personality Inventory) codetypes fail cognitive malingering instruments at an extremely high rate (68% of their sample); most notably, this was in the absence of clear indicators of invalid performance on the validity scales of the MMPI. Thus, symptom presentation in somatization/ conversion disorders (where there is a high preponderance of medically unexplained physical symptoms) can also extend to presentation with noncredible cognitive impairment.

A growing body of research suggests the influence of psychological factors on neuropsychological test performance; some of these factors may even be amenable to treatment or intervention. For example, Grace et al. (1999) reported that many of their participants with fibromyalgia discontinued the Paced Auditory Serial Addition Test due to high anxiety. Others have explored the concept of pain-related fear (or cogniphobia) and its potential contribution to poor test performance (Crombez et al., 1999; Martelli, Zasler, Grayson, & Liljedahl, 1999; van der Werf et al., 2002). The concept of cogniphobia is related to the widely studied phenomenon of kinesophobia, in which patients' fears about activity exacerbating pain symptoms are more strongly related to disability than the actual pain symptoms induced by engaging in that activity. Cogniphobia extends this concept to cognitive symptoms: the fear that engaging in cognitively effortful tasks will exacerbate pain symptoms (such as headache), thus patients will avoid putting forth too much effort into cognitive tasks. These psychological contributions to test behavior remain understudied and undermeasured, despite their potential for guiding treatment in these disorders.

Yet another psychological variable possibly contributing to poor neuropsychological test performance is the role that negative expectations can play in test performance. Smith and Sullivan's (2003) study, described earlier, is an excellent example of the role that expectations can play in cognitive test performance. Our laboratory has documented the effect of negative expectations on test performance in mild head injury (Suhr & Gunstad, 2002, 2005), and others (Mittenberg, Tremont, Zielinski, Ficheras, & Rayls, 1996) have demonstrated that acute interventions to address expectations for recovery after mild head injury are beneficial for long-term functional outcome. We are currently conducting a study of the effect of negative expectations in cognitive performance of persons with chronic headache; preliminary results suggest that memory test performance is diminished in individuals with chronic headache exposed to negative expectations about cognitive performance in headache disorders.

What such studies suggest is that neuropsychologists should "keep the psychology in neuropsychology" by (1) including psychological assessment and interpretation in their neuropsychological evaluations, which would include not only measures of poor effort but measures of other possible contributors to poor performance on effort tests, and (2) considering recommendations for intervention when psychological contributions are apparent.

Use of Effort Instruments in Medical Neuropsychological Referrals

Utilization of effort measures in individuals with medical conditions who have cognitive complaints offers the potential for more accurate and objective evaluation of the patient's cognitive strengths and weaknesses and more effective and equitable allocation of limited financial resources for treatment, rehabilitation, and disability support (Gervais et al., 2004). It would be poor clinical practice to ignore the role poor effort may play in such conditions and instead attribute these symptoms solely to disease or injury. If substantial variance in a patient's performance can be attributed to poor effort, it must be taken into consideration.

Although some studies have used effort measures in such populations, the number of studies remains sparse and offers little guidance to selection of the appropriate effort tests for such samples. Gervais et al. (2004) suggest that some tests are more sensitive to others in detecting poor effort. Specifically, consistent with other research in other populations (Gervais et al., 1999; Green et al., 2000), they found that not all forced-choice-based effort tests are created equal; the TOMM was less sensitive to malingering than the CARB or the WMT. Green (2001) suggests a plausible explanation for this finding. The TOMM uses visuospatial stimuli, rather than verbal stimuli, and patients generally tend to self-report verbal memory problems than they do other types of memory problems; thus verbally based forced-choice tasks may be viewed as more "face-valid" reflections of the area of complaint. In any event, such findings add weight to Gervais et al.'s (2004) recommendation to use more than one effort test in the clinical setting. Another consideration is the use of non-forced-choice-based effort tests, such as those presented in Meyer's research (Meyers & Diep, 2000; Meyers & Volbrecht, 2003) or Suhr's (2003). Such tests are based on patterns of test performance within standard clinical instruments and thus could provide additional information about poor effort without added time to the standard assessment.

Another issue is that most effort measures focus on memory, because memory complaints are the most common. However, non-memory-based effort tests might be needed, as one of the more consistent neuropsychological findings in medical disorders is related to slowed psychomotor speed. However, some initial attempts to develop indicators of poor effort from existing measures of psychomotor speed have not been successful. For example, although some early work suggested that using a ratio of Trailmaking Test A and B scores (time to completion) might be useful in detection of poor effort (Ruffolo, Guilmette, & Willis, 2000; Lamberty, Putnam, Chatel, Bieliauskas, & Adams, 1994), more recent work has suggested that this ratio is not effective in effort assessment (Iverson, Lange, Green, & Franzen, 2002; Martin, Hoffman, & Donders, 2003; O'Bryant, Hilsabeck, Fisher, & McCaffrey, 2003). However, some recently developed effort measures, such as the Dot Counting Test (Boone, Lu, & Herzberg, 2002a) and the b Test (Boone et al., 2002b), the Finger Tapping Test (Arnold et al., 2005) and adaptations of Digit Span (Babikian et al., 2006) incorporating a time component, may have particular potential for the assessment of non-memory-based effort in fatigue and pain populations. Additional timed techniques, such as analysis of Paced Auditory Serial Addition Test patterns, reaction time with graded complexity, combinations of various motor function test scores, and reaction time on symptom validity tests may prove useful in identifying noncredible performance in these patient groups.

Further, given that another common complaint in chronic pain disorders is nondermatomal sensory dysfunction (Fishbain, Goldberg, Rosomoff, & Rosomoff, 1991), effort indices examining credibility of sensory processing may be particularly effective in this population. For example, Greve, Bianchini, and Ameduri (2003) reported three case studies of patients with injury-associated sensory loss and chronic pain who failed a forced-choice symptom validity test of tactile discrimination at below-chance levels. The use of non-memory-based effort tests remains understudied in general yet may be crucial to examination of poor effort in medical disorders.

Implications for Neuropsychological Research

The foregoing review raises serious concerns about the role of poor effort in explaining cognitive test results in existing medical neuropsychology literature. If substantial variance in neuropsychological test outcomes can be accounted for by poor effort, then cognitive symptoms previously believed to be reflective of central nervous system-related disease were misattributed. Furthermore, the presence of so much error variance in the data may hide a clear pattern of neuropsychological findings or obscure a meaningful relationship between physiological factors and cognitive performance, which could better guide treatment efforts. From a research perspective, any assessment that does not employ effort testing procedures to screen medical patients for poor effort runs the risk of drawing conclusions based on invalid test data or questionable self-reported symptoms and limitations. Hartman (2002) dreams of the day when research omitting effort tests will come to be considered "unpublishable and uninterpretable" (p. 713). Our review demonstrates that unfortunately we have not yet reached that day.

REFERENCES

Aaron, L. A., & Buchwald, D. (2001). A review of the evidence for overlap among unexplained clinical conditions. *Annals of Internal Medicine, 134*, 868–881.

Ahles, T. A., Khan, S. A., Yunus, M. B., Spiegel, D. A., & Masi A. T. (1991). Psychiatric status of patients with primary fibromyalgia, patients with rheumatoid arthritis, and subjects without pain: A blind comparison of DSM-III diagnoses. *American Journal of Psychiatry, 148*, 1721–1726.

Arnold, G., Boone, K. B., Lu, P., Dean, A., Wen, J., Nitch, S., et al. (2005). Sensitivity and specificity of finger tapping scores for the detection of suspect effort. *The Clinical Neuropsychologist, 19*, 105–120.

Arnold, M. C., Papanicolaou, D. A., O'Grady, J. A., Lotsikas, A., Dale, J. K., Straus, S. E., et al. (2002). Using an interleukin-6 challenge to evaluate neuropsychological performance in chronic fatigue syndrome. *Psychological Medicine, 32*, 1075–1089.

Babikian, T., Boone, K. B., Lu, P., & Arnold, G. (2006). Sensitivity and specificity of various Digit Span scores in the detection of suspect effort. *The Clinical Neuropsychologist, 20*, 145–159.

Barrash, J., Suhr, J., & Manzel, K. (2004). Detecting poor effort and malingering with an expanded version of the Auditory Verbal Learning Test (AVLTX): Validation with clinical samples. *Journal of Clinical and Experimental Neuropsychology, 26*, 125–140.

Bell, B. D., Primeau, M., Sweet, J. J., & Lofland, K. R. (1999). Neuropsychological functioning in migraine headache, nonheadache chronic pain, and mild traumatic brain injury patients. *Archives of Clinical Neuropsychology, 14*, 389–399.

Bell, I. R., Baldwin, C. M., & Schwartz, G. E. (1998). Illness from low levels of environmental chemicals: Relevance to chronic fatigue syndrome and fibromyalgia. *American Journal of Medicine, 105*(Suppl. 3a), 74S–82S.

Bennett, R. M. (1996). Fibromyalgia and the disability dilemma. A new era in understanding a complex, multidimensional pain syndrome. *Arthritis and Rheumatism, 39*, 1627–1634.

Binder, L. M., Storzbach, D., Campbell, K. A., Rohlman, D. S., & Anger, W. K. (2001). Neurobehavioral deficits associated with chronic fatigue syndrome in veterans with Gulf War unexplained illnesses. *Journal of the International Neuropsychological Society, 7*, 835–839.

Boone, K. B., & Lu, P. H. (1999). Impact of somatoform symptomatology on credibility of cognitive performance. *Clinical Neuropsychologist, 13*, 414–419.

Boone, K., Lu, P., & Herzberg, D. (2002a). *The Dot Counting Test.* Los Angeles: Western Psychological Services.

Boone, K., Lu, P., & Herzberg, D. (2002b). *The b Test.* Los Angeles: Western Psychological Services.

Busichio, K., Tiersky, L. A., DeLuca, J., & Natelson, B. H. (2004). Neuropsychological deficits in patients with chronic fatigue syndrome. *Journal of the International Neuropsychological Society, 10*, 278–285.

Christodoulou, C., DeLuca, J., Lange, G., Johnson, S. K., Sisto, S. A., Korn, L., et al. (1998). Relation between neuropsychological impairment and functional disability in patients with chronic fatigue syndrome. *Journal of Neurology, Neurosurgery and Psychiatry, 64*, 431–434.

Cote, K. A., & Moldofsky, H. (1997). Sleep, daytime symptoms and cognitive performance in patients with fibromyalgia. *Journal of Rheumatology, 24*, 2014–2023.

Crombez, G., Eccleston, C., Baeyens, F., Van Houdenhove, B., & Van Den Broeck, A. (1999). Attention to chronic pain is dependent upon pain-related fear. *Annelies Journal of Psychosomatic Research, 47*, 403–410.

de Gier, M., Peters, M. L., & Vlaeyen, J. W. S. (2003). Fear of pain, physical performance, and attentional processes in patients with fibromyalgia. *Pain, 104*, 121–130.

de Lange, F. P., Kalkman, J. S., Bleijenberg, G., Hagoort, P., van den Werf, S. P., Van der Meer, J. W. M., et al. (2004). Neural correlates of the chronic fatigue syndrome—an fMRI study. *Brain: A Journal of Neurology, 127*, 1948–1957.

DeLuca, J., Christodoulou, C., Diamond, B. J., Rosenstein, E. D., Kramer, N., Ricker, J. H., et al. (2004). The nature of memory impairment in chronic fatigue syndrome. *Rehabilitation Psychology, 49*, 62–70.

Dick, B., Eccleston, C., & Crombez, G. (2002). Attentional functioning in fibromyalgia, rheumatoid arthritis, and musculoskeletal pain patients. *Arthritis and Rheumatism-Arthritis Care and Research, 47*, 639–644.

Dobbs, B. M., Dobbs, A. R., & Kiss, I. (2001). Working memory deficits associated with chronic fatigue syndrome. *Journal of the International Neuropsychological Society, 7*, 285–293.

Fiedler, N., Kipen, H. M., DeLuca, J., Kelly-McNeil, K., & Natelson, B. (1996). A controlled comparison of multiple chemical sensitivities and chronic fatigue syndrome. *Psychosomatic Medicine, 58*, 38–49.

Fishbain, D. A., Goldberg, M., Rosomoff, R. S., & Rosomoff, H. (1991). Chronic pain patients and the nonorganic physical sign of nondermatomal sensory abnormalities (NDSA). *Psychosomatics: Journal of Consultation Liaison Psychiatry, 32*, 294–303.

Gervais, R., Green, P., & Allen, L. M. (1999). Differential sensitivity to symptom exaggeration of verbal, visuospatial, and numerical symptom validity tests. *Archives of Clinical Neuropsychology, 14*, 746–747.

Gervais, R. O., Rohling, M. L., Green, P., & Ford, W. (2004). A comparison of WMT, CARB, and TOMM failure rates in non-head injury disability claimants. *Archives of Clinical Neuropsychology, 19*, 475–487.

Gervais, R., Russell, A., Green, P., Allen, L., Ferrari, R., & Pieschl, S. (2001). Effort testing in patients with fibromyalgia and disability incentives. *Journal of Rheumatology, 28*, 1892–1899.

Glass, J. M., & Park, D. C. (2001). Cognitive dysfunction in fibromyalgia. *Current Rheumatology Reports, 3*, 123–127.

Gordon, D. A. (1999). Chronic widespread pain as a medico-legal issue. *Baillieres Best Practices and Research Clinical Rheumatology, 13*, 531–543.

Grace, G. M., Nielson, W. R., Hopkins, M., & Berg, M. A. (1999). Concentration and memory deficits in patients with fibromyalgia syndrome. *Journal of Clinical and Experimental Neuropsychology*, *21*, 477–487.

Grafman, J., Schwartz, V., Dale, J. K., Scheffers, M., Houser, C., & Straus, S. E. (1993). Analysis of neuropsychological functioning in patients with chronic fatigue syndrome. *Journal of Neurology, Neurosurgery, and Psychiatry*, *56*, 812–815.

Green, P. (2001). Why clinicians often disagree about the validity of test results. *NeuroRehabilitation*, *16*, 231–236.

Green, P., Berendt, J., Mandel, A., & Allen, L. M. (2000). Relative sensitivity of the Word Memory Test and the Test of Memory Malingering in 144 disability claimants. *Archives of Clinical Neuropsychology*, *15*, 841.

Greve, K. W., Bianchini, K. J., & Ameduri, C. J. (2003). Use of a forced-choice test of tactile discrimination in the evaluation of functional sensory loss: A report of 3 cases. *Archives of Physical and Medical Rehabilitation*, *84*, 1233–1236.

Grisart, J., Van der Linden, M., & Masquelier, E. (2002). Controlled processes and automaticity in memory functioning in fibromyalgia patients: Relation with emotional distress and hypervigilance. *Journal of Clinical and Experimental Neuropsychology*, *24*, 994–1009.

Hart, R. P., Martelli, M. F., & Zasler, N. D. (2000). Chronic pain and neuropsychological functioning. *Neuropsychology Review*, *10*, 131–149.

Hartman, D. E. (2002). The unexamined lie is a lie worth fibbing. Neuropsychological malingering and the Word Memory Test. *Archives of Clinical Neuropsychology*, *17*, 709–714.

Iverson, G. L., King, R. J., Scott, J. G., & Adams, R. L. (2001). Cognitive complaints in litigating patients with head injuries or chronic pain. *Journal of Forensic Neuropsychology*, *2*, 19–30.

Iverson, G. L., Lange, R. T., Green, P., & Franzen, M. D. (2002). Detecting exaggeration and malingering with the Trailmaking Test. *The Clinical Neuropsychologist*, *16*, 398–406.

Iverson, G. L., & McCracken, L. M. (1997). "Postconcussive" symptoms in persons with chronic pain. *Brain Injury*, *11*, 783–790.

Jamison, R. N., Sbrocco, T., & Parris, W. C. (1988). The influence of problems with concentration and memory on emotional distress and daily activities in chronic pain patients. *International Journal of Psychiatry in Medicine*, *18*, 183–191.

Johansson, G., Risberg, J., Rosenhall, U., Orndahl, G., Svennerholm, L., & Nystrom S. (1995). Cerebral dysfunction in fibromyalgia: Evidence from regional cerebral blood flow measurements, otoneurological tests and cerebrospinal fluid analysis. *Acta Psychiatrica Scandinavica*, *91*, 86–94.

Johnson, S. K., DeLuca, J., Diamond, B. J., & Natelson, B. H. (1998). Memory dysfunction in fatiguing illness: Examining interference and distraction in short-term memory. *Cognitive Neuropsychiatry*, *3*, 269–285.

Joyce, E., Blumenthal, S., & Wessely, S. (1996). Memory, attention, and executive function in chronic fatigue syndrome. *Journal of Neurology, Neurosurgery and Psychiatry*, *60*, 495–503.

Kaplan, R. F., Meadows, M. E., Vincent, L. C., Logigian, E. L., & Steere, A. C. (1992). Memory impairment and depression in patients with Lyme encephalopathy: Comparison with fibromyalgia and nonpsychotically depressed patients. *Neurology*, *42*, 1263–1267.

Komaroff, A. L., & Goldenberg, D. (1989). The chronic fatigue syndrome: Definitions, current studies, and lessons for fibromyalgia research. *Journal of Rheumatology, 16,* 23–27.

Labarge, A. S., & McCaffrey, R. J. (2000). Multiple chemical sensitivity: A review of the theoretical and research literature. *Neuropsychology Review, 10,* 183–211.

Lamberty, G. J., Putnam, S. V., Chatel, D. M., Bieliauskas, L. A., & Adams, K. M. (1994). Derived Trailmaking Test indices: A preliminary report. *Neuropsychiatry, Neuropsychology, and Behavioral Neurology, 7,* 230–234.

Landro, N. I., Stiles, T. C., & Sletvold, H. (1997). Memory functioning in patients with primary fibromyalgia and major depression and healthy controls. *Journal of Psychosomatic Research, 42,* 297–306.

Lawrie, S., MacHale, S. M., Cavanagh, J. T. O., O'Carroll, R. E., & Goodwin, G. M. (2000). The difference in patterns of motor and cognitive function in chronic fatigue syndrome and severe depressive illness. *Psychological Medicine, 30,* 433–442.

Lawrie, S. M., MacHale, S. M., Power, M. J., & Goodwin, G. M. (1997). Is the chronic fatigue syndrome best understood as a primary disturbance of the sense of effort? *Psychological Medicine, 27,* 995–999.

Mahurin, R. K., Claypoole, K. H., Goldberg, J. H., Arguelles, L., Ashton, S., & Buchwald, D. (2004). Cognitive processing in monozygotic twins discordant for chronic fatigue syndrome. *Neuropsychology, 18,* 232–239.

Marcel, B., Komaroff, A. L., Fagioli, L. R., Kornish, R. J., & Albert, M. S. (1996). Cognitive deficits in patients with chronic fatigue syndrome. *Biological Psychiatry, 40,* 535–541.

Martelli, M. F., Zasler, N. D., Bender, M. C., & Nicholson, K. (2004). Psychological, neuropsychological, and medical considerations in assessment and management of pain. *Journal of Head Trauma Rehabilitation, 19,* 10–28.

Martelli, M. F., Zasler, N. D., Grayson, R., & Liljedahl, E. L. (1999). Kinesiophobia and cogniphobia: Assessment of avoidance conditioned pain related disability (ACPRD). *www.angelfire.com/va/MFMartelliPhD/nanposters.html*

Martin, T. A., Hoffman, N. M., & Donders, J. (2003). Clinical utility of the Trailmaking Test ratio score. *Applied Neuropsychology, 10,* 163–169.

Meyers, J. E., & Diep, A. (2000). Assessment of malingering in chronic pain patients using neuropsychological tests. *Applied Neuropsychology, 7,* 133–139.

Meyers, J. E., & Volbrecht, M. E. (2003). A validation of multiple malingering detection methods in a large clinical sample. *Archives of Clinical Neuropsychology, 18,* 261–276.

Michiels, V., Cluydts, R., & Fischler, B. (1998). Attention and verbal learning in patients with chronic fatigue syndrome. *Journal of the International Neuropsychological Society, 4,* 456–466.

Michiels, V., Cluydts, R., Fischler, B., & Hoffmann, G. (1996). Cognitive functioning in patients with chronic fatigue syndrome. *Journal of Clinical and Experimental Neuropsychology, 18,* 666–677.

Michiels, V., de Gucht, V., Cluydts, R., & Fischler, B. (1999). Attention and information processing efficiency in patients with chronic fatigue syndrome. *Journal of Clinical and Experimental Neuropsychology 21,* 709–729.

Mittenberg, W., Patton, C., Canyock, E. M., & Condit, D. C. (2002). Base rates of malingering and symptom exaggeration. *Journal of Clinical and Experimental Neuropsychology, 24,* 1094–1102.

Mittenberg, W., Tremont, G., Zielinski, R. E., Fichera, S., & Rayls, K. R. (1996). Cognitive behavioral prevention of postconcussive syndrome. *Archives of Clinical Neuropsychology*, *11*, 139–145.

Morriss, R. K., Robson, M. J., & Deakin, J. F. (2002). Neuropsychological performance and noradrenaline function in chronic fatigue syndrome under conditions of high arousal. *Psychopharmacology*, *163*, 166–173.

Mountz, J. M., Bradley, L. A., Modell, J. G., Alexander, R. W., Triana-Alexander, M., Aaron, L. A., et al. (1995). Fibromyalgia in women. Abnormalities of regional cerebral blood flow in the thalamus and the caudate nucleus are associated with low pain threshold levels. *Arthritis and Rheumatism*, *38*, 926–938.

Nicholson, K., & Martelli, M. F. (2004). The problem of pain. *Journal of Head Trauma Rehabilitation*, *19*, 2–9.

O'Bryant, S. E., Hilsabeck, R. C., Fisher, J. M., & McCaffrey, R. J. (2003). Utility of the Trailmaking Test in the assessment of malingering in a asample of mild traumatic brain injury litigants. *The Clinical Neuropsychologist*, *17*, 69–74.

Park, D. C., Glass, J. M., Minear, M., & Crofford L. J. (2001). Cognitive function in fibromyalgia patients. *Arthritis and Rheumatism*, *44*, 2125–2133.

Ross, S., Fantie, B., Straus, S. F., & Grafman, J. (2001). Divided attention deficits in patients with chronic fatigue syndrome. *Applied Neuropsychology*, *8*, 4–11.

Ruffolo, L. F., Guilmette, T. J., & Willis, W. G. (2000). Comparison of time and error rates on the Trailmaking Test among patients with head injuries, experimental malingerers, patients with suspect effort on testing, and normal controls. *The Clinical Neuropsychologist*, *14*, 223–230.

Schmand, B., Lindeboom, J., Schagen, S., Heijt, R., Koene, T., & Hamburger, J. L. (1998). Cognitive complaints in patients after whiplash injury: The impact of malingering. *Journal of Neurology, Neurosurgery and Psychiatry*, *64*, 339–342.

Schnurr, R. F., & MacDonald, M. R. (1995). Memory complaints in chronic pain. *Clinical Journal of Pain*, *11*, 103–111.

Sephton, S. E., Studts, J. L., Hoover, K., Weissbecker, I., Lynch, G., Ho, I., et al. (2003). Biological and psychological factors associated with memory function in fibromyalgia syndrome. *Health Psychology*, *22*, 592–597.

Short, K., McCabe, M., & Tooley, G. (2002). Cognitive functioning in chronic fatigue syndrome and the role of depression, anxiety, and fatigue. *Journal of Psychosomatic Research*, *52*, 475–483.

Sletvold, H., Stiles, T. C., & Landro, N. I. (1995). Information processing in primary fibromyalgia, major depression, and healthy controls, *Journal of Rheumatology*, *22*, 137–142.

Smith, S., & Sullivan, K. (2003). Examining the influence of biological and psychological factors on cognitive performance in chronic fatigue syndrome: A randomized double-blind, placebo-controlled, crossover study. *International Journal of Behavioral Medicine*, *10*, 162–173.

Sparks, P. J. (2000). Idiopathic environmental intolerance: Overview. *Occupational Medicine: State of the Art Reviews*, *15*, 497–510.

Suhr, J. A. (2003). Neuropsychological impairment in fibromyalgia: Relation to depression, fatigue, and pain. *Journal of Psychosomatic Research*, *55*, 321–329.

Suhr, J. A., & Gunstad, J. (2002). Postconcussive symptom report: The relative influence of head injury and depression. *Journal of Clinical and Experimental Neuropsychology*, *24*, 981–993.

Suhr, J. A., & Gunstad, J. (2005). Further exploration of the effect of "diagnosis threat" on cognitive performance in individuals with mild head injury. *Journal of the International Neuropsychological Society, 11,* 23–29.

Suhr, J. A., Gunstad, J., Greub, B., & Barrash, J. (2004). Exaggeration index for an expanded version of the Auditory Verbal Learning Test: Robustness to coaching. *Journal of Clinical and Experimental Neuropsychology, 26,* 416–427.

Tiersky, L., Matheis, R. J., DeLuca, J., Lange, G., & Natelson, B. H. (2003). Functional status, neuropsychological functioning and mood in chronic fatigue syndrome: Relationship to psychiatric disorder. *Journal of Nervous and Mental Disorders, 191,* 324–331.

van der Werf, S. P., de Vree, B., van der Meer, J. W. M., & Bleijenberg, G. (2002). The relations among body consciousness, somatic symptom report, and information processing speed in chronic fatigue syndrome. *Neuropsychiatry, Neuropsychology, and Behavioral Neurology, 15,* 2–9.

van der Werf, S. P., Prins, J. B., Jongen, P. J. H., van der Meer, J. W. M., & Bleijenberg, G. (2000). Abnormal neuropsychological findings are not necessarily a sign of cerebral impairment: A matched comparison between chronic fatigue syndrome and multiple sclerosis. *Neuropsychiatry, Neuropsychology, and Behavioral Neurology, 13,* 199–203.

Vercoulen, J. H. M. M., Bazelmans, E., Swanink, C. M. A., Galama, J. M. D., Fennis, J. F. M., van der Meer, J. W. M., et al. (1998). Evaluating neuropsychological impairment in chronic fatigue syndrome. *Journal of Clinical and Experimental Neuropsychology, 20,* 144–156.

Wallace, D. J. (1997). The fibromyalgia syndrome. *Annals of Medicine, 29,* 9–21.

White, K. P., & Harth, M. (1999). The occurrence and impact of generalized pain. *Baillieres Best Practice Research in Clinical Rheumatology, 13,* 379–389.

Wolfe, F., Ross, K., Anderson, J., Russell, I. J., & Hebert, L. (1995). The prevalence and characteristics of fibromyalgia in the general population. *Arthritis and Rheumatism, 38,* 19–28.

CHAPTER 13

The Impact of Psychiatric Disorders on Cognitive Symptom Validity Test Scores

Hope E. Goldberg
Carla Back-Madruga
Kyle Brauer Boone

Relatively few studies have been conducted to determine whether patients with depressive, psychotic, or other psychiatric disorders perform differently than normative groups on cognitive symptom validity tests (e.g., Ashendorf, Constantinou, & McCaffrey, 2004; Back et al., 1996; Lee et al., 2000; Suhr, Tranel, Wefel, & Barrash, 1997). This deficiency in the literature is problematic and has led some clinicians to assert that failed effort test performance can be due to depression or other psychiatric conditions. If the presence of psychiatric disorders confounds accurate interpretation of cognitive symptom validity test scores, conclusions drawn from such results would be invalid, and decisions based on those conclusions would be flawed. Therefore, determining the impact of psychiatric illness or symptomatology on performance on effort and symptom validity tests is a critical area of scientific inquiry.

This chapter contains a review of the extant literature on the impact of psychiatric disorders on cognitive effort test performance. To reduce confounds, *studies were selected only if the research contained scores on symptom validity tests from discrete psychiatric illness groups comprised of patients with no motive to feign cognitive symptoms.* These criteria resulted in a somewhat narrowed literature, as studies could not be included that examined patient groups comprised of heterogeneous psychiatric disorders (e.g., Barrash, Suhr, &

Manzel, 2004), nor could data be used from effort tests employed as criterion variables to exclude suspect patients in compensation-seeking circumstances (i.e., the Computerized Assessment of Response Bias, [CARB]; Allen, Conder, Green, & Cox, 1997, cited in Rohling, Green, Allen, & Iverson, 2002). However, the stringent criteria were necessary to obtain a clear picture of how *specific* psychiatric disorders affect scores on symptom validity tests (SVT) under *nonsuspect circumstances* and to determine whether unacceptably high false-positive rates are likely to occur as a function of psychiatric status alone.

The chapter is organized into sections for each effort test, with tests presented in order on the basis of the most to least amount of available data. In descending order, the tests are Digit Span Age Corrected Scaled Scores and Reliable Digit Span, Warrington Recognition Memory Test—Words, Dot Counting, Digit Memory Test/Hiscock Forced-Choice, Test of Memory Malingering, Rey 15-Item, Finger Tapping, b Test, 21-Item, Letter Memory Test, Word Memory Test, and the Victoria Symptom Validity Test. Relevant research for each test is briefly outlined, findings are summarized, and data from the studies are reproduced in tables. Conclusions are provided at the end of the chapter, areas of weakness are noted, and recommendations are made for further research. The authors of this chapter assume a working familiarity with these symptom validity tests.

DIGIT SPAN TESTS

A review of the existing literature found six published studies (Butler, Jenkins, Sprock, & Braff, 1992; Boone et al., 1994; Boone et al., 1995; Meyers & Volbrecht, 2003; Palmer et al., 1996; Suhr et al., 1997) that contained performance data on Digit Span age corrected scaled scores (DS ACSS) or Reliable Digit Span (RDS) in depression samples, although three of the studies contained overlapping data (Boone et al., 1994; Boone et al., 1995; Palmer et al., 1996). In addition, single studies provided Digit Span data on patients with schizophrenia (Butler et al., 1992), somatoform disorder (Suhr et al., 1997), late-life psychosis (Miller et al., 1991), late-life psychotic depression (Lesser et al., 1991), and obsessive–compulsive disorder (Boone, Ananth, Philpott, Kaur, & Djenderedjian, 1991).

In the Butler et al. (1992) and Suhr et al. (1997) studies, score frequencies were not available; thus, it is unclear precisely how many subjects in each sample fell below the recommended DS ACSS cutoff of ≤ 5 (Babikian, Boone, Lu, & Arnold, 2006). However, the reported means and standard deviations (reproduced in Table 13.1a) do provide gross estimates as to the proportion of each sample that might have scored below the cutoff. The raw data from the Boone et al. (1991; Boone et al., 1994; Boone et al., 1995), Palmer et al. (1996), Miller et al. (1991), and Lesser et al. (1991) studies were

TABLE 13.1a. Digit Span ACSS and Reliable Digit Span: Means, Standard Deviations, and Ranges

Study	n	Age	Education	Symptom measure(s)	Digit Span ACSS score[a]	Reliable DS[b]
		Mean (SD)				
Boone et al. (1994)						
Depression groups by age				HAM-D		
46–59	36	54.31 (3.26)	14.11 (3.66)	18.57 (4.55)	10.42 (2.61)	
60–69	23	64.44 (2.76)	15.61 (2.59)	21.39 (5.91)	10.35 (2.62)	
70–85	14	74.50 (5.05)	15.29 (2.81)	19.07 (4.75)	9.21 (2.72)	
Boone et al. (1995)						
Depression severity				HAM-D		
Mildly depressed	37	60.54 (9.19)	15.30 (2.60)	15.60	10.43 (2.67)	
Moderately depressed	36	62.22 (7.94)	14.39 (3.72)	23.61	9.89 (2.62)	
Butler et al. (1992)				SADS		
Affective Disorder	18	31.2 (9.2)	13.6 (2.0)	Not reported	8.3 (3.2)	
Schizophrenia groups				SANS SAPS		
More perseverative	22–24[c]	35.4 (7.0)	12.0 (1.6)	28.1 (18.8) 26.0 (16.5)	6.5 (2.2)	
Less perseverative	18–20[c]	27.3 (6.7)	11.9 (1.6)	26.6 (19.9) 30.1 (21.1)	8.2 (2.8)	
Meyers et al. (2003)						
Depression	25	45.28 (12.4)	13.56 (2.6)	Medical records[d]		9.66 (1.55)[e]
Palmer et al. (1996)						
Depression type				HAM-D		
Psychological	14	59.7 (4.9)	14.7 (2.3)	18.7 (4.6)	11.1 (3.6)	
Vegetative	22	62.1 (8.5)	14.3 (2.5)	20.5 (4.5)	9.6 (1.9)	
Suhr et al. (1997)						
Depression	30	41.4 (13.8)	12.6 (2.7)	DSM[f]	8.7 (2.9)	
Somatization	29	39.3 (12.3)	12.1 (2.3)		8.9 (3.4)	

[a] WAIS-R Digit Span Age Corrected/Correlated SS;

[b] DS ACSS recommended cutoff < 5 (Babikian et al., 2006). Reliable DS recommended cutoff < 6 (Babikian et al., 2006).

[c] Range.

[d] See text for detail.

[e] Scores ranged from 7 to 13 (100% specificity).

[f] DSM-III-R (1987) or DSM-IV (1994) criteria.

accessed for the purposes of this chapter to compute RDS (Greiffenstein, Baker, & Gola, 1994) scores and to obtain score frequencies to determine how many patients fell below the DS ACSS cutoff of ≤ 5 and the RDS cutoff of ≤ 6 (Babikian et al., 2006). Table 13.1b presents these raw frequency data.

The Butler et al. (1992) study contained DS ACSS scores from 48 inpatients. Patients were included if their medical history and scores on the Schedule for Affective Disorders and Schizophrenia (SADS; Spitzer & Endicott, 1975) met research diagnostic criteria for either chronic or subchronic paranoid schizophrenia. Patients with other psychotic disorder diagnoses were excluded. A second psychiatric group from the same facility (n = 18) consisted of inpatients diagnosed with only affective disorders including depression (n = 7), bipolar disorder (n = 7), posttraumatic stress disorders (PTSD) (n = 2), and unspecified (n = 2). Symptom measures

TABLE 13.1b. Digit Span ACSS and Reliable Digit Span: Harbor–UCLA Medical Center Unpublished Frequency Data

Scaled score	Digit Span ACSS LLP (n = 28)	LOPD (n = 15)	MD (n = 109)	OCD (n = 43)	Reliable Digit Span LLP (n = 27)	LOPD (n = 15)	MD (n = 109)	OCD (n = 43)	Sum of digits
19			1						19
18			1	1					18
17			1						17
16			4				2	1	16
15			4	1	1		4		15
14	1		6	4			2	1	14
13	1		10	8	1		7	7	13
12			11	9	1		7	6	12
11	3	1	24	1	1	1	20	10	11
10		4	11	7	3	2	17	5	10
9	6	1	13	3	5	3	22	7	9
8	4	5	13	5	7	5	18	3	8
7	2		6	3	4	1	10	3	7
6	6	1	3	1	4	2	1		6
5	3					1			5
4	1	3							4
3									3
2									2
Specificity	86%	80%	100%	100%	85%	80%	99%	100%	

Note. LLP, late-life psychosis (Miller et al., 1991); LOPD, late-onset psychotic depression (Lesser et al., 1991); MD, major depression; OCD, obsessive–compulsive disorder. Dashed lines indicate recommended cutoffs: DS ACSS ≤ 5, Reliable Digit Span ≤ 6 (Babikian et al., 2006).

included the Scale for the Assessment of Negative Symptoms (SANS; Andreasen, 1984a) and Scale for the Assessment of Positive Symptoms (SAPS; Andreasen, 1984b). The patients with schizophrenia were subgrouped on the basis of their Wisconsin Card Sorting Task (WCST) perseverative response scores, using a cutoff of 30 (approximately 2 SD > the manual's normative group mean; Heaton, 1981) to form cognitively impaired (more perseverative) versus unimpaired (less perseverative) groups. The mean DS ACSS for the less perseverative group (8.2, SD = 2.8) was similar to that of the affective disorder group (mean = 8.3, SD = 3.2) and likely within accepted specificity values using the recommended cutoff of ≤ 5, while the mean score for the more perseverative group was nearly 2 points lower than the others (6.5, SD = 2.2) and reflects an increased risk of false-positive identifications for schizophrenia patients when cognitive impairment is present.

The Boone et al. (1994) study provided DS ACSS data from well-educated, fluent English-speaking, middle-aged and older patients with major depression, by age group (46–59, 60–69, and 70–85). Patients' depressive symptoms were assessed with the Hamilton Rating Scale for Depression (HAM-D; Hamilton, 1960), and all patients met criteria for major depression according to DSM-III-R (American Psychiatric Association, 1987) criteria. Exclusion criteria included psychotic symptoms, history of a manic or hypomanic episode, drug or alcohol abuse, electroconvulsive therapy (ECT), stroke, epilepsy, Parkinson's disease, or evidence of hemiparesis or hemisensory deficits. All participants were studied when they were off psychotropic medications; those who had been on medications were tested after a washout period of at least 2 weeks. In 1995, Boone et al. examined data on the impact of level of depression on DS ACSS. Subjects, who included patients from the 1994 study, were divided into two groups (i.e., mild or moderate depression), for comparison to controls. Severity of depression was measured with the HAM-D and exclusion criteria were the same as in the 1994 study. The same dataset was again employed by Palmer et al. (1996), with patients grouped by depressive symptom type: either primarily vegetative (somatic) or psychological (cognitive). Examination of the unpublished frequency data for both Digit Span ACSS and RDS from the entire group of patients from the three studies (n = 109) revealed 100% specificity for the recommended cutoffs on both Digit Span effort indices, indicating that major depression does not result in false-positive identifications on these measures, and that older age, depressive symptom subtype, and increasing severity do not alter specificity levels.

Meyers and Volbrecht (2003) collected RDS data on adult patients with depressive disorder (n = 25) as part of a larger study (n = 796) assessing the validity of using various effort indicators derived from existing neuropsychological tests. The depressed patients were receiving mental health treatment for a depressive disorder of sufficient severity to warrant either inpatient or partial hospitalization treatment. No exclusion criteria were described other than involvement in litigation. None in the depression group obtained a RDS score of ≤ 6 (100% specificity).

Suhr et al. (1997) obtained DS ACSS scores from patients with depressive (n = 30) and somatoform (n = 29) disorders. Both groups were diagnosed according to criteria outlined in DSM-III-R (American Psychiatric Association, 1987) or DSM-IV (American Psychiatric Association, 1994). Exclusion criteria for both groups included a history of premorbid neurological conditions that would impact test performance, substance abuse, or learning disability. Both groups averaged DS ACSS of nearly 9, with a standard deviation of approximately 3, suggesting that only a relatively small proportion may have obtained ACSS ≤ 5.

Miller et al. (1991) provided data on cognitive functioning of inpatients and outpatients whose psychotic symptoms developed after age 45 (late-life psychosis or LLP). Specific diagnoses included schizophrenia, delusional disorder, schizophreniform disorder, and psychosis not otherwise specified based on initial clinical presentation and assessment, and Structured Clinical Interview for DSM-III-R (SCID; Spitzer & Williams, 1986). Mean severity of psychotic symptoms was 22.9 (SD = 8.5) months as measured by the Brief Psychiatric Rating Scale (BPRS; Overall & Gorham, 1962) and mean duration of illness was 19.9 (SD = 29.4) months. Patients' mean Mini-Mental State Examination (MMSE; Folstein, Folstein, & McHugh, 1975) score was 28.0 (SD = 2.2). Exclusion criteria included MMSE scores of less than 24, history of drug or alcohol abuse, stroke, epilepsy, Parkinson's disease, and hemiparesis or hemisensory deficits. The majority of patients had been on neuroleptic medications for days to weeks prior to the assessment. Of the 28 LLP patients, 4 scored below the recommended DS ACSS cutoff of ≤ 5 (86% specificity). Of the 27 patients with data on RDS, 4 scored below the recommended RDS cutoff of ≤ 6 (85% specificity). These specificity levels indicate that 14–15% of psychotic patients in this study would have been misidentified as exerting suboptimal effort on the Digit Span indicators.

In a companion study, Lesser et al. (1991) assessed the cognitive functioning of inpatients and outpatients with late-onset psychotic depression (LOPD) who had no history of psychotic or affective disorder prior to age 45 (n = 15). Diagnostic process and exclusion criteria were the same as noted in the Miller et al. (1991) study discussed previously. Patients' mean HAM-D score was 27.1 (SD = 10.5), average duration of illness was 17.8 months (range 2–48 months), and mean MMSE score was 28.1 (SD = 2.3). All patients were on either antipsychotic and/or antidepressant medications at the time of the study. Three of 15 patients fell below both ACSS and RDS cutoffs, indicating that 20% would have been misclassified as displaying suspect effort (80% specificity).

Boone et al. (1991) reported DS ACSS data on 20 patients diagnosed with obsessive–compulsive disorder (OCD) based on DMS-III criteria and whose score was ≥ 10 on the Obsessions and Compulsions items of the Yale–Brown Obsessive–Compulsive Scale (Goodman et al., 1989). Patients' mean length of illness was 17.54 (*SD* = 9.55) years. Patients with coexisting psychiatric conditions including affective, psychotic, paranoid, schizoid, and organic mental disorders were excluded. Additional exclusion criteria were history of alcohol or drug abuse, head injury, seizure disorder, cerebral vascular disease or stroke, psychosurgery, ECT within the past 3 months, or renal, hepatic, or pulmonary disease. Patients were medication free for at least 4 weeks prior to testing, and none had ever required medications on a regular basis. In addition to these 20 subjects, unpublished Digit Span data were available on an additional 23 patients who met the same diagnostic, inclusion, and exclusion criteria as described above, but who were receiving medications for treatment of OCD. Examination of DS ACSS and RDS score frequencies showed that no patient scored below cutoffs for either ACSS or RDS, indicating 100% specificity in this population, regardless of medication status.

In summary, patients with depression, obsessive–compulsive, and somatoform conditions do not appear to fall below the DS ACSS and RDS cutoffs recommended to detect suboptimal effort, and in the depression samples, older age, increasing severity of depression, and symptom subtype do not appear to increase the likelihood of false positive identifications. In contrast, scores below the recommended cutoffs occur in up to 20% of patients with psychotic disorders, or when psychosis is comorbid in depressive disorder, suggesting that use of the currently recommended Digit Span cutoffs results in an unacceptably high rate of false positives in these populations.

WARRINGTON RECOGNITION MEMORY TEST—WORDS

A review of the existing literature found four studies (Boone et al., 1994; Boone et al., 1995; Egeland et al., 2003; Palmer et al., 1996; Rohling et al., 2002) that provided Warrington Recognition Memory Test—Words scores from depressed patient groups of varying symptom severity and age, one study that investigated patients with schizophrenia (Egeland et al., 2003) and two studies that presented WRMT data on patients with LLP (Miller et al., 1991) and LOPD (Lesser et al., 1991). Score frequencies were not reported in the Rohling et al. (2002) and Egeland et al. (2003) studies; thus, it is unclear precisely how many subjects in each group fell below the recommended WRMT cutoff of < 33 (Iverson & Franzen, 1994) for detection of suspect effort. However, the reported means and standard deviations reproduced in Table 13.2a do provide gross estimates as to the proportion of the sample that might have scored below the cutoff. Raw data from the Boone et al. (1991; Boone et al., 1994; Boone et al., 1995), Palmer et al. (1996), Miller et al. (1991), and Lesser et al. (1991) studies were accessed for the purposes

TABLE 13.2a. Warrington Recognition Memory Test-Words: Means and Standard Deviations

			Mean (SD)		
Study	n	Age	Education	Symptom measure(s)	Warrington RMT–Words
Boone et al. (1994)				HAM-D	
Depression groups by age					
46–59	36	54.31 (3.26)	14.11 (3.66)	18.57 (4.55)	47.03 (2.61)
60–69	23	64.44 (2.76)	15.61 (2.59)	21.39 (5.91)	45.61 (4.42)
70–85	14	74.50 (5.05)	15.29 (2.81)	19.07 (4.75)	43.36 (6.99)
Boone et al. (1995)				HAM-D	
Depression severity					
Mildly depressed	37	60.54 (9.19)	15.30 (2.60)	15.60	46.92 (2.71)
Moderately depressed	36	62.22 (7.94)	14.39 (3.72)	23.61	44.81 (5.60)
Egeland et al. (2003)				HAM-D	
Major depression	50	35.1 (8.7)	13.9 (2.9)	22.4 (4.3)	48.1 (3.1)
Schizophrenia	53	31.5 (8.4)	13.3 (3.1)	BPRS 51.9 (16.9)	45.9 (4.8)
Palmer et al. (1996)				HAM-D	
Depression type					
Psychological[a]	14	59.7 (4.9)	14.7 (2.3)	18.7 (4.6)	47.1 (2.4)
Vegetative[b]	22	62.1 (8.5)	14.3 (2.5)	20.5 (4.5)	45.2 (4.2)
Rohling et al. (2002)[c]				BDI	
Depression severity					
Low depression	79	41.4 (13.8)	12.6 (2.7)	5.9 (3.1)	45.7 (4.4)
High depression	82	39.3 (12.3)	12.1 (2.3)	31.2 (6.1)	45.4 (4.7)

[a] Thinking/perceiving.
[b] Somatic.
[c] Demographic and depression score means from larger samples: low depression patients (n = 115); high depression patients (n = 112).

of this chapter to obtain WRMT score frequencies that were not included in the published articles. Table 13.2b illustrates the number of patients whose scores fell below the cutoff of 33 (Iverson & Franzen, 1994).

In the Boone et al. (1994) study previously described in the Digit Span section, depressed patients were grouped by age range: 45–59, 60–69, and 70–85. All participants were studied off psychotropic medications or after a washout period of ≥ 2 weeks. In a subsequent publication (Boone et al., 1995), the same sample was used to investigate the impact of level of depression on neuropsychological test scores, including the WRMT. Severity of depression was measured with the HAM-D, and subjects were divided into groups with mild or moderate depression. The same sample was again used by Palmer et al. (1996) to determine whether cognitive scores varied as a

TABLE 13.2b. Warrington Recognition Memory Test—Words: Harbor–UCLA Medical Center Unpublished Frequency Data

Number of items recalled	LLP (n = 23)	LOPD (n = 14)	MD (n = 108)	Number of items recalled
50		2	14	50
49	1		16	49
48	1	2	10	48
47	2	2	18	47
46	3	1	16	46
45	2	1	9	45
44		1	5	44
43	3	1	2	43
42	2		5	42
41		1	6	41
40	2		3	40
39		1		39
38	4		1	38
37	2		1	37
36				36
35			1	35
34				34
33				33
32				32
31			1	31
30				30
29		1		29
28				28
27	1			27
26				26
25			1	25
Specificity	96%	93%	98%	

Note. LLP, late-life psychosis (Miller et al., 1991); LOPD, late-onset psychotic depression (Lesser et al., 1991); MD, major depression. Dashed line indicates recommended cutoff: < 33 correct (Iverson & Franzen, 1994).

function of type of depressive symptomatology, categorized as either primarily vegetative (somatic) or primarily psychological (cognitive). Examination of unpublished frequency data for WRMT scores from the entire group of patients from all three studies (n = 108) revealed 98% specificity for the recommended cutoff of < 33, indicating that major depression does not result in excessive false-positive identifications, and that older age, depressive symptom subtype, and increasing depression severity do not appear to alter specificity levels.

Effects of depression severity on cognition were also examined in the Rohling et al. (2002) study. The initial sample included all patients referred to a private practice for compensation-seeking disability claims. Two tests were used to identify suspect effort. Patients whose scores were < 89% correct on the CARB, or whose scores were < 83% correct on immediate or delayed recognition from the Word Memory Test (Green, 2003; Green, Allen, & Astner, 1996) were not included in the study. Patients who passed these cutoffs were divided into two depression subgroups: low depression (n = 115) and high depression (n = 112), as determined by their quartile scores (first and fourth, respectively) on the Beck Depression Inventory (BDI; Beck & Steer, 1993; Beck, Steer, & Brown, 1996). Although it is possible that the CARB did not successfully screen out all individuals who were deliberately underperforming, both groups' mean WRMT scores were ≥ 45 (2½ standard deviations above the cutoff of < 33), indicating that few or no subjects fell below the cutoff, regardless of depression severity.

The Egeland et al. (2003) study investigated memory impairment among Norwegian adult inpatients (n = 72) and outpatients (n = 31) diagnosed with schizophrenia (n = 53) or recurrent major depressive disorder (n = 50). Diagnoses were established and agreed on by five senior university-based psychiatrists, using the Structured Clinical Interview for DSM-IV Axis I Disorders (SCID-I, version 2.0; First, Spitzer, Gibbon, & Williams, 1995). Symptom ratings were documented on a number of instruments, including the HAM-D and the Extended BPRS (Lukoff & Ventura, 1986). The schizophrenia group included 43 paranoid, 3 disorganized, 1 catatonic, 2 residual, and 4 undifferentiated patients. Of the 53 schizophrenic patients, 11 were on typical neuroleptics, 36 on atypical medications, and 2 on both. All 50 patients in the depression group had a minimum score of 18 on the HAM-D at the time of assessment and 5 also had psychotic symptoms. Of the 46 depressed patients receiving antidepressant medications, 28 were using selective serotonin reuptake inhibitors (SSRIs) and 11 also used neuroleptics. Exclusion criteria for all participants included a history of head trauma, neurological disorder, or developmental dysfunction, present alcohol or substance abuse, or medical disease that might impact central nervous system function; depressed patients with any history of hypomanic symptoms were also excluded. Although specific score distributions on the WRMT were not disclosed, scores for both clinical groups were both well above (i.e., > 2.5

*SD*s) the recommended cutoff of < 33, suggesting that specificity in both groups was high.

Miller et al. (1991) included WRMT scores from patients with LLP. Diagnostic, symptom severity, inclusion, and exclusion criteria were described previously in the Digit Span section. Of the 23 patients from whom WRMT scores were obtained, no patients scored below the recommended cutoff of < 33 (100% specificity). In a second study described previously, Lesser et al. (1991) gathered data from patients with LOPD; only 1 of 14 scored below 33 (93% specificity) on the WRMT.

In summary, available data were consistent in showing no impact of depression on WRMT performance, with scores substantially above cutoff scores used to detect noncredible performance. Further, the specificity rates available for psychotic patients were high (93–100%). Although these findings should be replicated, they suggest that in contrast to Digit Span cutoff scores, the currently recommended cutoff on WRMT may be used with depressed and/or psychotic patients without risking an unacceptable level of false positive identifications.

DOT COUNTING TEST

Four publications (Back et al., 1996; Boone et al., 2001; Boone, Lu, & Herzberg, 2002b; Lee et al., 2000) provided data for the Dot Counting Test (DCT; Boone, Lu, & Herzberg, 2002b) on distinct psychiatric groups (depression and schizophrenia); means and standard deviations for DCT scores are provided in Table 13.3.

Back et al. (1996) examined DCT performance of 30 outpatients and inpatients whose symptomatology met DSM-III-R criteria for a chronic schizophrenic disorder, and who spoke fluent English. Exclusion criteria included history of neurological disorder or positive findings on a neurological exam. The severity of psychotic symptoms, as measured by the BPRS, was generally in the moderate range. Using the cutoff criteria of mean grouped dot counting time of > 4.8 seconds and a ratio (mean ungrouped dot counting time divided by grouped dot counting time) of < 2 seconds, approximately 13% of schizophrenic patients were misidentified as possible malingerers. The authors reported that within the subset who failed the test, 75% evidenced cognitive impairment as measured by the MMSE (i.e., < 24) and 75% were over the age of 40. Results of hierarchical regression analyses indicated that MMSE scores and age were the only significant predictors of performance (other examined predictors were educational level and severity of psychiatric disturbance).

Lee et al. (2000) investigated the effect of level of depression (mild, moderate, severe) on DCT scores. The 64 participants were fluent English-speaking, adult outpatients with major depression diagnoses and are de-

TABLE 13.3. Dot Counting Tests: Means, Standard Deviations, and Ranges

Study	n	Age	Education	Symptom measure(s)	Rey Dot Counting Test scores (seconds) Mean (SD) Range			DCT E-score
					Ungrouped	Grouped	Ratio UG/G	E-score
Back et al. (1996)				BPRS				
Schizophrenia groups								
Impaired (MMSE ≤ 24)	13	35.62 (10.79)	10.87(3.18)	40.67 (11.20)	7.76 (2.96)	4.61* (2.04)	1.96 (0.96)	
Unimpaired (MMSE > 24)	22	34.59 (8.89)	14.02(2.33)		6.42 (1.91)	2.73* (1.30)	2.67 (1.09)	
Lee et al. (2000)				HAM-D				
Depression severity								
Mild	22	61.91 (9.93)	14.96 (2.34)	15.64 (1.33)	5.2 (1.26) 3.6–8.6	2.0 (0.75) 1.0–4.3	2.8 (0.91) 1.4–4.5	
Moderate	31	58.39 (6.70)	15.48 (2.86)	20.32 (2.17)	5.7 (1.24) 4.0–8.7	2.1 (0.73) 1.3–3.8	2.8 (0.87) 1.3–5.1	
Severe	11	60.36 (5.87)	13.64 (2.38)	28.82 (4.31)	5.5 (1.26) 4.3–8.6	2.2 (0.78) 1.5–3.8	2.5 (0.59) 1.6–3.4	
Boone et al. (2001, 2002b)[a]				SCID[b]				E-score
Depression group	64	59.8 (7.8)	15.1 (2.7)	40.67 (11.20)		2.1 (0.7)	2.8 (0.8)	8.6 (2.0)
Schizophrenia group	28	35.3 (9.4)	13.1 (3.2)			3.3 (1.8)	2.5 (1.1)	12.7 (3.3)

[a] Recommended E-score cutoff (depression ≥ 13; Boone et al., 2002a); sensitivity 88%, specificity 95%; recommended E-score cutoff (schizophrenia ≥ 19; Boone et al., 2002a); sensitivity 72%, specificity 93%.
[b] Patients met diagnostic criteria for major depression.
* Groups differed significantly at $p < .005$.

scribed further in the Boone et al. (1994; Boone et al., 1995) and Palmer et al. (1996) studies. No patient committed > 3 errors on the DCT, and no patient obtained a mean grouped dot counting score that was equal to or greater than the mean ungrouped dot counting score, indicating that level of depression does not have an impact on DCT performance.

An equation incorporating time and errors (Dot Counting E score) was found to enhance DCT sensitivity and specificity (Boone et al., 2001; Boone et al., 2002b). Boone et al. (2001, 2002b) report E-score data for the same depression and schizophrenia samples described earlier (Back et al., 1996; Boone et al., 1994; Boone et al., 1995; Lee et al., 2000; Palmer et al., 1996). Optimal cutoffs were higher for schizophrenia patients (≥ 19; 93% specificity) than for depression patients (≥ 13; 95% specificity) and controls (≥ 13; 94% specificity), indicating that schizophrenia, but not depression, is associated with poorer performance on this effort measure. However, adjustment of cutoffs enables adequate specificity to be maintained in the schizophrenic group, albeit with some sacrifice in sensitivity.

In summary, across these studies, depression had no deleterious impact on DCT scores; however, cutoffs for patients with schizophrenia required adjustment to control for increased false-positive rates.

THE DIGIT MEMORY TEST/HISCOCK FORCED-CHOICE TEST

Four studies contained relevant data on various forms of the Digit Memory Test/Hiscock Forced-Choice Test (DMT/HFCT; Hiscock & Hiscock, 1989). Three (Guilmette, Hart, & Giuliano, 1993; Guilmette, Hart, Giuliano, & Leninger, 1994; Inman et al., 1998) examined the effects of depression severity and one (Back et al., 1996) investigated patients with diagnoses of schizophrenia. Table 13.4 reproduces test means, standard deviations, percent correct, and specificities.

Guilmette et al. (1993) assessed how 20 inpatients with diagnoses of major depression of moderate severity (BDI mean score = 22.1, range = 13–38) performed on the 72-item original version of the DMT/HFCT. Clinical diagnoses were made according to DSM-III-R (American Psychiatric Association, 1987) criteria by treating psychiatrists, and patients with known history of traumatic brain injury or other neurological disorder were excluded. Using a cutoff of < 90% correct, the depressed inpatients' mean score was 71.05 (98% correct). In a follow-up study, Guilmette et al. (1994) examined the performance of 20 randomly chosen inpatients with affective disorder diagnoses as determined by DSM-III-R criteria. Of the 20 inpatients, 19 were diagnosed with major depression; of these, four demonstrated psychotic features. One of the 20 patients was diagnosed with bipolar disorder. Exclusion criterion was the same as in the previous study. The patients' mean score on the BDI (29.6, *SD* = 7.8) categorized the group as severely depressed. In this

TABLE 13.4. Digit Memory Test Hiscock Forced-Choice Test: Means, Standard Deviations, Percent Correct

Study	n	Age	Education	Symptom measure(s)	Score	Percent correct[a]
				Mean (*SD*)		
Guilmette et al. (1993) Moderate depression	20	40.4 (16.6)	12.5 (2.1)	BDI 22.1	71.05 (2.0)	98%
Guilmette et al. (1994) Severe depression	20	40.9 (17.3)	13.0 (3.8)	BDI 29.6 (7.8)	35.5 (1.0)	> 98%
Back et al. (1996) Schizophrenia groups:				BPRS		
Cognitively impaired (MMSE ≤ 24)	8	35.62 (10.79)	10.87 (3.18)	40.67 (11.20)	15.25 (2.7)[b]	85%
Unimpaired (MMSE > 24)	22	34.59 (8.89)	14.02 (2.33)		17.54 (1.0)[c]	97%
Inman et al. (1998) Mild to moderate depression	18	31.6 (9.6)	13.1 (2.7)	BDI 26.5 (13.5)	Not reported	98%

[a] All studies used the cutoff of < 90% correct to detect suspect effort.
[b] Specificity 38%.
[c] Specificity 86%.

294

study, the investigators used an abbreviated version of the HFCT containing only half the original 72 items. The severely depressed patients in this study had a mean score of 35.5 (> 98% correct), consistent with previous findings (Guilmette et al., 1993) showing no deleterious effect of depression status on test scores.

Inman et al. (1998) assessed the performance of depressed outpatients (n = 18) recruited from private practices and clinics who reported no history of neurological disorder or significant substance abuse, and whose BDI scores at time of screening were primarily in the mild to moderate range (≥ 10; range = 12–56). These patients averaged 98% correct on the 36-item computerized version of the DMT, substantially above the recommended cutoff score of < 90% correct (Guilmette et al., 1994), indicating that mild to moderate depressive symptoms did not increase the risk of false positives on this version of the measure.

Back et al. (1996), in a previously described study, examined the performance of 30 patients with chronic schizophrenia using an 18-item version of the DMT/HFCT. Of concern, a cutoff of < 90% correct misidentified 27% of patients as possible malingerers. Within the group of eight patients who failed the forced-choice measure, five were from the cognitive impairment group (MMSE ≤ 24), and had made errors in the attention and concentration section of that measure. Results of hierarchical regression analyses indicated that cognitive impairment, as measured by the MMSE, was the only significant predictor of performance on this forced-choice measure (other examined predictors were age, education, and severity of psychiatric disturbance), accounting for 22% of the variance, and suggesting that the greater the level of cognitive impairment, the more likely the patient was to score poorly. Back et al. (1996) noted that 29 of 30 schizophrenics would have been correctly identified had a 70% correct cutoff been used, thus considerably increasing specificity for that patient group.

In summary, depression was not associated with lowered specificity levels for the DMT/HFCT; however more than one-quarter of patients with chronic schizophrenia were misidentified as noncredible using the cutoff of < 90% correct, primarily those patients with lowered cognitive function and concentration as measured by the MMSE. However, lowering the cutoff to < 70% raised specificity to acceptable levels (96%), and thus it is recommended that this cutoff be adopted in the differential diagnosis of actual versus feigned psychosis.

TEST OF MEMORY MALINGERING

Four studies (Ashendorf et al., 2004; Duncan, 2005; Rees, Tombaugh, & Boulay, 2001; Yanez, Fremouw, Tennant, Strunk, & Coker, 2006) were identified that examined false-positive rates on the Test of Memory Malingering

(TOMM; Tombaugh, 1996) in specific psychiatric groups. Table 13.5 contains test means, standard deviations, frequency distributions, false positives, and specificity rates.

Rees et al.'s (2001) study reported the effects of depression on TOMM scores. In this study participants were 26 consecutive inpatients from an affective disorder unit whose primary diagnosis, as determined by DSM criteria, was major depressive disorder. All patients were receiving treatment, including past or present ECT. Exclusion criteria were psychotic symptoms, significantly impaired attention, or nonfluent English-language ability. Depression scores on the BDI were in the moderate to severe range. Three of 26 patients scored < 45 on Trial 1, and no patients scored < 45 on either Trial 2 or the retention trial (all patients' scores on the latter two trials were ≥ 49).

In their study investigating the impact of depression and anxiety on TOMM scores, Ashendorf et al. (2004) utilized archival data from 72 community-dwelling older adults between the ages of 55 and 75. Subjects were classified into depression, or state or trait anxiety groups, based on scores from the BDI and State-Trait Anxiety Inventory (STAI; Spielberger, 1983). In the depression group, only patients with BDI scores ≥ 10 were included in the study (n = 31; range = 10–24). Patients with STAI scores ≥ 44 (n = 41) were divided into state (n = 23) or trait (n = 18) anxiety groups. Of the 31 patients in the depression group, 9 met criteria for membership in the state anxiety group, and 10 were in the trait anxiety group; 12 individuals were in both groups. Exclusion criteria were multiple sclerosis, stroke, Parkinson's disease, severe head injury, dementia, HIV/AIDS, substance abuse, reported current use of more than four alcoholic drinks per day, or current psychopharmacological or other therapeutic treatment for depression. Only 1 of the 72 subjects scored < 45 on Trial 1. Regardless of group membership, all patients' scores on Trial 2 were ≥ 48, which is comparable to those of non-clinical populations.

Yanez et al. (2006) examined the impact of severe depressive symptomatology on TOMM performance. Their clinical sample consisted of 20 adults with a current diagnosis of major depressive disorder (based on medical records) who had recently completed a Social Security Disability (SSD) evaluation at an outpatient clinic. The patients were recruited *after* the SSD evaluation and offered a $5 honorarium to participate in a brief, university-sponsored study. Potential recruits were informed that the study was "completely unrelated to the already completed disability assessment and that its purpose was to examine the potential effects of depressed mood on memory tasks." Of the 23 patients who were invited, 20 agreed to participate; age range was 22–52 and education level ranged from 8 to 14 years. Nineteen were currently on antidepressant medication, and 13 had been previously hospitalized for depression. A minimum score of 30 on the BDI-II (Beck et al., 1996) was required for inclusion. No other demographic or clinical exclusion criteria were described. Six patients scored < 45 on Trial 1, two

TABLE 13.5. Test of Memory Malingering: Means, Standard Deviations, Number of False Positives, and Specificities

Study	n	Age	Education	Symptom measure(s)	Mean (SD)			False positives[a] (specificity)
					Trial 1	Trial 2	Retention	
Rees et al. (2001)								
Moderate–severe depression	26	40.4 (11.2)	14.9 (2.8)	BDI 27.9 (13.9)	47.8 (2.9)	49.9 (0.2)	49.9 (0.3)	0 of 26 (100%)
No. of patients scoring < 45					3	0	0	
Ashendorf et al. (2004)								
Depression	31	64.57 (5.52)		BDI 13.0 (3.1)	48.9 (1.3)	49.9 (0.3)		0 of 31 (100%)
No. of patients scoring < 45					0	0		
State anxiety	23			STAI 48.3 (2.6)	48.3 (1.9)	49.8 (0.5)		0 of 23 (100%)
No. of patients scoring < 45					1	0		
Trait Anxiety	18			46.0 (1.8)	48.7 (1.5)	49.9 (0.3)		0 of 18 (100%)
No. of patients scoring < 45					0	0		
Duncan (2005)								
Psychotic disorder groups[b]								
Concentration Impaired	29	36.7 (12.0)	11.9 (2.1)	BPRS 51 (14.7)	42.9 (5.8)	48.4 (3.4)	48.6 (2.9)	3 of 29 (89%)
No. of patients scoring < 45					6	2	1	
Unimpaired[c]	21	36.5 (13.7)	11.8 (2.1)	45 (11.5)	46.0 (3.2)	50.0 (.22)	49.3 (1.2)	0 of 21 (100%)
No. of patients scoring < 45					1	0	0	
Yanez et al. (2006)								
Severe depression	20	39.1 (8.9)	11.2 (1.6)	BDI-II 43.2 (7.0)	44.5 (6.6)	48.0 (4.9)	48.6 (4.2)	3 of 20 (85%)
No. of patients scoring < 45					6	2	1	

[a] Failure criteria: Scores of < 45 on Trial 2 or Retention Trial.
[b] Impaired: CPT-II Concentration Impersistence Index score of ≥ 65%.
[c] Unimpaired: CPT-II Concentration Impersistence Index score of < 65%.

297

scored < 45 on Trial 2, and only one scored < 45 on the Retention Trial; thus, specificity for the latter two trials was ≥ 90%.

Duncan (2005) provided the rate of false positives on the TOMM in two groups of psychotic inpatients recruited from forensic and civil units. Only patients deemed credible based on their adjudication and clinical status were considered for inclusion in the study. Of these, only patients hospitalized for > 2 weeks, with no history of neurological injury/disorder, whose IQ scores were ≥ 70, and who met attending psychiatrists' criteria for psychotic disorder diagnoses were included. Study participants were classified into intact (n = 21) or impaired (n = 29) concentration groups as a function of their scores on the Concentration Impersistence Index (CII) of the Connors Continuous Performance Test-II (CPT-II, Connors, 2000); patients with CII scores ≥ 65% were assigned to the impaired group. To examine the possibility that concentration impairment status could impact false-positive rates on the TOMM, scores from the two groups were compared. While the group with concentration difficulties showed lowered performance on Trial 1 relative to the normal concentration group, means for both groups were above the cutoff of < 45 for Trial 2 and the retention trial. However, of the group with impaired concentration, 3 of 29 scored < 45 on Trial 2 and Retention Trials, which indicated that specificity for both trials in that group was reduced to 89%, compared to 100% for psychotic patients with unimpaired concentration.

In summary, the findings from these four studies suggest that the presence of mild to severe depression, anxiety, and psychosis with unimpaired concentration, are associated with excellent specificity rates on Trial 2 and Retention Trials of the TOMM (≥ 90%). In contrast, psychotic patients with concentration difficulties performed slightly less well on those trials (89% specificity).

REY 15-ITEM TEST

Three studies (Back et al., 1996; Guilmette et al., 1994; Lee et al., 2000) examined the effects of specific psychiatric illnesses on scores on the Rey-15 Item Test (Rey-15; Lezak, 1995). Inclusion and exclusion criteria for these studies were described in previous sections. Table 13.6 reproduces test means, standard deviations, false positives, and specificity rates.

Guilmette et al. (1994) reported Rey 15-Item performance of 20 randomly chosen inpatients with severe major depression. Using a cutoff of < 9 correct items, two patients were classified as false positives (90% specificity). In a larger study (n = 64), Lee et al. (2000) evaluated the effect of level of depression (mild, moderate, severe) on Rey 15-Item scores. Using a cut-score of < 9 total items correct, only three patients in this study failed the Rey 15-Item (95% specificity); between groups analysis found no significant relationship between depression severity and Rey 15-Item performance.

TABLE 13.6. Rey 15-Item Test: Means, Standard Deviations, Number of False Positives, and Specificities

Study	n	Mean (SD)				False positives[a] (specificity)
		Age	Education	Symptom measure(s)	Rey 15-Item	
Guilmette et al. (1994)						
Major depression	20	40.9 (17.3)	13.0 (3.8)	BDI 29.6 (7.8)	12.6 (2.8)	2 of 20 (90%)
Back et al. (1996)						
Schizophrenia groups				BPRS		
Impaired (MMSE $\leq$ 24)	8	35.6 (10.79)	10.87 (3.18)	40.67 (11.20)	10.12 (2.90)	4 of 30 (87%)
Unimpaired (MMSE > 24)	22	34.59 (8.89)	14.02 (2.33)		12.86 (2.78)	
Lee et al. (2000)				HAM-D		
Depression severity groups						
Mild	22	61.91 (9.93)	14.96 (2.34)	15.64 (1.33)	13.50 (1.99)	3 of 64 (95%)
Moderate	31	58.39 (6.70)	15.48 (2.86)	20.32 (2.17)	13.36 (2.39)	
Severe	11	60.36 (5.87)	13.64 (2.38)	28.82 (4.31)	12.27 (2.76)	

[a] All studies used a cutoff of < 9 total correct items.

The effect of chronic schizophrenia on Rey 15-Item scores was assessed in the Back et al. (1996) study. Using the cutoff of < 9 correct, 4 of 30 schizophrenic patients failed the Rey 15-Item (87% specificity). Results of hierarchical regression analyses indicated that educational level was the only significant predictor of performance (other examined predictors were age, cognitive impairment, and severity of psychiatric disturbance), accounting for 37% of the score variance.

In summary, adequate specificity values (i.e., ≥ 90%) were found for depressed patients on the Rey 15-Item; a slightly lower specificity rate (87%) was observed in patients with chronic schizophrenia which appeared to be mediated by educational level.

FINGER TAPPING TEST

Two studies (Arnold et al., 2005; Rohling et al., 2002) investigated the effect of psychiatric illness on the Finger Tapping Test (Mitrushina, Boone, Razani, & D'Elia, 2005). Table 13.7 reproduces test means and standard deviations.

Arnold et al. (2005) examined finger-tapping performance in patients with psychiatric diagnoses of depression or psychosis referred for neuropsychological evaluation at Harbor-UCLA. All patients included in these two groups were fluent English speakers, had no obvious motor problems, and were not involved in litigation or applying for disability income. The depression group (n = 42) was identified as having significant depressive symptoms according to the referral source, high scores on the Minnesota Multiphasic Personality Inventory-2 (MMPI-2; Butcher et al., 2001) Clinical Scale 2 (depression), and/or a history of diagnosis of depression; exclusion criteria included no history of neurological disorder, psychosis, dementia, or Full Scale IQ scores of ≤ 70. The psychosis group (n = 27) experienced hallucinations or delusions, determined either by patient or referral source report or through observation by the examiner. Psychotic patients were excluded if their symptoms were related to substance abuse, or if they had a history of dementia or other neurological disorder. In this study, evidence of a gender effect on tapping performance was found; mean tapping scores for males were significantly higher than those for females for dominant, nondominant, and both hands combined, requiring that tapping score cutoffs be calculated separately by gender. For example, mean dominant hand tapping scores were 3 points lower for depressed females as compared to depressed males, and more than 6 points lower for female psychotic patients than their male counterparts.

Within females, the dominant hand tapping score for depressed patients (n = 21) was comparable to that of healthy older controls (n = 8) and nearly 5 points higher than that of psychotic females (n = 17). Using a domi-

TABLE 13.7. Finger Tapping Studies: Means and Standard Deviations

Study	n	Handedness		Mean (SD)				
		R	L	Age	Education	Symptom measure(s)	Dominant hand[a]	Nondominant hand
Arnold et al. (2005)							Dominant hand	
Females						SCID[b]		
Depression	21	21	0	43.0 (13.6)	14.0 (2.4)		46.1 (8.1)	41.6 (6.5)
Psychosis	17	15	2	42.0 (13.6)	13.0 (2.7)		40.8 (10.3)	35.1 (11.5)
Males								
Depression	21	19	2	39.0 (14.3)	13.3 (3.0)		49.1 (7.1)	45.6 (6.7)
Psychosis	10	8	2	37.4 (13.0)	11.6 (1.6)		47.0 (7.0)	43.2 (14.3)
Rohling et al. (2002)						BDI	Right hand	Left hand
Low depression	115	94%	6%	43.6 (11.0)	13.7 (3.0)	5.9 (3.1)	47.9 (9.4)	44.9 (7.6)
High depression	112	89%	11%	41.0 (11.2)	13.0 (3.2)	31.2 (6.1)	46.9 (9.9)	44.2 (8.1)

[a] Specificity using a dominant hand cutoff of ≤ 38 for both genders:

Females	(Sensitivity 76%)	Depression	90%
		Psychosis	53%
Males	(Sensitivity 55%)	Depression	95%
		Psychosis	90%

Specificity using an adjusted cutoff of ≤ 28 for females:

(Sensitivity 61%)	Depression	95%
	Psychosis	88%

[b] Diagnostic criterion for both groups is described in greater detail in the text of the Finger Tapping study section.

nant hand cutoff of ≤ 38 yielded 76% sensitivity and 90% specificity for depressed females; however, the same cutoff yielded an unacceptably low specificity for psychotic females (53%). Lowering the dominant hand cutoff to ≤ 28 improved specificity to 88% for psychotic patients and to 95% for depressed patients, although with an accompanying decrease in sensitivity to 61%.

In males, the differential effect of psychosis versus depression on tapping performance was not as prominent; a dominant hand cutoff of ≤ 38 yielded 55% sensitivity, with 95% specificity, in depressed males ($n = 21$), and 90% specificity in psychotic males ($n = 10$). The mean score of depressed males was 3 points lower than older controls ($n = 10$) and 2 points higher than that of psychotic males.

The impact of depression severity on tapping performance was examined in the Rohling et al. (2002) study, which is further described in the WRMT–Words section. Patients were divided into two depression subgroups, low-depression ($n = 115$) and high depression ($n = 112$). Frequency data were not available, but the mean scores for both groups on dominant hand performance were within 1 point of each other, and nearly 1 standard deviation above the recommended cutoff of an average of ≤ 38 taps for the dominant hand in male and female depressed samples (Arnold et al., 2005).

The results of both of these studies suggest that depression does not appreciably lower finger tapping scores, but psychosis is associated with mild declines in performance (i.e., 10–15%), a finding which appears to be more pronounced in women, although this requires replication in larger samples. Use of gender and diagnosis-specific cutoffs are advised when using this measure to assess effort.

B TEST

Literature found on use of the b Test with psychiatric patients (Boone, Lu, & Herzberg, 2002a) was limited to validity research data published in the b Test manual. These data were obtained from studies described previously that examined patients with depression (Boone et al., 1994; Boone et al., 1995; Palmer et al., 1996) and chronic schizophrenia (Back et al., 1996). The patients with schizophrenia ($n = 28$) required a higher cutoff (i.e., ≥ 190) than the 38 depressed patients (i.e., ≥ 120) and older controls ($n = 26$; ≥ 100) to maintain adequate specificity (i.e., $\geq 90\%$), although this lowered sensitivity by one-third (54% vs. 74%). Poorer performance by patients with schizophrenia on this measure is not unexpected given that that the b Test is a continuous performance task, and patients with schizophrenia and active psychosis have been found to perform relatively poorly on such measures (Nelson, Sax, & Strakowski, 1998). Table 13.8 reproduces means, standard deviations, and other variables of interest extracted from the b Test manual.

TABLE 13.8. The b Test, the 21-Item Test, the Letter Memory Test (LMT), and the Word Memory Test (WMT): Means and Standard Deviations

				Mean (SD)			
	n	Age	Education	Symptom measure(s)	b Test	21-Item	LMT	WMT
Boone et al. (2002a) Psychiatric groups					E-scores			
Depression	38	60.9 (7.5) 51–81	14.3 (2.7) 10–21	SCID	73.2 (36.7)[a]			
Schizophrenia	28	35.3 (9.4) 22–56	13.1 (3.2) 6–21	BPRS 40.7 (11.2)	114.7 (110.8)[b]			
Inman et al. (1998)						Mean % correct (SD)		
Depression	18	31.6 (9.6)	13.1 (2.7)	BDI 26.5 (13.5) 12–56		90.5 (10.3)[c]	99.4 (1.3)[d]	
Gorrison et al. (2005)								Effort score
Schizophrenia	64	18–65	> 6 years	PANSS				79 (12.3)[e]

[a] Using recommended cutoff for Depression > 120 (Boone et al., 2002a): sensitivity 74%, specificity 90%.
[b] Using recommended cutoff for Schizophrenia > 180 (Boone et al., 2002a): sensitivity 56%, specificity 86%.
[c] Using recommended cutoff < 43% correct (Iverson et al., 1991): sensitivity 22% (specificity 100% for depressive and neurological patients).
[d] Using recommended cutoff < 93% correct (Inman et al., 1998): sensitivity 84% (specificity 100% for depressed and neurological patients).
[e] Using recommended cutoff < 83% correct (Green, 2003): 46 of 64 schizophrenia patients failed (specificity 28%).

LETTER MEMORY TEST

Research on the Letter Memory Test (LMT; Inman et al., 1998) in a psychiatric population was limited to one development and validation study (Inman et al., 1998). A depression group ($n = 18$) was recruited, as described earlier in the DMT/HFCT section. Using the cutoff score of < 93% correct, the authors reported that specificity was 100% and sensitivity was 84%, demonstrating no deleterious effect of depression on test performance. Table 13.8 includes means and standard deviations.

21-ITEM TEST

The 21-Item Test (Iverson, Franzen, & McCracken, 1991) was also included in the Inman et al. (1998) study summarized previously. The depression group ($n = 18$) averaged 90.5% correct, well above the cutoff of < 43%; use of this cutoff was associated with 100% specificity but only 22% sensitivity. Table 13.8 presents means, standard deviations, and other data.

WORD MEMORY TEST

Studies in which the Word Memory Test (WMT; Green, 2003) was used *only* as a criterion variable *to rule out suspect patients* could not be included in this section (e.g., Rohling et al., 2002). Only the Gorissen, Sanz, and Schmand (2005) investigation met all criteria for inclusion. This study (reproduced in Table 13.8) focused on WMT performance in 64 patients diagnosed with schizophrenia disorders according to DSM-IV-TR (American Psychiatric Association, 2000) criteria, including inpatients and outpatients from psychiatric hospitals and medical centers in Spain and the Netherlands. Patients were excluded if they had tardive dyskinesia, drug addiction, unspecified "concomitant somatic disease that might affect cognitive functioning," or less than 6 years of education. Clinical symptoms were operationalized using the Positive and Negative Syndrome Scale (PANSS; Kay, Opler, & Fiszbein, 1986). The performance of patients with schizophrenia was compared against that of a normal control group. Effort was deemed insufficient when a patient scored below the cutoff of < 82.5% correct on any of the three WMT effort measures: Immediate Recognition (IR), Delayed Recognition (DR), or Consistency score (CON). Nearly three-quarters (46 of 64; 72%) of schizophrenia patients failed the WMT (28% specificity), in contrast to none of the controls. The authors found that negative symptoms were correlated with poor performance on the WMT in these schizophrenia patients, raising the possibility that apathy may mimic psychometric signs of poor effort.

VICTORIA SYMPTOM VALIDITY TEST

Egeland et al. (2003), described in the section on the WRMT, investigated memory impairment among Norwegian adult inpatients (n = 72) and outpatients (n = 31) diagnosed with schizophrenia (n = 53) or recurrent major depressive disorder (n = 50). The first 16 exposures of the Victoria Symptom Validity Test (VSVT; Slick, Hopp, Strauss, & Thompson, 1997) were administered. Of the patients with schizophrenia, 95% performed in the valid range (> 12 of 16 correct), while 100% of patients with depression scored above the cutoff; no further information regarding VSVT scores was provided.

CONCLUSIONS

The purpose of this chapter was to consolidate and review results of research examining the impact of psychiatric illness on effort test performance in homogenous patient groups. Data from these studies were consistent in showing no impact of depression, including increasing severity of depression and depression subtypes, on 12 separate effort indicators: DS ACSS, Reliable DS, WRMT–Words, DCT, DMT/HFCT, TOMM, Rey 15-Item, FTT, b Test, 21-item Test, LMT, and VSVT. Although of limited quantity, data from patients with OCD, anxiety disorders, and somatoform conditions indicated these illnesses have no effect on Digit Span or TOMM scores.

In contrast, psychosis, including schizophrenia, LLP, and LOPD, was associated with modestly increased false-positive identifications of suspect effort, particularly in patients with negative symptoms, concentration difficulties, and lowered education. In these patients, specificity levels < 89% were found when using standard cutoffs for Digit Span scores, DMT/HFCT, DCT, Rey 15-Item, FTT, b Test, and the WMT. On these measures, cutoffs can be adjusted to maintain adequate specificity (≥ 90%), although at a cost in terms of test sensitivity. In contrast, available data suggest that performance on the WRMT–Words, TOMM, and VSVT are relatively unaffected by psychosis (i.e., specificity rates ≥ 89%) and argue that these tests are preferable in the differential between actual and feigned psychosis.

While information could be accessed regarding the effects of depression and psychosis on effort test performance, minimal or no information was available regarding the impact of other specific psychiatric conditions on effort test scores. In particular, no information was found regarding the effect of bipolar illness, personality disorder, or PTSD on effort test scores and, as noted earlier, our knowledge regarding the relationship between cognitive effort indicators and anxiety disorders, OCD, and somatoform conditions is limited. Finally, no published studies examining the impact of discrete psychiatric conditions in nonsuspect patients were found for some commonly used SVTs, such as the CARB, Portland Digit Recognition Test (Binder, 1993; Binder, & Willis, 1991), and the Validity Indicator Profile (Frederick, 1997). Clearly, more research is needed to replicate prior findings and to extend our knowledge of the effect of specific psychiatric disorders on false-positive rates in cognitive SVTs.

REFERENCES

Allen, L. M., Conder, R. L., Jr., Green, P., & Cox, D. R. (1997). *Computerized assessment of response bias.* Durham, NC: Cognisyst.

American Psychiatric Association. (1987). *Diagnostic and statistical manual of mental disorders* (3rd ed., rev.). Washington, DC: Author.

American Psychiatric Association. (1994). *Diagnostic and statistical manual of mental disorders* (4th ed.). Washington, DC: Author.

American Psychiatric Association. (2000). *Diagnostic and statistical manual of mental disorders* (4th ed., text rev.). Washington, DC: Author.

Andreasen, N. C. (1984a). *Schedule for the Assessment of Negative Symptoms (SANS).* Iowa City: University of Iowa Press.

Andreasen, N. C. (1984b). *Schedule for the Assessment of Positive Symptoms (SAPS).* Iowa City: University of Iowa Press.

Arnold, G., Boone, K. B., Lu, P., Dean, A., Wen, J., Nitch, S., et al. (2005). Sensitivity and specificity of Finger Tapping Test scores for the detection of suspect effort. *The Clinical Neuropsychologist, 19,* 105–120.

Ashendorf, L., Constantinou, M., & McCaffrey, R. J. (2004). The effect of depression and anxiety on the TOMM in community-dwelling older adults. *Archives of Clinical Neuropsychology, 19* 125–130.

Babikian, T., Boone, K. B., Lu, P., & Arnold, G. (2006). Sensitivity and specificity of various Digit Span scores in the detection of suspect effort. *The Clinical Neuropsychologist, 20,* 145–159.

Back, C., Boone, K. B., Edwards, C., Parks, C., Burgoyne, K., & Silver, B. (1996). The performance of schizophrenics on three cognitive tests of malingering, Rey 15-Item Memory Test, Rey Dot Counting, and Hiscock Forced-Choice Method. *Assessment, 3*(4), 449–457.

Barrash, J., Suhr, J., & Manzel, K. (2004). Detecting poor effort and malingering with an expanded version of the Auditory Verbal Learning Test (AVLTX): Validation with clinical samples. *Journal of Clinical and Experimental Neuropsychology, 26*(1), 125–140.

Beck, A., & Steer, R. (1993). *Beck Depression Inventory: Manual.* San Antonio, TX: Psychological Corporation.

Beck, A., Steer, R., & Brown, G. (1996). *Manual for Beck Depression Inventory–II.* San Antonio, TX: Psychological Corporation.

Binder, L. (1993). Assessment of malingering after mild head trauma with the Portland Digit Recognition Test. *Journal of Clinical and Experimental Neuropsychology, 15,* 170–182.

Binder, L., & Willis, S. (1991). Assessment of motivation after financially compensable minor head injury. *Psychological Assessment, 3,* 175–181.

Boone, K. B., Ananth, J., Philpott, L., Kaur, A., & Djenderedjian, A. (1991). Neuropsychological characteristics of nondepressed adults with obsessive–compulsive disorder. *Neuropsychiatry, Neuropsychology and Behavioral Neurology*, *4*, 96–109.

Boone, K. B., Lesser, I., Miller, B., Wohl, M., Berman, N., Lee, A., et al. (1994). Cognitive functioning in a mildly to moderately depressed geriatric sample: relationship to chronological age. *The Journal of Neuropsychiatry and Clinical Neurosciences*, *6*, 267–272.

Boone, K. B., Lesser, I. M., Miller, B. L., Wohl, M., Berman, N., Lee, A., et al. (1995). Cognitive functioning in older depressed outpatients: relationship of presence and severity of depression to neuropsychological test scores. *Neuropsychology*, *9*, 390–398.

Boone, K. B., Lu, P., Back, C., King, C., Lee, A., Philpott, L., et al. (2001). Sensitivity and specificity of the Rey Dot Counting test in patients with suspect effort and various clinical samples. *Archives of Clinical Neuropsychology*, *7*, 625–642.

Boone, K. B., Lu, P., & Herzberg, D. (2002a). *The b Test: Manual.* Los Angeles: Western Psychological Services.

Boone, K. B., Lu, P., & Herzberg, D. (2002b). *The Dot Counting Test: Manual.* Los Angeles: Western Psychological Services.

Butcher, J. N., Graham, J. R., Ben-Porath, Y. S., Tellegen, A., Dahlstrom, W. G., & Kaemmer, B. (2001). *Minnesota Multiphasic Personality Inventory-2 (MMPI-2): Manual for administration, scoring, and interpretation* (rev. ed.). Minneapolis: University of Minnesota Press.

Butler, R. W., Jenkins, M. A., Sprock, J., & Braff, D. L. (1992). Wisconsin Card Sorting Test deficits in chronic paranoid schizophrenia. *Schizophrenia Research*, *7*, 169–176.

Connors, C. K. (2000). *Connors continuous performance test manual* (2nd ed.). Toronto, Canada: Multi-Health Systems.

Duncan, A. (2005). The impact of cognitive and psychiatric impairment of psychotic disorders on the Test of Memory Malingering (TOMM). *Assessment*, *12*(2), 123–129.

Egeland, J., Sundet, K., Rund, B. R., Asbjørnsen, A., Hugdahl, K., Landrø, N. I., et al. (2003). Sensitivity and specificity of memory dysfunction in schizophrenia: a comparison with major depression. *Journal of Clinical and Experimental Neuropsychology*, *25*(1), 79–93.

First, M. B., Spitzer, R. L., Gibbon, M., & Williams, J. B. W. (1995). *Structured clinical interview for DSM-IV axis I disorders–Patient edition* (SCID I/P, version 2.0). New York: New York State Psychiatric Institute, Biometrics Research Department.

Folstein, M. F., Folstein, S. E., & McHugh, P. R. (1975). Mini-mental state: A practical method of grading the state of patients for the clinician. *Journal of Psychiatric Research*, *12*, 189–198.

Frederick, R. I. (1997). *Validity Indicator Profile Manual.* Minnetonka, MN: NCS Assessments.

Goodman, W. K., Price, L. H., Rasmussen, S. A., Mazure, C., Fleischmann, R. L., Hill, C. L., et al. (1989). The Yale–Brown Obsessive Compulsive Scale, I: Development, use, and reliability. *Archives of General Psychiatry*, *46*, 1006–1011.

Gorrison, M., Sanz, J. C., & Schmand, B. (2005). Effort and cognition in schizophrenia patients. *Schizophrenia Research*, *78*, 199–208.

Green, P. (2003). *The Word Memory Test.* Edmonton/Seattle: Green's Publishing.

Green, P., Allen, L. M., & Astner, K. (1996). *The Word Memory test: A user's guide to the oral and computer-administered forms, US Version 1.1.* Durham, NC: Cognisyst.

Greiffenstein, M. F., Baker, R., & Gola, T. (1994). Validation of malingered amnesia measures with a large clinical sample. *Psychological Assessment, 6,* 218–224.

Guilmette, T., Hart, K., & Giuliano, A. (1993). Malingering detection: The use of a forced-choice method in identifying organic versus simulated memory impairment. *The Clinical Neuropsychologist, 7*(1), 59–69.

Guilmette, T., Hart, K., Giuliano, A., & Leininger, B. (1994). Detecting stimulated memory impairment: Comparison of the Rey Fifteen-Item Test and the Hiscock Forced-Choice Procedure. *The Clinical Neuropsychologist, 8,* 283–294.

Hamilton, M. (1960). A rating scale for depression. *Journal of Neurology, Neurosurgery, and Psychiatry, 23,* 56–62.

Heaton, R. K. (1981). *A Manual for the Wisconsin Card Sorting Test.* Odessa, FL: Psychological Assessment Resources.

Hiscock, M., & Hiscock, C. (1989). Refining the forced-choice method for the detection of malingering. *Journal of Clinical and Experimental Neuropsychology, 11,* 967–974.

Inman, T. H., Vickery, C. D., Berry, D. T. R., Lamb, D. G., Edwards, C. L., & Smith, G. T. (1998). Development and initial validation of a new procedure for evaluating adequacy of effort given during neuropsychological testing: The Letter Memory Test. *Psychological Assessment, 10*(2), 128–139.

Iverson, G. L., & Franzen, M. D. (1994). The Recognition Memory Test, Digit Span, and Knox Cube Test as markers of malingered memory impairment. *Assessment, 1,* 323–334.

Iverson, G., Franzen, M., & McCracken, L. (1991). Evaluation of an objective assessment technique for the detection of malingered memory deficits. *Law and Human Behavior, 15,* 667–676.

Kay, S. R., Opler, L. A., & Fiszbein, A. (1986). *Positive and Negative Syndrome Scale (PANSS) rating manual.* New York: Albert Einstein College of Medicine.

Lee, A., Boone, K. B., Lesser, I., Wohl, M., Wilkins, S., & Parks, K. (2000). Performance of older depressed patients on two cognitive malingering tests: False positive rates for the Rey 15-Item Memorization and Dot Counting tests. *The Clinical Neuropsychologist, 14*(3), 303–308.

Lesser, I. M., Miller, B. L., Boone, K. B., Hill-Gutierrez, E., Mehringer, C. M., Wong, K., et al. (1991). Brain injury and cognitive function in late-onset psychotic depression. *The Journal of Neuropsychiatry and Clinical Neurosciences, 3,* 33–40.

Lezak, M. D. (1995). *Neuropsychological assessment* (3rd ed.). New York: Oxford University Press.

Luckoff, D. N. K. H., & Ventura, D. (1986). Manual for the expanded BPRS. Symptom monitoring in the rehabilitation of schizophrenic patients. *Schizophrenia Bulletin, 12,* 594–602.

Meyers, J. E., & Volbrecht, M. E. (2003). A validation of multiple malingering detection methods in a large clinical sample. *Archives of Clinical Neuropsychology, 18,* 261–276.

Miller, B. L., Lesser, I. M., Boone, K. B., Hill, E., Mehringer, C. M., & Wong, K. (1991). Brain lesions and cognitive function in late-life psychosis. *British Journal of Psychiatry, 158,* 76–82.

Mitrushina, M., Boone, K. B., Razani, J., & D'Elia, L. F (2005). *Handbook of normative data for neuropsychological assessment* (2nd ed.). New York: Oxford University Press.

Nelson, E. B., Sax, K. W., & Strakowski, S. M. (1998). Attentional performance in patients with psychotic and nonpsychotic major depression and schizophrenia. *American Journal of Psychiatry, 155,* 137–139.

Overall, J. R., & Gorham, D. R. (1962). The Brief Psychiatric Rating scale. *Psychological Reports, 10,* 799–912.

Palmer, B. W., Boone, K. B., Lesser, I. M., Wohl, M. A., Berman, N., & Miller, B. (1996). Neuropsychological deficits among older depressed patients with predominantly psychological or vegetative symptoms. *Journal of Affective Disorders, 41,* 17–24.

Rees, L. M., Tombaugh, T. N., & Boulay, L. (2001). Depression and the Test of Memory Malingering. *Archives of Clinical Neuropsychology, 16,* 501–506.

Rohling, M. L., Green, P., Allen, L. M., & Iverson, G. L. (2002). Depressive symptoms and neurocognitive test scores in patients passing symptom validity tests. *Archives of Clinical Neuropsychology, 17,* 205–222.

Slick, D., Hopp, G., Strauss, E., & Thompson, G. B. (1997). *Victoria Symptom Validity Test.* Lutz, FL: PAR.

Spielberger, C. (1983). *State–Trait Anxiety Inventory (Form Y).* Palo Alto, CA: Mind Garden.

Spitzer, R. L., & Endicott, J. (1975). *Schedule for Affective Disorders and Schizophrenia (SADS).* New York: State Psychiatric Institute, Biometrics Research.

Spitzer, R. L., & Williams, J. B. (1986). *Structured Clinical Interview for DSM-III-R.* New York: New York State Psychiatric Institute.

Suhr, J., Tranel, D., Wefel, J., & Barrash, J. (1997). Memory performance after head injury: Contributions of malingering, litigation status, psychological factors, and medication use. *Journal of Clinical and Experimental Neuropsychology, 19*(4), 500–514.

Tombaugh, T. N. (1996). *Test of Memory Malingering.* North Tonawanda, NY: Multi-Health Systems.

Warrington, E. K. (1984). *Recognition Memory Test Manual.* Windsor, UK: NFER-Nelson.

Yanez, Y. T., Fremouw, W., Tennant, J. Strunk, J., & Coker, K. (2006). Effects of severe depression on TOMM performance among disability seeking outpatients. *Archives of Clinical Neuropsychology, 21,* 161–165.

CHAPTER 14

Identification of Feigned Mental Retardation

Tara L. Victor
Kyle Brauer Boone

Individuals may choose to feign or exaggerate intellectual deficits for many reasons. External incentives might include receiving extra time on tests, monetary compensation, or evading occupational or military obligations, but in some cases the stakes are much higher. In the forensic arena, a defendant's competency to stand trial (CST) is, in part, determined by his or her intellectual ability. In fact, CST has been one of the most studied areas of mental health law since the case of *Jackson v. Indiana* in 1972 in which a mentally retarded defendant (who was also unable to speak, hear, read, or write) was charged with two robberies but found incompetent. Typically when this happens (e.g., as in the case of psychotic disturbance), the defendant is institutionalized with the goal of restoring competency and eventually trying the case in court; however, in this particular instance (i.e., a case of congenital mental deficiency), it was thought that competency would never be regained. As it was considered unconstitutional to institutionalize the defendant indefinitely, the court decided the defendant must either be released or committed in accordance with the general civil commitment provisions (see Schlesinger, 2003). Thus, the incentive for successful feigning of intellectual impairment is clear; it has the potential to allow a defendant to avoid the consequences of a major criminal offense, and in fact, the base rate for feigned cognitive impairment in a CST sample has been estimated at 13–17% (Heinze & Purisch, 2001; Frederick, 2000a, 2000b).

Compounding the need to accurately assess effort in forensic neuropsychological assessment is the fact that, as of 2002, successful feigning of intellectual and functional impairment may allow criminals to avoid the death penalty. More specifically, in the recent Supreme Court case of *Atkins v. Virginia* (2002), the Court determined in a 6–3 decision that executing the mentally retarded was "cruel and unusual" punishment and therefore prohibited by the Eighth Amendment (see Keyes, Edwards, & Perske, 1997; for an excellent description of case details, see Graue et al., in press). Given that defendants must have the capacity to assist their attorneys in their defense (American Bar Association, 1984) and there is evidence to suggest that MR individuals are more susceptible to making false confessions (Gudjonsson, 2002, as cited in Johnstone & Cooke, 2003), as well as inaccurate statements, during testimony (Everington & Fulero, 1999), a number of states had already outlawed this practice. The federal court majority, however, reportedly wanted to create greater consistency with their decision. It left the definition of mental retardation (MR) up to the states, most of which define a person with MR as having an IQ of 70 or lower and having two or more adaptive deficiencies, a topic that is addressed in more detail later.

Earlier reports suggested that approximately 16% of murder/insanity defendants were mentally retarded (Lanzkron, 1963). More recent estimates indicate that between 4% and 10% of the jail population in the United States comprises individuals with MR (Davis, 2000), and approximately 11% of inmates in maximum security and on death row meet criteria for the diagnosis (Everington & Keyes, 1999). While some writers have argued that inmates will want to mask their intellectual deficits given the assumed stigma associated with such a label, as well as the possibility that their disability might make them more vulnerable once they return to the general prison population (Dolan, 2005; Hawthorne, 2005), it is the opinion of others (and we agree) that the Supreme Court decision in 2002 will likely increase the number of assessments of MR in forensic settings and, consequently, the need for accurate assessment of malingering in such cases (Brodsky & Galloway, 2003). In fact, empirical research shows that criminal defendants facing serious charges are more likely to feign than those facing less serious charges (Weinborn, Orr, Woods, Conover, & Feix, 2003). This is of particular concern given that the MR population has been virtually ignored in the malingering literature and mentally retarded subjects are frequently excluded from validation studies of effort indices.

In sum, it is important to address the issue of noncredible cognitive test performance in the assessment of MR, as the incentive for feigning (at least in the forensic arena) is now literally a matter of life or death. However, the validity of using standard measures of effort with this population is unclear. With this in mind, the goals of this chapter are to (1) clarify the definition of MR and describe its general clinical characteristics; (2) identify the most common causes of MR and their specific neuropsychological correlates to guide predictions about this population's ability to pass standard effort test cutoffs; (3) present the results of a recent survey sent out to diplomates in forensic psychology regarding current practice in this area; (4) review the extant empirical literature with respect to the validity of such practice and present preliminary data from our lab on the use of common effort indicators in a low IQ sample; and, finally, (5) integrate this information in such a way as to stimulate and guide the emergence of future research. Each of these areas is addressed in turn.

DEFINITION AND CLINICAL CHARACTERISTICS OF MR

Prevalence

Based on the normal distribution, 2–3% of the population (or about 7 million people in the United States) would be expected to have an IQ less than 70 (Pulsifier, 1996). This is consistent with epidemiological studies estimating approximately 6.2 to 7.5 million individuals are mentally retarded in the United States, 26,500 to 32,500 of which are in prison or residential facilities (Davis, 2000). Epidemiological studies based solely on the criteria of IQ less than 70 indicate prevalence rates ranging from 0.8 to 1.2% with approximately 3–6 per 1,000 in mild range, 2 per 1,000 in the moderate range, 1.3 per 1,000 in the severe range, and finally, 0.4 per 1,000 who meet criteria for profound MR (McLaren & Bryson, 1987; Lipkin, 1991). As one author points out, however, when adaptive criteria are included in the definition, the prevalence slightly lowers (Pulsifier, 1996). Estimates are also lowered by premature mortality (especially in profound MR; Pulsifier, 1996).

Definitions

The aforementioned caveats surrounding estimations of prevalence highlight the fact that there are varying ways in which MR has been defined. The fourth edition, text revision of *Diagnostic and Statistical Manual of Mental Disorders* (DSM-IV-TR; American Psychiatric Association, 2000) defines MR as the presence of "subaverage intelligence" defined as an IQ less than or equal to 70 on the basis of formal testing or clinical judgment (i.e., in the case of an infant or an untestable subject) *and* "concurrent . . . impairments in present adaptive functioning" found in at least 2 of 11 areas of functional independence (i.e., communication, self-care, home living, social/interpersonal skills, use of community resources, self-direction, functional academic skills, work, leisure, health and safety) with onset before age 18 (p. 46). Here, adaptive functioning is defined as "the person's effectiveness in meeting the standards expected for his or her age and by his or her cultural group" (p. 46). DSM-IV-TR further classifies MR individuals by the IQ range within which they fall, the vast majority of cases falling into the category of mild MR:

Level of functioning	IQ range	% of all MR cases
Mild	50–55 to approximately 70	85%
Moderate	35–40 to 50–55	10%
Severe	20–25 to 35–40	3–4%
Profound	below 20–25	1–2%

The American Association on Mental Retardation (AAMR; 1992, 2002) has actually changed the definition of MR 10 times since 1908, in part spurred by a California class action lawsuit that found schools had placed a disproportionate number of black children in special programming for MR. For example, in 1973, an IQ of less than 85 was thought to be indicative of MR; however, this was eventually lowered to 70 and is now at 75 (allowing for a margin of error in testing). Notably, it has been suggested that this higher cutoff doubles the number of people eligible for diagnosis (Mash & Wolfe, 2002). Also, in contrast to DSM-IV-TR's focus on degree of impairment (i.e., mild, moderate, severe, and profound), the AAMR describes an individual's level of functioning in terms of his or her use of, and need for, external supports (i.e., intermittent, limited, extensive, or pervasive; Loveland & Tunali-Kotoski, 1998; Luckasson et al., 1992; also see www.aamr.org). Thus, the focus of this system of classification is on the individual's ability to function and required level of support as opposed to the degree of psychometric deficit found upon neuropsychological examination. Indeed, since the late 1970s and early 1980s, the importance of considering adaptive behavior (and not just IQ) in making the diagnosis has grown in awareness (DeVault & Long, 1988; Huberty, Koller, & Ten Brink, 1980). Authors have speculated several reasons for this, including (1) the identified need to evaluate such abilities in context (i.e., in the interaction between a person and their environment; Hawkins & Cooper, 1990); (2) an attempt to promote nondiscriminatory testing procedures, as low test scores are overrepresented in some minority groups (DeVault & Long, 1988; Everington & Keyes, 1999); (3) the ease with which identified needs for assistance can be translated into specific treatment goals (Mash & Wolfe, 2002); and finally (4) the general dissatisfaction with our existing practice of focusing solely on IQ and assumed disability versus actual need (see Bruininks, Thurlow, & Gilman, 1987, for a review of the evolution of including adaptive criteria). The last reason appears most strongly related to the fact that many mild MR individuals are capable of supporting themselves and living independently in the community (American Psychiatric Association, 2000); thus, psychometric deficit in these cases does not translate into actual adaptive deficit.

As defined by the American Association on Mental Deficiency (AAMD), deficits in adaptive functioning refer to "limitations in an individual's effectiveness in meeting the standards of maturation, learning, personal independence and/or social responsibility that are expected for his or her age level . . ." (Grossman, 1983, p. 11). Elsewhere in the literature, adaptive functioning has also been defined as "the extent to which an individual takes care of personal needs, exhibits social competence, and refrains from exhibiting problem behaviors . . ." (Bruininks, McGrew, & Maruyama, 1988, p. 266), abilities which undoubtedly depend on age (Bruininks, Thurlow, & Gilman, 1987):

Age level	Expected adaptive skills
Infancy/early childhood	Sensorimotor skills, communication skills, self-help skills and socialization
Childhood/early adolescence	Application of academic skills to daily life, application of reasoning and judgment to environmental situations, development of group and interpersonal social skills
Late adolescence/ adulthood	Vocational adjustment and performance as well as social adjustment in the community

Commonly used measures of adaptive functioning include the Vineland Adaptive Behavior Scales–II (VABS-II; Sparrow, Balla, & Cicchetti, 1984), the AAMD's Adaptive Behavior Scale (AAMD-ABS; Nihira, Foster, Shellhaas, & Leland, 1974), and the Adaptive Behavior Scale (ABS; Fogelman, 1975; Nihira, Leland, & Lambert, 1993), and literature focused on the assessment of adaptive behavior specifically in defendants charged with capital murder is emerging (Stevens & Randall, 2006).

General Clinical Characteristics

Mental retardation occurs more often in men than women by a ratio of approximately 1.6 to 1.0 (see Pulsifier, 1996), and can occur through a number of varied etiologies, including "infection and intoxication, trauma or physical agents, disorders of metabolism or nutrition, gross prenatal brain disease, unknown prenatal factors, chromosomal abnormalities, gestational disorders, environmental factors, secondary to psychiatric conditions, and other conditions" (McCaffrey & Isaac, 1985, p. 63). Early research did not differentiate between groups of varying etiology and instead simply investigated the characteristics of samples of individuals with similar IQ (e.g., Roszkowski & Snelbecker, 1981). This early research hypothesized that individuals with MR had most difficulty with what was referred to at the time as short-term memory (Ellis, 1963) but what today would be referred to as attention and speed of information processing. For example, Sprague and Quay (1966) factor-analyzed the performance of a heterogeneous group of subjects with MR on the Wechsler Adult Intelligence Scale (WAIS) and identified four factors, including what the authors referred to as a trace factor (arithmetic, digit span and digit symbol) on which the subjects with MR performed the worst. More recently, MacKenzie and Hulme (1987) found significantly lower than expected digit spans (relative to mental age), and significantly slowed development of digit span as mental age increased over time, in a group with severe MR relative to controls. In addition, adults with MR were found to demonstrate slower mental speed measured through analysis of eye gaze, eye movement, and orientation as compared to controls (Nettelbeck, 1986).

Other research using similar samples and research methodology demonstrated deficits in other cognitive domains, such as executive/frontal dysfunction, including deficits in planning and regulation of simple behavioral tasks (McCaffrey & Isaac, 1985). This finding is of particular note, as adaptive functions are thought to be most strongly related to the cognitive domain of executive function in an MR population (Edgin, 2003). Limitations of this work, however, include not only the fact that MR etiology went unaccounted for but also that this particular study included an extremely small sample size ($n = 10$). Other cognitive profiles emerging from this literature include greater difficulty with arithmetic as compared to reading (see Pulsifier, 1996) and a marked discrepancy between Verbal and Performance IQs, the former of which was found to be significantly lower than the latter (Calvert & Crozier, 1978). Taken together, the above-mentioned findings led researchers to believe the primary neuropsychological difficulty in MR is in sequential information processing, which involves primarily attention, processing speed, and planning abilities. This type of processing would be in contrast to what is known as simultaneous processing, relying more on perceptual integration and spatial skills (Pulsifier, 1996).

Previous research has also documented deficits in motor speed, grip strength, and sensory function within this population. For example, subjects with mild and moderate MR were found to exhibit slower physical speed than controls in one study (Lin & Zhang, 2002) and slower physical speed was highly related to IQ in 245 mentally retarded individuals assigned to groups on the basis of IQ (Black & Davis, 1966). Further, decreased grip strength was found in children with mild to severe MR when compared to a non-mentally retarded group (Iki & Kusano, 1986). Finally, both visual and hearing impairments have been documented in MR samples (Pulsifier, 1996).

Although these general profiles have emerged, as mentioned earlier, the etiology of MR is quite diverse. More recent research has investigated the possibility that the neuropsychological profiles of groups of varying etiology may differ as well. Indeed, emerging from this literature is evidence to suggest the existence of different cognitive profiles and neuroanatomical deficits associated with the different causes of MR.

CAUSES OF MR AND THEIR NEUROPSYCHOLOGICAL CORRELATES

The patterns of cognitive and adaptive functioning deficits and/or relative strengths found in MR (as well as unique patterns of neuroanatomical abnormalities) differ as a function of the etiological mechanism (see Pennington & Bennetto, 1998; Pulsifier, 1996). In other words, individuals with MR do not form a homogeneous group with respect to neuropsychological development or adaptive functioning (Loveland & Tunali-Kotoski, 1998).

Genetic/Organic MR

Evidence suggests that at least 50% of intelligence can be explained by heredity, and there are now over 1,000 different known organic causes of MR (Mash & Wolfe, 2002); however, the eight most common (in order of prevalence) are fetal alcohol syndrome, Down syndrome, fragile X, autism spectrum disorder, phenylketonuria, William syndrome, Prader–Willi syndrome, and Angelman syndrome. The first three causes together comprise approximately 33% of the total cases of MR with identifiable causes, and the scope of this chapter is therefore limited to a discussion of the neuropsychological profiles associated with these conditions. An excellent, comprehensive review of each of these causes and their neuropsychological sequalae can be found elsewhere in the literature (see Pulsifier, 1996). Following is a condensed summary of this work.

Fetal Alcohol Syndrome

Fetal alcohol syndrome (FAS) is reportedly the leading single cause of MR (see Pulsifier, 1996). The syndrome is caused and defined by maternal alcohol use during pregnancy and is characterized by stunted growth, unusual physical features (e.g., characteristic facies) and central nervous system (CNS) dysfunction that usually includes, but is not limited to, MR. Other CNS abnormalities that can occur include delay in reaching developmental milestones, microencephaly, muscular hypotonia, and hyperactivity. "Fetal alcohol effects" is the term used when full criteria for the syndrome are not met.

Associated neuropsychological deficits appear to be dose related. More specifically, the literature suggests that low doses of in uterine exposure can lead to slower mental and motor speed, behavioral impulsivity, and less complex play, while higher doses (i.e., ≥ two to three drinks per day) are associated with reduced fine motor coordination and sustained attention. Exposure to alcohol in the womb has also been shown to lead to abnormalities in language function (e.g., articulation disorders), certain aspects of executive function (i.e., abstract thinking, problem-solving, and judgment), grip strength, attention, arithmetic, and short-term memory. Overall IQ in children exposed to more than one-fifth ounces of alcohol per day *in utero* was found to be about 5 points below controls by age 4 in one study (see Mash & Wolfe, 2002). In general, Verbal IQ is also found to be generally below Performance IQ in this group.

In terms of adaptive functioning, individuals with FAS typically function well in daily living skills but are not as successful in demonstrating adequate social function (see Pulsifier, 1996). Further, this group is known for its persisting behavior difficulties that manifest in problems with feeding and sleeping, irritability, overactivity and distractability in school, difficulties with speech, social and emotional problems, and stereotypical behavior, such as head and body rocking or nail biting. Some of these individuals eventually meet criteria for conduct disorder, displaying antisocial behavior and later being at risk for alcohol abuse themselves. However, as a group, they are generally able to live independently with only limited support.

Down Syndrome

Affecting chromosome 21, Down syndrome (DS) is the most common genetic cause of MR, accounting for one-third of all moderate to severe MR in the world (Pulsifier, 1996). The syndrome is characterized by physical abnormalities including microcephaly, upward-slanting eyes, a broad neck, and hands that are small with in-curving fifth fingers. These individuals are also usually shorter in height than their non-DS counterparts, and obesity is common, as well as changes in hair, skin elasticity, motor skills, and skeletal structure that mimic an early aging process. In fact, some research suggests these individuals might be at higher risk for the later development of Alzheimer's disease.

Neuropsychologically, these individuals manifest severe language impairment, including deficits in articulation, phonology, and expressive syntax. In fact, their phrase structure may not exceed the 2nd-grade level in some cases. This is in contrast to their relatively preserved visuospatial abilities (Pezzini, Vicari, Volterra, Milani, & Ossella, 1999; Edgin, 2003). A related dissociation also occurs between visual and auditory sequential processing and memory, with specific sparing of the former; in particular, individuals with DS display difficulty recalling auditorily presented material. As in FAS, individuals with DS also display delayed motor abilities (e.g., with abnormally slower performance on Finger Tapping than comparison groups; Frith & Frith, 1974, and lack of expected hand asymmetry in dominant and nondominant hands upon finger tapping; Madhavan & Narayan, 1988), as well as motor clumsiness. They also do *not* show improvement on pursuit rotor tracking in contrast to the marked improvement seen in severe MR autistic groups and controls. These findings are consistent with neuroanatomical studies demonstrating that DS groups have smaller cerebellums compared to normals and relative to the rest of their own brains.

Adaptively, these individuals function higher than their cognitive abilities would suggest, with particular strengths in daily living and socialization skills relative to communication on the VABS (see Pulsifier, 1996). Further, they display higher than expected levels of social maturity/social adaptiveness given their mental age or IQ as compared to language-communication abilities. However, the relationship between adaptive skills and intelligence may differ with chronological age, with relative weakness in language and communication increasing with age but with eventual improvement in daily life skills (see Loveland & Tunali-Kotoski, 1998, for a review). Behaviorally, individuals with DS tend to function fairly well with low incidence of comorbid psychiatric illness. They are often able to live in group settings with limited support and are able to work in supported employment situations (Pulsifier, 1996).

Fragile X

Fragile X is the most common inherited cause of MR with a very distinct physical phenotype (at least in males) that emerges near puberty marked by macrocephaly, an elongated face, prominent jaw, long protruding ears, and macroorchidism (i.e., enlarged testicles) in adulthood. Similar changes occur in females as well, but to a much lesser extent. Males show developmental delays in sitting, walking, and speaking and are more often found to be hypotonic and temperamentally difficult. Intellectually, fragile X males usually present with moderate to severe MR, but a range is present, accompanied by primary neuropsychological deficits in attention, visual and verbal short-term memory, visual–spatial functioning (e.g., Block Design tends to be one of their lowest scores), and mental speed. Academic achievement tends to be better than expected given IQ level; however, math is a clear weakness. Males with fragile X demonstrate relative strengths in expressive and receptive vocabulary, as well as verbal comprehension; however, their speech is often marked by articulation problems and tends to be echolalic, perseverative, and dysfluent. In contrast to individuals with DS of similar intelligence, fragile X males display poorer conversational skills as well as abnormalities in the pragmatics of language (e.g., they will often avert their gaze when talking to another person; Pulsifier, 1996).

The adaptive profile of a male with fragile X on the VABS is one of relative strength in daily life skills, particularly personal and domestic skills. Relative weaknesses lie in socialization skills and communication abilities. Behaviorally, these individuals often engage in self-stimulatory behaviors, such as hand flapping, and self-injurious behaviors, such as head banging. They have also been found to be energetic, impulsive and inattentive, with most meeting criteria for attention-deficit/hyperactivity disorder (ADHD). A smaller subgroup of these individuals show autistic behavior, while others are anxious.

Females with fragile X present quite differently. First, only about half of these individuals have MR, and it is usually less severe than in males with the disorder (i.e., mild to moderate). While no initial developmental delays are evident, over time difficulties with attention, speech, and the pragmatics of language can emerge, and some of these females are diagnosed with learning disorders. However, many display no cognitive impairment at all, although typically there are relative weaknesses in visual–spatial skills and arithmetic, and behaviorally, these individuals tend to be shy and withdrawn with more frequent diagnoses of avoidant personality disorder or mood disorders when compared to non-fragile X females of similar IQ. Overall level of adaptive skills tends to be commensurate with the level of their intellectual development (Pulsifier, 1996).

Ideopathic/Cultural–Familial MR

Unlike the disorders mentioned earlier, there is no identifiable cause for MR in the majority of cases, especially milder forms (Mash & Wolfe, 2002). Ideopathic or cultural–familial MR is the "catchall" category used to describe lowered intelligence due to unidentified neurological and genetic disorders, as well as those cases of MR that are environmentally determined, collectively representing about one-half of all mild MR (see Pulsifier, 1996) and about 15–20% of MR in general (Mash & Wolfe, 2002). Ziegler and Hodapp (1986) posit subtypes, including the "familial retarded" in which at least one parent is also mentally retarded, the "polygenic isolates" in which parents are of average intelligence and provide generally nurturant environments, and finally, the "environmentally deprived" subtype in which poverty, parental neglect and/or psychopathology, or inadequate child care/educational experiences were experienced.

Physically, these individuals are frequently normal in appearance and health and have a mortality rate comparable to that of the general population. However, they may display mild physical abnormalities (e.g., abnormal skull shape). They are also usually from lower socioeconomic backgrounds and have relatives who are mentally retarded. Neuropsychologically, although there is some evidence to suggest these individuals display weakness in sequential as compared to simultaneous processing, slightly reduced achievement scores in arithmetic compared to reading, and better visual short-term memory compared to those with organic MR, there reportedly exists no distinct neuropsychological profile. Likewise, neuroanatomical variations found upon magnetic resonance imaging (MRI) scanning of children with idiopathic MR show only normal brain variations. Adaptively, these individuals generally live independently with minimal support and are able to integrate into the community. More than 80% find employment and 80% will marry (Pulsifier, 1996).

In sum, MR can occur in the context of several biological and/or environmental causes, each with a neuropsychological profile of relative strengths and weaknesses. Likewise, the organization of adaptive behavior also varies to some degree by etiology. Recall, for example, that while individuals with FAS, fragile X and DS all have relative strengths in daily living skills, FAS and fragile X individuals are much weaker in socialization skills as compared to the DS group. Thus, while some commonalities in MR can be discerned, there are also many differences. Further, there are numerous other conditions not reviewed here (e.g., 9p monosomy) that can be associated with MR and that have specific neuropsychological sequelae (see McSweeny, Wood, Chessare, & Kurczynski, 1993). Complicating matters even further is that the relationship between intellectual impairment and adaptive impairment varies by etiology (e.g., IQ is more strongly related to adaptive functioning in DS as compared to some of the other syndromes; Loveland, Tunali-Kotoski, 1998), and often individuals with mild MR (as documented by psychometric testing) are able to function well, all of which must be considered in the assessment of malingering in this population.

Given known prevalence rates, it is likely that the majority of cases seen in clinical practice are idiopathic in nature (and therefore cases of mild MR) or the result of FAS (and therefore mild to moderate MR). Thus, using the neuropsychological profiles associated with these two categories of MR to guide initial hypotheses about ability to pass effort tests is potentially the most productive course of action and would be summarized as follows:

Relative weaknesses	Relative strengths
Verbal IQ	Performance IQ
Auditory short-term memory	Visual short-term memory
Sequential processing	Simultaneous processing
Mental and physical speed	
Fine motor coordination	
Grip strength	
Simple and sustained attention	
Arithmetic	
Language function (e.g., articulation disorders)	
Abstract thinking, problem solving and judgment	

This profile raises the question as to whether an individual with MR would be able to pass standard effort test cutoffs. For example, given its reliance on sustained attention, would an individual with MR be able to pass the b Test? Likewise, given an MR individual's difficulty in arithmetic skills, would he/she be able to use multiplication necessary for successful passing of the Dot Counting Test? Further, while the field is moving in the direction of incorporating indices of response time to detect suboptimal effort in the general population (Victor & Abeles, 2004), is it likely that this method will be ineffective in population with MR given its members' slower mental and physical speeds? Would it be best to use only visual tests of effort given the relative strength in visual processing and memory in mentally retarded individuals?

To determine how practitioners are navigating the issue of effort testing in the differential diagnosis of actual versus feigned MR, we surveyed experts conducting these types of evaluations, the results of which are presented below.

SURVEY OF CURRENT PRACTICES IN FORENSIC PSYCHOLOGY

In January 2005, a confidential survey was sent to diplomates of the American Board of Forensic Psychologists (ABFP) to investigate current practices in detecting suspect effort in the context of forensic MR assessment. Of the 212 surveys distributed through a combination of electronic and land mail, 53 were completed and returned. However, three respondents indicated that they did not conduct medicolegal or criminal assessment and were therefore deemed inappropriate for the survey, rendering a final sample of 50.

Sample demographics are presented in Table 14.1. Notably, the sample was very sophisticated, with a mean of 23 years of experience in forensic work (consisting of an average 24% in medicolegal and 50% in criminal work). Further, 90% indicated they had testified or had their reports used in the context of a legal case over 100 times. Ninety percent also said they had been involved in a legal case in which they were asked to evaluate a litigant or criminal defendant for MR (constituting an average 10% of their total workload), with over half of the sample having experience with this 20 or more times in the context of forensic MR assessment.

Table 14.2 summarizes the current practice of respondents in relation to forensic MR assessment. The sample indicated that approximately 9% of the individuals assessed in the last year were faking MR. The most frequently used measures to assess feigned *intellectual* (vs. Axis I) deficits in MR evaluations were the following (in order of frequency): (1) Test of Memory Malingering (Tombaugh, 1996; 64%), (2) the Validity Indicator Profile (Frederick, 1997; 50%), (3) the Rey 15-Item Test (Rey, 1964, in Lezak, 2004; 44%), (4) the Structured Inventory of Reported Symptoms (Rogers, Bagby, & Dickens, 1992; 30%), (5) Word Memory Test (Green, Allen & Astner, 1996; Green & Astner, 1995; 14%), and finally, (6) the Dot Counting Test (Rey, 1941, in Lezak, 2004; Boone, Lu, et al., 2002; 10%). All but one respondent was aware of the Supreme Court's 2002 decision regarding execution of individuals with MR, and 96% of the sample felt that the problem of detecting feigned intellectual impairment was "very important" or "extremely important." Further, over half of the sample (i.e., 60%) felt "very confident" or "extremely confident" about their ability to accurately detect feigned MR. This is in spite of the paucity of research validating the use of these tests in samples with

TABLE 14.1. Demographics of Survey Respondents

Variable	Number	%	Mean	SD
Age			53.2	9.2
Gender				
Male	42	84%		
Female	8	16%		
Employment[a]				
Private practice	45	90%		
Academic	17	34%		
Jail/prison	4	6%		
Other	1	2%		
Retired	8	16%		
Geographic region				
Northeast	15	30%		
Southeast	19	38%		
Northwest	0	0%		
Southwest	8	16%		
Midwest	7	14%		
Did not respond		2%		
Forensic experience				
% medicolegal work		24%		
% criminal work		50%		
Number of years	23			
Number of times testified				
<10	0	0%		
10–50	2	4%		
51–99	3	6%		
>100	45	90%		
Experience with MR assessment				
Proportion of workload		10%		
Number of times testified				
<5	5	10%		
5–10	7	14%		
10–20	5	10%		
>20	33	66%		

Note. n = 50.
[a] Some respondents indicated more than one employment type.

TABLE 14.2. Practices of Survey Respondents

Variable	Number	%
Tests used to assess MR		
WAIS	48	96%
Other intelligence test	17	34%
Vineland		
ABS		
Other adaptive	11	22%
Projectives	1	2%
Use of collateral data	18	36%
% time use adaptive measures		57%
Tests used to assess feigned intellectual deficit		
TOMM	32	64%
VIP	25	50%
Rey 15-Item	22	44%
SIRS	15	30%
WMT	7	14%
Miller Forensic Assessment of Symptoms Test	6	12%
DCT	5	10%
Computerized Assessment of Response Bias	2	4%
VSVT	1	2%
Portland Digit Recognition Test	1	2%
MACT	1	2%
Importance of topic		
Not very important	0	0%
Somewhat important	1	2%
Very important	27	54%
Extremely important	21	42%
Confidence in detecting feigned MR		
Not at all confident	0	0%
Somewhat confident	16	32%
Very confident	24	48%
Extremely confident	6	12%
Depends on case	2	4%
Awareness of court decision	49	98%

Note. n = 50.

MR. Following is a review of how well these more popular tests stand up to empirical scrutiny.

FEIGNED MR: CAN WE ACCURATELY DETECT IT?

Mentally retarded and lower intelligence individuals (not to mention other important clinical samples) are typically excluded from effort test validation samples, which are instead normed on individuals with "normal" intelligence (Tombaugh, 2002; Weinborn et al., 2003). There is also surprisingly little in the general literature addressing the issue of using our effort measures with individuals of lowered intelligence. Our review uncovered only a handful of investigations examining the validity of widely used effort tests in this population.

Test of Memory Malingering

The suggestion that standard Test of Memory Malingering (TOMM; Tombaugh, 1996) cutoffs may be inappropriate for use with mentally retarded individuals has been made in the literature. For example, Weinborn et al. (2003) attempted to validate the TOMM in the context of a differential prevalence design examining factors that might have influenced subject performance (overall N = 61), including (but not limited to) MR (18% of sample) and borderline intellectual functioning (15% of sample). While the results provided general support for use of the TOMM, subjects with low intelligence were not segregated from those of normal intelligence. Analysis of the false positives (of which there were three) revealed they were all subjects with MR (two moderate and one mild). Given that there were 11 subjects with MR in total, 27% of subjects with MR were therefore misclassified by the TOMM, suggesting that the TOMM may not be appropriate for use with mentally retarded individuals. However, there were too few subjects to thoroughly evaluate this hypothesis, and it was concluded by the authors that "the performance of individuals with mental retardation or borderline intellectual functioning on the TOMM has not been [adequately] evaluated" (Weinborn et al., 2003, p. 981).

Recently, Hurley and Deal (2006) examined the false-positive rate of the TOMM in a sample of subjects with known MR (i.e., they were living in residential facilities for individuals with MR and none of them had prior legal involvement; N = 39, mean age = 44.9, 96% Caucasian, Full Scale IQs ranging from 50 to 78) and found that standard TOMM cutoffs (< 45 on Trial 2) misclassified 41% of the sample. Similarly, Graue et al. (in press) compared a group of individuals with mild MR (with prior diagnosis, history of special education, currently in day-treatment programs, and *not* in litigation; N = 26) to demographically comparable community volunteers who were instructed to fake MR (N = 25), and they found that the TOMM misclassified 31% of their subjects with MR. However, Hurley and Deal (2006) noted that analyzing the change scores from Trial 1 to Trial 2 may provide important information, as about 85% of their sample with MR showed improvement.

Other studies have suggested that established TOMM cutoffs are appropriate for use with an MR sample. For example, Heinze and Purisch (2001) found the TOMM and other effort tests to be valid in a criminal population suspected of feigning incompetence to stand trial (many of whom were likely mentally retarded; N = 57); however, the authors suggested that not one of the tests alone was sufficiently sensitive. Unfortunately, there was no true MR comparison group so specificity, or the rate of false-positive identifications, could not be estimated. Preliminary data in a separate study using a sample of patients with known MR seen in the context of social security disability evaluation (N = 19; age range 18 to 60; WAIS-III Full Scale IQs range 57 to 70) indicated that the TOMM demonstrated 100% specificity (zero false positives) (Drwal, personal communication, October 2005).

Still other findings suggest that the TOMM cutoffs may be inappropriate only for use with samples of moderate (vs. mild) MR. Specifically, use of the TOMM was investigated with a sample of 60 psychiatric inpatients (mean age = 38, SD = 10.9, mean Full Scale IQ = 62.2, SD = 5.1; 68% male): (1) 29 psychiatric inpatients with MR (26 mild and 3 moderate); (2) two patients with MR without psychiatric illness (one mild, one moderate); and (3) 29 psychiatric patients of low intellectual functioning related to psychiatric disorder. Results indicated a moderate and significant correlation between Full Scale IQ and TOMM Trial 2 (r = .55, p < .01). In addition, there were only six failures (i.e., < 45 on Trial 2 and Retention), two of which were the individuals diagnosed with moderate MR. Given the calculated specificity of 90% for subjects with mild MR, the authors concluded that the TOMM was appropriate for use with these individuals but questioned its validity for use with individuals with moderate MR. Limitations of the study, however, include the confound of major mental illness in addition to the fact that some subjects were in litigation at the time of evaluation, including four of the six who failed the TOMM (Kennedy et al., 2005).

Validity Indicator Profile

Of note, there were no empirical data available for review of the Validity Indicator Profile (VIP) in a MR sample with the exception of that presented in the test manual, which provides data on 40 subjects with MR that were included in the validation sample. The test authors specifically state, "Most of the people (95%) with mental retardation were classified as invalid, supporting the caveat [that] the VIP test should not be administered to persons with obvious history of mental retardation" (Frederick, 1997, p. 8).

Rey 15-Item Test

In every investigation identified for this review, the validity of using standard cutoffs for the Rey 15-Item Test (Rey, 1964) with a MR population was called into question and a recent meta-analysis concluded that "one should use [the Rey-15] only with those who do *not* have mental retardation . . ." (Reznick, 2005, p. 542; italics added). The earliest study was that of Goldberg and Miller (1986) who administered the test to 50 acute psychiatric adult patients and 16 "intellectually deficient" adults (i.e., IQs ranging from 40 to 69 based on standard intelligence testing). While the psychiatric group all recalled at least 9 of the 15 items (and 92% recalled 11 or more), 37.5% of the mentally retarded group recalled 8 or fewer items and 0% recalled all 15. Citing the above-mentioned study in their review, Schretlen, Brandt, Krafft, and van Gorp (1991) noted that there was a paucity of literature examining the usefulness of the Rey 15-Item Test with individuals of low IQ, and they found a significant, modest correlation between total recall on the test and IQ in their own mixed sample of neurological, psychiatric and control subjects (N = 193; r = .55, p < .001). This is consistent with at least two other known investigations of IQ and Rey 15-Item Test performance (N = 213; r = .53, p < .00; Speigel, 2006; also see Hays, Emmons, & Lawson, 1993). Schretlen and his colleagues (2003) also observed that the number of repeated items on the tests correlated with IQ in the expected direction (r = −.29, p < .001). Further, although there was no strictly mentally retarded comparison group, the severe psychiatric group had the lowest IQ (mean = 73.6, SD = 9.3), and this group also performed the worst on the test, on the whole scoring below the standard cutoff (i.e., < 9 items).

Similarly, Hayes, Hale, and Gouvier (1997) investigated the utility of the Rey 15-Item Test (along with two other effort indicators) for predicting the malingering status of mentally retarded defendants (N = 37), including (1) 13 pretrial nonmalingerers with MR, (2) 18 subjects with MR found not guilty by reason of insanity (NGBRI), and (3) six malingerers with MR (as determined by treatment teams using stringent DSM-IV criteria and observation of inconsistent behavior). Results showed that the malingerers produced better memory scores than the groups with true MR, leading the authors of this paper to conclude that the Rey 15-Item Test should not be used among defendants with MR. Further, in a separate study of three groups of mentally retarded criminally insane men (9 malingerers, 12 nonmalingerers, and 18 dissimulators; mean IQ across groups = 62.4, mean SD = 5.6), when the Rey 15-Item Test was included in a discriminant function analysis along with two other effort indicators, the results were significant; however, only a little over half of the cases were correctly classified across groups, with unacceptable rates of specificity (i.e., over 25% of the nonmalingerers were incorrectly classified; Hayes, Hale, & Gouvier, 1998). Finally, a dissertation in progress examining Rey 15-Item performance (using standard cutoffs) in a sample without identified incentive to feign cognitive impairment revealed specificity estimates of 69% and 77% for individuals with Full Scale IQs in the mentally retarded (i.e., less than 70; $N = 39$) and borderline (i.e., IQs between 70 and 79; $N = 49$) ranges of intellectual functioning, respectively. In addition, IQ subgroups (from borderline to high average) differed significantly (after controlling for the effects of education) on test performance; specifically, patients in the borderline range scored significantly lower than the low average ($p < .01$), average ($p < .01$) and high average ($p < .01$) groups (overall ratio $F = 14.48$; $N = 147$). Given that approximately one-third of the sample fell within the borderline or mentally retarded IQ ranges, the author suggested that the test was not appropriate (especially for exclusive use as an effort indicator) in the type of ethnically diverse, low socioeconomic status, urban population from which the sample was drawn (Speigel, 2006).

All the above-mentioned study designs were confounded by psychiatric and/or neurological impairment. There are only two studies to our knowledge that examined an uncontaminated sample of MR subjects. Marshall and Happe (in press) examined the performance of 100 patients with MR (WAIS-III Full Scale IQs ranged from 51 to 74), referred for standard clinical neuropsychological assessment, on five commonly used malingering tests, including the Rey 15-Item Test (cutoff < 9; Lezak, 2004) and the revised Rey 15-Item Test with recognition trial (cutoff < 20; Boone, Salazar, Lu, Warner-Chacon, & Razani, 2002). Subjects had a history of confirmed MR based on intelligence testing and a history of special education in school with no identified reason to feign cognitive impairment (i.e., they were already receiving support services from a county developmental disabilities division and had no reason to believe they were in danger of losing such services). Further, they were in good health with no drug, psychiatric, or medical history that might negatively affect their cognition. Results indicated that over half failed the recall portion of the test (mean recall = 7.5, $SD = 3.6$, $N = 69$) and over 80% failed the combined recall/recognition trial (mean combination score = 11.9, $SD = 7.2$, $N = 69$), further invalidating their use with this population and isolating the impact of IQ on effort test performance in a way that previous investigations had not. These results are consistent with the results of the Hurley and Deal (2006) study described earlier ($N = 39$ known subjects with MR), demonstrating that nearly 80% of their sample were misclassified by the Rey-15 Item Test using the < 9 cutoff.

Structured Interview of Reported Symptoms

In one of the same studies cited earlier, Hayes, Hale, and Gouvier (1998) tested three groups of men with MR from a state facility for the criminally insane ($N = 39$). Group 1 consisted of 12 pretrial nonmalingerers, Group 2 of 9 pretrial malingerers (as determined by an interdisplinary team), and

Group 3 consisted of 18 individuals faking good who were originally found to be NGBRI but desired release at the time of evaluation. Discriminant function analysis revealed that the Structured Interview of Reported Symptoms (SIRS; Rogers et al., 1992) alone produced a rate of 95% overall classification accuracy. However, methodological limitations included the fact that the sample was a mixed group with various comorbid psychiatric conditions, and group status was defined solely by an interdisciplinary team assessment of self-reported symptoms and behaviors. Further, the malingerers were likely feigning psychosis as well as MR, limiting the generalizability of these findings to settings in which only MR is being feigned.

In the Hurley and Deal (2006) sample of known individuals with MR, the SIRS misclassified 53.8% of the sample using the total score cutoff (> 76), 30.8% of the sample using one definite scale cutoff (≤ 1), and 30.8% of the sample using three probable scales cutoff (≥ 3). Curiously, however, the authors found no relationship between the SIRS total score and subject IQ (r = .03). The authors speculated that this finding may be a function of test structure, specifically that "yes" responses produce higher scores on the SIRS, and individuals with MR may be more likely to display this type of response bias (consistent with their tendency to make false confessions, recall Everington & Fulero, 1999).

Word Memory Test

The Word Memory Test (WMT; Green et al., 1996; Green & Astner, 1995) is the only effort test that includes in its manual validation data for an adult population with MR, specifically demonstrating that adults with Verbal IQs in the MR range (i.e., ≤ 70; mean Verbal IQ = 64) scored a mean of 96% (SD = 5) on the WMT, which is well above the standard cutoff of 85% (Green, 2003); however, specificity rates were not reported, and the authors specifically state that "future studies should determine WMT scores for motivated individuals of given VIQ ranges [as]. . . . Some adjustment to cut-off scores might be needed for people of very low VIQ" (Green et al., 1996, p. 13).

VIQ was also not found to significantly predict WMT performance in children and adults who had at least a third-grade reading level (Green & Flaro, 2003; Green, Lees-Haley, & Allen, 2002, respectively). In addition, children of lower intelligence reportedly passed a shorter version of the test, the Memory and Concentration Test (MACT; Green, 2004). More specifically, in a sample of 33 children, including 3 subjects with MR and 7 subjects with FAS, given the oral version of the MACT, all but one child passed the primary effort measures. However, the sample size used in this analysis was inadequate and the one false positive was a 17-year-old boy with a Full Scale IQ of 56, suggesting that while individuals with mild MR might be able to successfully complete the task, those bordering moderate levels of MR might have difficulty.

Dot Counting Test

The DOT Counting Test (DCT) combination E-score (Rey, 1941, in Lezak, 2004; Boone, Lu, et al., 2002) has proven to be inadequately specific when used with a MR sample seen for social security disability evaluations. Specifically, in a sample of 24 known MR subjects (based on prior intelligence testing) ranging in age from 18 to 60 (mean = 31.8; SD = 11.9) with WAIS-III Full Scale IQs ranging from 57 to 70 (mean = 65.4; SD = 3.6), there were 11 false positives using the E-score's generic cutoff of greater than or equal to 17, which corresponds to a specificity rate of only 54% (Drwal, personal communication, October 2005). Behavioral observations suggested that patients had particular difficulty applying multiplication skills to the task and instead required lengthy periods of time to individually count grouped dots. Limitations of this analysis include the fact that subjects had motive to feign; however, several indices were used to exclude malingerers, such as inconsistencies found between two IQ tests administered the same day (e.g., between the Kaufman Brief Intelligence Test [K-Bit; Kaufman & Kaufman, 1990] and the WAIS-III) or inconsistent reports (e.g., a patient stating he could not work secondary to depression but could find the energy to volunteer at church 40 hours per week); however, the exact number of those individuals excluded was not reported.

Likewise, use of the DCT was found inadequate in both defendants with MR and a sample of screened subjects with MR (i.e., without comorbid substance abuse, or psychiatric or neurological condition). Specifically, in one of the same studies cited previously, Hayes et al. (1997) investigated the utility of the DCT (along with the Rey 15-Item Test and another effort indicator) for predicting the malingering status of defendants with MR (N = 37) and found that the malingerers made fewer dot-counting errors than the other two groups with true MR, leading the authors of this paper to conclude that the DCT should not be used among defendants with MR. The DCT E-score (cutoff ≤ 17; Boone, Lu, et al., 2002) was also included in the Marshall and Happe (in press) study of effort test performance in a sample of 100 subjects with MR (WAIS-III Full Scale IQs ranged from 51 to 74). Results indicated that 70% failed (mean total score = 25.8, SD = 9.6, N = 69), invalidating use of standard DCT indices with this population.

However, use of only the total time to complete score from the DCT may be useful with a mentally retarded population. Hurley and Deal (2006) found that while their 39 known subjects with MR made errors on the test, they were (for the most part) able to complete a six-card version of the test in 180 or less seconds, a recommended cutoff from Paul, Franzen, Cohen, and Fremouw (1992) (i.e., only one subject exceeded this cutoff). Limitations of this study, however, includes the fact that it was conducted with a predominantly Caucasian sample, and that performance at different levels of IQ (mild, moderate, etc.) was not examined.

Other Free-Standing Effort Indicators

Malingering Scale

Schretlen and Arkowitz (1990) compared five different groups ($N = 20$ in each), including two groups of prison inmates instructed to fake insanity or MR and three comparison groups (psychiatric inpatients, adults with MR [mean IQ = 47, $SD = 12$] and prison inmate controls) on the Minnesota Multiphasic Personality Inventory (MMPI), the Bender Gestalt Test, and the Malingering Scale (MaS), a 90-item experimental measure partially adapted from existing intelligence scales and designed by the authors to measure malingered cognitive symptoms. While those instructed to fake MR obtained significantly lower scores on the MaS (mean = 46, $SD = 21$) than the inmate controls (mean = 84, $SD = 4$), the true MR group scored the worst (mean = 63, $SD = 9$), suggesting that this is not a test that true MR individuals can pass.

Victoria Symptom Validity Test

Loring, Lee, and Meador (2005) investigated the validity of established cut-off scores for the Victoria Symptom Validity Test (VSVT; Slick, Hopp & Strauss, 1995) in a clinical sample of epileptic patients and found that of the 15 subjects with low intellectual functioning (i.e., WAIS-III Full Scale IQs between 60 and 69), 9 subjects either scored in the normal range or perfectly on the test. These authors concluded that low intelligence will not by itself cause failure on the VSVT, although their data suggest an un-acceptably low specificity level (i.e., 60%) in the subjects with MR as a group.

Digit Memory Test and the Letter Memory Test

Graue et al. (in press) also investigated the Digit Memory Test (DMT; Guilmette, Hart, Guiliano, & Leininger, 1994; cutoff < 90%) and the Letter Memory Test (LMT; Inman et al., 1998; cutoff < 93%) in their groups of indi-viduals with mild MR and laboratory simulators and found that while the DMT produced close to acceptable levels of predictive accuracy (i.e., specific-ity = 85%; sensitivity = 76%), the LMT misclassified 42% of their mentally retarded sample.

Standard Cognitive Effort Indicators

Many investigators have recommended that standard cognitive tests (vs. free-standing indicators) be used to detect noncredible test performance to both decrease overall administration time and lessen the potential impact of coaching (e.g., Sherman, Boone, Lu, & Razani, 2002). What is known about the performance of individuals with MR on these indicators is summarized below.

Digit Span

Babikian, Boone, Lu, and Arnold (2006) investigated the use of the Digit Span (DS) age corrected scaled score (ACSS) and Reliable Digit Span (RDS; i.e., the sum of the longest string of digits repeated without error over two trials under both forward and backward conditions) for detecting suspect effort in three groups of patients: (1) a noncredible group ($N = 66$); (2) a credible mixed clinic group ($N = 56$); and (3) a control group ($N = 32$). Individuals with MR were included in the analyses. Using the recommended standard cutoff for ACSS (i.e., ≤ 5; found to have the best predictive accuracy by the authors in their sample), there were three false positives, all averaging a FSIQ approximately 18 points lower than patients above the cutoff (i.e., Full Scale IQ = 73.7 vs. 91.2). Similarly, the recommended cutoff for RDS (i.e., ≤ 6) yielded two false positives who had a mean Full Scale IQ approximately 15 points lower than patients above the cutoff (i.e., Full Scale IQ = 74.5 vs. 90.7). Collectively, these findings predict that use of the ACSS and RDS with individuals of borderline or MR-range IQ leads to unacceptable rates of false-positive error. Similarly, Marshall and Happe's (in press) analysis of 100 nonpsychiatric, healthy subjects with MR (described in more detail previously) found that 69% failed RDS (using a cutoff of ≤ 7; Greiffenstein, Baker, & Gola, 1994), and (even more striking) Graue et al. (in press) found that using the same RDS cutoff and a cutoff of ≤ 5 for ACSS misclassified 85% and 81% of their mentally retarded sample, respectively, providing fairly clear evidence to suggest DS scores are invalid for use in an MR population.

Finger Tapping Test

Arnold et al. (2005) investigated the use of the Finger Tapping Test (FTT) (three trials alternating between hands) in multiple clinical comparison groups, including a low IQ sample of 17 adults (i.e., IQ ≤ 70) with no history of neurological disorder. Results suggested standard cutoffs were inadequate and that there was a need for adjusted cutoffs with this group. Using a cutoff of ≤ 33 for dominant hand performance resulted in 89% specificity and 43% sensitivity in men with MR (mean = 41.5, $SD = 6.3$, $N = 9$), while dominant hand performance ≤ 28 was associated with 87% specificity and 61% sensitivity in women with MR (mean = 40.8, $SD = 6.0$, $N = 8$), suggesting that this effort indicator may show promise in the differentiation of feigned versus actual mental retardation. However, sensitivity was compromised at these cutoffs, and limitations of this study include the fact that dividing the sample by gender led to small subsamples that affected the stability of specificity values and therefore requires replication.

Wechsler Adult Intelligence Scale—Third Edition

Graue et al. (in press) investigated both the Wechsler Adult Intelligence Scale–Third Edition (WAIS-III) Vocabulary–Digit Span index (Iverson & Tulsky, 2003; Greve, Bianchini, Mathias, Houston, & Crouch, 2003; cutoff ≥ 4) and the Mittenberg Disciminant Function (Mittenberg et al., 2001; cutoff > .21) in their sample of subjects with mild MR and simulators. Results demonstrated that the simulators were able to produce overall WAIS-III scores comparable to the group with MR, and that neither of the aforementioned derived effort indicators were effective in discriminating the two groups. The latter misclassified 35% of the subjects with MR and the former, while associated with no false-positive identification, detected 0% of the laboratory simulators.

California Verbal Learning Test and Wechsler Memory Scale— Third Edition

Marshall and Happe (in press) included in their analysis the performance of their 100 mentally retarded subjects (see details of sample above) on the California Verbal Learning Test (CVLT) forced-choice recognition test (CVLT-FCR; Delis, Kramer, Kaplan, & Ober, 2000; cutoff < 3 correct; Millis, Putnam, Adams, & Ricker, 1995) and the Wechsler Memory Scale–Third Edition (WMS-III) Rarely Missed Items (RMI) index (WMS-III RMI cutoff ≤ 136; Killgore & DellaPietra, 2000). Notably, 89% of their subjects reportedly passed the CVLT-FCR and 91% passed the RMI using standard cutoffs, suggesting that they may be particularly promising for use with this population. However, the typical trouble with the former is that using significant below-chance cutoffs results in poor sensitivity; unfortunately, in the Marshall and Happe (in press) study there was no malingering comparison group in which to evaluate this measure of predictive accuracy. With regard to the latter, Killgore and DellaPietra (2000) report sensitivity and specificity estimates of 97% and 100%, respectively in their RMI validation sample of simulated malingerers ($N = 36$) and bona fide brain-damaged subjects ($N = 51$; 12% mentally retarded), suggesting that use of this index may provide protection against false-positive error while still preserving its ability to detect true feigning in this population. Additional support for use of the RMI was found by Leduc (2005) in a sample of individuals applying for Social Security Disability Insurance, many of whom are often mentally retarded.

MMPI-2

One article discussed the use of the MMPI-2 for identifying malingered MR. It concluded that the test would be inappropriate to use for this purpose for a number of reasons, including the fact that many individuals with MR never reach the eighth-grade reading (or oral comprehension) level required for assurance of understanding of test items. Keyes (2004) also points out that the test manual specifically states that the "usefulness of the information obtained by the MMPI-2 depends heavily on the ability of test subject to understand the test instructions, to comply with the requirements of the task, to comprehend and interpret the content of the items as they relate to him or her, and to record these self-attributions in a reliable way" (Hathaway & McKinley, 1989, p. 13). Keyes (2004) argues that an individual with MR would not have the level of concentration or verbal comprehension abilities required to complete the 567-item test. He further argues that the language of the test manual suggests results should never be used to provide the state with evidence that could or would result in execution of a criminal defendant. This is alarming, as the author points out, given that the Mississippi Supreme Court has apparently ruled that the MMPI-2 is required to rule out malingering in the assessment of inmates up for the death penalty (Keyes, 2004).

In sum, there is little research investigating the use of our standardly employed effort indicator cutoff scores in a population with MR, and much of research that is available is plagued with methodological limitations (inadequate sample sizes; contamination of samples; incentives to feign; lack of comparison groups, etc.) that limit the reliability and generalizability of findings. In spite of this, the results of the survey we conducted suggest that forensic neuropsychological assessments are conducted on a regular basis with this population, and of particular concern is the fact that over half of the survey sample respondents (i.e., 60%) felt "very confident" or "extremely confident" about their ability to accurately detect feigned MR. Further, our review of the available literature revealed unacceptable specificity rates (i.e., < 90%; Millis, 1992) for the use of some of the more commonly used effort indicators (i.e., VIP, Rey 15-Item Test, and DCT).

Preliminary Data from Our Lab

In an attempt to address some of these methodological limitations and to provide preliminary data concerning how our effort tests behave in a low IQ population, we present preliminary data examining the false-positive rates of several effort indicators in a selected sample of patients with (1) no motive to feign (i.e., they were not applying for disability compensation and not in litigation at the time of evaluation), (2) no history of dementia or schizophrenia, and (3) an IQ of less than or equal to 75 based on the WAIS-III (i.e., they met AAMR psychometric criteria for MR). Forty-two subjects referred to one of two outpatient mental health clinics in southern California for neuropsychological evaluation met these criteria and all completed a full neuropsychological testing battery that included the following effort indicators: Rey

15-Item Test (Rey, 1964, in Lezak, 2004) with recognition trial (Boone, Salazar, et al., 2002a), DCT (Rey, 1941, in Lezak, 2004; Boone, Lu, et al., 2002), Warrington Recognition Memory Test—Words (WRMT-W; Iverson & Franzen, 1994; Millis, 1992; note: administration was altered to include having subjects read each word aloud upon presentation prior to making a decision regarding pleasantness—whether they liked the word, did not like the word, or felt neutral about it), Rey Word Recognition Test (Greiffenstein, Gola, & Baker, 1995), RDS (Babikian et al., 2006; Greiffenstein et al., 1994), WAIS-III DS ACSS (Iverson & Franzen, 1994; Iverson & Tulsky, 2003; Suhr, Tranel, Wefel, & Barrash, 1997), Rey–Osterreith Effort Equation (Lu, Boone, Cozolino, & Mitchell, 2003), Rey–Osterreith (R-O)/Rey Auditory Verbal Learning Test (RAVLT) discriminant function (Sherman et al., 2002) and the FTT (Arnold et al., 2005).

Subjects ranged in age from 19 to 60 (mean = 40.6; SD = 10.3); 64% were female. Various ethnic groups were represented, including 36% Hispanics, 31% African Americans, 26% Caucasians, 2% Asian, 2% Middle Eastern, and 2% identifying themselves as "other." Number of years of education ranged from 4 to 16 (mean = 11.6; SD = 2.3). WAIS-III Full Scale IQ scores ranged from 56 to 75 (mean = 69.2; SD = 4.9), and thus all subjects fell into the classification of mild MR.

Table 14.3 provides means, standard deviation and range values for subjects' performance on each of the indicators. Displayed in Table 14.4 is the degree of specificity of each indicator (cutoffs used for each measures are also noted in the table). Defining "acceptable" levels of specificity as $\geq$ 90% (i.e., $\leq$ 10% false-positive rate), adequate values were found for only the WRMT-W (95%). Marginally acceptable levels of specificity were found for the FTT (87%); however, this is not surprising given that the newly recommended cutoffs for patients with MR were employed in this analysis (i.e., $\leq$ 28 for women, $\leq$ 33 for men; Arnold et al., 2005). Varying degrees of inadequate specificity (i.e., < 90) were found for the remainder of the indicators, including the R-O/RAVLT Discriminant Function (87%), DCT (76%), the R-O Effort Equation (74%), DS ACSS (62%), RDS (62%), the Rey 15-Item Test plus recognition (59%), and Rey Word Recognition (37%), with false-positive rates ranging from 13% up to 63%, overall suggesting the standardly employed cutoffs for these indicators are not appropriate to use when attempting to identify inadequate effort in individuals who may be mentally retarded. Adjusted cutoffs to meet appropriate levels of specificity are also presented in the table; however, the degree to which lowering the cutoffs affects these indicators' sensitivity for detecting malingering is unknown and is a topic addressed in more detail later. Finally, noteworthy is the fact that, examined by IQ band, subjects with Full Scale IQs falling in the 70s failed one to two indicators on average, while subjects in the 60–69 IQ group failed an average of three indicators, and those with IQs in the 50–59 range failed a mean of four indicators.

TABLE 14.3. Performance of Subjects on the Effort Indicators

Effort indicator	n	Mean	SD	Min.	Max.
Recognition Memory Test[a]	19	43.5	5.7	32	50
Finger Tapping Test[b]	30	41.6	10.3	22	72
R-O/RAVLT Discriminant Function[c]	40	0.75	1.06	–3.00	2.31
DCT E-score[d]	33	14.9	5.5	6.7	32.6
R-O Effort Equation[e]	34	49.9	12.2	23.5	68
DS ACSS[f]	42	6.4	2.1	3	13
RDS[g]	39	7	2	2	11
Rey-15 Item plus recognition[h]	34	20.8	6.2	9	30
Rey Word Recognition[i]	19	6.5	3.3	1	13

Note. Total n = 42.
[a] Recognition Memory Test = total number correct out of 50.
[b] FTT = average with dominant hand across three trials.
[c] R-O/RAVLT discriminant function = (.006 × RAVLT Trial 1) – (.062 × R-O delay) + (.354 × RAVLT recognition) – 2.508.
[d] DCT E-score = Mean ungrouped dot counting time + Mean grouped dot counting time + number of errors.
[e] R-O Effort = Copy + [(recognition true positives – atypical false positives) × 3].
[f] DS ACSS = WAIS-III DS ACSS.
[g] RDS = Total number of digits recalled forwards and backwards on both trials.
[h] Rey 15-Item Test plus recognition = [recall correct + (recognition correct – false-positive errors)].
[i] Rey Word Recognition = Total recognition – number of false positives.

An Additional Consideration: The Co-Occurrence of MR and Malingering

Our discussion thus far has rested on the assumption that actual versus feigned MR are mutually exclusive categories. However, we recently assessed a 41-year-old criminal defendant with a Full Scale IQ of 58, which was documented at age 18 prior to any legal difficulties. He was charged in the death of an infant and was tested at the request of his defense attorney regarding competency to stand trial. On Trial I of the TOMM the defendant repeatedly indicated that he could not recall which items he had been shown. Trial 1 was discontinued and he was shown the stimulus pictures a second time. On TOMM Trial 2 he obtained a score of 4 out of 50, a score well below chance and suggestive of his awareness of the correct answers despite his responses to the contrary. In addition, his presentation was noteworthy for exceedingly long pauses in reciting digits forward (an average of 13.5 seconds to recite four digits; cutoff > 6 seconds; Babikian et al., 2006), particularly low dominant-hand finger tapping speed (24.6; cutoff ≤ 33; Arnold et al., 2005), and inability to reliably identify letters or compute the most basic single-digit addition calculations despite attending school for 12 years. Thus, it is apparent that feigning can occur in some individuals with MR, and this is yet another complicating consideration when conducting these types of assessments.

TABLE 14.4. False-Positive Rate Associated with the Use of Effort Tests in a Population of True MR Negatives

Effort indicator	Cutoff	No. of false positives	n	Specificity[a]	Adjusted cutoff[b]	Specificity[a] for adjusted cutoff
Recognition Memory Test[c]	< 33	1	19	95%	—	—
FTT[d]	≤ 33 (men) ≤ 28 (women)	4	30	87%	≤ 32 ≤ 27	90%
R-O/RAVLT Discriminant Function[e]	≤ -.40	5	40	87%	≤ -.70	90%
DCT E-score[f]	≥ 17	8	33	76%	≥ 23	92%
R-O Effort Equation[g]	≤ 47	9	34	74%	≤ 29	92%
DS ACSS[h]	≤ 5	16	42	62%	≤ 3	93%
RDS[i]	≤ 6	15	39	62%	≤ 4	90%
Rey 15-Item plus recognition[j]	≤ 20	14	34	59%	≤ 11	91%
Rey Word Recognition[k]	≤ 5 (men) ≤ 7 (women)	12	19	37%	≤ 1 (men) ≤ 3 (women)	90%

Note. Total $n = 42$.

[a] Specificity = the proportion of true negatives who were correctly classified.

[b] Adjusted cutoffs are associated with ≥ .90 levels of specificity.

[c] Recognition Memory Test = total number correct out of 50.

[d] FTT = average with dominant hand across three trials.

[e] R-O/RAVLT discriminant function = (.006 × RAVLT Trial 1) − (.062 × R-O delay) + (.354 × RAVLT recognition) − 2.508.

[f] DCT E-score = Mean ungrouped dot counting time + Mean grouped dot counting time + number of errors.

[g] R-O Effort = Copy + [(recognition true positives − atypical false positives) × 3].

[h] DS ACSS = WAIS-III DS subtest ACSS.

[i] RDS = Total number of digits recalled forwards and backwards on both trials.

[j] Rey 15-Item Test plus recognition = recall correct + (recognition correct − false positive errors).

[k] Rey Word Recognition = Total recognition − number of false positives.

336

SUMMARY, INTEGRATION, AND DIRECTIONS FOR FUTURE RESEARCH

There is now even greater incentive for individuals to feign intellectual deficits in the context of forensic neuropsychological assessment. However, our ability to accurately detect, or rule out, this behavior is complicated by several factors, including 1) the fact that MR is caused by a number of different conditions that are both biologically and environmentally determined and appear to have specific neuropsychological sequelae associated with them; (2) that subjects with MR are typically excluded from effort test validation samples; (3) that the extent of the neuropsychological deficits would suggest that standard effort test cutoffs may not be appropriate for use with this population; and, finally, (4) that the extant empirical literature addressing this issue is limited but would suggest great caution be used in effort test interpretation as the likelihood of false-positive error is probably quite high; individuals of borderline and MR levels of intelligence can fail on average one to four effort tests in a standard battery even when putting forth their full effort. Of further concern is the fact that these tests are being routinely used in a population with MR for the purposes of assisting legal decision makers without adequate empirical support for such practice. Based on these findings as reviewed previously, we provide the following preliminary suggestions regarding clinical practice and future research.

Significantly below-chance performance on forced-choice effort measures would appear to provide definitive evidence of feigning, even in individuals with MR (e.g., the CVLT forced-choice recognition test; Marshall and Happe, in press). However, sensitivity rates (i.e., correct identification of actual malingerers) are poor at these levels, necessitating that additional effort indices be examined. The available data suggests that the WRMT-W may have particular promise for the differential diagnosis of actual versus feigned MR, with specificity rates (i.e., nonmalingerers correctly identified as such) above 90% when using standard cutoffs that have been associated with acceptable sensitivity values (Iverson & Franzen, 1994; Millis, 1992). The R-O/RAVLT discriminant function (Sherman et al., 2002) produced a specificity rate approaching 90% and may also be valuable in this type of assessment. Also promising is the use of the WMS-III RMI, which has been found to have high specificity in individuals with MR, and the index's creators (Killgore & DellaPietra, 2000) report sensitivity and specificity estimates of 97% and 100%, respectively in their RMI validation sample of simulated malingerers ($N = 36$) and bona fide brain-damaged subjects ($N = 51$; 12% mentally retarded), suggesting that use of this index may provide protection against false-positive error while still preserving its ability to detect true feigning in this population. Finally, the WMT and the DMT may be helpful in assessing effort in this population, but additional data are needed.

In contrast, the use of standard cutoffs for the SIRS, the DCT, the Rey 15-Item Test, RDS, DS ACSS, the FTT, Vocabulary-Digit Span, Mittenberg Discriminant Function, and even the TOMM may lead to an unacceptable rate of false-positive identifications within MR samples. Use of derived effort indicators from the WAIS-III appears to be particularly contraindicated, a not unexpected finding given that the issue at hand is one of intelligence. Although it might seem practical to establish cutoffs specific to this population, as pointed out by Marshall and Happe (in press), it appears that MR individuals score so low on some of these tests that simply establishing new cutoffs is inadequate. For example, in their study, lowering the cutoff for the Rey 15-Item Test to < 3 still incorrectly classified 17% of their mentally retarded sample. Similarly, the cutoff for the DCT had to be raised to ≥ 38 to achieve acceptable levels of specificity (i.e., > .90). Using these cutoffs would improve specificity, but this would occur at the expense of sensitivity. This was most clearly demonstrated by Graue et al. (in press); lowering the cutoff for TOMM Trial 2 and Retention to 30 raised specificity from 69% to 96% but lowered sensitivities to 56% and 60%, respectively. However, these same authors reported that a revised cutoff score of < 80% for the DMT produced sensitivity of 72%, specificity of 95%, and a hit rate of 88%. Further, lowering the cutoff to < 70% on the LMT resulted in sensitivity of 76%, specificity of 96%, and a hit rate of 88%. Thus, sensitivity was not necessarily unacceptably compromised on these tests; however, as the authors point out, these cutscores require cross-validation as limitations of the study included small sample sizes, geographic restriction, and a simulation design.

It might also be useful to alter, or simplify, the tests given what we know about the ability of individuals with MR to successfully complete them. For example, it has been suggested that eliminating consideration of the time ratio between counting grouped and ungrouped dots on the DCT in individuals who may be mentally retarded is warranted given their difficulties employing multiplication strategies (Drwal, personal communication, October 2005). However, again this has a negative impact on sensitivity (i.e., consideration of errors alone, rather than a combination of errors and time, has been associated with lowered DCT sensitivity; Boone, Lu, et al., 2002).

It may also be useful to examine effort test scores in concert, rather than individually. Although it is fairly likely that an individual of lowered intelligence will fail one to four indicators, it is much less likely that such an individual will fail five or six according to our preliminary data. Hayes et al. (1998) found that the use of three effort indicators (the DCT, the Rey 15-Item Test, and the M Test) correctly classified 100% of their sample; however, the false-positive rates based on failure on at least one of the four effort indices (i.e., the SIRS, the DCT, the Rey 15-Item Test, and the M Test) ranged from 13% to 27%. Likewise, Graue et al. (in press) found that 69% of their participants with MR failed at least one of the multiple effort tests administered in their study. Discriminant function analyses may be useful in identifying weighted combinations of test results specific to individuals with actual MR.

Qualitative analysis of the types of responses or errors made by patients may also hold promise. For example, in the study by Marshall and Happe (in press), it was very rare for any of their subjects with MR to make even one dyslexic, false-positive recognition error on the Rey 15-Item plus recognition test. Further, there were some data to suggest that individuals with MR show a "yes" response bias (e.g., on Logical Memory recognition), that is not likely to be displayed by malingerers (Marshall & Happe, in press). In fact, it is this response bias that the authors believe underlies the ability of individuals with MR to pass the Logical Memory RMI of the WMS-III ("yes" is the correct answer to all six questions that comprise this test). Recall this was a speculation made by Hurley and Deal (2006) with regard to the high false-positive rate of subjects with MR on the SIRS. Development of tests that capitalize on unique response biases found in samples with MR may be a particularly promising area of future research. In addition, more creative and innovative paradigms are needed.

As in any case in which the individual is suspected of not putting forth adequate effort, observations of behavioral inconsistencies can be useful. It has been suggested that malingerers might hold inaccurate beliefs about the abilities of mentally handicapped, focusing only on achieving a low IQ with little consideration of other aspects of their presentation such as their behavioral, conversational, or social skills presentation (Johnstone & Crooke, 2003). Asking yourself, "Is the patient able to understand verbal instructions?" for example, or making note of the linguistical structure of their speech and any indication of an articulation disorder would also be informative. Listening and making note of language used during conversation can be a good indicator of whether a person's true ability exceeds test performance (Morrison, 1994). Further, it is always important to explore several sources of information (i.e., test scores, clinical interview, and collateral information from original judge, defense attorney, court records, and educational records) given that individuals with true MR are likely to have documentation of their mental functioning over time (Miller & Germain, 1988). Access to this information will likely enhance one's ability to identify feigning, although these data will never eclipse the need for objective effort measures specifically validated in a population with MR.

Ultimately, it may be that different effort tests are required for a population with MR, rather than simply importing for use tests developed on individuals of normal intelligence. It is likely that particular effort tests are effective in some IQ ranges and not others. Future research in this area is needed to examine the utility of primarily visual tests with use of unconfounded samples with MR (who have no incentive to feign) and appropriate comparison groups.

REFERENCES

American Association on Mental Retardation. (1992). *Mental retardation: Definitions, classification and systems of support* (9th ed.). Washington, DC: Author.

American Association on Mental Retardation. (2002). *Mental retardation: Definitions, classification and systems of support* (10th ed.). Washington, DC: Author.

American Bar Association. (1984). *Criminal Justice Mental Health Standards.* Retrieved August 31, 2005, from *www.abanet.org/crimjust/standards/mentalhealth_toc.html.*

American Psychiatric Association. (2000). *Diagnostic and statistical manual of mental disorders* (4th ed., text rev.). Washington, DC: Author.

Arnold, G., Boone, K., Dean, A., Wen, J., Nitch, S., Lu, P., et al. (2005). Sensitivity and specificity of finger tapping test scores for the detection of suspect effort. *The Clinical Neuropsychologist, 19,* 105–120.

Atkins v. Virginia, 536 U.S. 304, 153 L.Ed.2d 335 (2002).

Babikian, T., Boone, K. B., Lu, P., & Arnold, G. (2006). Sensitivity and specificity of various digit span scores in the detection of suspect effort. *The Clinical Neuropsychologist, 20,* 145–159.

Black, A. H., & Davis, L. J. (1966). The relationship between intelligence and sensorimotor proficiency in retardates. *American Journal of Mental Deficiency, 71,* 55–59.

Boone, K. B., Lu, P., Back, C., King, C., Lee, A., Philpott, L., et al. (2002). Sensitivity and specificity of the Rey Dot Counting Test in patients with suspect effort and various clinical samples. *Archives of Clinical Neuropsychology, 17,* 625–642.

Boone, K. B., Salazar, X., Lu, P., Warner-Chacon, K., & Razani, J. (2002). The Rey 15 item Recognition Trial: A technique to enhance sensitivity of the Rey 15-Item Memorization Test. *Journal of Clinical and Experimental Neuropsychology, 24,* 561–573.

Brodsky, S. L., & Galloway, V. A. (2003). Ethical and professional demands for forensic mental health professionals in post-Atkins era. *Ethics and Behavior, 13,* 3–9.

Bruininks, R. H., McGrew, K., & Maruyama, G. (1988). Structure of adaptive behavior in samples with and without mental retardation. *American Journal on Mental Retardation, 93,* 265–272.

Bruininks, R. H., Thurlow, M., & Gilman, C. J. (1987). Adaptive behavioral and mental retardation. *The Journal of Special Education, 21,* 69–88.

Calvert, E. J., & Crozier, W. R. (1978). An analysis of verbal–performance intelligence quotient discrepancies in the Wechsler Adult Intelligence Scale results of mentally subnormal hospital patients. *Journal of Mental Deficiency Research, 22,* 147–153.

Davis, L. A. (2000). *People with mental retardation in the criminal justice system.* Retrieved July 27, 2006, from *www.thearc.org/faqs/crimjustice.doc.*

Delis, D. C., Kramer, J. H., Kaplan, E., & Ober, B. A. (2000). California Verbal Learning Test (2nd ed.). San Antonio, TX: Psychological Corporation.

DeVault, S., & Long, D. (1988). Adaptive behavior, malingering and competence to waive right: A case study. *American Journal of Forensic Psychology, 6,* 3–15.

Dolan, M. (2005, February 11). Inmates can appeal based on their IQ: State justices define mental disability, giving dozens on death row a chance for life terms. *The Los Angeles Times,* pp. A1, A31.

Edgin, J. O. (2003). A neuropsychological model for the development of the cognitive profiles in mental retardation syndromes: Evidence from Down syndrome and Williams syndrome. *Dissertation Abstracts International: Section B: The Sciences and Engineering, 64,* 1522.

Ellis, N. R. (1963). The stimulus trace and behavioral inadequacy. In N. R. Ellis (Ed.), *Handbook of mental deficiency* (pp. 134–158). New York: McGraw-Hill.

Everington, C., & Fulero, S. (1999). Competence to confess: Measuring understanding and suggestibility of defendants with mental retardation. *Mental Retardation, 37,* 212–220.

Everington, C., & Keyes, D. W. (1999). Mental retardation: Diagnosing mental retardation in criminal proceedings: The critical importance of documenting adaptive behavior. *Forensic Examiner, 8,* 31–34.

Fogelmann, C. J. (Ed.). (1975). *AAMD Adaptive Behavior Scale Manual.* Washington, DC: American Association on Mental Deficiency.

Frederick, R. I. (1997). *Validity Indicator Profile manual.* Minneapolis, MN: National Computer Services.

Frederick, R. I. (2000a). Mixed group validation: A method to address the limitations of criterion group validation in research on malingering detection. *Behavioral Sciences and the Law, 18,* 693–718.

Frederick, R. I. (2000b). A personal floor effect strategy to evaluate the validity of performance on memory tests. *Journal of Clinical and Experimental Neuropsychology, 22,* 720–730.

Frith, U., & Frith, C. D. (1974). Specific motor disabilities in Down's Syndrome. *Journal of Child Psychology and Psychiatry and Allied Disciplines, 15,* 293–301.

Goldberg, J. O., & Miller, H. R. (1986). Performance of psychiatric inpatients and intellectually deficient individuals on a task that assesses the validity of memory complaints. *Journal of Clinical Psychology, 42,* 797–795.

Graue, L. O., Berry, D. T. R., Clark, J. A., Sollman, M. J., Cardi, M., Hopkins, J., et al. (in press). Identification of feigned mental retardation using the new generation of malingering detection instruments: Preliminary findings. *The Clinical Neuropsychologist.*

Green, P. (2003). *Green's Word Memory Test (WMT) for Windows User's Manual* [Online]. Edmonton, Alberta, Canada: Green's Publishing. Available at *www.wordmemorytest.com.*

Green, P. (2004). *Green's Memory and Concentration Test (MACT) for Windows User's Manual* [Online]. Edmonton, Alberta, Canada: Green's Publishing. Available at: *www.wordmemorytest.com.*

Green, P., Allen, L., & Astner, K. (1996). *Manual for Computerised Word Memory Test, U.S. version 1.0.* Durham, NC: Cognisyst.

Green, P., & Astner, K. (1995). *The Word Memory Test.* Edmonton, Alberta, Canada: Neurobehavioural Associates.

Green, P., & Flaro, L. (2003). Word Memory Test performance in children. *Child Neuropsychology, 9,* 189–207.

Green, P., Lees-Haley, P., & Allen, L. (2002). The Word Memory Test and the validity of neuropsychological test scores. *Forensic Neuropsychology, 2,* 97–124.

Greiffenstein, M. F., Baker, W. J., & Gola, T. (1994). Validation of malingered amnesia measures with a large clinical sample. *Psychological Assessment, 6,* 218–224.

Greiffenstein, M. F., Gola, T., & Baker, W. J. (1995). MMPI-2 validity scales versus domain specific measures in detection of factitious traumatic brain injury. *Clinical Neuropsychologist*, *9*, 230–240.

Greve, K. W., Bianchini, K. J., Mathias, C. W., Houston, R. J., & Crouch, J. A. (2003). Detecting malingered performance on the Wechsler Adult Intelligence Scale: Validation of Mittenberg's approach in traumatic brain injury. *Archives of Clinical Neuropsychology*, *18*, 245–260.

Grossman, H. J. (Ed.). (1983). *Classification in mental retardation*. Washington, DC: American Association on Mental Deficiency.

Gudjonsson, G. H. (2002). *The psychology of interrogations and confessions: A handbook*. Chichester, UK: Wiley.

Guilmette, T. J., Hart, K. J., Guiliano, A. J., & Leininger, B. E. (1994). Detecting simulated memory impairment: Comparison of the Rey Fifteen-Item Test and the Hiscock Forced-Choice Procedure. *The Clinical Neuropsychology*, *8*, 283–294.

Hathaway, S. R., & McKinley, J. C. (1989). *Minnesota Multiphasic Personality Inventory–2*. Minneapolis: University of Minnesota Press.

Hawkins, G. D., & Cooper, D. H. (1990). Adaptive behavioral measures in mental retardation research: Subject description in AJMD/AJMR articles. *American Journal on Mental Retardation*, *94*, 654–660.

Hawthorne, X. (2005, February 4). State high court to rule on mental retardation case: Death row inmates seeking IQ review. *Los Angeles Times*, pp. A1, A24.

Hayes, J. S., Hale, D. B., & Gouvier, W. D. (1997). Do tests predict malingering in defendants with mental retardation? *Journal of Psychology*, *131*, 575–576.

Hayes, J. S., Hale, D. B., & Gouvier, W. D. (1998). Malingering detection in a mentally retarded forensic population. *Applied Neuropsychology*, *5*, 33–36.

Hays, J. R., Emmons, J., & Lawson, K. A. (1993). Psychiatric norms or the Rey 15-Item visual memory test. *Perceptual and Motor Skills*, *76*, 1331–1334.

Heinze, M. C., & Purisch, A. D. (2001). Beneath the mask: Use of psychological tests to detect and subtype malingering in criminal defendants. *Journal of Forensic Psychology Practice*, *1*, 23–52.

Huberty, T. J., Koller, J. R., & Ten Brink, T. D. (1980). Adaptive behavior in the definition of mental retardation. *Exceptional Children*, *46*, 258–261.

Hurley, K. E., & Deal, W. P. (2006). Assessment instruments measuring malingering used with individuals who have mental retardation: Potential problems and issues. *Mental Retardation*, *44*, 112–119.

Iki, H., & Kusano, K. (1986). Muscle strength training of mentally retarded children. *Japanese Journal of Special Education*, *24*, 20–26.

Inman, T. H., Vickery, C. D., Berry, D. T. R., Lamb, D., Edwards, C., & Smith, G. T. (1998). Development and initial validation of a new procedure for evaluating adequacy of effort during neuropsychological testing: The Letter Memory Test. *Psychological Assessment*, *10*, 128–139.

Iverson, G. L., & Franzen, M. D. (1994). The Recognition Memory Test, Digit Span, and Knox Cube Test as markers of malingered memory impairment. *Assessment*, *1*, 323–334.

Iverson, G. L., & Tulsky, D. S. (2003). Detecting malingering on the WAIS-III unusual Digit Span performance patterns in the normal population and in clinical groups. *Archives of Clinical Psychology*, *18*, 1–9.

Jackson v. Indiana, 406 U.S. 715, 32 L.Ed.2d 435 (1972).

Johnstone, L., & Cooke, D. J. (2003). Feigned intellectual deficits on the Wechsler Adult Intelligence Scale—Revised. *British Journal of Clinical Psychology, 42,* 303–318.

Kaufman, A. S., & Kaufman, N. L. (1990). *Kaufman Brief Intelligence Test.* Minneapolis, MN: NCS.

Kennedy, C. Shaver, S., Weinborn, M., Manley, J., Broshek, D., & Marcopulos, B. (2005, November). *Use of the Test of Memory Malingering (TOMM) in Individuals with FSIQ below 70.* Poster session presented at the 25th annual meeting of the National Academy of Neuropsychology (NAN), Tampa, FL.

Keyes, D. W. (2004). Use of the Minnesota Multiphasic Personality Inventory (MMPI) to identify malingering mental retardation. *Mental Retardation, 42,* 151–153.

Keyes, D., Edwards, W., & Perske, R. (1997). People with mental retardation are dying—Legally. *Mental Retardation, 35,* 59–63.

Killgore, W., & DellaPietra, L. (2000). Using the WMS-III to detect malingering: Empirical validation of the rarely missed index. *Journal of Clinical and Experimental Neuropsychology, 22,* 761–771.

Lanzkron, J. (1963). Murder and insanity: A survey. *American Journal of Psychiatry, 119,* 754–758.

Leduc, L. G. (2005). Detection of dissimulation among social security disability applicants using the WMS-III. *Dissertation Abstracts International: Section B: The Sciences and Engineering, 66,* 1723.

Lezak, M. (2004). *Neuropsychological Assessment* (4th ed.). New York: Oxford University Press.

Lin, Z., & Zhang, Z. (2002). Study on the speed of hand tapping in mentally retarded children [Abstract]. *Chinese Journal of Clinical Psychology, 10,* 230–231.

Lipkin, P. (1991). Epidemiology of the developmental disabilities. In A. J. Caputee & P. K. Accardo (Eds.), *Developmental disabilities in infancy and childhood* (pp. 43–63). Baltimore: Brookes.

Loring, D. W., Lee, G. P., & Meador, K. J. (2005). Victoria Symptom Validity Test performance in non-litigating epilepsy surgery candidates. *Journal of Clinical and Experimental Neuropsychology, 27,* 610–617.

Loveland, K. A., & Tunali-Kotoski, B. (1998). Development of adaptive behavior in persons with mental retardation. In R. M. Hodapp & J. A. Burack (Eds.), *Handbook of mental retardation and development* (pp. 521–541). New York: Cambridge University Press.

Lu, P. H., Boone, K. B., Cozolino, L., & Mitchell, C. (2003). Effectiveness of the Rey Osterreith Complex Figure Test and the Meyers and Meyers Recognition Trial in the detection of suspect effort. *The Clinical Neuropsychologist, 17,* 426–440.

Luckasson, R., Coulter, D. L., Polloway, E. A., Reiss, S., Schalock, R. L., Snell, M. E., et al. (1992). *Mental retardation: Definition, classification and systems of support.* Washington, DC: American Association on Mental Retardation.

MacKenzie, S., & Hulme, C. (1987). Memory span development in Down's syndrome severely subnormal and normal subjects. *Cognitive Neuropsychology, 4,* 303–319.

Madhaven, T., & Narayan, J. (1988). Manual asymmetries in persons with Down's syndrome. *Indian Journal of Psychiatry, 30,* 193–195.

Marshall, P. S., & Happe, M. (in press). The performance of individuals with mental retardation on cognitive tests assessing effort and motivation. *The Clinical Neuropsychologist.*

Mash, E. J., & Wolfe, D. A. (2002). *Abnormal child psychology* (2nd ed.). Belmont, CA: Wadsworth.

McCaffrey, R. J., & Isaac, W. (1985). Preliminary data on the presence of neuropsychological deficits in adults who are mentally retarded. *Mental Retardation, 23,* 63–66.

McLaren, J., & Bryson, S. E. (1987). Review of recent epidemiological studies of mental retardation: Prevalence, associated disorders and etiology. *American Journal of Mental Retardation, 92,* 243–254.

McSweeny, A. J., Wood, G. L., Chessare, J. B., & Kurczynski, T. W. (1993). Cognitive and language anomalies in two brothers with a rare form of genetic abnormality (deletion of 9p24). *Clinical Neuropsychologist, 7,* 460–466.

Miller, R. D., & Germain E. J. (1988). The retrospective evaluation of competency to stand trial. *International Journal of Law and Psychiatry, 11,* 113–125.

Millis, S. R. (1992). The recognition memory test in the detection of malingered and exaggerate memory deficits. *Clinical Neuropsychologist, 6,* 406–414.

Millis, S. R., Putnam, S. H., Adams, K. N., & Ricker, J. H. (1995). California Verbal Learning Test in the detection of incomplete effort in neuropsychological evaluation. *Psychological Assessment, 7,* 463–471.

Mittenberg, W., Theroux, S., Aguila-Puentas, G., Bianchini, K. J., Greve, K. W., & Rayls, K. (2001). Identification of malingered head injury on the Wechsler Adult Intelligence Scale–3rd Edition. *The Clinical Neuropsychologist, 15,* 440–445.

Morrison, M. W. (1994). The use of psychological tests to detect malingered intellectual impairment. *American Journal of Forensic Psychology, 12,* 47–54.

Nettelbeck, T. (1986). Inspection time as mental speed in mildly mentally retarded adults: Analysis of eye gaze, eye movement and orientation. *American Journal of Mental Deficiency, 91,* 78–91.

Nihira, K., Foster, R., Shellhaas, M., & Leland, H. (1974). *AAMD Adaptive Behavior Scale Manual.* Washington, DC: American Association on Mental Deficiency.

Nihira, K., Leland, H., & Lambert, N. (1993). *AAMR Adaptive Behavior Scale–Residential and Community* (2nd ed.). Austin, TX: Pro-Ed.

Paul, D., Franzen, M. D., Cohen, S. H., & Fremouw, W. (1992). An investigation into the reliability and validity of two tests used in the detection of dissimulation. *International Journal of Neuropsychology, 14,* 1–9.

Pennington, B. F., & Bennetto, L. (1998). Toward a neuropsychology of mental retardation. In J. A. Burack, R. M. Hodapp, & E. Zigler (Eds.), *Handbook of mental retardation and development* (pp. 80–114). New York: Cambridge University Press.

Pezzini, G., Vicari, S., Volterra, V., Milani, L., & Ossella, M. T. (1999). Children with Williams Syndrome: Is there a single neuropsychological profile? *Developmental Neuropsychology, 15,* 141–155.

Pulsifier, M. B. (1996). The neuropsychology of mental retardation. *Journal of International Neuropsychological Society, 2,* 159–176.

Rey, A. (1964). *The clinical exam in psychology.* Paris: Presses Universitaries de France.

Reznick, L. (2005). The Rey 15-Item Memory Test for malingering: A meta-analysis. *Brain Injury, 19,* 539–543.

Rogers, R., Bagby, R. M., & Dickens, S. E. (1992). *Structured Interview of Reported Symptoms.* Odessa, FL: Psychological Assessment Resources.

Roszkowski, M. J., & Snelbecker, G. E. (1981). Configuration of WAIS subtest scores in mental retardation: Further evidence. *Psychological Reports, 48,* 1006.

Sattler, J. (1988). *Assessment of children* (3rd ed.). San Diego, CA: Sattler.

Schlesinger, L. B. (2003). A case study involving competency to stand trial: Incompetent defendant, incompetent examiner, or "malingering by proxy"? *Psychology, Public Policy and Law, 9,* 381–399.

Schretlen, D., & Arkowitz, H. (1990). A psychological test battery to detect prison inmates who fake insanity or mental retardation. *Behavioral Sciences and the Law, 8,* 75–84.

Schretlen, D., Brandt, J., Krafft, L., & van Gorp, W. (1991). Some caveats in using the Rey 15-Item Memory Test to detect malingered amnesia. *Psychological Assessment: A Journal of Consulting and Clinical Psychology, 3,* 667–672.

Sherman, D. S., Boone, K., Lu, P., & Razani, J. (2002). Re-examination of the Rey Auditory Verbal Learning Test/Rey Complex Figure discriminant function to detect suspect effort. *The Clinical Neuropsychologist, 16,* 242–250.

Slick, D., Hopp, G., & Strauss, E. (1995). Victoria Symptom Validity Test. Odessa, FL: Psychological Assessment Resources.

Sparrow, S. S., Balla, D., & Cicchetti, D. V. (1984). *Vineland Adaptive Behavior Scales* (Survey ed.). Circle Pines, MN: American Guidance Service.

Speigel, E. (2006). *The Rey 15-Item Memorization Test: Performance in under-represented populations in the absence of obvious motivation to feign neurocognitive symptoms.* Unpublished doctoral dissertation, Fuller Theological Seminary, Pasadena, CA.

Sprague, R. L., & Quay, H. C. (1966). A factor analytic study of the responses of mental retardates. *American Journal of Mental Deficiency, 70,* 595–600.

Spreen, O., & Strauss, E. (1998). *A compendium of neuropsychological tests: Administration, norms and commentary* (2nd ed.). New York: Oxford University Press.

Stevens, K. B., & Randall, J. (2006). Adaptive behavior, mental retardation and the death penalty. *Journal of Forensic Psychology Practice, 6,* 1–29.

Suhr, J., Tranel, D., Wefel, J., & Barrash, J. (1997). Memory performance after head injury: Contributions of malingering, litigation status, psychological factors, and medication use. *Journal of Clinical and Experimental Neuropsychology, 19,* 500–514.

Tombaugh, T. N. (1996). *Test of Memory Malingering.* Toronto, Ontario, Canada: Multi-Health Systems.

Tombaugh, T. N. (2002). The Test of Memory Malingering (TOMM) in forensic psychology. *Journal of Forensic Neuropsychology, 2,* 69–96.

Victor, T., & Abeles, N. (2004). Coaching clients to take psychological and neuropsychological tests: A clash of ethical obligations. *Professional Psychology: Research and Practice, 35,* 373–379.

Weinborn, M., Orr, T., Woods, S. P., Conover, E., & Feix, J. (2003). A validation of the Test of Memory Malingering in a forensic psychiatric setting. *Journal of Clinical and Experimental Neuropsychology, 25,* 979–990.

Ziegler, E. & Hodapp, R. M. (1986). *Understanding mental retardation.* Boston: Cambridge University Press.

CHAPTER 15

Symptom Validity Tests in the Epilepsy Clinic

David J. Williamson
Daniel L. Drane
Elizabeth S. Stroup

Symptom validity testing (SVT) of numerous forms has been employed in patients with seizures since the early years of the last decade (Abubakr, Kablinger, & Caldito, 2003; Binder, Salinsky, & Smith, 1994). This is a natural fit: Neuropsychologists have been lending their skills to help quantify aspects of cognitive ability and impairment to the field of epilepsy for decades. Likewise, discriminating symptoms that result primarily from neurological disease from symptoms that result primarily from psychiatric disease has been a pressing matter in the field of epileptology since its beginnings.

Research into SVT with patients with epilepsy has generally evolved along similar themes, such that three central questions have driven empirical efforts:

1. Given the established prevalence of cognitive difficulties in patients with epilepsy as a group, how does this population perform on various forms of SVT?
2. Can these tests help clinicians discriminate patients with epilepsy from patients who suffer from psychogenic nonepileptic seizures (PNES)?
3. What do these tests tell us about the nature of the cognitive deficits seen in patients with epilepsy or in patients with PNES?

When exploring these issues, it is important to remain cognizant of distinct and potentially relevant ways in which patients in epilepsy clinics differ from the patients upon which SVT have been developed (e.g., those with mild traumatic brain injury):

- *Most patients with epilepsy are not in litigation.* The questions, "Are there any deficits, and if so, who is to blame?" are rarely as charged, if indeed they are present at all, as one finds in populations such as those who have suffered mild traumatic brain injuries. Many patients with epilepsy receive compensation in the form of disability payments, but the cognitive deficits revealed on neuropsychological evaluation are far less frequently the focus of decisions about disability status. Consequently, conclusions about the types of behavior driving poor performance on SVT (e.g., potential for financial gain) are quite different than in other populations.
- *A "gold standard" for diagnosis exists.* Although the etiology of a given patient's seizures may be questioned, no one questions the validity of epilepsy as a chronic neurological disease. Likewise, there is wide consensus that video electroencephalography (EEG), wherein an individual's behavior can be videotaped and matched second for second with ongoing EEG recordings, is a defensible method of determining whether the disease is present, even in cases that are clinically indeterminant (Cascino, 2002). Although 25–30% of patients seen at an epilepsy center will remain indeterminant following a single monitoring study, the majority of cases receive a definitive diagnosis. The number of indeterminant cases can be decreased by repeat monitoring. At our center, an indeterminant study is one in which the patient (1) experienced no spells, (2) experienced episodes that are not typical for the individual, or (3) experienced episodes characterized solely by subjective symptoms (e.g., a "funny feeling") without any accompanying electrophysiological changes, as our neurologists are not comfortable ruling out the possibility of simple partial events in such cases. All the studies reviewed herein used video EEG to help classify their patients.

These questions and differences set the context for the relatively small literature that has developed in this area. We review the existing literature in the hopes that a more unified presentation of these findings will drive continued examination of the many questions regarding the utility of SVT in the epilepsy clinic that remain unanswered.

QUESTION 1: HOW DOES THIS POPULATION PERFORM ON SVT?

The first study in this literature (Lee, Loring, & Martin, 1992) examined the validity of the Rey 15-Item test in patients with epilepsy. The "Rey 15," sometimes called the Rey 3×5, is an array of 15 items arranged in three columns and five rows that a subject is instructed to learn during a 10-second exposure. The items are so easily recognizable and so redundant that all but the most severely impaired patients perform extremely well. In fact, the test is so easy that research performed since this study was first published suggests that the Rey 15 is among the least sensitive (but among the most specific) tests of poor effort (McCaffrey, O'Bryant, Ashendorf, & Fisher, 2003). Lee, Loring, and Martin (1992) compared a group of 100 inpatients with temporal lobe epilepsy (TLE), 16 outpatients in litigation, and 40 outpatients not in litigation. Laterality of seizure focus was not discussed. None of the patients with epilepsy were in litigation, and all of them had demonstrated memory impairment as indexed by performance below the 5th percentile on at least one of four standardized memory tests. All patients completed the Rey 15 as part of a comprehensive neuropsychological evaluation.

Patient demographics and Rey 15 results are depicted in Appendix 15.1. Ninety-six percent of the memory-impaired patients with epilepsy obtained scores above 7, with 42% of them obtaining perfect scores. Ninety-five percent of the nonlitigating outpatients scored above 7 as well; however, only 67.5% of the litigating patients performed this well. Thus, the investigators concluded that (1) patients with confirmed epilepsy who have known memory impairment are quite capable of performing well on the Rey 15, and (2) scores below 7 on the Rey 15 raise the index of suspicion for poor effort, even in neurological populations with demonstrated memory impairment.

Grote, Kooker, Nyenhuis, Smith, and Mattingly (2000), in a manner similar to Lee et al. (1992), compared a nonlitigating group of patients with video EEG-confirmed epilepsy to a compensation-seeking group composed primarily of mild traumatic brain injury in order to cross-validate the Victoria Symptom Validity Test (VSVT). The investigators sought not only to validate the use of the VSVT in a clearly identified "neurological" group but also to examine (1) the extent to which previously published decision rules meant to differentiate valid from invalid data generalized to this population and (2) the extent to which these rules could differentiate patients seeking compensation from those not seeking compensation. Unlike Lee et al. (1992), the extent to which this group with epileptic seizures (ES) had previously or concurrently established memory deficits was not noted. Demographics are noted in Appendix 15.1.

Grote et al. (2000) found that non-compensation-seeking patients with epilepsy performed well on the VSVT relative to published norms and outperformed litigating patients on average. Patients with epilepsy obtained better scores on measures of memory, response speed, and consistency of effort than did patients seeking compensation. The investigators proposed a number of cutoff scores to help the clinician differentiate patients seeking compensation from those not seeking compensation.

Loring, Lee, and Meador (2005) investigated the cutoff scores suggested by Grote et al. (2000) in a retrospective clinical sample of patients with epilepsy who had not been screened for compensation-seeking status. Of the 120 patients studied, 97 had focal seizure onset, 6 had generalized onset, and 17 had undefined seizure onset. Mean age was 34.5 (SD = 11.1), education was 12.6 (SD = 2.2), and mean Wechsler Adult Intelligence Scale–III (WAIS-III) Full Scale IQ was 83.0 (SD = 14.3). No comparison group was included.

This sample performed well on the VSVT in general, although 12% of the patients obtained scores suggestive of symptom exaggeration. The authors noted that this is consistent with the 8% rate of symptom exaggeration found in medical patient evaluations more generally (Mittenberg, Patton, Canyock, & Condit, 2002). VSVT performance was significantly related to most cognitive measures administered; however, the authors noted that, of the 15 patients with WAIS-III Full Scale IQs between 60 and 69, 6 obtained scores in the normal range as defined by Grote et al. (2000), and 3 of these obtained perfect scores.

Unexpectedly, VSVT performance correlated with age, with younger patients outperforming older patients. Grote et al. (2000) also reported a significant effect of age on these measures when examining their entire sample, although these relationships failed to reach statistical significance when each group (compensation seeking and non-compensation seeking) was analyzed separately. Interestingly, the age effect was noted in both studies despite (1) a substantial difference between the two samples in terms of Full Scale IQ and (2) the fact that Grote et al. (2000) always administered the VSVT first in their battery, whereas Loring et al. (2005) administered it at the conclusion of testing. Thus, it is difficult to argue that fatigue can account for this observation.

Loring et al. (2005) concluded that patients with epilepsy tend to perform well on the VSVT and that intellectual disability in isolation (at least as defined by an IQ between 60 and 69) is insufficient to cause SVT failure. However, there likely remains a minority of patients (around 10%) who will perform in such a way that their results underestimate their true ability. Unfortunately, as the sample was selected without reference to compensation-seeking status, it is impossible to know the extent to which this variable may have contributed to these findings.

Answer to Question 1

Patients with epilepsy, even those with confirmed memory deficits, are capable of performing quite well on the two forms of SVT examined in the population to date (i.e., VSVT and Rey 15). The extent to which age may play a moderating role on VSVT performance in this population remains an open question, as there is some suggestion that older patients may perform worse.

Regardless, one would not expect increased age or a diagnosis of epilepsy in and of themselves to invalidate the use of SVT in this population if the goal is to distinguish trustworthy neurocognitive data from suspect performance, assuming that there is no obvious neurological reason for such results.

QUESTION 2: CAN EPILEPSY BE DISCRIMINATED FROM PNES?

Question 2 has been important to the field of epilepsy for many years. The medical treatment of epilepsy has its own inherent risks, including side effects of medications and, in extreme cases, intubation for status epilepticus. Likewise, a diagnosis of epilepsy carries lifestyle and societal implications, from disability to removal of driving privileges (Morrell, 2002). As PNES cannot be effectively treated with antiepileptic drugs (and, in fact, one of the features that often distinguishes PNES from epilepsy is a refractory response to antiepileptic drugs), understanding the extent to which a patient's spells are a function of epilepsy versus some other etiology is critical in treatment planning. Although video EEG performs this discrimination very accurately, it is not always available for a number of patients. Neuropsychological testing and SVT may have their greatest potential for adding valuable diagnostic information in situations that remain unclear based on the other available information.

In understanding this topic, it is important to understand that epilepsy has a number of imitators (Gates, 2000). We focus our discussion on discrimination of ES from PNES, as this is the most common imitator of epilepsy as well as the area in which neuropsychologists are most likely to be of assistance. Also, as other authors in this volume have noted, these tests offer the most insight when one knows (1) the diagnostic characteristics of given tests, and (2) the base rates of the assessed phenomenon in the setting in which those techniques will be employed. We will try to make these attributes as explicit as possible given the available data.

We also acknowledge that "patients with epilepsy" and "patients with PNES" are not mutually exclusive. However, the prevalence of this comorbidity is lower than was once believed, with current estimates ranging from 10% to 30%. More recent studies employing the most sensitive and specific electrodiagnostic techniques and clear definitions of what constitutes a "seizure" typically find PNES/ES comorbidity near the lower end of this range (Benbadis, Agrawal, & Tatum, 2001; Benbadis & Hauser, 2000; Martin et al., 2003). Given these findings and the fact that relatively few empirical investigations have specifically targeted the ES + PNES group, this discussion proceeds with the admittedly artificial consideration of the ES and PNES groups as independent. This heuristic serves as a frame for discussion of the current findings and will, it is hoped, be altered as more data become available.

The important task of distinguishing epilepsy from seizures of non-epileptic origin has received quite of a bit of attention. Two recent reviews provide insight into the array of techniques that have been used and the sensitivity and specificity of these techniques according to each review's criteria for inclusion (Cragar, Berry, Fakhoury, Cibula, & Schmitt, 2002; Cuthill & Espie, 2005). At first glance, one might assume that patients with PNES, who generally have less objectively verifiable evidence of neuropathology than do patients with epilepsy (Dworetzky et al., 2005), would consistently outperform patients with epilepsy on neurocognitive testing. This has not proven to be the case (Binder, Kindermann, Heaton, & Salinsky, 1998; Dodrill & Holmes, 2000; Hill, Ryan, Kennedy, & Malamut, 2003; Risse, Mason, & Mercer, 2000; Swanson, Springer, Benbadis, & Morris, 2000). Consequently, the flag bearer in this endeavor for neuropsychologists has been the Minnesota Multiphasic Inventory/Minnesota Multiphasic Inventory–II (MMPI/MMPI-2).

Wilkus and Dodrill (1984) suggested that PNES should be suspected when one of three MMPI configural patterns is present: (1) scale 1 or 3 exceeds 69 and is one of the two most elevated scales, disregarding scales 5 and 0, (2) scale 1 or 3 exceeds 79 regardless of whether either is a high point, or (3) both 1 and 3 exceed 59, and both are at least 10 points higher than scale 2. These rules have been generalized to the MMPI-2, with corresponding point lowering of cutoffs to account for the rescaling of T-scores on the MMPI-2 relative to the MMPI (Warner, Wilkus, Vossler, & Dodrill, 1996). Other configural patterns have been suggested as well (Derry & McLachlan, 1996). Dodrill and Holmes (2000) reviewed nine studies examining the performance of the MMPI/MMPI-2 in this role and found an overall accuracy of 71%. Table 15.1 provides operating characteristics based on these data. Essentially, if a patient with seizures of uncertain etiology meets these criteria, he or she is approximately five times more likely to be diagnosed with PNES than with epilepsy. Other results have been reported (Cragar et al., 2003), but the review by Dodrill and Holmes (2000) remains the most comprehensive in the literature to date.

A more recently designed personality inventory, the Personality Assessment Inventory (PAI), has recently been used in epilepsy clinics as well. The PAI has four validity scales and a number of other scales sensitive to a variety of personality and psychological adjustment variables (Morey, 2003). Wagner, Wymer, Topping, and Pritchard (2005) studied a group of patients referred to a clinic for refractory epilepsy. Of 61 consecutive admissions, 26 patients with PNES and 15 patients with epilepsy met inclusion and exclusion criteria. Patients with mixed PNES and epileptic seizures were excluded, as were those failing to meet criteria on the validity indicators. No indication was given as to the diagnoses of those patients who were excluded. The authors used an "NES indicator" by subtracting the t-score of the Health

TABLE 15.1. Operating Characteristics of Different Techniques in Distinguishing Patients with Epilepsy from Patients with Psychogenic Nonepileptic Seizures (PNES)

Study	Test	N	% of PNES in sample	Sensitivity	Specificity	PPV	NPV	Accuracy	OR	OR CI
Dodrill and Holmes (2000)	MMPI Wilkus Dodrill criteria	741 (review)	37	64	75	60	78	71	5.3	3.8–7.5
Wagner et al. (2005)	PAI NES indicator	41	63	84	73	84	73	80	15.1	2.6–97.0
Bortz et al. (1995)	CVLT negative response bias	41	44	61	91	85	75	78	16.5	2.5–173.5
Binder et al. (1998)	Discriminant function with MMPI or MMPI-2 + PDRT	60	42	73	84	73	84	80	14.2	3.4–62.7
Hill et al. (2003)	TOMM failure of trial 2 or retention	105	55	9	96	71	53	50	2.2	0.3–24.1
Williamson et al. (2004)	WMT	113	32	53	72	47	77	66	3.0	1.2–7.4

Concerns subscale from the t-score of the Conversion subscale: patients with positive and negative scores on this index were classified as having PNES and ES, respectively. In this relatively small sample, this index performed quite well, with those patients obtaining positive scores on this index being 15 times more likely to be diagnosed with PNES than with ES. This compares quite favorably to the Wilkus-Dodrill criteria and could prove quite useful if it can be replicated in a larger sample.

Research into the extent to which SVT can distinguish these two groups began with Binder et al.'s (1994) investigation. These investigators noted the consistency of some of the findings between patients with PNES and patients with other forms of conversion disorder or who were seeking compensation for neurological injuries. They examined the extent to which a combination of neurocognitive and psychological self-report variables would discriminate patients with PNES from patients with ES. This study also made a specific point to examine the extent to which disability-seeking status varied according to group. The types of seizures suffered by the ES group are not detailed, though it is stated that patients with co-occurring ES and PNES were excluded. Appendix 15.1 notes patient demographics.

The investigators found that 19 PNES patients differed significantly from 34 ES patients on the Portland Digit Recognition Test (PDRT), a recognition memory test shown to be sensitive to poor effort in patients seeking compensation for mild traumatic brain injuries (Binder, 2002). The PDRT had a larger effect size (Cohen's $h = 1.3$) than the MMPI, disability status, and performance on either of two sensory tests (Face Hand test and Finger Agnosia). However, of the four measures, the MMPI most accurately discriminated between the groups. Operating characteristics for the MMPI in this sample were sensitivity, 71%; specificity, 65%; PPV (positive predictive value), 50%; and NPV (negative predictive value) 81%. Overall accuracy was 67%. Unfortunately, data were not provided that would allow the calculation of operating characteristics and odds ratios for other measures, including the PDRT. Although a greater proportion of patients with PNES were actively seeking disability (47% vs. 17%), the low absolute numbers of patients in these groups precluded statistical comparison of the performances of patients with PNES seeking disability from the performances of those PNES patients who were not seeking disability.

This study was the first to document that patients with PNES perform very differently than patients with ES on SVT. However, the findings introduce the theme that relying on the results of SVT in isolation may not be the best way to help the clinician discriminate between a patient with epilepsy and a patient with PNES.

In addition to SVT designed specifically to quantify the validity of one's effort on neurocognitive testing, other techniques have been demonstrated to be sensitive to poor effort as well, such as inconsistency of performance across time on tests that are typically stable, or extremely atypical performance on some aspects of established neurocognitive tests (Sweet, 1999). One of the most robust techniques of this type is pattern of performance on the recognition component of list learning tasks, such as the California Verbal Learning Test (CVLT) (Coleman, Rapport, Millis, Ricker, & Farchione, 1998; Millis, Putnam, Adams, & Ricker, 1995; Slick, Iverson, & Green, 2000; Sweet et al., 2000). Bortz, Prigatano, Blum, and Fisher (1995) compared the types of errors made by patients with epilepsy on this portion of the CVLT to those made by patients with PNES. Twenty-three patients with focal temporal lobe seizure onset (12 left, 11 right) and 18 patients with PNES completed the CVLT as part of a comprehensive neuropsychological evaluation. The compensation-seeking/receiving status of patients in this study was not noted. Appendix 15.1 summarizes demographics.

The PNES patients in this sample recognized fewer words on the recognition component of the CVLT than either of the TLE groups, although the difference between the right TLE (RTLE) and PNES groups did not reach statistical significance in this small study. In comparing their results to those of a group of 10 randomly selected patients with traumatic brain injury (not otherwise described) and to another group's published sample of patients pre- and posttemporal lobectomy (Hermann, 1993), Bortz et al. (1995) found that the PNES group was the *only* group to demonstrate a negative response bias. Notably, the original RTLE, left TLE (LTLE), and PNES groups did not differ on gross measures of immediate or delayed recall.

Table 15.1 provides operating characteristics of using a negative response bias on the CVLT to differentiate these groups in this sample. Overall accuracy was an impressive 78%, with an odds ratio suggesting that a patient from this sample who obtained a negative response bias was 16.5 times more likely to be diagnosed with PNES than with ES.

Binder et al. (1998) extended their investigation of neurocognitive performance in patients with PNES. The sample studied overlapped substantially (68%) with this group's 1994 sample. In this study, 30 patients with epilepsy (13 with generalized seizures), 42 patients with PNES, and 47 normal control subjects from a separate database matched for gender, age, and education were compared on a variety of cognitive measures. Appendix 15.1 reports demographics.

Control subjects outperformed both seizure groups on most measures, whereas the ES and PNES groups differed little. The differences between the ES and PNES groups on SVT first described in 1994 were replicated. In addition, PDRT performance correlated significantly with performance on measures of memory and sensory performance in the PNES group, whereas no such relationship existed in the ES group. The investigators found no significant relationships between PDRT performance and elevation of individual scales on the MMPI or MMPI-2.

The investigators also examined the ability of a discriminant function combining MMPI/MMPI-2 results (specifically, elevations on scales 1 and 2) and PDRT performance to differentiate patients with ES from patients with PNES. This function performed very well, correctly classifying 80% of patients (see Table 15.1). A patient with PNES was 14.4 times more likely to be classified as having PNES by this equation than a patient with ES. It is unclear whether this was significantly more accurate than the MMPI/MMPI-2 using the Wilkus–Dodrill criteria alone. The data that would allow for the calculation of operating characteristics of the PDRT in isolation were not provided. The authors noted that only three patients with PNES fell below cutoffs for motivational impairment, suggesting that most of the variance between the two groups occurred in the range not suggestive of poor effort. Thus, it may be that the PDRT in isolation may be quite specific but relatively insensitive to poor effort in this population, at least as defined by the 1994 cutoffs.

Thus, Binder et al.'s (1998) report replicated previous findings that (1) patients with ES and PNES cannot be reliably separated on the basis of traditional neurocognitive measures and (2) patients with ES significantly outperform patients with PNES on the PDRT. Other findings of note included (1) PDRT performances of patients with PNES correlated more highly with performance on measures of memory and learning and sensory skills than did the performances of patients with epilepsy, and (2) ES or PNES group membership could be predicted fairly accurately with a combination of SVT and MMPI/MMPI-2 data.

Hill et al. (2003) compared 48 patients with temporal lobe epilepsy (27 left-sided focus, 21 right-sided) to 57 patients with PNES on another SVT, the Test of Memory Malingering (TOMM). All patients underwent video EEG. All patients with TLE had demonstrated memory impairment (not specifically defined) on one or more measures. Patients with Full Scale IQ less than 70 were excluded. Appendix 15.1 describes demographics.

Of the 39 comparisons of performances on neurocognitive measures and scales of the Personality Assessment Inventory (PAI) that were performed, two were significant at the $p < .01$ level (Wechsler Memory Scale–Revised Delayed Memory Index and PAI Somatization). The groups' mean scores on the TOMM did not differ significantly. Despite the authors' noting that more PNES patients obtained scores in the invalid range, the overall ability of the TOMM to discriminate these groups was quite poor. Overall accuracy was only 50%, and the odds ratio suggested that passing or failing the test was not significantly more likely for one group than another ($p = .45$). These results are consistent with reports of the TOMM being quite specific but not as sensitive as other measures in identifying patients who are putting forth suboptimal effort (Gervais, Rohling, Green, & Ford, 2004).

Williamson, Drane, Stroup, Miller, and Holmes (2003) examined the ability of the Word Memory Test (WMT) to distinguish between patients with epilepsy and those with PNES. The data reported in 2003 can be supplemented by additional subjects found in this group's 2004 investigation of the role of effort in moderating neurocognitive performance more broadly (see below). Using the 2004 data, this group compared the WMT performances of 77 patients with epilepsy to those of 36 patients with PNES. These were consecutive referrals, considered without regard to compensation-seeking status, established level of disability, or Full Scale IQ. Appendix 15.1 lists demographic characteristics of the sample.

In this sample of patients, patients could be accurately characterized as ES or PNES 66% of the time on the basis of WMT results alone, as patients with PNES were nearly three times more likely to score in the invalid range than patients with epilepsy (p = .01). As with the other SVT techniques reviewed, the WMT appears to be relatively more specific than sensitive in this population when used for the purpose of classifying patients into ES or PNES categories.

Answer to Question 2

Patients with epilepsy outperform patients with PNES on some forms of SVT (PDRT, recognition component of CVLT, WMT), whereas the groups perform much more similarly on others (e.g., TOMM). SVT based on verbal stimuli rather than graphic stimuli appear to be more sensitive in general (Gervais et al., 2004); thus, the differential sensitivity of these techniques is most likely a broader issue that extends beyond these specific groups.

Although levels of performance consistently vary between groups on verbally based SVT, the extent to which results of SVT may be used to either supplant or complement the results of the MMPI/MMPI-2 (or, possibly, the PAI) in distinguishing patients with ES from patients with PNES remains an open question. Only Binder et al. (1998) examined the diagnostic performance of a combination of an SVT (PDRT) and the MMPI/MMPI-2, and they did not provide enough data to get a complete picture of the performance of the PDRT alone. Likewise, they did not report the incremental gain in diagnostic accuracy obtained by adding the PDRT to the MMPI/MMPI-2. From the investigators' discussion, it appears that the PDRT, like the TOMM, is very specific but not very sensitive to differences between the two groups, at least if one employs the cutoffs employed by Binder et al. (1994). The negative response bias index on the CVLT appears promising (Bortz et al., 1995), but this finding should be replicated in a larger sample. The WMT does not appear to outperform the MMPI/MMPI-2, although the two have yet to be directly compared in the same sample. Likewise, the extent to which the WMT or the CVLT negative response bias may add meaningful incremental utility to the discriminatory power of the MMPI/MMPI-2 or PAI has not yet been examined.

Thus, the best answer to Question 2, though admittedly still tenuous, is that some forms of SVT appear likely to contribute useful information when used in conjunction with other information.

QUESTION 3: HOW DO THESE TESTS DESCRIBE DEFICITS?

Binder et al. (1998) delved into this question when they examined the extent to which the different groups' PDRT performance predicted performance on neurocognitive tests. The PDRT performance of the patients with PNES, but not that of patients with ES, correlated significantly with measures of memory and sensory abilities.

Drane et al. (2006) examined the extent to which the lack of difference between the groups in terms of overall neurocognitive performance could be explained on the basis of effort, as quantified by the WMT. These investigators compared the neurocognitive performances of 36 patients with PNES (including four patients with both ES and PNES) and 77 patients with epilepsy. Overall cognitive performance was indexed by the Dodrill Discrimination Index (DDI), a validated measure of the proportion of 16 neuropsychological tests that fall outside the normal range (Dodrill, 1978). The two groups did not differ significantly on DDI when the scores were compared without reference to WMT performance. However, once performance on the DDI was stratified according to WMT performance, the PNES patients who scored in the valid range significantly outperformed all other groups (Figure 15.1). In fact, this group's overall DDI fell within the range expected from a historical control sample of normal adults. In contrast, within the sample of patients with epilepsy, the DDI did not differ significantly in subgroups stratified on WMT performance.

Answer to Question 3

The answers to question 3 have the potential to provide us with novel insights into the relationship between PNES, epilepsy, and cognition. Previous efforts have demonstrated that at the group level, patients with epilepsy and patients with PNES do not differ reliably on neurocognitive testing. Binder et al. (1998), Bortz et al. (1995), and Drane et al. (2006) demonstrate that these groups do differ significantly on some aspects of their performances on SVT; however, these differences may not be sufficient to reliably differentiate between the two groups, at least when the measures are used in isolation. Drane et al.'s (2006) findings suggest that that these differences may be extremely valuable in guiding a reexamination of the lack of neurocognitive differences seen between the two groups. These findings suggest that rather than the two groups performing equivalently, one actually sees the PNES group split into one group that performs substantially better on neurocognitive testing (in or near the normal range, in fact) and another that performs substantially worse than patients with epilepsy, despite a lack of findings on physical exam, video EEG, or imaging that could account for such differences. Thus, if these findings are replicated, approximately 50%

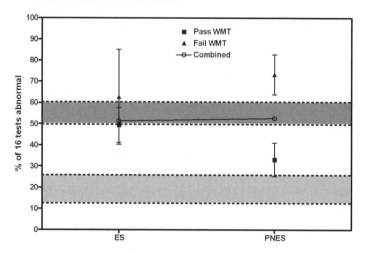

FIGURE 15.1. Mean Dodrill Discrimination Index (DDI) and 95% confidence intervals for patients with epileptic seizures (ES) and psychogenic nonepileptic seizures (PNES), stratified by performance on the effort-sensitive measures of the Word Memory Test (WMT). A higher DDI value indicates more impairment. The dotted line depicts the mean level of performance for each group before stratifying for WMT performance. The uppermost (darkly) shaded area is the 95% confidence interval of the DDI performance of 100 epilepsy patients (4), whereas the lower (lightly) shaded area is the 95% confidence interval around the DDI performance of 50 normal control subjects (18). From Drane et al. (2006). Copyright 2006 by Blackwell. Reprinted by permission.

of patients with PNES may perform on neurocognitive testing in ways that overestimate their level of impairment. By extension, it is the performances of these patients that drive overestimation of cognitive impairment in PNES groups more broadly.

In attempting to answer the three central questions that have driven this literature to date, we now understand that (1) in most cases, the cognitive deficits associated with epilepsy do not invalidate the use of SVT in this population, (2) it does not appear that SVT can reliably discriminate epilepsy from PNES in isolation, but some techniques may assist in this discrimination when used in conjunction with other predictors, and (3) the oft-replicated finding that patients with epilepsy and patients with PNES score similarly on neurocognitive batteries may well be largely due to the confound of effort. It appears that once one controls for effort, the PNES group bifurcates into groups that perform significantly better and significantly worse on neurocognitive measures, respectively, than patients with epilepsy.

HOW CAN I PUT THESE FINDINGS INTO PRACTICE TOMORROW?

When you obtain a score on a validated SVT that suggests poor effort, you must take the entire clinical context into account. The first and most obvious implication is that in the absence of clearly documented brain pathology and obvious dependence on others to handle at least some aspects of daily life, one must doubt the extent that the neurocognitive data obtained from the evaluation are a valid reflection of a patient's true capabilities. Patients are obviously capable of performing *at least* as well as they perform on a given neuropsychological battery, but "failure" on SVT without an obvious explanation suggests that at least some performances significantly underrepresent true neurocognitive ability. There may well be instances in which knowing a minimum level of performance can be diagnostically helpful; thus, SVT failure in and of itself does not necessarily mean that there is no useful information to be extracted from other performances. Rather, any conclusions based on such data must be interpreted very conservatively as only the minimum performances of which a patient is capable, and few, if any, conclusions may be drawn from the pattern of performance within or across measures.

In this population in particular, confidence in one's neurocognitive data is critical. Decisions about the nature and advisability of neurosurgical intervention can be swayed by these data, as can prognostic expectations, particularly with regard to results of memory testing (Westerveld, 2002). As performance on memory tests is perhaps the domain of neuropsychological assessment most susceptible to change as a function of effort, it is critical to understand the impact that effort may have had on a given patient's performance.

As other authors in this volume have noted, however, SVT performance rarely tells one *why* a patient performs in such a manner as to compromise the interpretability of test results. Besides malingering, which does not appear to be a major contributor to the SVT failures seen in the PNES population, there are a number of factors that are sometimes considered to have the potential to impact SVT performance in a more general sense. These include severe fatigue, depression or psychiatric symptomatology, pain, and side effects of medications. We know that pain and depression do not necessarily lead to poorer SVT performance (Gervais et al., 2004; Gervais, Russell, Green, Allen, & Ferrari, 2001; Rohling, Green, Allen, & Iverson, 2002), and there is no evidence to date that antiepileptic drugs (AEDs) impair cognitive performance to such an extent as to cause SVT failure. However, careful examination of the impact of specific AEDs on performance on specific SVTs has yet to be reported, so this cannot be assumed to be a settled matter. Likewise, patients with epilepsy sometimes experience epileptiform discharges that do not manifest themselves in visible behavioral changes but may have effects on cognition (Aldenkamp & Arends, 2004); the extent to which such discharges may affect SVT performance has yet to be carefully examined. Given our current state of knowledge, then, all factors that could theoretically suppress optimal effort for reasons other than volition need to be carefully considered in each individual case. It may well be that, in this population, there are patients who produce neurocognitive data that portray an inaccurately poor depiction of their true capabilities yet whose suboptimal performances are driven by causes other than explicit motivation.

These findings have implications in the research setting as well. A small percentage of patients with epilepsy demonstrate suboptimal effort on neurocognitive measures, even when controlling for false-positive results (Abubakr et al., 2003; Loring et al., 2005; Williamson et al., 2004); thus, it is likely that invalid data are currently contaminating research exploring the base rates of neurocognitive deficits in various epilepsy syndromes and the outcome of surgical intervention. Even a few negatively skewed results due to the impact of variable effort could significantly alter group data used in these areas. It is essential to employ SVT with these populations if one plans to use neuropsychological test performance as a marker for brain impairment or if one seeks to characterize or compare the level or pattern of neurocognitive performance of one or more diagnostic groups.

WHAT NEXT?

That we can comprehensively review each study in this literature speaks to its small size—clearly many questions remain to be answered. Replication is essential. Most of these studies are quite small, and most of the findings are based on posthoc analyses with questionable power, given the ratio of number of statistical tests performed to number of subjects examined. Interesting hypotheses have been raised, but the conclusions that one can draw based on these findings would be enhanced significantly with larger samples and prospectively designed trials.

In addition, a number of questions remain unexplored. For instance, as noted earlier, *are there transient disruptions of function associated with epilepsy that may interfere with SVT performance?* The impact of acute seizure activity or interictal epileptiform discharges are just two of the many factors potentially contributing to temporary and intermittent cognitive dysfunction in patients with epilepsy.

• *Who are the patients who "fail" SVT, either with or without PNES?* As a number of patients with chronic epilepsy experience profound cognitive and functional impairment related to traumas and neurological conditions (e.g., stroke, tumor, and encephalitis) that are causing their epileptiform discharges, it is to be expected that some patients with epilepsy will not be capable of passing even simple effort measures. When such individuals are unable to function in an independent fashion, it appears reasonable to consider failed SVT performances as "false positives." These scores fall in the range suggestive of suspect effort yet the results likely provide an accurate indication of the patient's true level of neurocognitive function. Some individuals from the PNES group will also fall into this category, as PNES sometimes occurs in extremely low functioning individuals, perhaps as a means of exerting some minimal control over their environments (e.g., PNES events occurring in a developmentally delayed, severely mentally retarded individual when faced with an undesired activity in the setting of a group home). Patients with severe cognitive and functional limitations may yet be capable of performing suboptimally in a purposeful fashion, but the ability to disentangle intent from profound impairment can prove impossible on the basis of behavioral data alone.

Assuming the findings of Drane et al. (2006) can be replicated, approximately 50% of patients with PNES perform in a manner that leads to overestimation of their true level of cognitive impairment. However, this obviously implies that approximately 50% of patients with PNES do *not* perform in such a manner. Do these groups differ in systematic ways that can help us understand their presentation or, better yet, help predict the extent to which they may respond to intervention?

• *What is the best way to go about collecting historical, neurocognitive, or psychological data to help guide the diagnosis and treatment of PNES?* To date, it does not appear that SVT in isolation discriminates PNES from ES as well as the MMPI or MMPI-2. The work of Binder et al. (1998) suggests, however, that combining SVT with psychological information may be of benefit, and a number of studies have identified behavioral and historical signs that aid in discrimination of the disorders (Benbadis, 2005; Cragar et al., 2002). The potential utility of other MMPI-2 scales that have demonstrated utility in identifying patients whose effort or presentation may be driven more powerfully by psychiatric factors, such as Lees-Haley's Fake Bad Scale (Greiffenstein, Baker, Axelrod, Peck, & Gervais, 2004; Larrabee, 1998, 2003a, 2003b), has yet to be explored. Optimal combinations of these predictors need to be examined, as well as the possibility that the best combination may vary according to setting (e.g., tertiary epilepsy clinic vs. outpatient neurology office).

This is an area of study that remains wide open to energetic and creative researchers. Such individuals have already provided some guidance about the potential utility of SVT in the epilepsy clinic and the lessons that such tests may provide in understanding neurocognitive scores produced by these groups. We look forward to following the development of this literature as it instructs us how best to help those who come to us for assistance.

REFERENCES

Abubakr, A., Kablinger, A., & Caldito, G. (2003). Psychogenic seizures: Clinical features and psychological analysis. *Epilepsy and Behavior*, *4*(3), 241.

Aldenkamp, A., & Arends, J. (2004). The relative influence of epileptic EEG discharges, short nonconvulsive seizures, and type of epilepsy on cognitive function. *Epilepsia*, *45*(1), 54–63.

Benbadis, S. R. (2005). A spell in the epilepsy clinic and a history of "chronic pain" or "fibromyalgia" independently predict a diagnosis of psychogenic seizures. *Epilepsy and Behavior*, *6*(2), 264–265.

Benbadis, S. R., Agrawal, V., & Tatum, W. O. (2001). How many patients with psychogenic nonepileptic seizures also have epilepsy? *Neurology*, *57*(5), 915.

Benbadis, S. R., & Hauser, W. A. (2000). An estimate of the prevalence of psychogenic non-epileptic seizures. *Seizure*, *9*(4), 280.

Binder, L. M. (2002). The Portland Digit Recognition Test: A review of validation data and clinical use. *Journal of Forensic Neuropsychology*, *2*(3–4), 27.

Binder, L. M., Kindermann, S. S., Heaton, R. K., & Salinsky, M. C. (1998). Neuropsychologic impairment in patients with nonepileptic seizures. *Archives of Clinical Neuropsychology*, *13*(6), 513.

Binder, L. M., Salinsky, M. C., & Smith, S. P. (1994). Psychological correlates of psychogenic seizures. *Journal of Clinical and Experimental Neuropsychology*, *16*(4), 524.

Bortz, J. J., Prigatano, G. P., Blum, D., & Fisher, R. S. (1995). Differential response characteristics in nonepileptic and epileptic seizure patients on a test of verbal learning and memory. *Neurology*, *45*(11), 2029.

Cascino, G. D. (2002). Video-EEG monitoring in adults. *Epilepsia*, *43*(Suppl. 3), 80–93.

Coleman, R. D., Rapport, L. J., Millis, S. R., Ricker, J. H., & Farchione, T. J. (1998). Effects of coaching on detection of malingering on the California Verbal Learning Test. *Journal of Clinical and Experimental Neuropsychology*, *20*(2), 201.

Cragar, D. E., Berry, D. T. R., Fakhoury, T. A., Cibula, J. E., & Schmitt, F. A. (2002). A review of diagnostic techniques in the differential diagnosis of epileptic and nonepileptic seizures. *Neuropsychology Review*, *12*(1), 31.

Cragar, D. E., Schmitt, F. A., Berry, D. T. R., Cibula, J. E., Dearth, C. M. S., & Fakhoury, T. A. (2003). A Comparison of MMPI-2 Decision Rules in the Diagnosis of Nonepileptic Seizures. *Journal of Clinical and Experimental Neuropsychology*, *25*(6), 793.

Cuthill, F. M., & Espie, C. A. (2005). Sensitivity and specificity of procedures for the differential diagnosis of epileptic and non-epileptic seizures: A systematic review. *Seizure*, *14*(5), 293–303.

Derry, P. A., & McLachlan, R. S. (1996). The MMPI-2 as an adjunct to the diagnosis of pseudoseizures. *Seizure*, *5*, 35–40.

Dodrill, C. B. (1978). A neuropsychological battery for epilepsy. *Epilepsia*, *19*(6), 611.

Dodrill, C. B., & Holmes, M. D. (2000). Psychological and neuropsychological evaluation of the patient with non-epileptic seizures. In J. R. Gates & A. J. Rowan (Eds.), *Non-epileptic seizures* (2nd ed., pp. 169–181). Boston: Butterworth-Heinemann.

Drane, D. L., Williamson, D. J., Stroup, E. S., Holmes, M. D., Jung, M., Koerner, E., et al. (2006). Cognitive impairment is not equal in patients with epileptic and psychogenic nonepileptic seizures. *Epilepsia*, *47*(11), 1879–1886.

Dworetzky, B. A., Strahonja-Packard, A., Shanahan, C. W., Paz, J., Schauble, B., &

Bromfield, E. B. (2005). Characteristics of male veterans with psychogenic nonepileptic seizures. *Epilepsia, 49*(9), 1418–1422.

Gates, J. R. (2000). Epidemiology and classification of non-epileptic events. In J. R. Gates & A. J. Rowan (Eds.), *Non-epileptic seizures* (2nd ed., pp. 3–14). Boston: Butterworth-Heinemann.

Gervais, R. O., Rohling, M. L., Green, P., & Ford, W. (2004). A comparison of WMT, CARB, and TOMM failure rates in non-head injury disability claimants. *Archives of Clinical Neuropsychology, 19*(4), 475.

Gervais, R. O., Russell, A. S., Green, P., Allen, L. M., & Ferrari, R. P., Pieschl, S.D. (2001). Effort testing in patients with fibromyalgia and disability incentives. *Journal of Rheumatology, 28*, 1892–1899.

Greiffenstein, M. F., Baker, W. J., Axelrod, B. N., Peck, E. A., & Gervais, R. (2004). The Fake Bad Scale and MMPI-2 F-family detection of implausible psychological trauma claims. *The Clinical Neuropsychologist, 18*(4), 573–590.

Grote, C. L., Kooker, E. K., Nyenhuis, D. L., Smith, C. A., & Mattingly, M. L. (2000). Performance of compensation seeking and non-compensation seeking samples on the Victoria Symptom Validity Test: Cross-validation and extension of a standardization study. *Journal of Clinical and Experimental Neuropsychology, 22*(6), 709–719.

Hermann, B. P. (1993). Neuropsychological assessment in the diagnosis of non-epileptic seizures. In A. J. Rowan & J. Gates (Eds.), *Non-epileptic seizures* (pp. 21-30). Stoneham, MA: Butterworth-Heinemann.

Hill, S. K., Ryan, L. M., Kennedy, C. H., & Malamut, B. L. (2003). The relationship between measures of declarative memory and the Test of Memory Malingering. *Journal of Forensic Neuropsychology, 3*, 1–18.

Larrabee, G. J. (1998). Somatic malingering on the MMPI and MMPI-2 in personal injury litigants. *The Clinical Neuropsychologist, 12*(2), 179.

Larrabee, G. J. (2003a). Detection of symptom exaggeration with the MMPI-2 in litigants with malingered neurocognitive dysfunction. *The Clinical Neuropsychologist, 17*(1), 54.

Larrabee, G. J. (2003b). Exaggerated MMPI-2 symptom report in personal injury litigants with malingered neurocognitive deficit. *Archives of Clinical Neuropsychology, 18*(6), 673.

Lee, G. P., Loring, D. W., & Martin, R. C. (1992). Rey's 15-Item Visual Memory Test for the detection of malingering: Normative observations on patients with neurological disorders. *Psychological Assessment, 4*(1), 43.

Loring, D. W., Lee, G. P., & Meador, K. J. (2005). Victoria Symptom Validity Test Performance in Non-Litigating Epilepsy Surgery Candidates. *Journal of Clinical and Experimental Neuropsychology, 27*(5), 610.

Martin, R., Burneo, J. G., Prasad, A., Powell, T., Faught, E., Knowlton, R., et al. (2003). Frequency of epilepsy in patients with psychogenic seizures monitored by video-EEG. *Neurology, 61*(12), 1791.

McCaffrey, R. J., O'Bryant, S. E., Ashendorf, L., & Fisher, J. M. (2003). Correlations among the TOMM, Rey-15, and MMPI-2 validity scales in a sample of TBI litigants. *Journal of Forensic Neuropsychology, 3*(3), 45.

Millis, S. R., Putnam, S. H., Adams, K. M., & Ricker, J. H. (1995). The California Verbal Learning Test in the detection of incomplete effort in neuropsychological evaluation. *Psychological Assessment, 7*(4), 463.

Mittenberg, W., Patton, C., Canyock, E. M., & Condit, D. C. (2002). Base rates of malingering and symptom exaggeration. *Journal of Clinical and Experimental Neuropsychology, 24*(8), 1094.

Morey, L. C. (2003). *Essentials of PAI assessment.* Hoboken, NJ: Wiley.

Morrell, M. J. (2002). Stigma and epilepsy. *Epilepsy and Behavior, 3,* 521–525.

Risse, G. L., Mason, S. L., & Mercer, D. K. (2000). Neuropsychological performance and cognitive complaints in epileptic and nonepileptic seizure patients. In J. Gates & A. J. Rowan (Eds.), *Non-epileptic seizures* (2nd ed., pp. 139–150). Boston: Butterworth-Heinemann.

Rohling, M. L., Green, P., Allen, L. M., & Iverson, G. L. (2002). Depressive symptoms and neurocognitive test scores in patients passing symptom validity tests. *Archives of Clinical Neuropsychology, 17*(3), 205.

Slick, D. J., Iverson, G. L., & Green, P. (2000). California Verbal Learning Test indicators of suboptimal performance in a sample of head-injury litigants. *Journal of Clinical and Experimental Neuropsychology, 22*(5), 569.

Swanson, S. J., Springer, J. A., Benbadis, S. R., & Morris, G. L. (2000). Cognitive and psychological functioning in patients with non-epileptic seizures. In J. Gates & A. J. Rowan (Eds.), *Non-epileptic seizures* (2nd ed., pp. 123–137). Boston: Butterworth-Heinemann.

Sweet, J. J. (1999). Malingering: Differential diagnosis. In J. J. Sweet (Ed.), *Forensic neuropsychology: Fundamentals and practice* (pp. 255–285). New York: Swets & Zeitlinger.

Sweet, J. J., Wolfe, P., Sattlberger, E., Numan, B., Rosenfeld, J. P., Clingerman, S., et al. (2000). Further investigation of traumatic brain injury versus insufficient effort with the California Verbal Learning Test. *Archives of Clinical Neuropsychology, 15*(2), 105.

Wagner, M. T., Wymer, J. H., Topping, K. B., & Pritchard, P. B. (2005). Use of the Personality Assessment Inventory as an efficacious and cost-effective diagnostic tool for nonepileptic seizures. *Epilepsy and Behavior, 7,* 301–304.

Warner, M. H., Wilkus, R. J., Vossler, D. G., & Dodrill, C. B. (1996). MMPI-2 profiles in differential diagnosis of epilepsy vs. psychogenic seizures. *Epilepsia, 37*(Suppl. 5), 19.

Westerveld, M. (2002). Inferring function from structure: Relationship of magnetic resonance imaging-detected hippocampal abnormality and memory function in epilepsy. *Epilepsy Currents, 2*(1), 3–7.

Wilkus, R. J., & Dodrill, C. B. (1984). Intensive EEG monitoring and psychological studies of patients with pseudoepileptic seizures. *Epilepsia, 25,* 100–107.

Williamson, D. J., Drane, D. L., Stroup, E. S., Miller, J. W., & Holmes, M. D. (2003). Most patients with psychogenic seizures do not exert valid effort on neurocognitive testing. *Epilepsia, 44*(Suppl. 8).

Williamson, D. J., Drane, D. L., Stroup, E. S., Miller, J. W., Holmes, M. D., & Wilensky, A. J. (2004). Detecting cognitive differences between patients with epilepsy and patients with psychogenic nonepileptic seizures: Effort matters. *Epilepsia, 45*(Suppl. 7), 179.

APPENDIX 15.1. DEMOGRAPHIC CHARACTERISTICS OF CITED SAMPES

	N	% female subjects	Age	Education	IQ
Lee, Loring, and Martin (1992)					
TLE	100	41	30.0 (9.6)	11.0 (2.0)	82.4 (11.7)
Litigating Outpatient	16	19	35.4 (9.8)	9.8 (2.4)	77.1 (15.4)
Nonlitigating outpatient	40	35	38.4 (16.0)	11.3 (2.3)	86.7 (12.8)
Binder, Salinsky, and Smith. (1994)					
ES	34	38	35.5 (11.1)	12.2 (2.8)	*
PNES	19	47	36.9 (9.3)	12.6 (3.1)	*
Bortz, Prigatano, Blum, and Fisher (1995)					
Right TLE	12	57	36.8 (8.6)	12.8 (2.9)	93.3 (14.2)
Left TLE	11	37	31.1 (12.2)	13.3 (2.1)	92.6 (10.7)
PNES	18	72	33.6 (11.3)	12.3 (2.7)	91.3 (10.4)
Binder, Kinderman, Heaton, and Salinsky (1998)					
ES	42	36	35.2 (11.5)	12.3 (2.8)	90.6 (15.3)
PNES	30	47	36.0 (9.8)	12.3 (2.6)	92.0 (14.3)
Control	47	34	36.1 (12.7)	12.7 (2.7)	102.1 (15.4)
Grote, Kooker, Nyerhuis, Smith, and Mattingly (2000)					
ES	30	43	33.4 (10.6)	14.0 (2.6)	95.7 (15.8)
Compensation seeking	53	41	46.2 (10.9)	13.3 (2.6)	93.0 (15.3)
Hill, Ryan, Kennedy, and Malamut (2003)					
TLE	48	48	37.1 (10.8)	12.7 (1.7)	88.5 (9.0)
PNES	57	72	36.8 (12.0)	13.2 (2.7)	89.8 (12.0)
Williamson et al. (2004)					
ES	77	43	35.2 (12.4)	12.2 (2.4)	*
PNES	36	75	38.5 (10.6)	12.2 (2.7)	*
Wagner, Wymer, Topping, and Pritchard (2005)					
ES	15	*	*	*	82.4 (15)
PNES	26	*	*	*	92.6 (16)
Drane et al. (2006)					
ES	41	46	36.9 (14.4)	12.6 (2.3)	*
PNES	43	79	40.6 (10.2)	12.4 (2.6)	*

Note. *, not provided.

CHAPTER 16

The Use of Effort Tests in the Context of Actual versus Feigned Attention-Deficit/Hyperactivity Disorder and Learning Disability

Kimberly Alfano
Kyle Brauer Boone

At first glance, one might find it surprising to discover a chapter addressing feigning of learning disability (LD) or attention-deficit/hyperactivity disorder (ADHD). In part, this may be because these disorders originate in childhood in contrast to the acquired injuries neuropsychologists typically see in litigation. Therefore, LD and ADHD are typically thought of as "childhood" disorders that are not typically "malingered." Recent research, however, has shown that malingered cognitive symptoms can occur in children (Stutts, Hickey, & Kasdan, 2003; Lu & Boone, 2002). In adult populations, neuropsychologists no longer think twice before considering the likelihood of symptom fabrication or exaggeration, given the estimated base rate of malingering in a forensic context. For example, recent estimates of base rates for probable malingering for a variety of presumptive diagnoses have ranged from 29% and 30% in personal injury and disability cases, while some authors have reported a 40% base rate of malingered head injury in personal injury cases (Larrabee, 2003; Mittenberg, Patton, Canyock, & Condit, 2002).

Although the literature is now burgeoning with articles on malingering within the workers' compensation and personal injury realm of neuropsychological practice, the possibility of malingered symptoms of ADHD and/ or LD by adult students has generally been ignored. In contrast to the monetary incentives for malingering in litigation suits, adult students with ADHD/ LD may exaggerate or fabricate cognitive deficits and symptoms in order to receive special accommodations such as being awarded extra time on tests as mandated under the Americans with Disabilities Act (U.S. Department of Justice, 2004), and/or to obtain stimulant medications. Despite the very tangible benefits to academic performance provided by feigning of ADHD or LD, many clinicians and academicians view malingering in this context as rare. In the *UCLA Daily Bruin* in December 2004 (Miller, 2004), a clinical psychology graduate student who conducted psychological evaluations at the UCLA Psychology Clinic was quoted as claiming, "Not to sound arrogant but I don't think you could fool me. Students can read about psychological testing methods on the Internet but there are some things they don't know." Similarly, a professor of pediatrics and child study at the Yale School of Medicine was cited in *yalesdailynews.com* in April 2006 as concluding that "there's a great suburban myth that students or parents pretend they might have dyslexia. People talk about it but there are no reports and it's very, very rare that you can find a case." Further, in the same news source, the director of Yale's Resource Office on Disabilities was reported as asserting that it is difficult to cheat on standardized tests used to determine the presence of reading disorder: "You can shop doctors but you can't fool the tests."

However, emerging data are troubling. According to ABC News, of 300,000 students taking the Scholastic Aptitude Test (SAT), a college admissions test, in April 2006, 10% were provided special accommodations. However, it is estimated that less than 2% of high school students in fact have learning disabilities. In 2000, the office of the California State Auditor reviewed the cases of 330 public school students who had received accommodations and found the basis for accommodations questionable in 60 (18%).

Further, the inflated rate of accommodations is disproportionately found in affluent, white, private school students, namely, those who have the discretionary family income to pay for independent psychoeducational testing used to document need for accommodations. The 2000 California State Auditor report found that the ethnic composition of students receiving special accommodations for a yearly standardized achievement test (STAR) (which has no bearing on college admissions) matched that of students enrolled in special education classes for learning disabilities. However, on the SAT, although 38% of students taking the test identified themselves as white, 56% of students receiving test accommodations were white. Only 12% of students taking the test indicated that family income was greater than $100,000, although 29% of students receiving accommodations indicated that family income fell in this category. Students in private schools were twice as likely to receive accommodations as public school students, and those students in private schools with family income greater than $100,000 were three times as likely to receive accommodations as public school students with the same family income.

Osmon and Mano (personal communication, May 17, 2006) in fact documented a 31% effort test failure in their university learning disorder clinic, a prevalence comparable to that reported in personal injury litigants and disability claimants (Mittenberg et al., 2002), and Osmon and Mano suggest that this may actually be an underestimate given that the effort test employed in their clinic (Word Memory Test) is designed to detect memory difficulties, not reading disorder or other learning disabilities. They conclude that "the greatest current lack in LD assessment technology is an instrument demonstrated to detect malingering and poor effort."

Despite the clear motives for malingering in adult students, there is a dearth of literature investigating symptom feigning in this population. In fact, a review of the literature identified only four studies on malingered ADHD symptoms, with one publication consisting of a brief cautionary note rather than a formal study (Conti, 2004; Henry, 2005; Leark, Dixon, Hoffman, & Huynh, 2002; Quinn, 2003), and only two investigations addressing malingered reading disability (Lu, Boone, Jimenez, & Razani, 2004; Osmon, Plambeck, Klein, & Mano, 2006).

STUDIES OF FEIGNED ADHD

Conti (2004) cautioned that ADHD could be easily simulated in attempts to obtain stimulant medications due to the accessibility of information regarding ADHD symptoms on the Internet or other forms of public media, and the fact that it is not difficult to maintain fabricated ADHD symptoms over a short duration of observation, such as that which occurs during brief visits to a general practitioner. Conti also noted that, in particular, adolescents may be able to readily fabricate ADHD symptoms due to the subjective nature of the symptoms, in addition to the fact that teenagers are typically able to directly observe peers who may genuinely have ADHD, and they freely share symptom information with each other when confined (i.e., in a juvenile detention facility). Conti's comments highlight the need for thorough evaluations which incorporate behavioral observations, objective test results, and background information regarding onset of symptoms and presence across a variety of settings, as well as contact with objective collateral sources regarding current functional ability; reliance on brief observations of behavior when the student is aware he or she is being observed or self-report symptom questionnaires are likely to be highly susceptible to symptom feigning. However, it is possible that even comprehensive ADHD evaluations may not be "foolproof," necessitating the development of indices that objectively identify noncredible performance in this context.

Conti (2004) notes that it is generally accepted that no single test procedure in isolation is adequate for making a diagnosis of ADHD; however, continuous performance tests (CPTs) have received wide acceptance. A meta-analysis of 26 CPT studies showed that ADHD samples displayed twice as many missed targets and false hits as non-ADHD groups (Losier, McGrath, & Klein, 1996). Subsequently, Forbes (1998) demonstrated the clinical utility of the Test of Variables of Attention (TOVA) in distinguishing between clinically referred children with ADHD and those diagnosed with other clinical conditions. He noted that use of the criterion of any one TOVA variable greater than 1.5 standard deviation from age- and sex-adjusted means correctly identified 80% of the sample with ADHD. Similarly, the Integrated Visual and Auditory (IVA) CPT, developed by Sandford and Turner (1995), has been reported to achieve excellent sensitivity (92%) and specificity (90%) as well as good concurrent validity with other CPTs (e.g., TOVA; Forbes, 1998).

Sattler (1988) suggested that lack of internal consistency in CPT scores may be indicative of malingering, and Quinn (2003) specifically hypothesized that excessive between item variance and reaction time variance on CPTs may be particularly sensitive to malingering. Quinn further predicted that ADHD could not be effectively simulated on a CPT but could be faked on traditionally used rating scales of ADHD symptoms because the latter provide cues as to what symptoms should be endorsed to simulate ADHD. To test this hypothesis, she compared performance of 16 undergraduates with ADHD with that of 42 volunteer undergraduates drawn from psychology courses and randomly assigned to either a control ($n = 19$) or a simulated malingerer ($n = 23$) condition. The ADHD students were recruited through the University Office for Students with Disabilities and had previously been diagnosed with ADHD by a trained psychiatrist in accordance with DSM-IV (American Psychiatric Association, 1994) criteria; 4 were diagnosed with primarily inattentive type and 12 were diagnosed with the combined type. The Behavior Checklist (Murphy & Barkley, 1996), used to obtain both current and childhood symptoms, and the IVA CPT were administered. The IVA CPT uses both auditory and visual stimuli and has two global scales: the Full Scale Response Control (a measure of impulsivity as assessed by commission errors) and the Full Scale Attention Quotient (a measure of attending as documented by omission errors). There are also six subscales: Prudence, Consistency, Stamina, Vigilance, Focus, and Speed. All scores are reported separately for both the auditory and visual modalities as well as in a combined score. Other scores are also calculated, including a comprehension score which measures idiopathic errors of commission and omission. The simulator group was asked to complete the CPT and checklist while playing the role of an adult with ADHD and were admonished to make their symptoms realistic by not faking in an obvious manner.

No significant differences were found between malingerers and ADHD subjects on any of the ADHD Behavior Checklist scales. Quinn (2003) concluded that malingerers were able to successfully fake reports of childhood symptoms of ADHD and easily met DSM-IV criteria for this condition. Interestingly, the ADHD Behavior Checklist—Current scale mean scores for the actual ADHD group did not fall in the clinical range using DSM-IV criteria for these adults, whereas the mean scores for malingerers did meet these criteria.

On the IVA CPT, malingerers scored significantly poorer than controls and ADHD subjects on the Full Scale Attention Quotient, Auditory Attention Quotient, Visual Attention Quotient, and the auditory and visual versions of the Consistency, Focus, Prudence, Vigilance, and Comprehension subscales; malingerers significantly differed from the other groups on 81% of the IVA's subscales. Using a cutoff of Full Scale Response Control < 75 + Full Scale Attention Quotient < 37 (for a combined score of < 112), sensitivity was .81 and specificity was .91. Slightly higher sensitivity rates were found when only results for auditory scores were employed; Auditory Response Control < 74 + Auditory Attention Quotient < 44 (for a combined score < 118) was associated with .94 sensitivity and .91 specificity.

Quinn (2003) concluded that fraudulent claims of ADHD can be identified through the inclusion of CPTs during assessment of adult ADHD. She noted that the IVA is calibrated to a mean of 100, with a score of 80 (1.5 standard deviations below the mean) determined to be clinically significant, and she suggested that "scores in the 50s [i.e., < 3sd below control means] and below are typical of malingerers."

Subsequent analyses were conducted to determine which strategies malingerers used to fake ADHD. In general, all participants used more than one strategy with the most commonly employed approach that of faking general inattention (61%), followed by ignoring visual (43%) and auditory stimuli (17%). Analysis of error types revealed that most malingerers produced commission errors (57%), with approximately one-third reporting deliberate omission errors (35%), and a limited number using a random response strategy (9%). In addition, several reported that they "double-clicked the mouse" to demonstrate symptoms of hyperactivity (30%), while a minority produced generalized "fidgeting behaviors" (13%).

Leark et al. (2002) used the visual stimulus version of the TOVA to investigate the effect of test-taking bias in a simulation study of 36 non-LD and non-ADHD college students. The TOVA is a computer-based CPT which requires that the subject press a button when the target appears on the screen. In the first half of the test, the target is infrequent (3.5:1 nontarget to target ratio), and in the second half of the test, the target is frequent (3.5:1 target to nontarget ratio). Four types of scores (percentage of omission errors, percentage of commission errors, mean response time and variability of response time) are provided for each quarter, both halves, and for the total test. Subjects were administered the test twice: once under standard instructions and once with the instructions to simulate difficulties with attention and impulse control.

Under instructions to fake ADHD, subjects made significantly more errors of commission and omission; in fact, when instructed to fake, subjects exhibited nearly four times the number of missed targets. Of note, when there were more "nontargets" on the TOVA than "targets," more errors of commission were made in the faking bad condition; conversely, when there were more "targets" than "nontargets," more errors of omission were committed. In addition, when malingering, subjects were slower across the entire test (although particularly for those quarters when there were fewer targets than nontargets) and also showed more variability in time scores. Leark et al. (2002) concluded that test-taking bias should be considered in the presence of grossly elevated TOVA performances.

While the Leark et al. (2002) study suggested how individuals faking symptoms of ADHD might perform on the TOVA, because there was no comparison group of individuals with actual ADHD, it was unclear whether the "malingering pattern" identified by Leark and colleagues was specific to simulators.

In a recent study, Henry (2005) investigated the performance of actual malingerers using the TOVA. Subjects consisted of 52 adults who had undergone neuropsychological evaluations in personal injury litigation; 26 were classified as definitive or probable malingerers based on scores below cutoffs on at least one measure of effort such as the Test of Memory Malingering (TOMM), the Word Memory Test (WMT), or the Computerized Assessment of Response Bias (CARB), and if they met Slick, Sherman, and Iverson's (1999) malingered neurocognitive dysfunction criteria (definite or probable). Subjects identified as definite/probable malingerers performed significantly worse than the remaining subjects on all TOVA variables including errors of commission and omission, as well as mean response times and response time variability. Response time variability and response time, but particularly errors of omission, were statistically significant predictors of group membership. A cutoff of > 7 omission errors resulted in sensitivity of 69% at acceptable specificity levels (i.e., 92%); 89% of the malingerers generated > 3 omission errors while 81% of the nonmalingerers produced < 3 omission errors.

The lowered TOVA scores documented in the noncredible group were comparable to the omission errors, slower response times, and greater variability of scores described by Leark et al. (2002) in their subjects instructed to feign ADHD. However, the studies differed in that in the Leark et al. (2002) investigation, subjects in the simulation condition exhibited significantly more errors of commission, an observation not corroborated in the real-world probable malingerers in the Henry (2005) study, which raises some concerns regarding the generalizability of simulation studies.

It is of note that the TOVA was sensitive to feigned cognitive symptoms in the Henry (2005) study, despite the fact that the litigants were not specifically alleging ADHD but rather cognitive changes secondary to acquired brain injury. These observations suggest that individuals feigning effects of alleged brain injury may display noncredible attentional impairments, and that the "malingering pattern" on the TOVA appears to be effective in detecting feigned cognitive symptoms in general. Taken as a whole, the data from the Henry (2005) and Leark et al. (2002) studies on the TOVA corroborate the Quinn (2003) findings on the IVA showing underperformance in malingerers relative to actual subjects with ADHD, and they provide further support that CPT measures have utility in the detection of malingered cognitive symptoms.

STUDIES OF FEIGNED LD

Lu et al. (2004) investigated the use of the Stroop test in a case report of six individuals in litigation (criminal or civil) who alleged complete inability to read. These individuals claimed that they could not read the words "red," "green," and "blue" on the word-reading card of the Comalli Stroop Test, but on the interference trial they were observed to make errors of reading (failure to inhibit a reading response), thereby providing incontrovertible evidence of malingering (i.e., they were observed performing a task they claimed they could not do). These findings suggest that the Stroop test may be the instrument of choice for the determination of feigned complete inability to read: however, admittedly, this is a rare situation (i.e., most malingerers are not claiming total illiteracy).

Osmon et al. (2006) reported findings of their investigation of a newly developed Word Reading Test (WRT) for measurement of effort in simulated learning disability. In their study, 60 non-learning disabled and non-ADHD college students were randomly assigned to either a normal effort, reading simulator, or speed simulator group and were then administered the WMT followed by the WRT. The WRT is a computerized forced-choice measure in which, for each trial, a word is shown followed by the target and a foil having a characteristic consistent with a layperson's knowledge of dyslexia, such as a nonsense word beginning with the "mirror image" letter of the target word (e.g., "develop" vs. "bevelop"), additions/deletions of letters ("through" and "thorough"), and homophones ("too" vs. "two") The reading simulator group was instructed to "pretend that you are being evaluated for reading problems because you are concerned about your performance in college and want to receive accommodations in the classroom . . . you should try to perform on these tests the way you think someone with dyslexia might perform. . . ." In contrast, the mental speed simulators were told to "pretend that you are being evaluated for slowed thinking associated with learning disability because you have noticed being the last to finish exams and having to take longer to learn than your college classmates . . . you should try to perform on these tests the way you think someone with learning disability might perform. . . ."

Simulators differed from controls on all WMT scores, although the two simulating groups did not differ from each other. With WMT failure defined by a below-cutoff performance on any WMT score, specificity was high (96%) but sensitivity was only moderate (65%).

On the WRT accuracy score, all groups significantly differed from each other, with nonsimulators performing best, speed simulators performing intermediately, and reading simulators performing worst. In contrast, for the WRT speed score, controls and reading simulators performed comparably, and the speed simulators scored significantly lower than the two other groups. No nonsimulators made more than three errors, while 28/31 reading simulators and 20/27 speed simulators made four or more errors. A cutoff of ≥ 4 errors was associated with 90% sensitivity for reading simulators and 74% sensitivity for speed simulators at 100% specificity.

Osmon et al. (2006) concluded that the WRT error score was more effective than the WMT in detecting feigned learning disability. They suggested that their results support the validity of the WRT and provide evidence that effort in specific populations is best detected by tests designed to address layperson notions of the deficits associated with that population's disorder. While promising, the results of this initial investigation require corroboration to determine whether the WRT can be used to capture feigned reading deficits in a real-world population of individuals feigning reading disability. In addition, it is unknown how adult students with a confirmed diagnosis of reading disorder perform on the WRT and whether the test can accurately discriminate between genuine and feigned reading disability.

Fortunately, some data, reproduced below, are available regarding false-positive identification rates in subjects with LD for other effort indicators.

EFFORT TEST PERFORMANCE IN SUBJECTS WITH LD

Warner-Chacon (1994) hypothesized that adults with genuine LD might be at particular risk for poor performance on some commonly used tests of effort as these procedures may require cognitive abilities which are impaired in this population. As such, her study was undertaken for the following purposes: (1) to determine the false-positive rates on commonly used cognitive tests of effort in a population of genuine students with LD, and (2) to ascertain which cognitive skills are associated with performance on each test by examining the relationship between effort test scores and measures of intellectual and academic functioning.

Four cognitive effort tests were investigated in this study: the Rey 15-Item Memory Test (Lezak, 1995), the Dot Counting Test (Boone, Lu, et al., 2002; Lezak, 1995), Forced-Choice Method (Hiscock & Hiscock, 1989), and the Rey Word Recognition Test (Lezak, 1983). The initial sample consisted of 40 fluent English-speaking adult students with LD over the age of 18 who were recruited from the California State University, Northridge, Office of Disabled Student Services (ODSS). Subjects were eligible to participate in the study if they were currently enrolled in the university, had already participated in the screening process by the ODSS for the evaluation of LD based on 6–7 hours of diagnostic testing by ODSS LD specialists, had confirmed LD, and were actively receiving services through the ODSS. Subjects with a history of significant head trauma, alcohol or drug abuse, psychotic or bipolar illness, or neurological disorder were excluded. (It is noteworthy that one student with LD had to be excluded from the study due to evidence of noncooperation on two cognitive malingering tests [e.g., reproduced the bottom row on the 15-Item Test in reverse order; miscounted eight dots as four on the Dot Counting Test].) Ultimately 34 subjects were included in the study. Subjects averaged 30.71 (SD = 12.70, range = 19–72) years of age and 15.44 (SD = 1.01, range = 13–18) years of education. Eighteen subjects were females and 16 were males. Fifty-nine percent were Caucasian, 32% were Latino, 6% were African American, and 3% were designated "other."

Participants were individually administered the four effort tests. In addition, archival data for the Wechsler Adult Intelligence Scale–Revised (WAIS-R) and Woodcock–Johnson–Revised Psychoeducational Battery were available for 16 students. The following test scores were used for statistical analyses: (1) Rey 15-Item total correct, spatial score (number of symbols accurately placed within a row), and adjusted spatial score (number of symbols accurately placed within a row minus intrusions) (Greiffenstein, Baker, & Gola, 1996); (2) Dot Counting Test errors, mean ungrouped time, mean grouped time, and mean ungrouped/grouped time; (3) Rey Word Recognition Test total, total minus false positives, and total minus Rey Auditory Verbal Test [RAVLT] Trial 1; (4) Forced-Choice Test total correct; (5) WAIS-R Verbal IQ, Performance IQ, and individual subtest scaled scores measuring attention (Digit Span), information processing speed (Digit Symbol), math skills (Arithmetic), language knowledge (Vocabulary), visual perception (Picture Completion), visual sequencing (Picture Arrangement), and visuoconstructional skill (Block Design; Object Assembly); and (6) Woodcock–Johnson–Revised Passage Comprehension, Applied Problems, and Letter–Word Identification.

False-Positive Rates

No subject failed the Rey 15-Item Memory Test using the cutoff of < 9 total items or < 9 spatial score, although two subjects fell below the cutoff of < 8 adjusted spatial score. Two subjects also failed the Rey Dot Counting Test using the cutoff of > 3 errors, but only one subject obtained a mean grouped dot counting score ≥ mean ungrouped dot counting score, and no subject exceeded an ungrouped time of 62 seconds (mean of 10.2 seconds) or a grouped time of 38 seconds (mean of 7 seconds). No subject failed the Forced-Choice task (using a cutoff of < 90% correct trials).

On the Rey Word Recognition Test, three subjects failed using the criterion of RAVLT Trial 1 recall ≥ recognition, and two subjects obtained a recognition score < 6. Only one subject obtained a recognition score minus false positives < 5. Examination of the performances of the individuals "failing" the Rey Word Recognition test revealed that while three of 34 subjects technically showed recognition ≤ RAVLT Trial 1 recall, in two of the three cases, recall on the first trial of the RAVLT was 10 of 15. One of these subjects also obtained a Word Recognition score of 10, and the other obtained a score of 8. Because the Recognition scores were equal to or lower than the first trial RAVLT score, these subjects were judged to have "failed" the Recognition task. However, a score of 10 on the first trial of the RAVLT is unusual and rarely attained even in a normal control population (cf. Mitrushina, Boone, & D'Elia, 1999). This considerably elevated score would not be consistent with an intention to fake cognitive impairment. Exclusion of those subjects whose Trial 1 RAVLT scores are above control means (i.e., a score of 7 or higher) would have dropped the false-positive rate to 3%. Thus, the test specificity rates (% of subjects correctly identified as not malingering) ranged from 94% to 100%. Tabulation of failure rates across the four tasks indicated that while 24% (8 of 34) subjects failed one effort test using at least one of the aforementioned criteria, only one subject (3%) fell below cutoffs on two separate tests (Word Recognition, Dot Counting); no subject failed more than two tests.

Correlational Analyses

Results of correlational analyses revealed that the various cognitive malingering tests have differing associations with IQ and achievement tasks. Rey 15-Item total score is related to basic attention (Digit Span, $r = .40$, $p = .09$) and visuospatial ability (Object Assembly, $r = .52$, $p = .03$). Rey 15-Item adjusted spatial scores were also correlated with visuospatial ability (Object Assembly, $r = .52$, $p = .03$), while 15-item spatial scores and adjusted spatial scores were both significantly related to visual sequencing ability (Picture Arrangement, $r = .51$, $p = .03$). These results reflect the fact that spatial and adjusted spatial scores require correct sequencing of items in a row whereas this is not required for total score. The documentation of a relationship between 15-Item total score and Digit Span confirms the assertion of Greiffenstein et al. (1996) that 15-Item performance taps immediate memory skills analogous to Digit Span.

Mean grouped and ungrouped dot counting performance appeared to be related to different cognitive abilities. Speed in counting of grouped dots was associated with math skills (Arithmetic, $r = -.63$, $p = .004$; Applied Problems, $r = -.59$, $p = .02$), visuospatial ability (Block Design, $r = -.54$, $p = .02$), basic attention (Digit Span, $r = -.60$, $p = .01$), and nonverbal intellectual skills (Performance IQ, $r = -.54$, $p = .03$). In contrast, counting of ungrouped dots was related, at a trend level, to visuospatial ability (Block Design, $r = -.45$, $p = .06$) and information-processing speed (Digit Symbol, $r = -.41$, $p = .08$). Decreases in grouped dot counting time require efficient use of multiplication skills, processing of the visuospatial (i.e., grouped) configuration of the dots, and basic working memory (i.e., adding the sums of each group); thus, the fact that math, visuospatial abilities, and attention were closely related to grouped dot counting time is not surprising. The finding that mean ungrouped dot counting time was related to information-processing speed and visuospatial skills is also expected in that rapid counting of ungrouped, random dots would appear to primarily require processing of a visuospatial array and speed in executing a rote task. Number of errors was not significantly related to any IQ or achievement score. Similar to our findings, Youngjohn, Burrows, and Erdal (1995) also documented an association between Dot Counting performance and Performance IQ but found Dot Counting performance to be unrelated to Verbal IQ, mental speed, and divided attention.

Number of words recognized on the Rey Word Recognition Test was significantly associated with overall verbal intellectual skills (Verbal IQ, $r = .60$, $p = .01$), vocabulary range (Vocabulary, $r = .56$, $p = .02$), and reading skills (Revised Passage Comprehension, $r = .45$, $p = .08$).

Because of the lack of variability in Forced-Choice scores, correlations could not be computed with IQ and achievement scores.

The small sample size on which correlational analyses were based raises the possibility of Type II error, specifically, that additional relationships exist between IQ/achievement scores and malingering test performance which were not detected due to lack of power. Thus, our findings may not accurately reflect all associations between these two sets of test scores. However, our data have identified the intellectual and achievement skills which account for 16% or more of malingering test score variance.

Means and standard deviations for scores on the cognitive malingering tests, the WAIS-R, and the Woodcock–Johnson–Revised battery are presented in Tables 16.1 and 16.2.

In summary, while performance on three tests of effort was found to be correlated with some intellectual and achievement skills, the amount of effort score variance accounted for by the intellectual and achievement scores was moderate at most (16% to 37%). In addition, as discussed earlier, a very low effort test failure rate was documented in our sample. Thus, while differing cognitive abilities are involved in performance on the various tests of effort, the deficient cognitive skills found in LD rarely impact effort test score performance to the extent that a task is actually failed. The findings do

TABLE 16.1. Means and Standard Deviations for Effort Test Scores

	Means + *SD*	Range
Cognitive malingering test scores		
Rey 15-Item		
• Total score	14.06 ± 1.46	10–15
• Spatial score	13.29 ± 2.08	9–15
• Adjusted spatial score	13.12 ± 2.41	7–15
Rey Dot Counting		
• Errors	1.21 ± 1.20	0–4
• Mean ungrouped time	6.02 ± 1.75	2.80–10.20
• Mean grouped time	2.66 ± 1.32	1.20–6.30
• Mean ungrouped/grouped	2.65 ± 1.18	.98–5.90
Word Recognition Test		
• Total	9.83 ± 2.34	5–15
• Total minus False Positive	8.68 ± 2.38	4–15
• Total minus RAVLT Trial 1	3.65 ± 2.46	–2–9
Forced Choice		
• Total	17.94 ± .24	17–18

TABLE 16.2. Means and Standard Deviations for WAIS-R IQ, Subtest Scaled Scores, and Achievement Scores

	Means + *SD*	Range
WAIS-R		
• Full Scale IQ	97.31 ± 7.98	82–108
• Verbal IQ	99.31 ± 8.62	84–114
• Performance IQ	95.50 ± 11.07	77–112
• Digit Span	7.74 ± 2.05	4–11
• Vocabulary	9.83 ± 2.15	7–14
• Arithmetic	9.05 ± 2.53	6–14
• Picture Completion	8.56 ± 2.06	5–11
• Picture Arrangement	9.44 ± 2.36	5–15
• Block Design	9.61 ± 2.79	5–16
• Object Assembly	9.17 ± 2.81	5–13
• Digit Symbol	8.79 ± 2.30	6–12
Woodcock–Johnson–Revised Psychoeducational Battery		
• Letter–Word Identification	105.06 ± 13.83	80–128
• Passage Comprehension	105.81 ± 12.63	89–128
• Calculations	108.44 ± 14.50	86–136
• Applied Problems	99.00 ± 9.30	85–121

suggest, however that should a specific patient have a marked disability in a particular cognitive skill (e.g., math), more emphasis should be given to those effort tasks that do not strongly involve the compromised skill, and that several different effort tests be administered to lower the possibility of false-positive identification; none of our subjects failed more than two tests.

In conclusion, while it was suspected that a population with LD might be at particular risk of failure on the cognitive malingering tests due to the impact of the disabilities on task execution, this hypothesis was not confirmed. However, a concern regarding the findings is that the sample may not be representative of the entire adult population with LD. Although the subjects in this study were identified as LD by campus LD specialists, and were receiving services through the campus disabled student agency, their achievement scores as a group were within the average range. One explanation is that ceiling effects on achievement tests may limit their usefulness for detection of disabilities in college students (Hughes & Smith, 1990). In addition, it is likely that the population was only mildly to moderately disabled in that there appears to be a self-selection process such that individuals with LD who attend college are less disabled than those individuals who do not attempt college. College students with LD have significantly higher reading and math achievement scores than students with LD who do not attend college (Hughes & Smith, 1990; Miller, Snider, & Rzonca, 1990). As a group, college students with LD have been reported to perform within the average range (i.e., within 1 standard deviation of the normative mean) on achievement testing (Cordoni & Snyder, 1981; Morris & Leuenberger, 1990). It is relevant to note that the Woodcock–Johnson–Revised Psychoeducational scores of this sample are virtually identical to those reported in literature on college students with LD (Gajar, Salvia, Gajria, & Salvia, 1989). The higher Verbal IQ relative to Performance IQ observed in the sample has also been reported in other college-level subjects with LD (Blalock, 1987; Gajar, Murphy, & Hunt, 1982; Minskoff, Hawks, Steidle, & Hoffman, 1989). This sample is likely representative of the college population with LD but may differ from adult individuals with LD who have not attempted post-high school education. As such, conclusions regarding effort test performance may only apply to the former group. Additional research is needed to determine whether individuals with more severe LD with less than a college education show similar false-positive rates and comparable relationships between IQ/achievement scores and malingering test performance.

The dataset from this investigation was subsequently employed in validation studies of the Dot Counting Test (Boone, Lu, & Herzberg, 2002b), the b Test (Boone et al., 2000; Boone, Lu, & Herzberg, 2002a), the Rey 15-Item Test plus recognition trial (Boone, Salazar, et al., 2002), and Rey Word Recognition Test (Nitch, Boone, Wen, Arnold, & Alfano, 2006). Examination of scores specific to these later publications shows that two subjects fell below the cutoff of < 20 for the Rey 15-Item equation incorporating recall plus recognition minus false positives (94% specificity). No subject exceeded the Dot Counting Test E-score cutoff of ≥ 17, and use of a cutoff of ≥ 13 was associated with adequate specificity (≥ 90%). On the b Test, no subject committed more than three "d" commission errors, committed more than four commission errors in general, or required more than 750 seconds to complete the b Test, although the E-score cutoff had to be raised to ≥ 140 to maintain specificity of ≥ 90%. On the Rey Word Recognition Test, no male subject obtained a score of < 5 and no female subject obtained a score < 7, and no male subject obtained a weighted recognition score (i.e., recognition minus false positives plus the first eight words on the list recognized) ≤ 7 and no female subject obtained a score ≤ 10. Thus, these cutoffs appear appropriate for use in the differential diagnosis of actual versus feigned LD.

CASE: MALINGERING IN A PATIENT WITH LD

A 28-year-old male patient with 12 years of education underwent neuropsychological testing at a community mental health clinic for the purposes of determining employability. He complained of poor memory for recent events and conversations, as well as word-finding difficulty and problems with concentration. He indicated that his symptoms developed subsequent to an assault 5 years previously which was not associated with loss of consciousness or posttraumatic amnesia and for which the patient did not seek medical attention. The patient also reported difficulties in reading, writing, and spelling dating from grade school, although as a student he had refused to undergo formal testing to ascertain the nature and extent of his learning disability. His poor academic skills had a substantial impact on his subsequent occupational functioning as a security guard (e.g., he had difficulty with report writing and copied reports of coworkers). During the examination, the patient was judged to have put forth inadequate effort as demonstrated by failed performance on 4 effort indicators, including the TOMM (Trial 1 = 13, Trial 2 = 17, Retention = 20), the b Test (E-score = 777), the Dot counting Test (E-score = 25), and Reliable Digit Span (5; cutoff ≤ 6; Babikian, Boone, Lu, & Arnold, 2006), although he passed the Rey 15-Item plus recognition trial (23; cutoff < 20; Boone, Salazar, et al., 2002), a RAVLT effort equation (15; cutoff ≤ 12; Boone, Lu, & Wen, 2005), a Rey–Osterrieth effort equation (53; cutoff ≤ 47; Lu et al., 2003), and dominant hand finger tapping (43.4; cutoff ≤ 35 for men; Arnold et al., 2005). Results of neuropsychological testing revealed borderline to impaired scores (i.e., ≤ 8th percentile) on the majority of measures, and both Verbal and Performance IQ were with the extremely low/mentally retarded range (Verbal IQ = 61; Performance IQ = 68).

Six weeks after initial testing, the patient was referred for evaluation at the neuropsychology service at Harbor–UCLA Medical Center by an attorney representing the patient in an attempt to obtain disability compensation. The patient denied undergoing any previous cognitive testing, which suggested that he had received feedback that his performance was not credible. On second exam, nine effort indicators were administered, all of which the patient passed, including the Rey 15-Item Test plus recognition trial (28), the b Test (E-score = 40), the Dot Counting Test (E-score = 13), the Warrington Recognition Memory Test (42; cut-off < 33; Iverson & Franzen, 1994), the Rey–Osterrieth (RO) effort equation (55), Reliable Digit Span (7), a RAVLT/RO discriminant function (1.343; cutoff ≤ -.40; Sherman, Boone, Lu, & Razani, 2002), finger tapping dominant (36); and Rey Word Memory Test (11; cutoff for men ≤ 5; Nitch et al., 2006). Results of cognitive testing on this evaluation now revealed a Performance IQ in the low average range (Performance IQ = 81) while Verbal IQ was in the borderline range (Verbal IQ = 71), and the patient was demonstrating low average to average visual perceptual/spatial and constructional skills, visual memory, and executive abilities (9th–63rd percentiles). In contrast, deficits in language (3rd–4th percentiles) and attention (5th percentile) were still apparent; word list recall was borderline (7th percentile) while recall of story details was nearly average (24th percentile); and word reading speed had improved by nearly 50% although it was still impaired (< 1st percentile). Thus, on second testing, a test profile consistent with a language-based learning disability emerged.

Although conclusions should be drawn cautiously from a single case, the data do suggest that several effort indicators (b Test, Dot Counting, Reliable Digit Span, Forced-Choice paradigms) may be appropriate for use in individuals with substantial language-based learning disability in that they detected non-credible performance when it was present but were passed when the patient with LD performed with adequate effort.

CONCLUSIONS

The possibility of feigned LD and/or ADHD in older adolescents and adults has been underappreciated and understudied, although emerging prevalence data suggest that malingered LD and/or ADHD, at least in the context of university learning disorder clinics, may be as common as that found in personal injury litigants and disability seekers.

The minimal data available for subjects with LD suggest that standard effort tests are generally passed by individuals with actual disability and thus are likely appropriate for clinical use in the differential diagnosis of actual versus feigned LD. However, LD false-positive rates are not available for all effort measures, and false-positive rates may differ based on specific learning disability subtype; therefore, specificity data are needed for additional effort measures and in homogeneous subgroups of subjects with LD. In addition, the available effort test data have been obtained on college student subjects with LD who may represent the mild end of the LD continuum; effort test false-positive rates need to be assessed in subjects with more severe LD. Finally, emerging evidence suggests that effort tests specifically designed to detect LD may be more effective than standard effort indices that target feigned memory symptoms.

Regarding ADHD, some standard CPT measures appear to have potential not only to detect feigned attentional disorders per se but also to identify feigned cognitive symptoms such as those claimed by brain injury patients, although these data require replication. Of concern, no information is currently available on effort test false-positive rates in subjects with actual ADHD, raising concerns regarding the use of these measures in subjects with claimed attentional symptoms.

REFERENCES

American Psychiatric Association. (1994). *Diagnostic and statistical manual of mental disorders* (4th ed.). Washington, DC: Author.

Arnold, G., Boone, K. B., Lu, P., Dean, A., Wen, J., Nitch, S., & McPherson, S. (2005). Sensitivity and specificity of finger tapping test scores for the detection of suspect effort. *The Clinical Neuropsychologist, 19,* 105–120.

Babikian, T., Boone, K. B., Lu, P., & Arnold, B. (2006). Sensitivity and specificity of various Digit Span scores in the detection of suspect effort. *The Clinical Neuropsychologist, 20,* 145–159.

Blalock, J. W. (1987). Intellectual levels and patterns. In D. J. Johnson & J. W. Blalock (Eds.), *Adults with learning disabilities: Clinical studies* (pp. 47–66). Orlando, FL: Grune & Stratton.

Boone, K. B., Lu, P., Back, C., King, C., Lee, A., Philpott, L., et al. (2002). Sensitivity and specificity of the Rey Dot Counting Test in patients with suspect effort and various clinical samples. *Archives of Clinical Neuropsychology, 17,* 625–642.

Boone, K. B., Lu, P., & Herzberg, D. (2002a). *The b Test.* Los Angeles: Western Psychological Services.

Boone, K. B., Lu, P., & Herzberg, D. (2002b). *The Dot Counting Test.* Los Angeles: Western Psychological Services.

Boone, K. B., Lu, P., Sherman, D., Palmer, B., Back, C., Shamieh, E., et al. (2000). Validation of a new technique to detect malingering of cognitive symptoms: The b test. *Archives of Clinical Neuropsychology, 15,* 227–241.

Boone, K. B., Lu, P., & Wen, J. (2005). Comparison of various RAVLT scores in the detection of noncredible memory performance. *Archives of Clinical Neuropsychology, 20,* 310–319.

Boone, K. B., Salazar, X., Lu, P., Warner-Chacon, K., & Razani, J. (2002). The Rey 15-Item recognition trial: A technique to enhance sensitivity of the Rey 15-Item memorization test. *Journal of Clinical and Experimental Neuropsychology, 24,* 561–573.

Conti, R. (2004). Malingered ADHD in adolescents diagnosed with conduct disorder: A brief note. *Psychological Reports, 94,* 987–988.

Cordoni, B. K., & Snyder, M. K. (1981). A comparison of learning disabled college students' achievement from WRAT and PIAT grade, standard, and subtest scores. *Psychology in the Schools, 18,* 28–34.

Forbes, G. (1998). Clinical utility of the test of variables of attention (TOVA) in the diagnosis of attention deficit hyperactivity disorder. *Journal of Clinical Psychology*, *54*(4), 461–476.

Gajar, A., Murphy, J., & Hunt, F. (1982). A university program for learning disabled students. *Reading Improvement*, *19*, 282–288.

Gajar, A., Salvia, J., Gajria, M., & Salvia, S. (1989). A comparison of intelligence achievement discrepancies between learning disabled and non-learning disabled college students. *Learning Disabilities Research*, *4*, 119–124.

Greiffenstein, M. F., Baker, W. J., & Gola, T. (1996). Comparison of multiple scoring methods for Rey's malingered amnesia measures. *Archives of Clinical Neuropsychology*, *11*, 283–293.

Henry, G. K. (2005). Probable malingering and performance on the test of variables of attention. *The Clinical Neuropsychologist*, *19*, 121–129.

Hiscock, M., & Hiscock, C. K. (1989). Refining the forced method for the detection of malingering. *Journal of Clinical and Experimental Neuropsychology*, *11*, 967–974.

Hughes, C. A., & Smith, J. O. (1990). Cognitive and academic performance of college students with learning disability: A synthesis of the literature. *Learning Disability Quarterly*, *13*, 66–79.

Iverson, G. L., & Franzen, M. D. (1994). The Recognition Memory Test Digit Span and Knox Cube Test as markers of malingered memory impairment. *Assessment*, *1*, 323–334.

Larrabee, G. (2003). Detection of malingering using atypical performance patterns on standard neuropsychological tests. *The Clinical Neuropsychologist*, *17*, 410–425.

Leark, R. A., Dixon, D, Hoffman, T., & Huynh, D. (2002). Fake bad test response bias effects on the test of variables of attention. *Archives of Clinical Neuropsychology*, *17*, 335–342.

Lezak, M. D. (1983). *Neuropsychological assessment* (2nd ed.). New York: Oxford University Press.

Lezak, M. D. (1995). *Neuropsychological assessment* (3rd ed.). New York: Oxford University Press.

Losier, B., McGrath, P., & Klein, R. (1996). Error patterns on the Continuous Performance Test in non-medicated and medicated samples of children with and without ADHD: A meta-analytic review. *Journal of Child Psychology and Psychiatry and Allied Disciplines*, *37*, 971–987.

Lu, P. H., & Boone, K. B. (2002). Suspect cognitive symptoms in a 9-year-old child: Malingering by proxy? *The Clinical Neuropsychologist*, *16*(1), 90–96.

Lu, P., Boone, K. B., Jimenez, N., & Razani, J. (2004). Failure to inhibit the reading response on the Stroop Test: A pathognomonic indicator of suspect effort. *Journal of Clinical and Experimental Neuropsychology*, *26*, 180–189.

Miller, D. (2004, December 6). Difficult for test-takers to fake learning disabilities. *Daily Bruin*.

Miller, R. J., Snider, B., & Rzonca, C. (1990). Variables related to the decision of young adults with learning disabilities to participate in postsecondary education. *Journal of Learning Disabilities*, *23*, 349–354.

Minskoff, E. H., Hawks, R., Steidle, E. F., & Hoffman, F. J. (1989). A homogenous group of persons with learning disabilities: Adults with severe learning disabilities in vocational rehabilitation. *Journal of Learning Disabilities*, *22*, 521–528.

Mitrushina, M. N., Boone, K. B., & D'Elia, L. F. (1999). *Handbook of normative data for neuropsychological assessment.* New York: Oxford University Press.

Mittenberg, W. M., Patton, C., Canyock, E. M., & Condit, D. C. (2002). Base rates of malingering and symptom exaggeration. *Journal of Clinical and Experimental Neuropsychology, 24*(8), 1094–1102.

Morris, M., & Leuenberger, J. (1990). A report of cognitive, academic, and linguistic profiles for college students with and without learning disabilities. *Journal of Learning Disabilities, 23*, 355–385.

Murphy, K., & Barkley, R. A. (1996). Attention deficit hyperactivity disorder in adults: Comorbidities and adaptive impairments. *Comprehensive Psychiatry, 37*, 393–401.

Nitch, S., Boone, K. B., Wen, J., Arnold, G., & Alfano, K. (2006). The utility of the Rey Word Recognition Test in the detection of suspect effort. *The Clinical Neuropsychologist, 20*, 873–887.

Osmon, D. C., Plambeck, E., Klein, L., & Mano, Q. (2006). The word reading test of effort in adult learning disability: A simulation study. *The Clinical Neuropsychologist, 20*, 315–324.

Quinn, C. A. (2003). Detection of malingering is assessment of adult ADHD. *Archives of Clinical Neuropsychology, 18*, 379–395.

Sandford, J. A., & Turner, A. (1995). *Intermediate visual and auditory continuous performance test interpretation manual.* Richmond, VA: Braintrain.

Sattler, J. M. (1988). *Clinical and forensic interviewing of children and families–Guidelines for mentally health, education, pediatric, and child maltreatment fields.* San Diego: Author.

Sherman, D. S., Boone, K. B., Lu, P., & Razani, J. (2002). Re-examination of a Rey auditory verbal learning test/Rey complex figure discriminant function to detect suspect effort. *The Clinical Neuropsychologist, 16*(3), 242–250.

Slick, D. J., Sherman, E. M. S., & Iverson, G. L. (1999). Diagnostic criteria for malingered neurocognitive dysfunction: Proposed standards for clinical practice and research. *The Clinical Neuropsychologist, 13*, 545–561.

Stutts, J. T., Hickey, S. E., & Kasdan, M. L. (2003). Malingering by proxy: A form of pediatric condition falsification. *Developmental and Behavioral Pediatrics, 24*(4), 276–278.

U.S. Department of Justice. (2004). *A guide to disability rights laws.* Washington, DC: Civil Rights Division Disability Rights.

Warner-Chacon, K. (1994). *The performance of adults with learning disabilities on cognitive tests of malingering.* Unpublished doctoral dissertation, California School of Professional Psychology.

Youngjohn, J. R., Burrows, L., & Erdal, K. (1995). Brain damage or compensation neurosis? The controversial post-concussion syndrome. *The Clinical Neuropsychologist, 9*, 112–123.

CHAPTER 17

Cognitive Complaints in Multiple Chemical Sensitivity and Toxic Mold Syndrome

Robert J. McCaffrey
Christine L. Yantz

Conditions with unexplained symptoms, such as multiple chemical sensitivity and toxic mold syndrome, have received much attention, despite controversy surrounding the supporting research. Although there have been studies demonstrating correlations between the health impairments and the presence of low levels of chemicals and various toxigenic molds or mycotoxins, the current research on these topics cannot support a causal link between exposure to these "toxicants" and subsequent impairments or complaints. Psychological factors appear to play a role in the symptoms associated with both of these syndromes. This chapter provides background on both of these diagnoses, detailing the research that has focused on neuropsychological correlates of the conditions. We also discuss methods that can be used to clarify the nature of these conditions, including the use of controlled experimentation and the inclusion of symptom validity tests in future studies of these populations.

MULTIPLE CHEMICAL SENSITIVITY

Multiple chemical sensitivity (MCS; also sometimes referred to as idiopathic environmental intolerance) has been defined as a disorder with a range of somatic, cognitive, and affective symptoms alleged to result from exposure to extremely low levels of various chemicals. Symptoms frequently associated with MCS are headache, fatigue, confusion, depression, shortness of breath, arthralgia, myalgia, nausea, dizziness, memory difficulties, and gastrointestinal and respiratory problems (Labarge & McCaffrey, 2000). A main controversy surrounding the existence of MCS concerns the extent to which psychological factors play a role in symptom manifestation. In fact, individuals whose occupations expose them to chemicals (e.g., construction and manufacturing) are less likely to have been diagnosed with MCS than are people in low-chemical-exposure settings (e.g., education, health care; Cullen, Pace, & Redlich, 1992; Ross, 1992). Researchers frequently have reported that people who have received a diagnosis of MCS have a higher than expected level of psychiatric problems. For example, one study of 264 "environmental patients" found that 75% met DSM-IV criteria for at least one psychiatric disorder, and in only five cases were toxic chemicals determined to be the most probable cause of the presented symptoms (Bornschein, Hausteiner, Zilker, & Forstl, 2002). Similarly, Simon, Daniell, Stockbridge, Claypoole, and Rosenstock (1993) documented that 44% of their sample of 41 MCS patients had a depressive or anxiety disorder, and that 25% met criteria for somatization disorder *prior to* the chemical sensitivity. The potential somatoform nature of MCS was illustrated by case of a woman with a 10-year history of disability attributed to MCS and who complained of chemical-elicited seizures but was shown to have no electroencephalograph (EEG) abnormalities when seizures were experimentally induced by presentation of fragrances (Staudenmayer & Kramer, 1999).

Recent research has focused on the role of learning and sensitization in the symptom presentation of MCS. Specifically, the conceptualization framework used to understand anxiety disorders, such as posttraumatic stress disorder and panic disorder, has been applied to MCS (Devriese et al., 2000; Sorg & Newlin, 2002; Van den Bergh, Winters, Devriese, & Van Diest, 2002). One study found that persons with MCS had higher self-reported scores of agoraphobia, anxiety, and stress compared to normal controls (Poonai et al., 2001). Three separate investigators have each described cases of women with MCS symptom complaints suspected to be related to long-standing anxiety-based disorders (Black, 2002; Stenn & Binkley, 1998; Temple, 2003). After treatment targeting the anxiety disorder, chemical sensitivity reactions were markedly reduced in all three cases. This success of psychological interventions in reducing MCS symptomatology is a strong indicator that psychological factors are at play in individuals with a diagnosis of MCS. Furthermore, these studies suggest that persons diagnosed with MCS may misattribute their symptoms to chemical exposure and not to their preexisting anxiety disorder.

Several studies of MCS have used a double-blind, placebo-controlled challenge test method, in which participants are exposed to either a "placebo" or a chemical to which they are reportedly sensitive (Leznoff, 1997;

Rea et al., 1990; Staudenmayer, Selner, & Buhr, 1993). If the sensitivity exists, the individual would be expected to react to the chemical and not the placebo. For the greatest level of experimental control, the double-blind condition requires that both the experimenter and the participant are blind to the sample's status (i.e., chemical or placebo). There are some difficulties in applying this procedure to MCS studies, including the difficulty in masking differences between placebos and test chemicals (often with distinct odors) and the requirement of a controlled test environment without any other substances to which the participants may potentially react. Because of these limitations, the results from these studies are still somewhat equivocal; however, the null results of the Staudenmayer et al. (1993) study (i.e., persons with MCS responded similarly to either chemical or placebo) has been used as evidence of the dissociation between chemical exposure and reported symptoms. As further confirmation, Simon et al. (1993) found that immunological testing (autoantibody titers, lymphocyte surface markers, and interleukin-1 generation by monocytes) did not differentiate MCS patients from controls.

Despite the controversial nature of the diagnosis, some within the general public and legal system have been premature in viewing the alleged condition as a credible disorder, which has led to some absurd situations. In a 2003 Associated Press article, it was reported that prosecutors had charged a woman with aggravated battery for "dousing herself with perfume, spraying the house with bug killer and disinfectant, and burning scented candles in an attempt to seriously injure her chemically sensitive husband" who allegedly had developed his symptoms secondary to exposure to toxic mold and hazardous chemicals during his employment as a construction worker. He had been awarded $150,000 in workers' compensation benefits but refused to give his estranged wife half of his settlement, prompting her actions. However, the wife's attorney claimed, "The guy's a faker. He just wanted to gain an advantage in the divorce case" (Associated Press, 2003).

MCS and Neuropsychological Performance

Several studies have examined the neuropsychological performances of persons with a diagnosis of MCS. Fiedler, Maccia, and Kipen (1992) reported that 4 of 11 MCS patients showed lowered cognitive scores when compared to normative standards; however, in a subsequent study (Fiedler, Kipen, Deluca, Kelly-McNeil, & Natelson, 1996) examining 23 MCS patients compared against normal controls and chronic fatigue patients, the MCS patients were only lower than controls on a single test score (false positives on the Continuous Visual Memory Test) and scored comparably to chronic fatigue patients. Simon et al. (1993) compared cognitive performance of 41 MCS patients against that of 34 controls and found lowered scores in the MCS sample on immediate recall/learning of verbal information (Rey Auditory Verbal Learning Test [RAVLT], Weschsler Memory Scale [WMS] Paired Associates) but after control for anxiety and depression as measured by the Symptom Checklist 90–Revised (SCL-90-R), group differences disappeared. Bolla (1996) compared 17 self-referred individuals with a diagnosis of MCS, 16 chemically exposed patients with no symptoms of MCS, and 126 healthy controls on tests of verbal and visual learning and memory, executive functioning, and psychomotor functioning (RAVLT, Symbol Digit, Digit Symbol, Trailmaking Test A and B, and visual reaction time). MCS subjects only scored significantly below controls on Symbol Digit, whereas the chemically exposed subjects without MCS scored significantly below controls on Symbol Digit, Digit Symbol, Trailmaking Test B, and visual reaction time, leading Bolla to conclude that patients with MCS do not show evidence of compromised central nervous system function. Similarly, Osterberg, Orbaek, and Karlson (2002) compared 17 individuals with a diagnosis of MCS to 34 matched controls on Digit Symbol and tests of verbal memory, reaction time, complex and sustained attention, and executive function. Groups significantly differed on only one of 17 test scores, leading the authors to conclude that the MCS patients showed "a basically normal pattern of results across the neuropsychological tests. . . . (The) single deviation can hardly be taken as evidence of an organic brain dysfunction in MCS patients" (p. 144).

In contrast to the foregoing studies which found virtually no cognitive abnormalities in MCS subjects, Ziem and McTamney (1997) reported prominent neuropsychological impairment in 13 MCS patients assessed with the Halstead–Reitan Neuropsychological Battery (HRNB) and the Wechsler Adult Intelligence Scale–Revised (WAIS-R). Six subjects were reported to have a Verbal IQ > Performance IQ split, and impairment rates of > 40% were cited for six HRNB subtests (Category Test, Tactual Performance Test, Seashore Rhythm Test, Speech Sounds Perception Test, Finger Tapping, and Trailmaking). However, no control group was used, only subjects reporting cognitive symptoms were tested, and an unspecified number of the larger pool of MCS patients recruited were in litigation. Further, personality test data were apparently not collected, which would be especially important for the interpretation of these results, given that Ziem and McTamney (1997) report that fibromyalgia and chronic fatigue syndrome were common among their patients (at levels of 75% and 85%, respectively). Of most concern, no symptom validity tests were administered to verify that patients were, in fact, performing with adequate effort. In fact, examination of embedded effort indices contained within the tests administered showed that 5 of 13 subjects failed at least one (i.e., one patient failed five indicators, one failed four, one failed three, one failed two, and two failed one). Specifically, four patients made ≥ 8 errors on the Seashore Rhythm Test (Trueblood & Schmidt, 1993), three required ≥ 63 seconds to complete Trailmaking Test A (Iverson, Lange, Green, & Frazen, 2002), two obtained Digit Span Age Correlated Scaled Scores ≤ 5 (Babikian, Boone, Lu, &

Arnold, 2006), two scored ≤ 28 on Finger Tapping dominant hand (Arnold et al., 2005), two obtained a Vocabulary minus Digit Span difference score of ≥ 6 (Iverson & Tulsky, 2003; Miller, Ryan, Carruthers, & Cluff, 2004), and one made more than 17 errors on the Speech Sounds Perception Test (Trueblood & Schmidt, 1993).

Of relevance, two recent publications utilizing the Minnesota Multiphasic Personality Inventory–2 (MMPI-2) in MCS claimants reported elevated Fake Bad Scale scores (e.g., mean of 27; Binder, Storzbach, & Salinsky, 2006; Staudenmayer & Phillips, 2007) in their samples, a pattern of performance reflective of the presence of non-credible physical complaints (Larrabee, 1998).

The available data would suggest that individuals claiming MCS show only isolated lowered scores which may simply reflect the impact of concurrent depression, inflated type I error due to multiple comparisons, or normal variability (75% of normal individuals administered a neuropsychological battery obtained one borderline or impaired score [≤ 5th percentile], and 20% obtained two lowered scores [Palmer, Boone, Lesser, & Wohl, 1998]). From their review of MCS, Labarge and McCaffrey (2000) concluded that "there is insufficient evidence to conclusively settle the question of the etiology of the variety of symptom pictures that are classified as MCS, [but] there does not appear to be compelling evidence to suggest that MCS results solely from toxic effects of chemical exposure" (p. 204).

TOXIC MOLD SYNDROME

Like exposure to high levels of certain chemicals, high-level exposure to mycotoxins is known to have health-related consequences. Mycotoxicosis is an accepted, uncontroversial disease associated with acute ingestion or inhalation of toxins produced by mold (mycotoxins). The three undisputed categories of disease that are caused by molds are allergy, infection, and ingestion toxicity (Chapman, Terr, Jacobs, Charlesworth, & Bardana, 2003; Hardin, Kelman, & Saxon, 2003; Terr, 2004). Some persons routinely exposed to moisture-damaged and moldy environments, most frequently homes or workplaces, experience an increase in subjective health complaints, including upper respiratory and gastrointestinal symptoms (Kuhn & Ghannoum, 2003). Similar to MCS, however, speculation about health and cognitive risks of low levels of environmental mold exposure has led to the controversial "toxic mold syndrome." Reported symptoms associated with toxic mold syndrome include headache, cough, dyspnea, diarrhea, nausea, vomiting, memory loss, weakness, and mood variations (Lee, 2003; Nordness, Zacharisen, & Fink, 2003; Platt, Martin, Hunt, & Lewis, 1989; Santilli, 2002; Sudakin, 1998). Interestingly, it has been argued that the toxigenic fungus need not be present for the mycotoxins to produce symptoms (Fung, Clark, & Williams, 1998).

Popular media has sensationalized the idea that exposure to moldy buildings or moldy surfaces can have dire consequences. In 2001, a cover of the *New York Times Magazine*, titled "Lurking, Choking, Toxic Mold," showed a woman in a home wearing a gas mask (Belkin, 2001). A recent, informal internet search of *ABCnews.com* and *CNN.com* for news stories released in the last 4 years revealed seven separate stories with titles suggesting toxic mold has negative health consequences. One effect of high public interest in toxic mold is an increased number of mold-related lawsuits and subsequently raised insurance costs (Barrett, 2003). One lawyer, Edward H. Cross (1999), states that "the new developing area of microbial contamination litigation promises to be a dynamic area of practice—for both experts and lawyers, who can make lasting impressions on juries about novel scientific concepts" (p. 602).

One species of fungi, *Stachybotrys chartarum* (previously referred to as *Stachybotrys atra*), receives the most attention when considering correlations between mold exposure and health impairments. Samples of this genera of *Stachybotrys* fungi are found worldwide, growing in soil and cellulose-rich materials (Fung et al., 1998). This black mold has been found in many of the moisture- and mold-damaged buildings that are alleged to be the environmental causes of health symptoms. Research supporting the disease-producing nature of this fungus is not compelling, although some correlation-based research tends to link the two (Hossain, Ahmed, & Ghannoum, 2004; Kuhn & Ghannoum, 2003). Other toxigenic molds have been suggested to cause health impairments, including *Aspergillus fumigatus*, *Aspergillus versicolor*, *Fusarium incarnatum*, and various *Penicillium* species (Auger et al., 1999; Sobotka, Brodie, & Spaid, 1978).

The majority of the research investigating the effects of toxic mold exposure has focused on physical health, primarily respiratory symptoms. The inhalation of spores or mycotoxins has been associated with allergic alveoliti, or hypersensitivity pneumonitis (Apostolakos, Rossmoore, & Beckett, 2001; Nordness et al., 2003). Symptoms that accompany exposure include a dry cough, dyspnea, high fever, chills, myalgias, and malaise that are alleviated within hours after initial exposure. A correlational study by Terr (2004) found that an increased mold spore level was associated with an increased rate of asthma-related deaths. Infants and young children are suspected to be at greater risk for negative health consequences due to mold exposure. The American Academy of Pediatrics issued a statement recommending the avoidance of exposing infants to chronically moldy environments, due to studies showing a *trend* for idiopathic pulmonary hemorrhage to occur more frequently among mold-exposed infants (Etzel et al., 1998). Respiratory symptoms are also common health complaints of older children and adults who have been exposed to moldy environments; however, psychological factors may play a role in these reports. A recent study by Handal, Leiner, Cabrera, and Straus (2004) examined the level of symptom complaints of children before and after mold status of a school was publicized. These investigators found that the perceptions of coughing and wheezing, headaches, and joint pains increased when it was reported that the school had a mold contamination problem.

Toxic Mold and Neuropsychological Studies

To date, a few studies have attempted to demonstrate a relationship between environmental mold exposure and neuropsychological functioning. In one of the first studies to examine cognitive abilities, Hodgson et al. (1998) found that 26 mold-exposed subjects, some of whom were seeking workers' compensation benefits, actually outperformed controls on the California Verbal Learning Test (CVLT) and Grooved Pegboard.

Gordon, Johanning, and Haddad (1999) assessed the cognitive functioning of 20 mold-exposed individuals who were complaining of cognitive decline; information on the litigation status of the participants was not provided. Using the WAIS-R, WMS-R, CVLT, and Booklet Category Test, six criteria to define cognitive impairment were created: Verbal IQ > Performance IQ by 10 points, WMS Visual Memory Index > Verbal Memory Index by 10 points, WMS General Memory Index > Attention/Concentration Index by 10 points, total responses on the CVLT > 1 standard score below age and gender mean, CVLT Trials 1 and 5 scores both > 1 standard score below age and gender mean, and inability to complete the Booklet Category test or score < 1st percentile. The number of total symptoms (44 possible) reported by the mold-exposed group (93% of the sample had more than 13) was much greater than the amount of symptoms reported by a control sample ($n = 278$, only 4% of which had more than 13 symptoms). All the mold-exposed individuals met at least one criterion for cognitive impairments, and 13 of the 20 met three or more of the criteria, leading the authors to conclude "these findings strongly suggest that long-term exposure to toxigenic molds results in cognitive impairment in some people" (p. 97). However, only the last criterion constructed by the authors for their study would be considered an actual "impairment"; other scores were likely within normal limits. For example, while half of the sample obtained Verbal IQ > Performance IQ by 10 points, mean Performance IQ for the group was average (109), and while the WMS-R Verbal Memory Index was more than 10 points lower than the Visual Memory Index in 60% of the sample, the sample's mean was also average (104). Further, the inconsistent nature of the impairment criteria (i.e., Verbal IQ > Performance IQ, but Visual Memory Index > Verbal Memory Index) suggests that the criteria were selected after performances were scrutinized for patterns, rather than based on a priori hypotheses. In fact, Attention/Concentration Index (ACI) < General Memory Index (GMI) is a marker of poor effort and not a pattern found in true brain dysfunction. Mittenberg, Azrin, Millsaps, and Heilbronner (1993) reported that a GMI/ACI difference score of 9 to 12 is associated with a 60% to 65% probability of malingering, and that attention worse than memory is nonsensical in that "one cannot remember what is not first attended to" (p. 37).

In a follow-up study, Gordon et al. (2004) examined neuropsychological test performance of 31 mold-exposed individuals (29 of whom were in litigation). The Test of Memory Malingering (TOMM) and Rey 15-Item Test were used to rule out malingering and symptom exaggeration. The scores of the mold-exposed patients as a group were within the normal range with the exception of some lowered performances on the CVLT, although > 70% were reported as showing impairments on at least one measure; lowered memory scores were the most common followed by executive disturbances (e.g., reduced scores on the Booklet Category Test and Watson–Glaser Test).

Baldo, Ahmad, and Ruff (2002) studied the neuropsychological performance of 10 people involved in litigation and claiming exposure to varying species of mold in their homes or workplaces for variable lengths of time. The data from these mold-exposed subjects were compared to those of a matched sample of litigants with mild traumatic brain injuries (MTBI). Cognitive complaints included attentional problems, memory loss, and slowed mental processing, but subjects also claimed depressed mood, anxiety, and increased emotionality (e.g., anger and crying more often). The Rey 15-Item Test and the Rey Dot Counting Test were used to rule out malingering, and all subjects were described as having performances within the normal limits. Between one and five mold-exposed patients were reported as scoring < 10th percentile on 16 of 17 cognitive scores, with the most frequent lowered scores noted for visuospatial learning and short-term memory (Rey–Osterrieth Complex Figure Test 3-minute delay, Ruff–Light Trail Learning Test, Block Tapping Test), verbal learning (Selective Reminding Test), and psychomotor speed (Ruff 2 & 7 Selective Attention Test), with scores similar to those found in the MTBI group with the exception of higher Stroop performance in the mold-exposed patients. However, some mold-exposed patients had a number of cognitive deficits while others had fewer problems, with no consistent symptom pattern across the group.

Kilburn (2003) compared 65 self-referred individuals who had mold identified in their homes to 202 subjects who had no known mold or chemical exposures on performance of neurobehavioral tasks. Litigation status was not reported, but all mold-exposed subjects had "consulted the author" regarding their mold exposure. Group comparisons were conducted using "percent predicted" rather than actual test scores. The mold-exposed group was reported to score significantly lower on grip strength, grooved pegboard, Trailmaking A and B, and several subtests of the WAIS-R and WMS-R (Digit Symbol, Vocabulary, Information, Picture Completion, and Logical

Memory) than the control group. No differences between groups were found for fingertip number writing errors, WAIS-R Similarities test, or scores on a nonverbal, nonarithmetic intelligence test (Culture Fair). It was claimed (but not further explained) that recall of the Rey figure was used to rule out malingering. Psychiatric symptoms (all scales of the Profile of Mood States [POMS]) were found to be significantly higher in the mold-exposed group than the control group. Though antibody titers tended to show increased amounts of antibodies to mold and mycotoxins for the exposed group compared to the unexposed group, there was no significant correlation between antibody titer and neurobehavioral impairments. Repeat testing on eight subjects obtained 11 to 20 months after the initial evaluation showed that seven exhibited worse performance and one subject's scores remained unchanged, despite the fact that all eight had vacated their mold-exposed homes. The failure to use standard test scores, and the fact that subjects showed worse cognitive performance over time although they were no longer exposed to mold and that subjects had reduced performances on measures of "overlearned information" (i.e., vocabulary and fund of general information) raise questions regarding the regarding the reliability of the reported data.

Crago et al. (2003) reported that 182 mold-exposed individuals showed lower than expected scores as compared to normative data on the Color Word and Trailmaking subtests of the Delis–Kaplan Executive Function System (D-KEFS), and that several WAIS-III subtests were lower than expected in comparison to the Vocabulary subtest (e.g., attention, working memory, visual motor learning, speed, and visual scanning). While the authors describe the lowered scores as "impairment," in fact mean scores were within normal limits (i.e., ≥ 25th percentile). An unspecified number of subjects were in litigation, but no tests were administered to assess veracity of effort. The authors stated that only 3.8% of the sample reported premorbid psychiatric or neuropsychiatric problems, and they conceded that there were no attempts to validate the participants' self-report of this.

While the foregoing studies overall appear to represent accumulating evidence for the presence of cognitive dysfunction in those alleging exposure to toxic mold, closer examination of the studies reveals major methodological limitations in all. First, some studies failed to administer tests to verify adequacy of effort and to rule out malingering, which is of particular relevance given that most investigations included litigants in the samples (Baldo et al., 2002; Crago et al., 2003; Gordon et al., 2004; Hodgson et al., 1998). Gordon et al. (2004) and Baldo et al. (2002) did employ effort measures which subjects were reported as passing; however, the particular effort tests administered are associated with low sensitivity (i.e., percentage of noncredible subjects correctly identified). For example, the Rey 15-Item Test and TOMM may be associated with less than 50% sensitivity (Boone, Salazar, Lu, Warner-Chacon, & Razani, 2002; Gervais, Rohling, Green, & Ford,

2004), and the version of the Dot Counting Test employed by Baldo and colleagues also shows low effectiveness in identifying noncredible individuals (Vickery, Berry, Inman, Harris, & Orey, 2001). Crago et al. (2003) did not administer effort tests but did report the presence of discrepancies between WAIS Vocabulary and Digit Span subtests which have been found to be indicative of poor effort (Mittenberg et al., 2001). Kilburn (2003) claimed to use the Rey–Osterrieth Complex Figure Test to rule out malingering, but no further information is provided; this test, in its original format, has never been validated as an effort measure. Thus, suboptimal effort was not adequately ruled out in any of these studies.

Further, the presence of concurrent depression could explain any cognitive abnormalities detected. Baldo et al. (2002) reported that the majority (7 of 10) of their toxic mold-exposed patients were depressed (three severe, two moderate, one mild, one minimally) and severity of depression correlated with the number of cognitive impairments, leading the authors to conclude that "accompanying depression may have played a role in the presentation of cognitive deficits in our group of patients" (p. 200). Similarly, despite the fact that subjects with a psychiatric history had been excluded from the Gordon et al. (2004) study, the mean Beck Depression Inventory–II (BDI-II) score was elevated ($n = 20.18$, SD = 10.37), and BDI-II scores were related to the number of cognitive impairments as well as significantly correlated with CVLT scores and Trailmaking Test A performance. In the Crago et al. (2003) study, all SCL-90-R scales were described as significantly elevated, with the four highest scores appearing on the obsessive–compulsive, somatization, depression, and anxiety scales. Similarly, Kilburn (2003) described subjects as depressed based on POMS score. In the Baldo et al. (2002) study, some subjects showed elevations on the MCMI-III somatoform and histrionic scales; this, in conjunction with the Crago et al. (2003) observation of elevations on the SCL-90-R somatization scale, would indicate the frequent presence of a somatoform disorder, in addition to depression, in mold-exposed claimants.

Relevant to the above two points, in a recent report (Stone, Boone, Back-Madruga, & Lesser, 2006) of all mold litigants alleging cognitive dysfunction evaluated by the authors ($n = 6$), two patients were found to show evidence of malingering as demonstrated by failure on multiple cognitive effort tests, while four patients exhibited evidence for a somatoform disorder (as demonstrated by elevations on scales 1 and 3 of the MMPI-2, passed cognitive effort tests, and elevated Fake Bad Scale scores). In the four somatoform patients, cognitive abnormalities were only found in the two individuals who were also depressed.

Finally, additional methodological limitations of the existing empirical reports tying mold exposure to cognitive dysfunction are outlined by Fox, Greiffenstein, and Lees-Haley (2005) and McCaffrey and Yantz (2005), and which include (1) selection bias (i.e., subjects studied were those who presented with complaints rather than a sample of the larger pool of exposed individuals, leading to inherent bias to find deficits), (2) comparison of patient test scores with published normative data in lieu of use of demographically matched control groups (e.g., Gordon et al., 2004, Crago et al., 2003, Baldo et al., 2002) which "is considered a weak form of evidence-based analysis, little better than anecdote" (Fox et al., 2005, p. 131), (3) failure to consider the base rate of isolated low cognitive scores in the normal population (i.e., 98% of individuals administered 25 tests would be expected to perform poorly on one; on an empirical basis, 75% of normal individuals administered a neuropsychological battery obtained one borderline or impaired score [≤ 5th percentile], and 20% obtained two lowered scores; Palmer et al., 1998), (4) two studies (Baldo et al., 2002; Gordon et al., 2004) concluded that the cognitive abnormalities in mold-exposed individuals were comparable to those found in persons with MTBI; however, this is an odd comparison group given that there is extensive empirical evidence showing that any cognitive residuals associated with MTBI tend to disappear within weeks or months postinjury (Dikmen, Ross, Machamer, & Temkin, 1995; Gentilini et al., 1985; Goldstein, Levin, Goldman, Clark, & Altonen, 2001; Millis & Volinsky, 2001; Schretlen & Shapiro, 2003) and that the rate of cognitive symptom feigning in a litigating population with MTBI may approach 50% (Youngjohn, Burrows, & Erdal, 1995), and (5) use of problematic statistical analyses that inflated the Type 1 error rate, increasing the probability of detecting significant (but nonexistent) group differences.

CONCLUSIONS AND CONTROVERSIES REGARDING MCS AND TOXIC MOLD

Research on MCS and toxic mold exposure and their effects has been highly controversial. Some researchers do recommend the avoidance of reactive chemicals or prevention of mold growth but seem to be choosing to "err on the side of caution" rather than basing their conclusions on empirical evidence (King & Auger, 2002; Terr, 1993). Labarge and McCaffrey's (2000) review, as well as others, suggest that there is little evidence that MCS is an organic disorder (Hartman, 1998; Pankratz, 2002; Ross et al., 1999). Similarly, a large number of reviews on health symptoms and mold exposure do not find strong support for the link, besides those of infection, allergy, and ingestion toxicity (Assoulin-Dayan, Leong, Shoenfeld, & Gershwin, 2002; Burr, 2001; Chapman et al., 2003; Fung & Hughson, 2003; Hardin et al., 2003; Robbins, Swenson, Nealley, Gots, & Kelman, 2000; Terr, 2004; Verhoeff & Burge, 1997). Lees-Haley (2003) reached a similar conclusion about the lack of evidence that environmental mold exposure leads to cognitive and psychological outcomes, and Binder and Campbell (2004) classify symptoms associated with environmental mold exposure as lacking demonstrable pathophysiological causes, similar to syndromes such as chronic fatigue syndrome, nonepileptic seizure disorders, and MCS.

Procedures for measurement of toxic mold exposure and methodological flaws of available studies have contributed to discrepant findings across studies. Differing types of sampling methods for measuring fungal presence can result in enormous variations, and deciding what, where, and when to sample can be difficult (Dillon, Miller, Sorenson, Douwes, & Jacobs, 1999; Kuhn & Ghannoum, 2003). To compound this problem, "unhealthy" levels of mold have not been established, though < 1,000 spores/m^3 has been suggested (Santilli & Rockwell, 2003). A further difficulty is that environmental confounds, such as the type of carpeting or presence of a pet, can greatly influence the spore count (Kuhn & Ghannoum, 2003). Even if these factors are controlled, establishing causality between mold exposure and subsequent health complaints is difficult for a number of reasons. First, in water-damaged buildings, a number of potentially toxic microorganisms, not just molds, grow, and these other microorganisms could contribute to symptom presentation. In fact, one study demonstrated that bacteria can actually cause stronger inflammatory responses in human and mouse cells than mold spores (Huttunen, Hyvarinen, Nevalainen, Komulainen, & Hirvonen, 2003). Also, the damp environments that are ideal for fungal growth foster many species at once (Jarvis, 2002; Kuhn & Ghannoum, 2003), so that parsing out which, among various, potentially toxic species, seems to be linked with toxic mold syndrome would be impossible without using an experimental design. Despite this, sampling techniques commonly test preferentially for *Stachybotrys* species, while minimally examining the presence of other microorganisms, leading to the higher links of symptom complaints with this mold (Kuhn & Ghannoum, 2003). Finally, the presence of a potentially toxigenic fungus does not necessarily mean that mycotoxins have been formed, as mycotoxin production requires a specific balance of pH, moisture, nutrients, and temperature that varies between fungi strains (Kuhn & Ghannoum, 2003).

Another concern about attributing health consequences to exposure to chemical or mold exposure is that other forms of building pollution could be overlooked. Sabir, Shashikiran, and Kochar (1999) review different types of indoor pollutants, including smoke, nitrogen dioxide, carbon monoxide, biological agents (including mold), formaldehyde and other volatile organic compounds, and radon. All these pollutants can cause some of the symptomatology that some researchers suggest are related to MCS or toxic mold. Evacuating the problematic environment, the most frequent method of alleviating the symptoms, would relieve exposure to all these various pollutants. Therefore, exposure to all these other toxic substances must be ruled out before the causal nature of MCS or mold can be suggested.

Statistical analyses of studies have also been flawed. Two studies examining MCS and neuropsychological functioning and two others addressing toxic mold syndrome and its effects employed a "power inflating" sampling technique. For example, Bolla (1996) examined 7.4 times the number of controls relative to MCS subjects, and Osterberg et al. (2002) recruited 2 times the number of controls. Similarly, Kilburn's (2003) study of mold employed 3.2 times the number of controls while Gordon et al. (2004) included 13.9 times as many controls as mold-exposed individuals. These disproportionate control group-weighted designs are biased in terms of detecting differences that may not have any clinical significance. Further, many of the researchers studying the effects of MCS or mycotoxins use their results to imply the causal role of chemical or mold exposure on health impairments, when only correlational analyses or use of nonrandomized group methodology has been employed (Kuhn & Ghannoum, 2003; Reynolds, 1999). In their paper, "Statistical Methods in Psychology Journals: Guidelines and Explanations," Wilkinson and the Task Force on Statistical Inference (1999) comment that

> inferring causality from nonrandomized designs is a risky enterprise. Researchers using nonrandomized designs have an extra obligation to explain the logic behind covariates included in their designs and to alert the reader to plausible rival hypotheses that might explain their results. Even in randomized experiments, attributing causal effects of any one aspect of the treatment condition requires support form additional experimentation. (p. 600)

In addition, studies have used self-selected MCS or mold-exposed individuals, who are, by definition, the subset of people experiencing symptoms; there are much larger samples of exposed individuals who do not report symptoms and who are apparently asymptomatic. Also, the measurement of health effects as reported in studies is problematic, with most relying on retrospective and self-report questionnaires (Kuhn & Ghannoum, 2003; Labarge & McCaffrey, 2000). Lees-Haley and Brown (1992) described biases in perceiving and reporting reactions following "toxic" exposures and suggested that prior beliefs, influence of the media, self-perception, influence of others, and forensic environment may influence a person's symptom report following perceived exposure to a chemical. In addition, some literature has shown that personal injury claimants without a history of toxic exposure or central nervous system injury report high rates of the types of neuropsychiatric problems that have been alleged to be associated with toxic exposure (Dunn, Lees-Haley, Brown, Williams, & English, 1995). Of interest, one report of the mass psychosomatic presentation of illness symptoms in 58 (of 200) students immunized with tetanus toxoid, indicated that there was no organic basis for the symptoms of giddiness, headache, vomiting, and restlessness that were reported after immunization was administered, demonstrating the power of psychosocial factors in presentation of somatic symptoms (Gupta, Vohra, Madaan, & Gaur, 2001). Thus, the impact of suggestion may also play a role in the development of MCS and toxic mold syndrome.

Further, authors tend to report only postchemical or mold-exposure complaints, not participants' prior health, psychological, or cognitive status. A recent study of children exposed to mold-infested school buildings (measured with air, floor, and ventilation sampling techniques) found that these children had increased complaints of eye and throat irritation, headache, concentration problems, and dizziness as floor dust mold level increased (Meyer et al., 2004). However, logistic regression analyses revealed that presence of asthma, hay fever, recent respiratory infection, or psychosocial factors were stronger covariates than mold exposure. This study shows that although mold may be correlated with reported symptoms, premorbid and concurrent factors may contribute to reported abnormalities. Depression has also been shown to be related to symptom complaints and cognitive impairments (Gunstad & Suhr, 2004; Iverson & Lange, 2003; Sawchyn, Brulot, & Strauss, 2000; Suhr & Gunstad, 2002), strengthening the argument for a potential psychological underpinning for MCS and toxic mold syndrome complaints; in fact, depression has been found to be associated with cognitive performance in both of these syndromes (e.g., Baldo et al., 2002; Gordon et al., 2004; Labarge & McCaffrey, 2000).

In addition to these confounds, the frequent litigating status of chemical or mold-exposed subjects creates a strong impetus for these individuals to claim, and even fabricate, symptoms and impairments. Given this context, it is a particular concern that no studies of MCS and only some studies of toxic mold exposure have reported using any measures to assess for overreporting or exaggeration of symptom complaints, and the measures that have been used have been problematic, as discussed previously. A recent survey of the American Board of Clinical Neuropsychology members found that 27% of persons seeking financial compensation for neurotoxic disorders received a diagnosis of probable malingerer (Mittenberg, Patton, Canyock, & Condit, 2002). van Hout, Schmand, Wekking, Hageman, and Deelman (2003) recently examined performances of 185 patients with suspected chronic toxic encephalopathy on two symptom validity tests (the Amsterdam Short-Term Memory Test and the TOMM) and found that only 54% of the sample was determined to have adequate effort on both tests when using cutoff scores chosen for a specificity of 99%, suggesting that suboptimal effort may be problematic for this type of alleged toxicant-exposed sample. Similarly, Bianchini et al. (2003) demonstrated with four cases of suspected neurocognitive deficits following neurotoxic exposure that neuropsychological deficits could be attributed to inadequate effort, using the Slick criteria for malingered neurocognitive deficit (Slick, Sherman, & Iverson, 1999) and eight separate symptom validity measures.

These results indicate that use of symptom validity tests should be considered crucial in the assessment of neuropsychological status in chemical- and mold-exposed cases. Currently there are numerous, well-validated dedicated measures, as well as indices derived from standard cognitive tests,

many discussed in this book. In the Stone et al. (2006) case report of six litigating mold-exposed individuals, one identified malingerer failed 3 of 6 measures, while the second failed 8 of 12 measures, indicating that numerous
effort measures should be administered; if only one or two had been
obtained in these cases, malingering may not have been detected. Further,
rather than relying on self-report of psychiatric status, it is imperative that
objective, psychometrically sound personality inventories be administered to
assess the nature and extent of psychiatric conditions. In the Stone et al.
(2006) case series of somatoform and malingering toxic mold-exposed
patients, all subjects showed significant elevations on the hypochondriasis
and hysteria scales of the MMPI-2, and cognitive abnormalities were found
only in those credible subjects with concurrent depression. Recently, there
have been reports in the literature regarding the use of the Fake Bad Scale
(FBS), which was empirically derived from a subset of items on the MMPI-2
and has been demonstrated to be efficacious in the identification of
examinees who are exaggerating either cognitive/neuropsychological complaints or their degree of emotional distress (Lees-Haley, English, & Glenn,
1991). In the Stone et al. (in press) series of mold-exposed cases, five of six
had elevations on the FBS, consistent with either somatoform presentation
or malingering. Thus, it is recommended that the FBS also be included in
examination of mold and MCS claimants. Reliability of symptom report
should be further buttressed by obtaining a thorough medical and psychosocial history.

Until methodologically sound research is conducted and replicated that
reveals that chemical exposure causes MCS or that mold exposure causes
toxic mold syndrome, the best conclusion is that MCS and mold-related complaints are driven by psychological factors, or in the case of litigation, possible frank malingering.

REFERENCES

Apostolakos, M. J., Rossmoore, H., & Beckett, W. S. (2001). Hypersensitivity pneumonitis from ordinary residential exposures. *Environmental Health Perspectives*,
109, 979–981.

Arnold, G., Boone, K. B., Lu, P., Dean, A., Wen, J., Nitch, S., et al. (2005). Sensitivity
and specificity of Finger Tapping scores for the detection of suspect effort. *The
Clinical Neuropsychologist*, *19*, 105–120.

Associated Press. (2003, May 1). Wife arrested in aroma assault. *CNN News*.

Assoulin-Dayan, Y., Leong, A., Shoenfeld, Y., & Gershwin, M. E. (2002). Studies of
sick building syndrome. IV. Mycotoxicosis. *The Journal of Asthma*, *39*, 191–201.

Auger, P., Pepin, P., Miller, J. D., Gareis, M., Doyon, J., Bouchard, R., et al. (1999).
Chronic toxic encephalopathies apparently related to exposure to toxigenic
fungi. In E. Johanning (Ed.), *Bioaerosols, fungi and mycotoxins: Health effects, assessment, prevention and control* (pp. 131–138). Albany, NY: Boyd.

Babikian, T., Boone, K. B., Lu, P., & Arnold, B. (2006). Sensitivity and specificity of various Digit Span scores in the detection of suspect effort. *The Clinical Neuropsychologist, 20,* 145–159.

Baldo, J. V., Ahmad, L., & Ruff, R. (2002). Neuropsychological performance of patients following mold exposure. *Applied Neuropsychology, 9,* 193–202.

Barrett, J. R. (2003). Mold insurance: Crafting coverage for a spreading problem. *Environmental Health Perspectives, 111,* A100–A103.

Belkin, L. (2001, August 12). Haunted by mold. *The New York Times Magazine,* pp. 28–33, 48, 62–65.

Bianchini, K. J., Houston, R. J., Greve, K. W., Irvin, T. R., Black, F. W., Swift, D. A., et al. (2003). Malingered neurocognitive dysfunction in neurotoxic exposure: An application of the Slick criteria. *Journal of Occupational and Environmental Medicine, 45,* 1087–1099.

Binder, L. M., & Campbell, K. A. (2004). Medically unexplained symptoms and neuropsychological assessment. *Journal of Clinical and Experimental Neuropsychology, 26,* 369–392.

Binder, L. M., Storzbach, D., & Salinsky, M. C. (2006). MMPI-2 profiles of persons with multiple chemical sensitivity. *The Clinical Neuropsychologist, 20,* 848–857.

Black, D. W. (2002). Paroxetine for multiple chemical sensitivity syndrome. *American Journal of Psychiatry, 159,* 1436–1437.

Bolla, K. I. (1996). Neurobehavioral performance in multiple chemical sensitivities. *Regulatory Toxicology and Pharmacology, 24,* S52–S54.

Boone, K. B., Salazar, X., Lu, P., Warner-Chacon, K., & Razani, J. (2002). The Rey 15-Item Recognition Trial: A technique to enhance sensitivity of the Rey 15-Item Memorization Test. *Journal of Clinical and Experimental Neuropsychology, 24,* 561–573.

Bornschein, S., Hausteiner, C., Zilker, T., & Forstl, H. (2002). Psychiatric and somatic disorders and multiple chemical sensitivity (MCS) in 264 "environmental patients." *Psychological Medicine, 32,* 1387–1394.

Burr, M. L. (2001). Health effects of indoor molds. *Reviews on Environmental Health, 16,* 97–103.

Chapman, J. A., Terr, A. I., Jacobs, R. L., Charlesworth, E. N., & Bardana, E. J., Jr. (2003). Toxic mold: Phantom risk vs. science. *Annals of Allergy, Asthma, and Immunology, 91,* 222–232.

Crago, B. R., Gray, M. R., Nelson, L. A., Davis, M., Arnold, L., & Thrasher, J. D. (2003). Psychological, neuropsychological, and electrocortical effects of mixed mold exposure. *Archives of Environmental Health, 58,* 452–463.

Cross, E. H. (1999). Microbial contamination litigation: Expert witnesses and scientific evidence. In E. Johanning (Ed.), *Bioaerosols, fungi and mycotoxins: Health effects, assessment, prevention and control* (pp. 595–602). Albany, NY: Boyd.

Cullen, M. R., Pace, P. E., & Redlich, C. A. (1992). The experience of the Yale occupational and environmental medicine clinics with multiple chemical sensitivities. *Toxicology and Industrial Health, 8,* 15–19.

Devriese, S., Winters, W., Stegen, K., Van Diest, I., Veulemans, H., Nemery, B., et al. (2000). Generalization of acquired somatic symptoms in response to odors: A Pavlovian perspective on multiple chemical sensitivity. *Psychosomatic Medicine, 62,* 751–759.

Dikmen, S. S., Ross, B. L., Machamer, J. E., & Temkin, N. R. (1995). One year psychosocial outcome in head injury. *Journal of the International Neuropsychological Society*, *1*, 67–77.

Dillon, H. K., Miller, J. D., Sorenson, W. G., Douwes, J., & Jacobs, R. R. (1999). Review of methods applicable to the assessment of mold exposure to children. *Environmental Health Perspectives*, *107*(Suppl. 3), 473–480.

Dunn, J. T., Lees-Haley, P. R., Brown, R. S., Williams, C. W., & English, L. T. (1995). Neurotoxic complaint base rates of personal injury claimants: Implications for neuropsychological assessment. *Journal of Clinical Psychology*, *51*, 577–584.

Etzel, R. A., Balk, S. J., Bearer, C. F., Miller, M. D., Shannon, M. W., Shea, K. M., et al. (1998). Toxic effects of indoor molds. *American Academy of Pediatrics*, *101*, 712–714.

Fiedler, N., Kipen, H., Deluca, J., Kelly-McNeil, K., & Natelson, B. (1996). A controlled comparison of multiple chemical sensitivity and chronic fatigue syndrome. *Psychosomatic Medicine*, *58*, 38–49.

Fiedler, N., Maccia, C., & Kipen, H. (1992). Evaluation of chemically sensitive patients. *Journal of Occupational Medicine*, *34*, 529–538.

Fox, D. D., Greiffenstein, M. F., & Lees-Haley, P. R. (2005). Commentary on "Cognitive impairment associated with toxigenic fungal exposure." *Applied Neuropsychology*, *12*, 129–133.

Fung, F., Clark, R., & Williams, S. (1998). *Stachybotrys*, a mycotoxin-producing fungus of increasing toxicologic importance. *Journal of Toxicology: Clinical Toxicology*, *36*, 79–86.

Fung, F., & Hughson, W. G. (2003). Health effects of indoor fungal bioaerosol exposure. *Applied Occupational and Environmental Hygiene*, *18*, 535–544.

Gentilini, M., Nichelli, P., Schoenhuber, R., Bortolotti, P., Tonelli, L., Falasca, A., et al. (1985). Neuropsychological evaluation of mild head injury. *Journal of Neurology, Neurosurgery, and Psychiatry*, *48*, 137–140.

Gervais, R., Rohling, M., Green, P., & Ford, W. (2004). A comparison of WMT, CARB, and TOMM failure rates in non-head injury disability claimants. *Archives of Clinical Neuropsychology*, *19*, 475–487.

Goldstein, F. C., Levin, H. S., Goldman, W. P., Clark, A. N., & Altonen, T. K. (2001). Cognitive and neurobehavioral functioning after mild *versus* moderate traumatic brain injury in older adults. *Journal of the International Neuropsychological Society*, *7*, 373–383.

Gordon, W. A., Cantor, J. B., Johanning, E., Charatz, H. J., Ashman, T. A., Breeze, J. L., et al. (2004). Cognitive impairment associated with toxigenic fungal exposure: A replication and extension of previous findings. *Applied Neuropsychology*, *11*, 65–74.

Gordon, W. A., Johanning, E., & Haddad, L. (1999). Cognitive impairment associated with exposure to toxigenic fungi. In E. Johanning (Ed.), *Bioaerosols, fungi and mycotoxins: Health effects, assessment, prevention and control* (pp. 94–98). Albany, NY: Boyd.

Gunstad, J., & Suhr, J. A. (2004). Cognitive factors in postconcussion syndrome symptom report. *Archives of Clinical Neuropsychology*, *19*, 391–405.

Gupta, R., Vohra, A. K., Madaan, V., & Gaur, D. R. (2001). Mass hysteria among high school girls following tetanus toxoid immunisation. *Irish Journal of Psychological Medicine*, *18*, 90–92.

Handal, G., Leiner, M. A., Cabrera, M., & Straus, D. C. (2004). Children symptoms before and after knowing about an indoor fungal contamination. *Indoor Air, 14,* 87–91.

Hardin, B. D., Kelman, B. J., & Saxon, A. (2003). Adverse human health effects associated with molds in the indoor environment. *Journal of Occupational and Environmental Medicine, 45,* 470–478.

Hartman, D. E. (1998). Missed diagnoses and misdiagnoses of environmental toxicant exposure: The psychiatry of toxic exposure and multiple chemical sensitivity. *The Psychiatric Clinics of North America, 21,* 659–670.

Hodgson, M. J., Morey, P., Leung, W. Y., Morrow, L., Miller, D., Jarvis, B. B., et al. (1998). Building associated pulmonary disease from exposure to *Stachybotrys chartarum* and *Aspergillus versicolor*. *International Journal of Occupational Medicine and Environmental Health, 40,* 241–249.

Hossain, M. A., Ahmed, M. S., & Ghannoum, M. A. (2004). Attributes of *Stachybotrys chartarum* and its association with human disease. *The Journal of Allergy and Clinical Immunology, 113,* 200–208.

Huttunen, K., Hyvarinen, A., Nevalainen, A., Komulainen, H., & Hirvonen, M. R. (2003). Production of proinflammatory mediators by indoor air bacteria and fungal spores in mouse and human cell lines. *Environmental Health Perspectives, 111,* 85–92.

Iverson, G. L., & Lange, R. T. (2003). Examination of "postconcussion-like" symptoms in a healthy sample. *Applied Neuropsychology, 10,* 137–144.

Iverson, G. L., Lange, R. T., Green, P., & Frazen, M. D. (2002). Detecting exaggeration and malingering with the Trail Making Test. *The Clinical Neuropsychologist, 16,* 398–406.

Iverson, G. L., & Tulsky, D. S. (2003). Detecting malingering on the WAIS-III: Unusual Digit Span performance patterns in the normal population and in clinical groups. *Archives of Clinical Neuropsychology, 18,* 1–9.

Jarvis, B. B. (2002). Chemistry and toxicology of molds isolated from water-damaged buildings. *Advances in Experimental Medicine and Biology, 504,* 43–52.

Kilburn, K. H. (2003). Indoor mold exposure associated with neurobehavioral and pulmonary impairment: A preliminary report. *Archives of Environmental Health, 58,* 390–398.

King, N., & Auger, P. (2002). Indoor air quality, fungi, and health. How do we stand? *Canadian Family Physician, 48,* 298–302.

Kuhn, D. M., & Ghannoum, M. A. (2003). Indoor mold, toxigenic fungi, and *Stachybotrys chartarum*: Infectious disease perspective. *Clinical Microbiology Reviews, 16,* 144–172.

Labarge, A. S., & McCaffrey, R. J. (2000). Multiple chemical sensitivity: A review of the theoretical and research literature. *Neuropsychology Review, 10,* 183–211.

Larrabee, G. J. (1998). Somatic malingering on the MMPI and MMPI-2 in personal injury litigants. *The Clinical Neuropsychologist, 12,* 179–188.

Lee, T. G. (2003). Health symptoms caused by molds in a courthouse. *Archives of Environmental Health, 58,* 442–446.

Lees-Haley, P. R. (2003). Toxic mold and mycotoxins in neurotoxicity cases: *Stachybotrys, Fusarium, Trichoderma, Aspergillus, Penicillium, Cladosporium, Alternaria, Trichothecenes*. *Psychological Reports, 93,* 561–584.

Lees-Haley, P. R., & Brown, R. S. (1992). Biases in perception and reporting following a perceived toxic exposure. *Perceptual and Motor Skills, 75,* 531–544.

Lees-Haley, P. R., English, L. T., & Glenn, W. J. (1991). A fake bad scale on the MMPI-2 for personal injury claimants. *Psychological Reports, 68,* 203–210.

Leznoff, A. (1997). Provocative challenges in patients with multiple chemical sensitivity. *Journal of Allergy and Clinical Immunology, 99,* 439–442.

McCaffrey, R. J., & Yantz, C. L. (2005). "Cognitive impairment associated with toxigenic fungal exposure:" A critique and critical analysis. *Applied Neuropsychology, 12,* 134–137.

Meyer, H. W., Wurtz, H., Suadicani, P., Valbjorn, O., Sigsgaard, T., & Gyntelberg, F. (2004). Molds in floor dust and building-related symptoms in adolescent school children. *Indoor Air, 14,* 65–72.

Miller, L. J., Ryan, J. J., Carruthers, C. A., & Cluff, R. B. (2004). Brief screening indexes for malingering: A confirmation of Vocabulary minus Digit Span from the WAIS-III and the Rarely Missed Index from the WMS-III. *The Clinical Neuropsychologist, 18,* 327–333.

Millis, S. R., & Volinsky, C. T. (2001). Assessment of response bias in mild head injury: Beyond malingering tests. *Journal of Clinical and Experimental Neuropsychology, 23,* 809–828.

Mittenberg, W., Azrin, R., Millsaps, C., & Heilbronner, R. (1993). Identification of malingered head injury on the Wechsler Memory Scale—Revised. *Psychological Assessment, 5,* 34–40.

Mittenberg, W., Patton, C., Canyock, E. M., & Condit, D. C. (2002). Base rates of malingering and symptom exaggeration. *Journal of Clinical and Experimental Neuropsychology, 24,* 1094–1102.

Mittenberg, W., Theroux, S., Aguila-Puentes, G., Bianchini, K. J., Greve, K. W., & Rayls, K. (2001). Identification of malingered head injury on the Wechsler Adult Intelligence Scale—3rd Edition. *The Clinical Neuropsychologist, 15,* 440–445.

Nordness, M. E., Zacharisen, M. C., & Fink, J. N. (2003). Toxic and other non-IgE-mediated effects of fungal exposures. *Current Allergy and Asthma Reports, 3,* 438–446.

Osterberg, K., Orbaek, P., & Karlson, B. (2002). Neuropsychological test performance of Swedish multiple chemical sensitivity patients—An exploratory study. *Applied Neuropsychology, 9,* 139–147.

Palmer, B. W., Boone, K. B., Lesser, I. M., & Wohl, M. A. (1998). Base rates of "impaired" neuropsychological test performance among healthy older adults. *Archives of Clinical Neuropsychology, 13,* 503–511.

Pankratz, L. (2002). Hard times, dancing manias, and multiple chemical sensitivity. *The Scientific Review of Mental Health Practice, 1,* 62–75.

Platt, S. D., Martin, C. J., Hunt, S. M., & Lewis, C. W. (1989). Damp housing, mould growth, and symptomatic health state. *The British Medical Journal, 298,* 1673–1678.

Poonai, N. P., Antony, M. M., Binkley, K. E., Stenn, P., Swinson, R. P., Corey, P., et al. (2001). Psychological features of subjects with idiopathic environmental intolerance. *Journal of Psychosomatic Research, 51,* 537–541.

Rea, W. J., Ross, G. H., Johnson, A. R., Smiley, R. E., Sprague, D. E., Fenyves, E. J., et al. (1990). Confirmation of chemical sensitivity by means of double-blind inhalant challenge of toxic volatile chemicals. *Clinical Ecology, 6,* 113–118.

Reynolds, C. R. (1999). Inferring causality from relational data and designs: Historical and contemporary lessons for research and clinical practice. *The Clinical Neuropsychologist, 13,* 386–395.

Robbins, C. A., Swenson, L. J., Nealley, M. L., Gots, R. E., & Kelman, B. J. (2000). Health effects of mycotoxins in indoor air: A critical review. *Applied Occupational and Environmental Hygiene, 15,* 773–784.

Ross, G. H. (1992). History and clinical presentation of the chemically sensitive patient. *Toxicology and Industrial Health, 8,* 21–28.

Ross, P. M., Whysner, J., Covello, V. T., Kuschner, M., Rifkind, A. B., Sedler, M. J., et al. (1999). Olfaction and symptoms in the multiple chemical sensitivities syndrome. *Preventative Medicine, 28.*

Sabir, M., Shashikiran, U., & Kochar, S. K. (1999). Building related illnesses and indoor air pollution. *The Journal of the Association of Physicians of India, 47,* 426–430.

Santilli, J. (2002). Health effects of mold exposure in public schools. *Current Allergy and Asthma Reports, 2,* 460–467.

Santilli, J., & Rockwell, W. (2003). Fungal contamination of elementary schools: A new environmental hazard. *Annals of Allergy, Asthma, and Immunology, 90,* 203–208.

Sawchyn, J. M., Brulot, M. M., & Strauss, E. (2000). Note on the use of the postconcussion syndrome checklist. *Archives of Clinical Neuropsychology, 15,* 1–8.

Schretlen, D. J., & Shapiro, A. M. (2003). A quantitative review of the effects of traumatic brain injury on cognitive functioning. *International Review of Psychiatry, 15,* 341–349.

Simon, G. E., Daniell, W., Stockbridge, H., Claypoole, K., & Rosenstock, L. (1993). Immunologic, psychological, and neuropsychological factors in multiple chemical sensitivity. *Annals of Internal Medicine, 19,* 97–103.

Slick, D. J., Sherman, E. M. S., & Iverson, G. L. (1999). Diagnostic criteria for malingered neurocognitive dysfunction: Proposed standards for clinical practice and research. *The Clinical Neuropsychologist, 13,* 545–561.

Sobotka, T. J., Brodie, R. E., & Spaid, S. L. (1978). Neurobehavioral studies of tremorgenic mycotoxins Verruculogen and Penitrem A. *Pharmacology, 16,* 287–294.

Sorg, B. A., & Newlin, D. B. (2002). Sensitization as a mechanism for multiple chemical sensitivity: Relationship to evolutionary theory. *Scandinavian Journal of Psychology, 43,* 161–167.

Staudenmayer, H., & Kramer, R. E. (1999). Psychogenic chemical sensitivity: Psychogenic pseudoseizures elicited by provocation challenges with fragrances. *Journal of Psychogenic Research, 47,* 185–190.

Staudenmayer, H., & Phillips, S. (2007). MMPI-2 Validity, Clinical, and Content Scales and the Fake Bad Scale for personal injury litigants claiming idiopathic environmental intolerance (IEI). *Journal of Psychosomatic Research, 62,* 61–72.

Staudenmayer, H., Selner, J. C., & Buhr, M. P. (1993). Double-blind provocation chamber challenges in 20 patients presenting with "multiple chemical sensitivity." *Regulatory Toxicology and Pharmacology, 18,* 44–53.

Stenn, P., & Binkley, K. (1998). Successful outcome in a patient with chemical sensitivity: Treatment with psychological desensitization and selective serotonin reuptake inhibitor. *Psychosomatics, 39,* 547–550.

Stone, D., Boone, K. B., Back-Madruga, C., & Lesser, I. (2006). Has the rolling uterus finally gathered moss? Somatization and malingering of cognitive deficit in six cases of "toxic mold" exposure. *The Clinical Neuropsychologist, 20*, 766–785.

Sudakin, D. L. (1998). Toxigenic fungi in a water-damaged building: An intervention study. *American Journal of Industrial Medicine, 34*, 183–190.

Suhr, J. A., & Gunstad, J. (2002). Postconcussive symptom report: The relative influence of head injury and depression. *Journal of Clinical and Experimental Neuropsychology, 24*, 981–993.

Temple, S. (2003). A case of multiple chemical sensitivities: Cognitive therapy for somatization disorder and metaworry. *Journal of Cognitive Psychotherapy, 17*, 267–277.

Terr, A. I. (1993). Multiple chemical sensitivities. *Annals of Internal Medicine, 119*, 163–164.

Terr, A. I. (2004). Are indoor molds causing a new disease? *Journal of Allergy and Clinical Immunology, 113*, 221–226.

Trueblood, W., & Schmidt, M. (1993). Malingering and other validity considerations in the neuropsychological evaluation of mild head injury. *Journal of Clinical and Experimental Neuropsychology, 15*, 578–590.

Van den Bergh, O., Winters, W., Devriese, S., & Van Diest, I. (2002). Learning subjective health complaints. *Scandinavian Journal of Psychology, 43*, 147–152.

van Hout, M. S., Schmand, B., Wekking, E. M., Hageman, G., & Deelman, B. G. (2003). Suboptimal performance on neuropsychological tests in patients with suspected chronic toxic encephalopathy. *Neurotoxicology, 24*, 547–551.

Verhoeff, A. P., & Burge, H. A. (1997). Health risk assessment of fungi in home environments. *Annals of Allergy, Asthma, and Immunology, 78*, 544–554.

Vickery, C., Berry, D., Inman, T., Harris, M., & Orey, S. (2001). Detection of inadequate effort on neuropsychological testing: A meta-analytic review of selected procedures. *Archives of Clinical Neuropsychology, 16*, 45–73.

Wilkinson, L., & Task Force on Statistical Inference. (1999). Statistical methods in psychology journals: Guidelines and explanations. *American Psychologist, 54*, 594–604.

Youngjohn, J. R., Burrows, L., & Erdal, K. (1995). Brain damage or compensation neurosis? The controversial post-concussion syndrome. *The Clinical Neuropsychologist, 9*, 112–123.

Ziem, G., & McTamney, J. (1997). Profile of patients with chemical injury and sensitivity. *Environmental Health Perspectives, 105*(Suppl. 2), 417–436.

CHAPTER 18

The Use of Effort Tests in Ethnic Minorities and in Non-English-Speaking and English as a Second Language Populations

Xavier F. Salazar
Po H. Lu
Johnny Wen
Kyle Brauer Boone

Few would argue that the phenomenon of malingering exists across cultural and ethnic boundaries. The motives underlying the impetus for deception—including the lure of a large monetary award, the opportunity to improve life circumstances, and the avoidance of work, military duty, or criminal prosecution—are universal temptations. For example, Mayers (1995) reported three specific cases of Vietnamese, non-English-speaking individuals who presented with emotional disability as well as severe intellectual and memory deficits in the context of applying for social security disability (SSD) benefits. Each of these individuals also manifested numerous indicators of malingering. Similarly, Garcia and Juan (2003) presented a case study of a middle-age, non-English-speaking Spaniard seeking financial compensation for a work-related head injury. Although the patient complained of persistent and severe deficits in memory and attention, as well as emotional disturbance, a close examination of the case revealed conflicting collateral information, inconsistent medical history, and suspect performance on indicators of malingering.

In this chapter we focus on two of the largest cultural groups in the United States, Hispanics and Chinese. The U.S. Census Bureau (2003) estimates that of the more than 209 million adults in this country, 37 million speak a language other than English in their household. Of the latter group, it estimates that 21 million speak Spanish and nearly 2 million speak Chinese. Despite these numbers, there is a relative paucity of research addressing cognitive malingering in these populations. To date, a literature search on the general topic of malingering yielded over 200 pertinent peer-reviewed publications, with over half of these utilizing quantitative research designs in their methodology. In contrast, when cultural and ethnic filters, such as language or race were added (i.e., Chinese, Spanish, and Hispanic/ Latino), the results were reduced to 12. Seven of these studies (Chiu & Lee, 2002; Deng & Tang, 2002; Ding, Gao, & Liu, 2002; Gao, 2001; Gao, Li, & Chen, 2003; Gao, Liu, Ding, & Lu, 2002; Liu, Gao, & Li, 2001) focused on native Chinese individuals and their performance on measures designed to detect cognitive malingering. The remaining five studies analyzed Spanish-speaking participants and those of Latin descent. Of these five, the only one that addressed malingering of cognitive symptoms was the case study by Garcia and Juan (2003) described previously. The remaining four (DuAlba & Scott, 1993; Guy & Miller, 2004; Johnson & Torres, 1992; Lucio, Durán, & Graham, 2002) primarily examined feigned psychiatric symptoms on self-report inventory measures, such as the Minnesota Multiphasic Personality Inventory (MMPI; Butcher, Dahlstrom, Graham, Tellegen, & Kaemmer, 1989) and the Miller Forensic Assessment of Symptoms Test (MFAST; Miller, 2001). In the absence of more robust data, clinicians assessing minority populations are often forced to infer the validity, and justify the use, of common malingering instruments, based largely on their own unique experience and expertise with a specific cultural group.

Below we provide case examples illustrating the assessment of malingering with non-English-speaking populations, as well as summarize original empirical research that we hope will help clarify the use of existing malingering measures with diverse populations.

SPANISH-SPEAKING PATIENTS

In a study presented by Salazar, Lopez, Peña, and Mitrushina (2003) at the Spanish Language Association of Neuropsychology, the authors examined the reliability of two commonly used measures of malingering when applied to a male Hispanic population. All of the 108 participants were native Spanish speakers living in the greater Los Angeles area. All were male day laborers, with a mean age of 30.58 (SD = 11.37) years, a mean education level of 6.11 (SD = 2.55) years, and a mean length of residency in the United States of 44.34 (SD = 74.91) months. Exclusion criteria for the participants included a history of head injury, previous diagnosis of a cognitive disorder, and substance abuse.

The participants were administered in standard fashion, using translated Spanish instructions, the Dot Counting Test (DCT; Boone, Lu, & Herzberg, 2002) and the Rey 15-Item Test plus recognition (Rey 15-IR; Boone, Salazar, Lu, Warner-Chacon, & Razani, 2002). In the DCT, subjects are presented multiple cards (one card at a time) that contain a variable number of dots. On half of these cards the dots are arranged in a standardized random order, and on the remaining cards the dots are arranged in small, easily recognizable, symmetrical groups. Conversely, the Rey 15-IR is a two-part test consisting of a free recall and a recognition component. In the free recall trial, the patient is briefly exposed to a page containing 15 items (e.g., numbers, letter, and geometrical figures) and asked to reproduce the stimuli. In the recognition portion of the test, the patient is presented with a page containing all target items intermixed with 15 foils and asked to identify the former.

Results suggest that the performance of this Spanish-speaking sample was comparable to that of the published data on English speakers for the DCT; use of the standard E score cutoff of ≥ 17 was associated with specificity of 95.4%. DCT performance was not significantly related to age or educational level. However, the sample's performance on the Rey 15-IR was lowered relative to English speakers, and significantly related to educational level ($r = .21$ for free recall; $r = .30$ for recall plus recognition), but not age. Participants with less than 6 years of education scored on average 2 points lower than their more educated counterparts and the English-speaking normative sample. More significantly , while 86.4% of individuals with > 6 years of education scored above the standard cutoff of < 9 for free recall, only 67.2% of subjects with ≤ 6 years education obtained a score of 9 or higher. Furthermore, both educational groups scored below the normative sample on the more sensitive composite score, with the lower and higher education groups scoring on average 6 and 3 points below the normative sample, respectively. Use of the standard cutoff of < 20 for recall + (recognition minus false positives) was associated with 81% specificity in subjects with > 6 years or education, while in subjects with ≤ 6 years education, specificity was only 67.7%. Lowering the cutoff to < 17 resulted in adequate specificity in those with > 6 years of education (90.5%), but lowering the cutoff to 14 was still associated with less than optimal specificity in those with ≤ 6 years of education (82.3%).

The results suggest that existing paradigms for the detection of malingering may be successfully utilized with Spanish-speaking Hispanic patients in the United States. In particular, the standard DCT test cutoff can be used with monolingual Spanish speakers of low educational level with no loss in specificity; however, the Rey 15-Item Test cutoffs require adjustments to maintain acceptable specificity (i.e., $\geq 90\%$), resulting in some sacrifice in sensitivity. Additional empirical studies examining performance of monolingual Spanish speakers as a function of education on other effort measures are needed.

Following is a case presentation of a Hispanic male with a seizure disorder seeking to retain disability benefits but consistently demonstrating suspect effort and feigning of cognitive symptoms on testing. The case illustrates the use of the DCT as well as other indicators of suboptimal effort.

Case Example 1

The patient was a 55-year-old, right-handed, monolingual Spanish-speaking Hispanic male referred for neuropsychological assessment by a private physician as part of a comprehensive evaluation for dementia. The patient was born and raised in a Central American country and had 4 years of formal education. He immigrated to the United States 15 years prior to evaluation and lived in a single-family home with his wife and children. Since arriving in the United States, the patient worked in office janitorial services and prior to that he worked as a field laborer in his native country.

Thirteen years prior to evaluation the patient had experienced a grand mal seizure while at work and was transported to an emergency room. After several hours of observation, the patient was discharged. He denied any previous history of seizures and reported that since the foregoing incident he experienced memory difficulties, right-sided weakness, and periodic swelling in his legs for which he receives disability compensation. In addition, the patient endorsed nondescript visual hallucinations with onset following his seizure in 1993. No history of delusions was noted and the patient recalled only one additional partial seizure since the initial seizure. Two years after the first seizure, the patient was diagnosed with neurocysticercosis with secondary seizure disorder, and 3 months prior to the present neuropsychological evaluation, he was diagnosed with hypertension. Medications included phenobarbital, carbamazepine, dilantin, hytrin, claritin, hydrochlorothiazide, risperdal, and albuterol. The patient reported compliance with this medication regimen but noted that he required the assistance of family members. Medical records indicated that his seizure disorder and hypertension were well controlled.

A number of behavioral observations are noteworthy. The patient arrived on time to his appointment via transportation provided by the facility where he was evaluated. Use of the facility's transportation service was made at the request of the patient, as he reported that he could no longer drive and would have no other means of attending the appointment. He was casually dressed and groomed and carried a soft, medium-size, zippered lunch bag. Within minutes of his arrival, the patient made requests of nonmedical personnel to help him identify his hypertension medication from among the multiple bottles that filled the zippered container. After a nurse verified the correct medication, the patient took the stated dosage and requested to use the restroom. Verbal instructions directing him to the restroom were provided. The patient was able to navigate these directions and return to the waiting area without difficulty. Upon his return, he made a second request of the clerical staff, asking them to order a refill for a medication that had been prescribed by an outside physician. When staff personnel pointed out that the bottle was still half full, the patient succinctly explained that he took multiple doses of this medication throughout the day, and that he would consequently run out of medication prior to his next appointment at the end of the month. The patient spontaneously provided the exact date of the appointment without reference to any written reminder.

During the testing session, the patient was notably slowed, both in his gross motor movements and in the speed of his verbal responses. On a test battery comprised of 30 tasks and that typically requires 90 to 120 minutes to administer in its entirety, the patient was able to complete only nine tests in 2 hours. He obtained a score of 20/30 on the Mini-Mental State Exam (MMSE; Folstein, Folstein, McHugh, 1975). The patient misidentified the season, the state, the county, and the city in which the evaluation took place. He was able to recall only one of three words after a short delay and was unable to engage in mental reversal tasks, write a spontaneous sentence, or copy two interlocking pentagons. He was, however, able to repeat two simple sentences and follow a written command, as well as a three-step verbal command. His performance on the remaining tests ranged from the impaired to the borderline-impaired range.

While a score of 20 on the MMSE and an impaired neuropsychological profile would be indicative of marked cognitive decline, convergent evidence from multiple sources suggested that the patient was feigning his difficulties. The patient was administered two discreet measures of effort, the Test of Memory Malingering (TOMM; Tombaugh, 1996), and the DCT (Boone, Lu, & Herzberg, 2002). On the TOMM, which employs a binary forced-choice paradigm, he scored 36/50 and 39/50 on the first two trials, and a 39/50 on a retention trial administered following a 20-minute delay; the latter two performances fall below test cutoffs indicative of noncredible performance. These cutoff scores correctly classify 95% of nondemented patients and 93% of moderately to severely demented patients.

Similarly, the patient's performance was below expectation on the DCT (Boone, Lu, & Herzberg, 2002). The patient was observed to pause both at the start of each trial and prior to providing each response. Prompts for speed were minimally effective as the patient laboriously counted each dot individually, placing his index finger over each as he counted them. This behavior was observed on both the ungrouped and grouped trials. Of note, rather than lowering his mean time on the grouped dot trials, as is expected when full effort is exerted, the patient's time increased by 2%, and even at this slowed pace, he still committed two counting errors. His composite score (48.16) was nearly three times the suggested cutoff score of ≥ 17.

A collateral interview with the patient's wife revealed multiple behavioral inconsistencies as well. She reported that the patient is independent in all instrumental activities of daily living, including driving and administration of his medication regimen. This report is in conflict with the patient's insistence on the use of a transportation service due to his inability to drive and his endorsed need for assistance with his medication management. Behavioral observations at the time of exam were also contradictory. The patient initially sought the aid of clerical staff to help him select an appropriate medication from the multiple bottles in his bag. Moments later, however, he independently identified a second medication and requested a refill. Furthermore, the rationale that he presented during this request exceeded problem-solving abilities that would be expected from an individual with a psychometric profile spanning the borderline-impaired to impaired range. Specifically, the patient's logic required him to remember and track the various dosages of each medication, recall the date of his follow-up appointment, utilize simple arithmetic to project a shortage in his medication, and act proactively to avoid this outcome.

The patient's neuropsychological profile and his purported functional deficits were also inconsistent with radiological and neurological findings. On a computed tomography (CT) scan of the brain conducted approximately 12 months prior, it was noted that with the exception of a cysticercosis in the left parietal lobe, the remainder of the brain was unremarkable. No atrophy or suspect vascular accidents were identified. Similarly, the dictation of a neurological examination conducted 3 weeks prior to the foregoing evaluation noted no physical, motor, or sensory deficits and cranial nerves were grossly normal, although a decreased sensation to cold on the right face was noted. In contrast, the patient's neuropsychological performance was at the level of mid- to late-stage dementia. It would be exceedingly rare to find this degree of impairment without detectable physiological changes upon imaging of the brain or neurological evaluation. In fact, the above neurologist made note of the incongruent findings in her evaluation and the patient's presentation, describing the physical examination as "atypical" with "a great deal of behavior overlay with exaggeration of physical symptoms."

The aforementioned case demonstrates how information from a variety of independent sources—behavioral observations, formal measures of effort and motivation, collateral information, and medical history—can converge to provide compelling evidence of intentional suboptimal performance by a patient. The patient failed both effort tests administered (DCT, TOMM), and as discussed in the next case presentation, both of these measures were also effective in the detection of suboptimal effort during an evaluation of a monolingual Chinese patient.

CHINESE-SPEAKING PATIENTS

In 1983, a door-to-door survey conducted in China estimated that 56/ 100,000 persons per year suffer head trauma primarily from bicycle accidents (Wang et al., 1986). In a recent study conducted in Taiwan, Teng, Chang, Peng, and Yang (2004) reported that approximately 1,500 people each year suffer head injuries sustained from motor vehicle accidents. Given today's litigious society, it is not surprising that many of these individuals pursue legal action in order to secure financial compensation for their injuries. Gao (2001) called attention to the potential problem of malingering and exaggeration of cognitive impairments in personal injury cases in China, particularly in the context of head injury litigation, and reviewed possible strategies in assessing feigned cognitive deficits. The reports by Mayers (1995) and Gao (2001) urge health care professionals to be alert in recognizing the possibility of fabricated or exaggerated symptomatology when working with non-English-speaking patients and highlight the need to develop measures to objectively document suspect effort and noncredible cognitive impairment for these individuals. Next, we present the case of a Chinese male who was involved in litigation for a head injury and, on an exam conducted in Chinese, displayed consistent evidence of suspect effort and feigning of cognitive symptoms on testing.

Case Example 2

The patient was a 44-year-old, monolingual Mandarin-speaking Chinese male who was riding his bicycle when he struck a grate causing him to be thrown from his bike. His face hit the concrete ground and he consequently lost his front teeth and suffered lacerations to his upper lip and mucous membrane. He reported a brief loss of consciousness; upon waking, he recalled being helped up by a passing pedestrian who called 911. He also remembered that his lip was bleeding, and that he felt intense pain in his head and various parts of the body as well as dizziness and nausea. He was taken to the emergency room of a nearby hospital for examination and treatment. He received five stitches for his wounds, a tetanus shot, and x-rays for his skull and right elbow, which revealed no fractures, and was discharged.

Six months after the accident, the patient continued to experience persistent headaches and dizziness though with reduced intensity and frequency. He also reported worsening of short-term memory and difficulty with concentration, adding that he would write his name incorrectly and say things that he did not mean to say. Neurological examination did not find any physical, motor, or sensory deficit and cranial nerves were grossly normal. The patient was observed to be alert and oriented and his mental status and language ability, including comprehension and speech production, were judged to be within normal limits with good "memory of details." Medical examination conducted about a year post-accident revealed that most of his bodily injuries had resolved with multiple modalities of physical therapy and analgesics, though residual headache, dizziness, and neck pain remained. Of note, the patient's medical history was significant for a craniotomy approximately 2 years prior to the accident. A CT study of the brain revealed focal encephalomalacia in the right basal ganglia, right parietal region, and right occipital area related to prior surgery, possibly for hematoma evacuation.

Neuropsychological evaluation was initiated because the patient brought suit against the city in which the accident occurred, alleging unsafe conditions. The assessment was conducted approximately 18 months postinjury. On clinical interview, the patient reported daily headaches, pain in his right shoulder and right side of his neck, numbness in his right arm and hand, lower back pain, gastrointestinal symptoms, chest discomfort, and toothaches. From a cognitive perspective, the patient described short-term memory difficulties, characterized as a tendency to misplace documents and become lost in familiar places, as well as reduced reaction time and attention. These cognitive symptoms were reported to have worsened since the accident. The patient described his mood as depressed, which was directly attributed to his physical ailments and cognitive decline.

The patient was observed to be well groomed and appropriately attired. Speech characteristics were unremarkable except for sparse output and low volume. Thought processes were linear, well organized, and relevant. He was overtly cooperative but subdued. On the MMSE (Folstein et al., 1975), the patient was disoriented to date, day of the week, season, hospital, floor, city, and county. He required six trials to register three words and recalled none after a brief delay. He could not perform simple mental subtractions, follow a three-step command, repeat a phrase, or draw a simple line figure. His total score of 10 suggested severely impaired global cognitive ability. However, evidence emerged indicating that the patient was not exerting his best effort on the tasks. For example, on the TOMM (Tombaugh, 1996), he scored 15/50 and 14/50 on the first two trials, displaying significantly below chance performance on both occasions. The binary forced-choice paradigm of the TOMM dictates that even in the context of random guessing, the patient would be expected to garner approximately 50% correct responses given a sufficient number of trials (Guiterrez & Gur, 1998). Therefore, significantly below chance performance suggests that the individual was systematically selecting the incorrect response in order to demonstrate his or her supposed disability. After being exposed to the same stimuli the second time, the patient's performance actually declined; the probability of two consecutive below-chance performances is minuscule and would not occur even in the most amnestic patients, and is strongly suggestive of a deliberate attempt to choose the incorrect answer. The patient also failed the DCT (Boone, Lu, & Herzberg, 2002), another measure of effort and cooperation. Specifically, he frequently buried his head in his hands during the task, stating "I can't think!" Upon encouragement, he would count the dots extremely slowly; he had already exceeded the cutoff score threefold halfway through the task at which time the task was discontinued. Even at this laborious pace, he miscounted the number of dots on five of six trials.

In addition to psychometric indices, the patient also presented with multiple behavioral evidence of feigned cognitive impairment. Namely, the neuropsychological test results, which indicated profound global cognitive impairment, were not consistent with the severity of his head injury, which was mild at most. There were also marked inconsistencies in postinjury cognitive performance across separate testing evaluations. For example, neurological and medical examinations conducted 6 months to 1 year prior to the neuropsychological assessment found the patient to be alert and oriented with generally normal mental status, whereas he was disoriented to time and place during the neuropsychological evaluation and demonstrated severely impaired performance on the MMSE, a score consistent with mid- to late-stage dementia patients. Cognitive abilities either remain static or gradually improve after a brain injury and there would be no mechanism to explain a marked decline in performance 1½ years after the accident. This combination of an atypical neuropsychological profile and performance inconsistencies strongly indicates that the patient was not exerting his best effort on the tasks and was portraying himself as more cognitively impaired than was actually the case. In fact, the combination of the reported psychometric indices and behavioral indices would meet the criteria for definite neuro-cognitive malingering as described by Slick, Sherman, and Iverson (1999) and Rogers (1986).

The aforementioned case is contrasted with that of a 33-year-old, monolingual Mandarin-speaking Chinese male who presented for neuropsychological evaluation status post a self-inflicted gunshot wound to his head 5 months prior to the assessment. A craniotomy was performed to remove bullet and skull fragments but his postoperative recovery was complicated by altered mental status and fever. A head CT scan about a month postsurgery revealed intracranial abscess necessitating a second bifrontal craniotomy for evacuation of the abscess and removal of additional skull fragments. Neuropsychological assessment results revealed marked executive dysfunction, slowing in speed of information processing, and moderate deficits in visual–spatial ability. In contrast, basic attention, memory for auditory verbal information and simple line figures, language ability, and fund of general knowledge remained relatively preserved. This patient passed the same two measures specifically designed to discretely assess motivation and cooperation in the testing procedures. Specifically, he scored 48/50 on the first trial of the TOMM and performed the DCT efficiently, scoring far below the cutoff (E-score = 10). These two cases highlight the importance of documenting effort and cooperation through objective measures and suggest that nonverbal tests of malingering are not only sensitive in detecting noncredible/suboptimal effort in other ethnic and cultural populations but also possess good specificity and do not incorrectly misclassify true patients who are putting forth their best effort.

Groups of researchers in China and Hong Kong have recently begun to investigate the effectiveness of various detection techniques commonly used in the Northern American and European countries, particularly the forced-choice paradigm, in identifying noncredible effort. Liu, Gao, Li, and Lu (2001) found that the mean scores of the simulated malingering group (n = 42) were significantly lower than those of a control group (n = 58) on the Digit Memory Test (DMT), a forced-choice test developed by Hiscock and Hiscock (1989). Gao et al. (2003) administered this same instrument to 57 patients with accident-related brain damage who were seeking compensation and independently determined to be falsifying intellectual deficits. Their DMT performance was compared to 66 patients with brain damage and exhibiting normal effort. Significant group differences in scores were found with the latter group producing 92.7% to 100% correct responses relative to 0 to 7.3% accuracy rate in patients with suspect effort.

Chiu and Lee (2002) adopted and modified the DMT, to include two levels of difficulty. The foils in the easy condition were very different from the target digits (e.g., 42719 and 81359); in fact, recognition of the first digit is sufficient to discriminate between correct and incorrect responses. In the difficult condition, the foil was almost identical to the correct answer (e.g., 62866 and 62686). Even though the latter condition appears "difficult" at face value, it is in actuality a very easy task and yields a high rate of correct responding. The test was administered to 37 monolingual Chinese-speaking university students who participated in both simulated malingering and control conditions. Significantly poorer performance was observed for the malingering condition, but more important, classification accuracy markedly improved on the difficult trials (Chiu & Lee, 2002). Thus, tasks that convey an appearance of difficulty but are in fact very easy may have promise in producing greater separation between true and suspect effort.

In addition to the forced-choice paradigm, Ding et al. (2002) examined the effectiveness of Raven's Standard Progressive Matrices (RSPM; Ravens, 1958) in detecting suspect cognitive performance. Examination of the slope of the progressive decrease in scores across the five RSPM subtests effectively differentiated the malingering and nonmalingering head-injured patients, suggesting that the RSPM may aid in assessing validity of test performance (Ding et al., 2002).

The case examples and findings from the foregoing empirical studies confirm that patients from other cultural and ethnic groups are capable of feigning memory impairment and that the forced-choice format is as sensitive to detecting malingering in the Chinese population as North American and Europeans, suggesting some underlying similarity in this form of faking behavior across ethnic boundaries. Investigation of other nonverbal-based measures of effort in Chinese and other non-English-speaking populations would be needed to further verify this speculation.

A major limitation of the current studies is the use of the simulation design, which provides a convenient research sample and good internal validity but markedly reduces the generalizability of the results to real-world settings (Rogers, Harrell, & Liff, 1993). Replication of the above research on real-world, independently verified malingerers would be an important future research endeavor. Nevertheless, anecdotal and empirical evidence suggests that existing nonverbal instruments designed to detect malingering hold promise in effectively detecting malingering in Chinese and other ethnic populations.

THE IMPACT OF ETHNICITY AND LANGUAGE/CULTURE ON EFFORT INDICATORS

The few published studies and the case examples described previously suggest that standard cognitive effort indicators have the potential for appropriate use with non-English-speaking ethnic groups. However, no data are available regarding effort test performance in English-speaking ethnic minorities, or in individuals who speak English as a second language, and whether standard effort test cutoffs require adjustment in these groups to maintain test score specificity (i.e., ≤ 10% false-positive rates).

To address this issue, permission was obtained from the Institutional Review Board at Harbor–UCLA Medical Center to examine archival data from individuals referred for outpatient neuropsychological evaluation at this public hospital. Subjects who were in civil litigation for personal injury, attempting to obtain disability compensation, met criteria for dementia, or who had Wechsler Adult Intelligence Scale–Revised/Wechsler Adult Intelligence Scale–III (WAIS-R/III) Full Scale IQ < 70 were excluded from analysis. The final sample consisted of 168 subjects (75 male and 93 female); 82.7% were native English speakers (n = 139) and 16.7% spoke English as a second language (ESL; n = 28); 50.6% were Anglo-Caucasian (n = 85), 19.0% were African American (n = 32), 19.0% were Hispanic (n = 32), and 11.3% were Asian (n = 19). Table 18.1 reproduces demographic information for each ethnic group, as well as frequency of diagnoses.

The following effort measures and cutoffs were examined (1) Digit Span age corrected scaled score (DS ACSS) ≤ 5 (Babikian, Boone, Lu, & Arnold, 2006), (2) Reliable Digit Span (RDS) ≤ 6 (Babikian et al., 2006), (3) Rey 15-IR (recall plus [recognition minus false positives] < 20) (Boone, Salazar, et al., 2002), (4) Rey Auditory Verbal Learning Test (RAVLT) recognition ≤ 7 (Suhr, Tranel, Wefel, & Barrash, 1997), (5) RAVLT effort equation ≤ 12 (Boone, Lu, & Wen, 2005), (6) DCT E-score ≥ 17 (Boone, Lu, & Herzberg, 2002), (7) Warrington Recognition Memory Test–Words (WRMT-W) < 33 (Iverson & Franzen, 1994), (8) Rey–Osterrieth (RO) effort equation ≤ 47 (Lu, Boone, Cozolino, & Mitchell, 2003), and (9) RO/AVLT discriminant function ≤ –.40 (Sherman, Boone, Lu, & Razani, 2002).

Ethnic Group Comparisons

Groups significantly differed in age and education. Subsequent pair-wise comparisons failed to revealed significant group differences for age; however, Caucasians and Asians had significantly more education than Hispanics and African Americans, and African Americans had more education than Hispanics. Examination of correlations between effort test scores and age and education revealed that age was only significantly related to Rey 15-IR (Spearman r = –.183, p = .044), RAVLT effort equation (Spearman r = –.289, p = .0001), RAVLT recognition (Spearman r = –.244, p = .002), and RO effort equation (Spearman r = –.235, p = .007), while educational level was only significantly related to DS ACSS (Spearman r = .379, p = .0001), RDS (Spearman r = .325, p = .0001), and RO/AVLT discriminant function (Spearman r = –.194, p = .028).

TABLE 18.1. Demographic Information and Frequency of Diganosis by Ethnicity

	Caucasians	African Americans	Hispanics	Asians	F	p
n	85	32	32	19		
Age	48.18 (13.15)	40.75 (15.56)	41.19 (14.67)	47.32 (17.36)	3.177	.026
Education	13.93 (2.82)	12.28 (1.55)	10.03 (3.05)	14.42 (1.98)	20.36	.0001
Gender	40m/45f	13m/19f	11m/21f	11m/8f		
Diagnoses						
Depression	15 (17.7%)	3 (9.4%)	3 (9.4%)	2 (10.5%)		
Severe head injury	13 (15.3%)	3 (9.4%)	3 (9.4%)	2 (10.5%)		
Drugs/alcohol	13 (15.3%)	3 (9.4%)	4 (12.5%)	0		
Learning disability	5 (5.9%)	7 (21.9%)	2 (6.3%)	0		
Bipolar disorder	4 (4.7%)	0	1 (3.1%)	1 (5.3%)		
Psychosis	4 (4.7%)	6 (18.8%)	6 (18.8%)	2 (10.5%)		
Mild cognitive impairment	3 (3.5%)	2 (6.3%)	0	3 (15.8%)		
Tumor/cyst	3 (3.5%)	0	2 (6.3%)	0		
Multiple sclerosis	3 (3.5%)	0	0	0		
Stroke/aneurysm	3 (3.5%)	5 (15.6%)	5 (15.6%)	2 (10.5%)		
Seizures	3 (3.5%)	0	0	1 (5.3%)		
Attention deficit disorder	2 (2.4%)	0	0	0		
Panic/anxiety	2 (2.4%)	1 (3.1%)	1 (3.1%)	0		
Anoxia	2 (2.4%)	0	1 (3.1%)	1 (5.3%)		
Somatoform disorder	2 (2.4%)	1 (3.1%)	2 (6.3%)	1 (5.3%)		
HIV	2 (2.4%)	0	0	0		
Moderate head injury	1 (1.2%)	0	0	0		
Encephalitis	1 (1.2%)	0	0	0		
Asperger syndrome	1 (1.2%)	0	0	0		
Immune disorder	1 (1.2%)	0	0	0		
Klinefelter syndrome	1 (1.2%)	0	0	0		
Personality disorder	1 (1.2%)	0	0	0		
Hydrocephalus	0	1 (3.1%)	0	0		
Tourette syndrome	0	0	1 (3.1%)	0		
Carotid stenosis	0	0	1 (3.1%)	0		
Congestive heart failure	0	0	0	1 (5.3%)		
Mild head injury	0	0	0	1 (5.3%)		
Amnestic disorder	0	0	0	1 (5.3%)		
Ruled-out cognitive disorder	0	0	0	1 (5.3%)		

Group comparisons covarying for age (with the exception of DS ACSS which is already age-corrected) and education revealed significant group differences for DS ACSS ($F = 4.504$, $p = .005$), RDS ($F = 4.461$, $p = .005$), RAVLT recognition ($F = 3.761$, $p = .012$), RAVLT equation ($F = 2.922$, $p = .036$), RO equation ($F = 2.894$, $p = .038$), and RO/AVLT discriminant function ($F = 3.889$, $p = .011$), but not Rey 15-IR ($F = 2.048$, $p = .111$), DCT E-score ($F = 1.547$, $p = .206$), or WRMT-W ($F = .867$, $p = .464$). Pair-wise comparisons with Bonferroni adjustment showed that Caucasians scored significantly higher than Hispanics on DS ACSS and RDS, and higher than African Americans on RAVLT recognition, RAVLT recognition equation, the RO effort equation, and RO/AVLT discriminant function.

While data on group comparisons can be informative, they do not provide information on the classification accuracy of test cutoffs and whether adjustments are required to maintain specificity (i.e., the percentage of nonmalingering subjects correctly identified as not malingering). To this end, test frequency data within each ethnic group were examined. Table 18.2 reproduces specificity data for various test cutoffs in the four ethnic groups.

These data show that for Caucasians, some cutoffs can actually be made more stringent while still retaining adequate specificity; specifically DS ACSS can be lowered to ≤ 6 (specificity = 94.0%), the WRMT cutoff can be dropped to ≤ 39 (specificity = 96.6%), RAVLT recognition can be raised to ≤ 9 (91.1% specificity), the DCT E-score cutoff can be decreased to ≥ 15 (specificity = 91.8%), and the RO/AVLT discriminant function can be raised to $\geq -.19$. In contrast, the recommended cutoff of ≤ 12 for the RAVLT effort equation was associated with only 85.1% specificity; lowering the cutoff to ≤ 11 resulted in adequate specificity (90.5%).

In African Americans, standard test cutoffs for RDS ≤ 6, and DCT ≥ 17, are appropriate for use (i.e., specificity rates remained $\leq 90\%$ using these cutoffs), and WRMT cutoffs could even be raised to ≤ 37 to maintain acceptable specificity. Further, the Rey 15-IR and DS ACSS cutoffs only required minor adjustment (i.e., moving the cutoffs to < 18 and ≤ 4, respectively) to achieve $\geq 90\%$ specificity. However, the RO effort equation, RAVLT effort equation, RAVLT recognition, and RO/AVLT discriminant function scores were more problematic. For example, the RO effort equation standard cutoff of ≤ 47 resulted in specificity of only approximately 67%; the cutoff had to be reduced to < 34 in order to achieve a false-positive rate of < 10%. Similarly, the RAVLT effort equation cutoff required lowering to ≤ 2, the RAVLT recognition trial had to be dropped to ≤ 4, and the RO/AVLT discriminant function had to be decreased to ≤ -1.41 to achieve < 10% false-positive identifications.

In Hispanics, existing cutoffs for RAVLT recognition, RAVLT effort equation, WRMT-W, DCT, and RO/AVLT discriminant function are appropriate and can even be made more stringent without sacrificing specificity; specifically, the RAVLT recognition cutoff can be raised to ≤ 10 (93.1% spec-

TABLE 18.2. Specificity Data for Effort Tests in Ethnic and ESL Groups

	Caucasians	African Americans	Hispanics	Asians	ESL
DS ACSS	$n = 83$	$n = 31$	$n = 32$	$n = 19$	$n = 27$
≤ 3	100.0	100.0	100.0	100.0	100
≤ 4	100.0	100.0	93.7	100.0	96.3
≤ 5	98.8	93.5	87.5	100.0	88.9
≤ 6	94.0	80.6	59.4	84.2	63.0
≤ 7	71.1	54.8	37.5	78.9	48.1
Range	5–17	5–13	4–11	6–14	4–14
RDS	$n = 76$	$n = 30$	$n = 27$	$n = 16$	$n = 25$
≤ 4	100.0	100.0	100.0	100.0	100
≤ 5	100.0	100.0	96.3	100.0	96.0
≤ 6	100.0	93.3	81.5	93.7	84.0
≤ 7	82.9	80.0	44.4	87.5	52.0
≤ 8	63.2	40.0	11.1	50.0	24.0
≤ 9	42.1	23.3	11.1	18.7	8.0
Range	7–15	6–13	5–11	6–13	5–12
Rey 15-IR	$n = 56$	$n = 24$	$n = 29$	$n = 13$	$n = 23$
≤ 9	100.0	100.0	100.0	100.0	100.0
≤ 10	100.0	100.0	96.6	100.0	100.0
≤ 12	100.0	100.0	93.1	92.9	91.3
≤ 14	98.2	100.0	93.1	78.6	87.0
≤ 15	98.2	91.7	93.1	78.6	87.0
≤ 16	94.6	91.7	89.7	78.6	87.0
≤ 17	92.9	91.7	86.2	78.6	87.0
≤ 18	92.9	87.5	82.8	78.6	87.0
≤ 20	87.5	79.2	75.9	78.6	82.6
≤ 21	80.4	70.8	72.4	64.3	78.3
Range	14–30	15–30	10–30	12–30	12–30
RAVLT recognition	$n = 79$	$n = 30$	$n = 29$	$n = 17$	$n = 24$
≤ 2	100.0	100.00	100.0	100.0	100.0
≤ 3	100.0	96.7	100.0	100.0	100.0
≤ 4	100.0	93.3	100.0	100.0	100.0
≤ 5	98.7	86.7	100.0	100.0	100.0
≤ 6	98.7	86.7	100.0	88.2	95.8
≤ 7	97.5	86.7	100.0	82.4	95.8
≤ 8	94.9	83.3	96.6	76.5	91.7
≤ 9	91.1	80.0	93.1	76.5	91.7
≤ 10	84.8	66.7	93.1	76.5	91.7
≤ 11	75.9	56.7	89.7	76.5	91.7
≤ 12	62.0	50.0	75.9	64.7	79.2
Range	5–15	3–15	8–15	6–15	6–15
RAVLT equation	$n = 74$	$n = 29$	$n = 26$	$n = 15$	$n = 23$
≤ 1	98.6	93.1	100.0	100.0	100.0
≤ 2	98.6	89.7	100.0	100.0	100.0
≤ 4	97.3	89.7	100.0	100.0	100.0
≤ 5	97.3	89.7	100.0	93.3	95.7
≤ 6	97.3	89.7	100.0	86.7	95.7

(continued)

TABLE 18.2. *(continued)*

	Caucasians	African Americans	Hispanics	Asians	ESL
RAVLT equation *(continued)*					
≤ 7	97.3	86.2	100.0	86.7	95.7
≤ 8	95.9	82.8	100.0	86.7	95.7
≤ 9	94.6	79.3	100.0	86.7	95.7
≤ 10	91.9	79.3	96.2	86.7	95.7
≤ 11	90.5	75.9	92.3	86.7	95.7
≤ 12	85.1	72.4	92.3	86.7	95.7
≤ 13	75.7	72.4	92.3	86.7	95.7
≤ 14	66.2	58.6	69.1	86.7	78.3
Range	1–20	–2–20	10–20	5–19	5–20
WRMT-W	$n = 29$	$n = 13$	$n = 16$	$n = 7$	$n = 8$
≤ 35	100.0	100.0	100.0	100.0	100.0
≤ 36	100.0	100.0	100.0	85.7	100.0
≤ 37	100.0	92.3	100.0	85.7	100.0
≤ 38	100.0	84.6	100.0	85.7	100.0
≤ 39	96.6	84.6	100.0	85.7	100.0
≤ 40	89.7	84.6	100.0	85.7	100.0
≤ 41	86.2	84.6	87.5	57.1	87.5
Range	39–50	37–50	41–50	36–49	41–50
DCT E-score	$n = 49$	$n = 25$	$n = 27$	$n = 16$	$n = 22$
≥ 14	85.7	64.0	88.9	68.8	81.8
≥ 15	91.8	76.0	88.9	75.0	81.8
≥ 16	91.8	80.0	92.6	81.3	81.8
≥ 17	91.8	92.0	92.6	81.3	81.8
≥ 18	95.9	96.0	92.6	87.5	86.4
≥ 19	95.9	96.0	92.6	93.8	86.4
≥ 21	95.9	96.0	96.3	93.8	95.5
≥ 23	98.0	96.0	96.3	93.8	100.0
≥ 24	98.0	100.0	100.0	93.8	100.0
≥ 28	98.0	100.0	100.0	100.0	100.0
≥ 35	100.0	100.0	100.0	100.0	100.0
Range	6–35	8–24	6–23	4–27	6–23
RO effort equation	$n = 67$	$n = 24$	$n = 24$	$n = 16$	$n = 23$
≤ 29	100.0	100.0	100.0	100.0	100.0
≤ 30	100.0	95.8	100.0	100.0	100.0
≤ 31	100.0	91.7	100.0	100.0	100.0
≤ 34	98.5	91.7	100.0	100.0	100.0
≤ 35	98.5	87.5	100.0	100.0	100.0
≤ 36	97.0	79.5	100.0	100.0	100.0
≤ 37	97.0	79.5	100.0	100.0	100.0
≤ 39	97.0	79.5	100.0	100.0	100.0
≤ 41	95.5	75.0	100.0	100.0	100.0
≤ 42	95.5	70.8	100.0	100.0	100.0
≤ 43	95.5	66.7	91.7	100.0	100.0
≤ 44	95.5	66.7	91.7	93.7	95.5
≤ 45	95.5	66.7	87.5	93.7	90.9

(continued)

TABLE 18.2. *(continued)*

	Caucasians	African Americans	Hispanics	Asians	ESL
RO effort equation *(continued)*					
≤ 46	95.5	66.7	83.3	93.7	90.9
≤ 47	94.0	66.7	79.2	93.7	90.9
≤ 48	86.6	62.5	75.0	87.5	86.4
≤ 49	85.1	62.5	75.0	81.2	86.4
Range	34–72	30–66	43–70	44–70	44–72
RO/AVLT discriminant function	n = 67	n = 22	n = 24	n = 15	n = 21
−2.02	100.0	95.5	100.0	100.0	100.0
−1.41	100.0	90.9	100.0	100.0	100.0
−1.23	100.0	86.4	100.0	100.0	100.0
−1.07	100.0	86.4	95.8	100.0	100.0
−.94	98.4	86.4	95.8	100.0	100.0
−.91	98.4	86.4	95.8	93.3	100.0
−.86	98.4	81.8	95.8	93.3	100.0
−.83	98.4	81.8	95.8	86.7	95.2
−.63	97.0	81.8	95.8	86.7	95.2
−.48	95.5	81.8	95.8	86.7	95.2
−.38	94.0	81.8	95.6	86.7	95.2
−.34	92.5	81.8	95.8	86.7	95.2
−.19	91.0	81.8	95.8	86.7	95.2
−.06	89.6	81.8	95.8	86.7	95.2
−.03	88.1	81.8	95.8	86.7	95.2
.24	83.6	63.6	95.8	86.7	95.2
.27	83.6	63.6	91.7	86.7	95.2
.30	83.6	63.6	87.5	86.7	90.5

ificity), the RAVLT effort equation can be increased to ≥ 13 (92.3% specificity), DCT E-score can be lowered to ≥ 16 (92.6% specificity), WRMT-W cutoffs can be increased to ≤ 40 (100% specificity), and the RO/AVLT discriminant function can be raised to ≥ .27. However, the RO effort equation, Rey 15-IR, DS ACSS, and RDS cutoffs had to be decreased (to ≤ 44, ≤ 15, ≤ 4, and ≤ 5, respectively) to achieve acceptable specificity. The fact that educational level is significantly related to DS ACSS and RDS raises the possibility that the lowered specificity levels in the Hispanic, using established cutoffs, for these measures, could be an artifact of the lowered educational level of this group.

For Asians, recommended cutoffs for DS ACSS and RDS were appropriate, and the WRMT-W cutoff could be raised to ≤ 35 (100% specificity); however, six cutoffs required adjustment to maintain acceptable specificity: RAVLT effort equation ≤ 5, RAVLT recognition ≤ 5, Rey 15-IR ≤ 12, DCT E-score ≥ 19, RO effort equation ≤ 44, and RO/AVLT discriminant function ≥ −.86.

Native English-Speaking versus ESL Comparison

As shown in Table 18.3, ESL and non-ESL groups differed in education level but not age. Comparison of ESL and non-ESL groups, covarying for education, revealed that the native English speakers outperformed the ESL subjects in RDS ($F = 5.835$, $p = .017$), while the ESL group scored significant higher on RO effort equation ($F = 4.233$, $p = .042$); no significant group differences were observed for DS ACSS ($F = 3.550$, $p = .061$), RAVLT recognition ($F = .809$, $p = .370$), RAVLT effort equation ($F = .288$, $p = .592$), Rey 15-IR ($F = .411$, $p = .523$), DCT E-score ($F = .036$, $p = .850$), WRMT-W ($F = .135$, $p = .715$), and RO/AVLT discriminant function ($F = 1.200$, $p = .275$).

TABLE 18.3. Demographic Information and Frequency of Diagnosis for Native English-Speaking and ESL Groups

	Native English	ESL	t	p
n	139	28		
Age	45.07 (14.40)	45.75 (15.55)	−.224	.823
Education	13.23 (2.64)	11.64 (4.33)	2.572	.011
Gender	60m/79f	15m/13f		
Diagnoses				
Depression	20 (14.4%)	4 (14.3%)		
Severe head injury	19 (13.7%)	1 (3.6%)		
Drugs/alcohol	17 (12.3%)	3 (10.7%)		
Psychosis	12 (8.6%)	5 (17.9%)		
Learning disorder	12 (8.6%)	1 (3.6%)		
Stroke	10 (7.2%)	5 (17.9%)		
Mild cognitive impairment	7 (5.0%)	1 (3.6%)		
Bipolar	5 (3.6%)	1 (3.6%)		
Tumor/cyst	4 (2.9%)	1 (3.6%)		
Seizures	4 (2.9%)	0		
Panic/anxiety	4 (2.9%)	0		
Somatoform	4 (2.9%)	2 (7.1%)		
Multiple sclerosis	3 (2.2%)	0		
Anoxia	3 (2.2%)	1 (3.6%)		
HIV	2 (1.4%)	0		
Attention deficit disorder	2 (1.4%)	0		
Moderate head injury	1 (.7%)	1 (3.6%)		
Encephalitis	1 (.7%)	0		
Asperger syndrome	1 (.7%)	0		
Immune disorder	1 (.7%)	0		
Klinefelter syndrome	1 (.7%)	0		
Personality disorder	1 (.7%)	0		
Hydrocephalus	1 (.7%)	0		
Tourette syndrome	1 (.7%)	0		
Carotid stenosis	1 (.7%)	0		
Congestive heart failure	0	1 (3.6%)		
Mild head injury	0	1 (3.6%)		
Amnestic disorder	1 (.7%)	0		
Ruled-out cognitive disorder	1 (.7%)	0		

Examination of correlations between effort test scores and acculturation variables revealed that DS ACSS and RDS were significantly related to age at which English was learned (Spearman $r = -.248$, $p = .001$, and $r = -.290$, $p = .0001$, respectively). No effort test scores were significantly related to number of years in the United States (subtracted from total age) or number of years educated in the United States (subtracted from total education).

As shown in Table 18.2, examination of score frequencies suggested that established cutoffs for RAVLT recognition and RAVLT effort equation were appropriate for use in the ESL subjects, and for WRMT-W and RO/AVLT discriminant function the cutoffs could actually be made more stringent (i.e., ≤ 40 and $\leq. 30$, respectively) while still maintaining adequate specificity. However, for the remaining measures, the following cutoffs were required to maintain adequate specificity: DS ACSS ≤ 4 (96.3% specificity), RDS ≤ 5 (96.0% specificity), DCT E-score ≤ 19 (90.9% specificity), Rey 15-IR ≤ 12 (91.3% specificity), and RO effort equation ≤ 45 (90.9% specificity). The fact that educational level is significantly related to DS ACSS and RDS raises the possibility that the lowered specificity levels in the ESL sample, using established cutoffs for these measures, could be an artifact of the lowered educational level of this group.

DISCUSSION

The routine administration of effort measures, particularly in medical–legal and criminal cases, has become the standard of practice for neuropsychologists. However, the diversity of ethnicities in the United States and the variety of languages spoken by them has brought into question the utility of these measures with non-Caucasian and non-native English-speaking populations. Traditionally there has been little effort made to include these groups in normative samples of psychometric instruments (including measures of effort and motivation) and the literature addressing the utility of effort tests with non-Caucasians and individuals who speak other languages is sparse to nonexistent.

The information summarized in this chapter suggests that standard tests can be successfully used with ethnic minorities and those who do not speak English or speak it as a second language, but the impact of cultural and language variables requires adjustment in cutoffs on many of the measures to restrict false-positive identifications to acceptable levels (i.e., $\leq 10\%$). For example, cutoffs for the Rey 15-IR required lowering in all ethnic minorities and ESL speakers; DS ACSS and RDS cutoffs needed to be lowered in Hispanics and those who spoke English as a second language; the RAVLT recognition and RAVLT effort equation cutoffs necessitated lowering in African Americans and Asians; DCT required adjustments in Asians and those who spoke English as a second language; and RO effort equation cutoffs needed to be dropped for African Americans and Hispanics. These findings are not surprising given previously published data, including a manuscript incorporating many of the same subjects from the current study (Boone, Victor, Wen, Razani, & Ponton, in press), showing that Caucasians score higher than Hispanics on Digit Span and Boston Naming Test; score higher than African Americans on Digit Span, Trailmaking Test A, Boston Naming Test, RO copy, and Wisconsin Card Sorting Test categories; and higher than Asians on the Boston Naming Test.

Of note, the results of group comparisons did not completely mirror data from frequency analyses. For example, no differences were found between performance of Asians and other ethnic groups, yet examination of frequency counts showed that several standard test cutoffs required adjustment in Asians to prevent excessive false-positive identifications. Similarly, ESL patients only scored significantly below non-ESL patients on RDS, yet cutoffs required adjustments on several other measures to maintain specificity. These findings suggest that the use of group comparison data is not sufficient to identify which tests require adjustments to cutoffs, and that only examination of score frequencies can provide this information.

Failure to modulate cutoffs for ethnicity/language will cause some individuals to be inaccurately identified as not providing adequate effort on cognitive tasks. Recommended changes to cutoffs scores have been provided, although these should be viewed as preliminary due to the small sample sizes in some of the comparison groups. Also, given that the present data were derived from a heterogeneous clinical sample, diagnoses may not have been completely comparable across ethnic and language groups, thereby possibly introducing error into group comparisons. In addition, groups were not equated on educational level, and in particular, the required lowering of Digit Span cutoff scores may have been an artifact of lowered educational level in the Hispanic and ESL groups. Future research on larger samples with matched levels of cognitive impairment and comparable educational levels are needed. Finally, while data are presented here for several effort indices, research is lacking regarding the impact of culture/language on other commonly used effort indicators, and thus it is unknown to what extent cutoffs require adjustment on these other measures.

Caution should be taken in applying the results of the foregoing study to monolingual non-English-speaking patients. Individuals who speak English as a second language have, by definition, reached a minimum level of acculturation to their host country. Whether they acquire their English skills through academia in their home country or, as is most often the case, learn English over time through immersion in the dominant culture, they have been exposed, and if not adopted, at least become functionally familiar with the behavior, social expectations, and problem-solving strategies of this new culture. Bilingual individuals are therefore not the same as non-English-speaking monolingual immigrants who have been unable, been unwilling, or simply not had sufficient opportunity to reach a similar level of acculturation. How measures of effort would fare in the assessment of the latter group is still somewhat of an open question. The anecdotal evidence (i.e., case studies) found in the literature and presented in this chapter suggests that existing test of effort and motivation should provide comparable utility with this population as well. However, empirical studies employing sound experimental methodologies are still needed to explore this hypothesis.

In closing, we should address a final factor that has perhaps been implied but not explicitly stated regarding the assessment of non-native English speakers. Language is more than just the knowledge and use of a given cipher and grammatical structure. It is the communication of an idea through the selection of specific words, the cadence of speech, the intonation of one's voice, and the subtext that the combination of these conveys. Though often taken for granted when one has mastery over a specific language, expression via this mode is a complex and challenging endeavor, both for the message sender and for the recipient. When evaluating individuals who are monolingual in a foreign language, or have limited proficiency in English, it is imperative that the examiner have a comparable proficiency in the patient's preferred language. Artiola i Fortuni and Mullaney (1998), in fact, argued that evaluating a patient whose language the clinician does not know falls below the standard of practice for the profession. It is simply not possible for an individual unfamiliar with a language to capture the nuances essential to making fine discriminations leading to diagnosis or treatment. Though the techniques for the assessment of malingering that we discuss in this chapter are objective in their nature, and of invaluable utility to the clinician, they are not designed or intended to serve as finite determinants of a patient's mental state or overall abilities. The responsibility of this task continues to fall squarely on the clinician, who must use all information available, including that which is elusively found during interpersonal verbal communication, to render his or her expert opinion.

REFERENCES

Artiola i Fortuni, L., & Mullaney, H. A. (1998). Assessing patients whose language you do not know: Can the absurd be ethical? *The Clinical Neuropsychologist, 12,* 113–126.

Babikian, T., Boone, K., Lu, P., & Arnold, G. (2006). Sensitivity and specificity of various Digit Span scores in the detection of suspect effort, *The Clinical Neuropsychologist, 20*(1), 145–159.

Boone, K., Lu, P., & Herzberg, D. (2002). *The Dot Counting Test.* Los Angeles: Western Psychological Services.

Boone, K. B., Lu, P. H., & Wen, J. (2005). Comparison of various RAVLT scores in the detection of noncredible memory performance. *Archives of Clinical Neuropsychology, 20*(3), 301–319.

Boone, K., Salazar, X., Lu, P., Warner-Chacon, K., & Razani, J. (2002). The Rey 15-Item Recognition Trial: A technique to enhance sensitivity of the Rey 15-Item Memorization Test. *Journal of Clinical and Experimental Neuropsychology, 24*, 561–573.

Boone, K. B., Victor, T. L., Wen, J., Razani, J., & Ponton, M. (in press). The association between ethnicity and neuropsychological scores in a large patient population. *Archives of Clinical Neuropsychology*.

Butcher, J. N., Dahlstrom, W. G., Graham, J. R., Tellegen, A., & Kaemmer, B. (1989). *Manual for administration and scoring MMPI-2*. Minneapolis: University of Minnesota Press.

Chiu, V. W. Y., & Lee, T. M. C. (2002). Detection of malingering behavior at different levels of task difficulty in Hong Kong Chinese. *Rehabilitation Psychology, 47*, 194–203.

Deng, Y., & Tang, Q. (2002). The MMPI characteristics of somatoform disorders in general hospital. *Chinese Journal of Clinical Psychology, 10*(3), 179–180.

Ding, S-M, Gao, B., & Liu, R. (2002). The comparison of RSPM performances between the head injured patients with and without malingering. *Chinese Journal of Clinical Psychology, 10*, 97–99.

DuAlba, L., & Scott, R. L. (1993) Somatization and malingering for workers' compensation applicants: A cross-cultural MMPI study. *Journal of Clinical Psychology, 49*(6), 913–917.

Folstein, M. F., Folstein, S. E., & McHugh, P. R. (1975). "Mini-mental state." A practical method for grading the cognitive state of patients for the clinician. *Journal of Psychiatric Research, 12*, 189–198.

Gao, B. (2001). Assessment of malingering and exaggeration in patients involved in head injury litigation. *Chinese Journal of Clinical Psychology, 9*, 233–236.

Gao, B., Li, Z., & Chen, J. (2003). Binomial Forced-Choice Digit Recognition Test in identification of dissimulation of intelligent deficit in asking compensation after traffic accident. *Chinese Mental Health Journal, 17*(1), 50–53.

Gao, B., Li, Z., Chen, J., Liu, R., Ding, S., Li, Y., et al. (2003). Binomial forced-choice Digit Recognition Test in identification of dissimulation of intellectual deficit in asking compensation after traffic accident. *Chinese Mental Health Journal, 17*, 50–53.

Gao, B., Liu, R., Ding, S., & Lu, S. (2002). Application of the Binomial Forced-Choice Digit Memory Test in patients with compensable head trauma. *Chinese Journal of Clinical Psychology, 10*(4), 256–259.

Garcia, M., & Juan, J. (2003). Malingering on neuropsychological tests. *Anales de Psiquitría, 19*(8), 348–353.

Gutierrez, J. M., & Gur, R. C. (1998). Detection of malingering using forced-choice techniques. In C. R. Reynolds (Ed.), *Detection of malingering during head injury litigation* (pp. 81–104). New York: Plenum Press.

Guy, L. S., & Miller, H. A. (2004). Screening for malingered psychopathology in a correctional setting: Utility of the Miller-Forensic Assessment of Symptoms Test (MFAST). *Criminal Justice and Behavior, 31*(6), 695–716.

Hiscock, M., & Hiscock, C. K. (1989). Refining the forced-choice method of detection of malingering. *Journal of Clinical and Experimental Neuropsychology, 11,* 967–974.

Iverson, G., & Franzen, M. (1994). The recognition memory test, Digit Span and Knox Cube Test as markers of malingered memory impairment. *Assessment, 1,* 323–334.

Johnson, M. B., & Torres, L. (1992). Miranda, trial competency and Hispanic immigrant defendants. *American Journal of Forensic Psychology, 10*(4), 65–80.

Liu, R., Gao, B., Li, Y., & Lu, S. (2001). Simulated malingering: A preliminary trial on Hiscock's Forced-Choice Digit Memory Test. *Chinese Journal of Clinical Psychology, 9,* 173–175.

Lu, P., Boone, K., Cozolino, L., & Mitchell, C. (2003). Effectiveness of the Rey-Osterrieth Complex Figure Test and the Meyers and Meyers Recognition Trial in the detection of suspect effort. *The Clinical Neuropsychologist, 17,* 426–440.

Lucio, E., Durán, C., & Graham, J. R. (2002). Identifying faking bad on the Minnesota Multiphasic Personality Inventory–Adolescent with Mexican adolescents. *Assessment, 9*(1), 62–69.

Mayers, K. (1995). Faking it: Non-English speaking applicants for social security disability who falsify claims. *Journal of Forensic Psychology, 13,* 31–46.

Miller, H. A. (2001). *Miller-Forensic Assessment of Symptoms Test professional manual.* Odessa, FL: Psychological Assessment Resources.

Raven, J. C. (1958). *Standard progressive matrices, 1956 revision.* San Antonio, TX: Psychological Corporation.

Rogers, R. (1986). *Conducting insanity evaluations.* New York: Van Nostrand Reinhold.

Rogers, R., Harrell, E. H., & Liff, C. D. (1993). Feigning neuropsychological impairment: A critical review of methodological and clinical considerations. *Clinical Psychology Review, 13,* 255–274.

Salazar, X. F., Lopez, E., Peña, R., & Mitrushina, M. (2003, October). *Datos normativos y validez de tres pruebas para la evaluación de bajo esfuerzo/simulación en personas con educación limitada.* [Validation and preliminary normative data for three effort measures within a limited education, Spanish-speaking sample living in the United States]. Poster session presented at the annual international meeting of the Sociedad Latinoamericana de Neuropsicología, Montreal, Canada.

Sherman, D., Boone, K., Lu, P., & Ranzani, J. (2002). Re-examination of a Rey Auditory Verbal Learning Test/Rey Complex Figure discriminant function to detect suboptimal effort. *The Clinical Neuropsychologist, 16,* 242–250.

Slick, D. J., Sherman, E. M., & Iverson, G. L. (1999). Diagnostic criteria for malingered neurocognitive dysfunction: Proposed standards for clinical practice and research. *Clinical Neuropsychology, 13*(4), 545–561.

Suhr, J., Tranel, D., Wefel, J., & Barrash, J. (1997). Memory performance after head injury: Contributions of malingering, litigation status, psychological factors, and medication use. *Journal of Clinical and Experimental Neuropsychology, 19*(4), 500–514.

Teng, T-L., Change, F-A., Peng, C-P., & Yang, B-W. (2004). The study of head injury and neck injury in traffic accidents. *Journal of Applied Sciences, 4,* 449–455.

Tombaugh, T. N. (1996). *TOMM: Test of memory and malingering.* North Tonawanda, NY: Multi-Health Systems.

U.S. Census Bureau. (2003). *Statistical abstract of the United States: 2004–2005.* [Online]. Available: http//www.census.gov/compendia/statab/2006/population/pop.pdf

Wang, C. C., Schoenberg, B. S., Li, S. C., Yang, Y. C., Cheng, X. M., & Bolis, C. L. (1986). Brain injury due to head trauma. Epidemiology in urban areas of the People's Republic of China. *Archives of Neurology, 6,* 570–572.

CHAPTER 19

Assessment of Malingering in Criminal Forensic Neuropsychological Settings

Robert L. Denney

The practice of neuropsychology in the criminal setting is unique in a variety of ways, whether it is in the evaluation and/or treatment of pretrial defendants or sentenced inmates (Denney & Wynkoop, 2000). Evaluation and treatment often occur in an atypical environment that includes handcuffs, belly chains, law enforcement officers, and potentially aggressive violent offenders. While not all criminal forensic evaluees have a history of violence, they are, nonetheless, attempting to find their way through an adversarial system that may literally pose a risk of life or death to them (Rogers, 1990). Such a setting is rife with opportunity to exaggerate or, in some manner, to manipulate the neuropsychologist in an attempt to chart a safe course through these turbulent and dangerous waters. Some authors report that criminal defendants malinger in a more blatant fashion than civil litigants (Boone et al., 2002; Swanson, 1985), as predicted by Wynkoop and Denney (1999). The neuropsychologist functioning in the criminal justice system must remain mindful of the potential for symptom exaggeration and incorporate methods to identify disingenuous clinical presentation.

In this chapter, I discuss unique characteristics of criminal defendants and inmates as they relate to neuropsychological services and the different settings in which these services occur. I address the base rate of malingering

Opinions expressed in this chapter are those of the author and do not necessarily represent the position of the Federal Bureau of Prisons or the U.S. Department of Justice.

in criminal settings in regard to psychiatric and neurocognitive presentations, with an emphasis on complaints of remote memory loss. Competency to stand trial, and by extension related competency to proceed questions, are the issues most commonly addressed by mental health experts in this setting (Melton, Petrila, Poythress, & Slobogin, 1997). Complaints of memory loss have unique bearing on competency to proceed in criminal matters, as such the mental health case law will be reviewed. Finally, I address validity assessment as it relates to complaints of remote memory loss.

NEUROPSYCHOLOGICAL SERVICES IN CORRECTIONAL ENVIRONMENTS

It is commonly believed that the incarcerated population, particularly the male population, has a higher prevalence of neurocognitive compromise than does the nonincarcerated population. It is a logical conclusion given the increased incidence of traumatic brain injury-related emergency room visits among males (Langlois, Rutland-Brown, & Thomas, 2004), high rates of antisocial and psychopathic personalities in prisons (Hare, 1983; Robins, Tipp, & Przybeck, 1991), and elevated impulsive, sensation-seeking, and reckless behaviors characterized by these personalities (American Psychiatric Association, 2000; Hemphill & Hart, 2003). In fact, several different lines of research are converging to support this common understanding. Eighty-seven percent of a county jail population reported traumatic brain injury during their lifetime, and 36% reported brain injury in the year previous to incarceration; this subset showed a trend toward poorer cognitive test results and had a higher prevalence of psychiatric disorder and worse anger and aggression scores (Slaughter, Fann, & Ehde, 2003). Histories of significant brain injury were found to be more prevalent in men convicted of domestic violence than in nonoffenders, and domestic violence offenders/batterers scored significantly lower on executive, mental speed, and verbal memory measures (Turkstra, Jones, & Tolar, 2003; Westby & Ferraro, 1999; Cohen, Rosenbaum, Kane, Warnken, & Benjamin, 1999; Rosenbaum et al., 1994). Similarly, Galski, Thornton, and Shumsky (1990) identified a large percentage of 35 sex offenders as having evidence of cognitive dysfunction. Martell (1992) found at least one sign suggestive of neurocognitive compromise in 84% of 50 referrals to a maximum-security state hospital, and multiple signs were present in 64% of the sample. Examination of convicted murderers has shown that 18% have abnormal neuroimaging and 16% have Full Scale IQ < 70 (Frierson & Finkenbine, 2004). Reviews of the literature have shown a significant relationship between organic brain dysfunction and criminality (Martell, 1996), with neuroimaging revealing disruption of prefrontal–subcortical systems in violent offenders (Bassarath, 2001). The foregoing research indicates that neurocognitive dysfunction likely plays a part in at least some forms of criminal behavior and suggests that neuropsychologists may have a role to play in the assessment and management of criminal offenders.

While clinical and counseling psychologists are common in many correctional facilities (e.g., every prison in the Federal Bureau of Prisons [BOP] has psychologists as staff members), the presence of specialist clinicians, trained in neuropsychology, are predominantly relegated to medical referrals centers (e.g., there are three in the BOP, each at different medical centers). In these settings, neuropsychologists deal with a host of general medical and neurological concerns as well as pretrial and presentence court referrals. In both cases, symptom exaggeration and malingering are great concerns.

Sentenced inmates have motivation to exaggerate psychiatric and neurocognitive impairment in order to transfer to a medical center, where narcotic pain medication is more readily available and female staff are more numerous (e.g., nursing staff), and away from difficulties in the regular institution (e.g., gambling debts and gang-related violence). Often sentenced inmates also have legal appeals pending and perceive a mental illness or neurocognitive diagnosis as potentially helping their case. It has been my experience that some incarcerated individuals with little clear motivation to exaggerate their deficits even perform poorly out of disinterest, lack of motivation, or simply boredom. As illogical as this sounds, the behavior likely rises out of the impulsiveness and easily bored nature of many antisocial individuals. While sentenced inmates occasionally have motivation to perform poorly on neuropsychological testing, pretrial and presentence criminal defendants are clearly at a higher risk for malingering.

Base Rates of Symptom Exaggeration

Larrabee (2003), in an analysis of 11 different studies addressing negative response bias among civil forensic cases, reported rates which varied from 15% to 64.3% with an overall mean of 40%. Rates of malingering in the criminal arena are less clear, with most studies focusing on general psychiatric evaluations rather than neuropsychology specific referrals. For example, Rogers (1986) identified rates of 20% for suspected malingering of psychiatric symptoms and 4.5% for "definite malingering" among criminal defendants. Cornell and Hawk (1989) documented feigned psychosis among 8% of their pretrial criminal defendants. Lewis, Simcox, and Berry (2002) found that 31.4% of inpatient pretrial criminal defendants feigned psychiatric concerns based on results of the Structured Interview of Reported Symptoms (SIRS; Rogers, Bagby, & Dickens, 1992).

Data on the rate of feigned cognitive symptoms in a criminal population were contained in the results of a survey of members of the American Board of Clinical Neuropsychology who were asked to estimate the frequency of symptom exaggeration during the previous year of practice (Mittenberg, Patton, Canyock, & Condit, 2002). As one would expect, rates were higher for civil and criminal forensic cases compared to nonforensic, medical, or psychiatric cases. Only 4% of the total referrals to these clinicians were for criminal forensic cases, and of those, 68% were defense referrals; the estimate of probable malingering or symptom exaggeration in the criminal forensic sample was 22.78%.

The demographic characteristics of the survey respondents suggested that all these clinicians performed the criminal forensic evaluations on an outpatient basis. Data on feigning of psychiatric symptoms, summarized previously, suggest that higher rates of malingering are found in inpatients. Thus, the base rates of exaggerated neuropsychological concerns in a correctional population could be higher if limited to strictly inpatient referrals.

Frederick (2000a, 2000b) reported that 16% to 17% of a sample of over 600 incarcerated inpatients failed the Rey Word Recognition Test; however, he employed a low cut-score ($\leq$ 4; recommended cut-score for men $\leq$ 5; Nitch, Boone, Wen, Arnold, & Alfano, 2006) and not all defendants were specifically referred for competency to stand trial or sanity at the time of offense evaluations (other referrals were for risk assessment, general psychological evaluation regarding sentencing issues, and evaluation regarding treatment to restore competency to stand trial). Weinborn, Orr, Woods, Conover, and Feix (2003) documented that 44% of 25 inpatients referred for competency to stand trial or sanity at the time of offense failed the Test of Memory Malingering (TOMM) using standard cutoffs. However, this finding may still represent an underestimate of the prevalence of feigning in this population given data that the TOMM may have less than half the sensitivity rate of other effort measures (Gervais, Rohling, Green, & Ford, 2004).

Data from Ardolf, Denney, and Houston (in press) demonstrate a much higher prevalence of feigning of cognitive symptoms in an incarcerated population when multiple cognitive effort indicators are employed. These authors presented results of 105 serially referred inpatient neuropsychological evaluations on pretrial and presentence criminal defendants facing significant criminal charges. The evaluations were conducted over a 12-year period and included a wide variety of negative response bias indicators, some of which were dedicated malingering tests and others were indices within standard neuropsychological tests (Table 19.1). When there was more than one index within one instrument, only one of them was used to classify that entire test as positive.

Defendants experienced a variety of neuropathologies, some of which were severe; however, all evaluees were independent in their activities of daily living and were able to complete a lengthy neuropsychological test battery (Table 19.2). All referrals for neuropsychological consultation occurred because of the defendant's history of neurological condition or neurocognitive complaints.

TABLE 19.1. Cutoff Scores Used for Each Measure of Negative Response Bias

NRB measure	Cutoff criteria
Booklet Category Test	Number of criteria > 1 (Bolter, Picano, & Zych, 1985; Tenhula & Sweet, 1996)
Computerized Assessment of Response Bias (CARB)	< 89% (Allen, Conder, Green, & Cox, 1997)
Finger Oscillation Test (FOT)	< 63 total of mean scores (Larrabee, 2003)
Forced-Choice Test–Nonverbal (FCT-NV)	< 83 score & > −0.0041 consistency slope (Frederick, Sarfaty, Johnston, & Powel, 1994)
Halstead–Reitan Neuro-psychological Battery (HRNB)	> 0 Discriminant function score (Mittenberg, Rotholc, Russell, & Heilbronner, 1996)
Abbreviated Hiscock Digit Memory Test (Hiscock)	< 32 (Guilmette, Hart, Giuliano, & Leininger, 1994)
Minnesota Multiphasic Personality Inventory–2 (MMPI-2)	If male, score > 24 on FBS (Lees-Haley, 1992)
Rey 15-Item Memory Test (RMT)	< 9 Free recall correct items (Lezak, 1995); Total score < 20 (Boone, Salazar, Lu, Warner-Chacon, & Razani, 2003)
Rey Complex Figure Test	> 2 Atypical Recognition or Recognition Failure Errors (Meyers & Meyers, 1995)
Rey Dot Counting Test	Mean ungrouped time + mean grouped time + errors (i.e., no. of cards on which there was a miscount) (Bonne, Salazar, Lu, Warner-Chacon, & Razani, 2002)
Rey Word Recognition Test	< 23 (Greiffenstein, Baker, & Gola, 1996)
Test of Memory Malingering	< 33 on T^1, < 45 on T^2 or T^3 (Tombaugh, 1996)
Validity Indicator Profile	Irrelevant or suppressed response style (Frederick, 2004)
Victoria Symptom Validity Test	< 18 (Slick et al., 1997)
Wechsler Adult Intelligence Scale–R/III V-DS	V-DS > 1 (Mittenberg et al., 1995; Mittenberg et al., 2001)
Discriminant function	Discriminant function score > 0 (Mittenberg, Theroux-Fichera, Zielinski, & Heilbronner, 1995; Mittenberg et al., 2001)
Reliable Digit Span	Reliable Digit Span < 7 (Greiffenstein, Baker, & Gola, 1994; Mathias, Greve, Bianchini, Houston, & Crouch, 2002)
Wechsler Memory Scale–R	> 0 discriminant function score (Mittenberg, Azrin, Millsaps, & Heilbronner, 1993)
Wechsler Memory Scale–R (WMS-R) Forced Choice	< 19 forced-choice procedures (Denney, 1999)
Wechsler Memory Scale–III	< 137 Rarely Missed Index (Killgore & Dellapietra, 2000)
Word Memory Test	< 82.5% on IR, DR, or CNS (Green, 2003)

Note. IR, Immediate Recognition; DR, Delayed Recognition; CNS, Consistency. Adapted from Ardolf, Denney, and Houston (in press). Copyright by Taylor & Francis. *www.psypress.com/journals.asp*. Adapted by permission.

TABLE 19.2. Rates of Neuropathological Diagnosis/Conditions

Neuropathology	Frequency	%
Alzheimer's disease, Early	1	1.0
Capgras syndrome	1	1.0
Chronic fatigue syndrome	1	1.0
Cholestetoma	1	1.0
Cerebrovascular accident	5	4.8
Cerebrovascular disease	3	2.9
Alcohol dependence	7	6.7
Frontotemporal dementia, Early	1	1.0
Gunshot wound to brain	7	6.7
Inhalant dependence	2	1.9
Learning disability	2	1.9
Systemic lupus	1	1.0
Metabolic encephalopathy	1	1.0
Methamphetamine overdose	1	1.0
Mild traumatic brain injury	47	44.8
Moderate traumatic brain injury	13	12.4
Severe traumatic brain injury	2	1.9
Neurocysticosis	1	1.0
Nonspecific memory complaints	1	1.0
Polydrug dependence	2	1.9
Rocky Mountain spotted fever	1	1.0
Brain tumor	3	2.9
Vasculitis	1	1.0
Total	105	100

Note. From Ardolf, Denney, and Houston (in press). Copyright by Taylor & Francis. *www.psypress.com/journals.asp*. Reprinted by permission.

Over 89% of the sample demonstrated at least one positive indicator for negative response bias, while 70.5% had two or more indicators, and slightly more than half (53.3%) of the sample obtained three or more indicators. Table 19.3 shows other cutoff scores, and their corresponding rates. These numbers are striking and suggest that the rates of negative response bias may be higher in the criminal forensic population than in the civil forensic setting. However, these rates are not actual rates of negative response bias as it is unknown how many of these cases were truly positive. The results are also confounded by the presence of significant, and mixed, neuropathologies in the sample and use of less conservative cut off scores for several tests (e.g., Wechsler Adult Intelligence Scale [WAIS] discriminant function score > 0 and Vocabulary–Digit Span [V-DS] > 1). However, the rate of below-random-responding on forced-choice testing was 21.9%, indicating that this subset of the sample would be considered to have definite malingered neurocognitive dysfunction per criteria delineated by Slick, Sherman, and Iverson (1999). Table 19.4 reveals the rate of positive findings on each

TABLE 19.3. Rates of Negative Response Bias at Different Possible Cutoff Scores

Number of positive tests	% positive
≥ 1	89.5
≥ 2	70.5
≥ 3	53.3
≥ 4	34.3
≥ 5	29.5
≥ 6	20.0
≥ 7	16.2
≥ 8	6.7
> 9	4.8
>10	2.9
>11	1.0
Below random	21.0

Note. From Ardolf, Denney, and Houston (in press). Copyright by Taylor & Francis. *www.psypress.com/journals.asp.* Reprinted by permission.

index. One must keep in mind, however, that every evaluee did not receive every negative response bias measure. In this sense, results do not provide a head-to-head comparison of potential sensitivities between various measures.

To address the issue of mixed neuropathologies and potential impact of severe pathology on the test results, an updated version of the original database, which now includes 118 cases, was revisited. Of those 118, 67 (57%) were alleged to have experienced a mild to moderate closed head injury (22.4% moderate and 77.6% mild). The mean age of this subsample of head-injured men was 36.8 (SD = 9.9), mean education was 10.3 years (SD = 2.8); 53.7% were Caucasian, 26.9% were African American, 11.9% were Hispanic, 4.5% were Asian, and 3.0% were Native American. Mean IQ was 79.4 (SD = 12.2), although this was an underestimate due to the presence of a large number of probable and definite malingerers; when subjects were grouped using Slick et al. (1999) classification of valid, probable malingered neurocognitive dysfunction (PMND), and definite malingered neurocognitive dysfunction (DMND), mean IQs were 84.56 (SD = 9.8), 78.56 (SD = 10.33), and 71.86 (SD = 15.24), respectively. The difference in IQs between the valid and DMND group was statistically significant (F = 5.746, p = .005, Scheffe p = .006), but no significant difference was documented between IQs in the valid and PMND groups, or between IQs in the PMND and DMND group. Examination of the standard deviations shows progressively increasing variability in IQ scores from valid to PMND and DMND groups.

For this new sample, more recent and conservative cutoffs were used for the WAIS-R/III discriminant function (> .212) and V-DS (> 2) (Greve et al., 2003), and the Halstead–Reitan Neuropsychological Battery (HRNB) discriminant function cutoff was also increased from > 0 to > 0.2 (Mittenberg

TABLE 19.4. Rates and Percentage of Positive Findings

Test	% positive	No. positive/no. of administrations
HRNB DF	61.70	(29/47)
TOMM	61.54	(16/26)
WMT	60.61	(20/33)
CARB	60.00	(18/30)
WMS-R DF	58.33	(21/36)
WAIS DF, RDS, V-DS	55.17	(48/87)
BCT	54.76	(46/84)
DCT	47.82	(22/46)
MMPI-2 FBS	45.07	(32/71)
WRT	43.59	(17/39)
VSVT	40.00	(6/15)
FCT-NV	37.14	(13/35)
VIP-NV	31.82	(14/44)
VIP-V	29.73	(11/37)
DMT	28.00	(7/25)
FOT	27.54	(19/69)
Rey 15-Item	25.58	(22/86)
WMS-III Rare	21.21	(7/33)
RCFT	13.00	(3/23)
WMS-R FC	2.50	(1/40)

Note. All these measures are cited in Table 19.1. HRNB, Halstead–Reitan Neuropsychological Battery discriminant function; TOMM, Test of Memory Malingering; WMT, Word Memory Test; CARB, Computerized Assessment of Response Bias; WMS-R DF, Wechsler Memory Scale–Revised discriminant function; WAIS, WAIS-R or WAIS-III discriminant function; RDS, Reliable Digit Span; V-DS, Vocabulary-Digit Span; BCT, Booklet Category Test; DCT, Dot Counting Test; MMPI-2 FBS, Minnesota Multiphasic Personality Inventory-2 Fake Bad Scale; WRT, Word Recognition Test; VSVT, Victoria Symptom Validity Test; FCT-NV, Forced-Choice Test of Nonverbal Ability; VIP-NV, Validity Indicator Profile, nonverbal subtest; VIP-V, Validity Indicator Profile, verbal subtest; DMT, Abbreviated Hiscock Digit Memory Test; FOT, Finger Oscillation Test; WMS-III Rare, Wechsler Memory Test–III Rarely Missed Index; RCFT, Rey Complex Figure Test Atypical Recognition and Recognition Failure Errors. Based on Ardolf, Denney, and Houston (in press).

et al., 1996). The Rey 15-Item Test (Rey 15) results were divided into free recall criteria (< 9) and Boone et al.'s (2002) recall and recognition total score (< 20). For those few cases which included the Victoria Symptom Validity Test (VSVT), easy and hard items were treated separately as research demonstrates malingerers are prone to suppress hard items more than easy items (Slick, Hopp, Strauss, & Thompson, 1997). Table 19.5 provides the rate of positive findings for this dataset.

Table 19.6 reveals the percentage of cases positive for potential negative response bias based on the number of positive test findings. For this calculation, tests containing multiple negative response bias indices (e.g., WAIS and Rey 15) were counted positive if any of the instrument's indices were positive. The Booklet Category Test criteria remained > 1 of five indices positive. Fourteen of these criminal defendants (20.9%) scored below random (< .05,

TABLE 19.5. Rate and Percentages of Positive Findings for 67 Pretrial Criminal Defendants with Mild and Moderate Traumatic Brain Injury Referred for Neuropsychological Evaluation, in Descending Order

Test	% positive	No. positive/no. of administrations
WMT	72.0	(18/25)
CARB	60.0	(15/25)
TOMM	56.5	(13/23)
WRT	54.1	(13/24)
WMS-R DF	52.4	(11/21)
DCT	52.0	(13/25)
HRNB	51.6	(16/31)
VSVT	50.0	(3/6)
FCT-NV	45.5	(10/22)
BCT	45.2	(24/53)
MMPI-2 FBS	44.0	(22/50)
WAIS RDS	40.0	(22/55)
WAIS DF	34.0	(16/47)
DMT	33.3	(6/18)
FOT	29.8	(14/47)
VIP-NV	29.0	(9/31)
Rey 15 Total	26.0	(6/23)
Rey 15 Recall	23.7	(14/59)
VIP-V	19.2	(5/26)
RCFT	17.6	(3/17)
WAIS V-DS	13.5	(7/52)
WMS-III Rare	13.0	(3/23)

Note. WMT, Word Memory Test; CARB, Computerized Assessment of Response Bias; TOMM, Test of Memory Malingering; WRT, Word Recognition Test; WMS-R DF, Wechsler Memory Scale–Revised discriminant function; DCT, Dot Counting Test; HRNB, Halstead–Reitan Neuropsychological Battery discriminant function; VSVT, Victoria Symptom Validity Test; FCT-NV, Forced-Choice Test of Nonverbal Ability; BCT, Booklet Category Test; MMPI-2 FBS; Minnesota Multiphasic Personality Inventory–2 Fake Bad Scale; WAIs RDS, Reliable Digit Span; WAIS DF, WAIS-R or WAIS-III discriminant function; DMT, Abbreviated Hiscock Digit Memory Test; FOT, Finger Oscillation Test; VIP-NV, Validity Indicator Profile, nonverbal subtest; Rey 15 Total, Total score = recall correct + (correct recognition – recognition errors); Rey 15 Recall, Free recall correct; VIP-V, Validity Indicator Profile, verbal subtest; RCFT, Rey Complex Figure Test > 2 atypical errors; WAIS V-DS, Wechsler Adult Intelligence Scale–R or III Vocabulary–Digit Span; WMS-III Rare, Wechsler Memory Scale–III Rarely Missed Index.

one tail) on some form of two alternative, forced-choice testing; these individuals are considered to demonstrate definite negative response bias. Nearly 12% did not score positive on any malingering index. Twenty-seven percent scored positive on less than two indices, thereby classifying them as valid from testing alone (Slick et al., 1999, Criteria B only). In contrast, 73.1% had two or more positive indices (which included individuals with below-random performances). This score is slightly higher than the 70.48% found for the original 105 mixed neuropathology population (Ardolf et al., 2004). This finding was somewhat unexpected in that the data from the trau-

TABLE 19.6. Rates of Negative Response Bias at Different Possible Cutoff Scores for Pretrial Criminal Defendants with Mild and Moderate Traumatic Brain Injury Referred for Neuropsychological Evaluation

No. of tests positive	Frequency	%	Cumulative %
0	8	11.9	11.9
1	10	14.9	26.9
2	12	17.9	44.8
3	8	11.9	56.7
4	2	3.0	59.7
5	9	13.4	73.1
6	5	7.5	80.6
7	6	9.0	89.6
8	5	7.5	97.0
9	1	1.5	98.5
10	1	1.5	100.0
Total	67	100.0	

matic brain injury (TBI) subset were anticipated to be more conservative (i.e., less contaminated by false-positive identifications) given that each malingering index was designed to identify feigned or exaggerated TBI specifically and because the pathologies found in the brain injury group were less severe than those of many of the non-TBI subjects. However, as discussed below, the rate of noncredible cognitive symptoms may be particularly elevated in a head injury population. Overall, the data from the head injury sample and the unselected larger group shed light on the likely base rate of malingering in the inpatient population of pretrial criminal defendants referred for neuropsychological evaluation; specifically, that nearly three in four appear to be feigning or exaggerating cognitive impairment.

However, determination of malingering requires additional information beyond simply presence of negative response bias on testing. The Slick et al. (1999) diagnostic classification for PMND and DMND was also applied to the 67 mild and moderate TBI cases. This classification requires that all other neurological and psychiatric reasons for poor performance have been ruled out, and that performance was judged to have been consciously motivated by secondary gain. All these pretrial criminal defendants had substantial secondary gain as they were facing serious federal charges with substantial prison sentences. Also, malingered neurocognitive dysfunction can include individuals who only test positive on one, or even no, malingering indices yet present atypical and unlikely test results (Criteria B) or self-report (Criteria C).

Twenty-five of the brain trauma cases (37.3%) were considered valid. This group included eight individuals who scored negative on all malingering indices; they also demonstrated no positive indications of exaggeration on B and C criteria. Eight cases scored positive on only one malingering index (positive Criterion B2) but no other positive findings in B or C criteria. The remaining nine cases were considered valid, even though they scored positive on multiple indices (two indices, $n = 6$, 67%; three indices, $n = 2$, 22%; and four indices, $n = 1$, 11%). None of these cases produced positive findings on other B criteria or C criteria. Twenty-eight cases (41.8%) were considered to have PMND, and 14 (20.9%) were judged to have DMND due to below-random performance. In addition, two of the PMND cases were known malingerers because of instantaneous "recoveries" shortly after the judge found them competent to stand trial. This reassignment would result in a DMND total of 23.9%.

Combining PMND and DMND groups resulted in a total of 62.7%. This possible base rate is more conservative than the 73.1% rate of cases with two or more positive test indices. Likely the true base rate for malingered neurocognitive dysfunction lies between 63% and 73% for pretrial inpatient criminal defendants referred for neuropsychological evaluation although these findings require replication.

Importance of Base-Rate Information

Identifying the base rate for malingering among criminal defendants referred for neuropsychological evaluations is vital because it sheds light on the predictive value of any malingering detection method (Baldessarini, Finkelstein, & Arona, 1983). The Mittenberg et al. (2002) survey suggested the base rate for symptom exaggeration among this population was approximately 23% (corrected for influence of referral source). That base rate was based on clinicians' estimates of the rates of identification over the course of the most recent year rather than a case-by-case file review. It was not clear how thoroughly the clinicians evaluated for symptom exaggeration, although most respondents reported using multiple methods to detect negative response bias. Results from my data suggest the base rate in the criminal forensic population is actually much higher, even over 50%.

The importance of prevalence rates rising beyond 50% cannot be overstated. The difference in diagnostics certainly as it relates to classification accuracy between a low-base-rate phenomenon and a high-base-rate phenomenon can easily be demonstrated. We must keep in mind that test sensitivity (that is, cases with the diagnosis that have a positive test finding; also true positives/[true positives + false negatives]) and specificity (nonimpaired cases that have a negative test finding; also true negative/[true negatives + false positives]) are unique to the instrument and do not vary based on prevalence of disorder. The hit rate index identifies the overall correct classification ability of the instrument and is demonstrated with (true positives + true negatives)/N. Predictive value statistics, such as positive predictive value (PPV) and negative predictive value (NPV) incorporate the prevalence of disorder (Baldesserini et al., 1983). PPV is determined by true positives/(true positives + false positives) and NPV is determined by true negatives/(true negatives + false negatives). Baldesserini et al provide these formulas for computing PPV and NPV, incorporating test sensitivity (x), specificity (y), and base rate (prevalence, p):

$$PPV = (px)/[(px) + (1 - p)(1 - y)]$$
$$NPV = [(1 - p)y]/[(1 - p)y + p(1 - x)].$$

Let us assume the use of a well-validated, and very accurate, malingering instrument or combination of instruments that have a sensitivity of .80 and specificity of .90. In a base-rate setting of .20, PPV is .667, and NPV is .947. In this situation, one has much more diagnostic confidence in negative findings. The confidence significantly changes as the base rate changes, however. In a base-rate setting of .70, PPV is .949, and NPV is .659. Here one has much more confidence in positive findings and strikingly less confidence in negative findings. Knowledge of prevalence rates does not change the accuracy of the test; rather, the knowledge changes confidence in the test findings. My data suggest the base rate of malingered neurocognitive dysfunction among criminal defendants with neurocognitive concerns is over 50% (very possibly over the 70% rate). In this setting, positive findings on malingering indices have convincing determinative power, while negative malingering results need closer scrutiny.

Mittenberg et al. (2002) provide a cogent discussion regarding the importance of considering the base rates of actual neurocognitive impairment within the population in question. Referring to Larrabee's (2003) 40% estimate of malingering in personal injury litigation and the very low rate of impairment for individuals with mild TBI after 3 months (approximately 5%), Mittenberg et al. (2002) conclude that the likely true base rate for malingering in that population may actually approach 88%. Using that reasoning, the base rate for malingered neurocognitive dysfunction among criminal defendants with complaints based on mild TBI could be astoundingly high.

COMPLAINTS OF REMOTE MEMORY LOSS

Memory complaints are common after head injury and a wide number of other neuropathologies. Often, these complaints involve concentration, new learning, and occasionally remote memories (Hannay, Howieson, Loring, Fischer, & Lezak, 2004). Claims of remote memory loss involving specific events in the past beyond a period of retrograde amnesia are relatively uncommon in personal injury settings. Claims of remote memory loss, particularly for alleged criminal activity, are not unusual, however (Schacter,

1986). Rates appear higher for acts of violence; estimates have ranged from 23% to 65% for homicide cases (Bradford & Smith, 1979; Guttmacher, 1955; Leitch, 1948; Parwatikar, Holcomb, & Menninger, 1985). Hopwood and Snell (1933) reviewed the rates of amnesia among 100 criminal cases and found 90% of the claims pertained to murder or attempted murder. In contrast, only 8% of 120 cases of nonhomicide violent crimes claimed amnesia, and there were no claims of amnesia among 47 individuals charged with nonviolent crimes (Taylor & Kopelman, 1984).

Researchers have long held the perspective that a substantial number of amnestic claims for alleged criminal acts are feigned (Adatto, 1949; Bradford & Smith, 1979; Hopwell & Snell, 1933; Lynch & Bradford, 1980; O'Connell, 1960; Parwatikar et al., 1985; Power, 1977; Price & Terhune, 1919). In this regard, Schacter (1986) provided this summary:

> In the large majority of criminal cases that involve amnesia, the loss of memory either has a functional origin or concerns only a single critical event. I have found no cases in the literature in which a patient afflicted with chronic organic amnesia has come before the courts on a serious criminal matter that is related to his or her memory disorder. Organic factors may play a role when concussion, alcohol intoxication, or epileptic seizure occurs during a crime, with subsequent limited amnesia for the crime itself, but in these cases memory problems typically do not exist prior to the crime. (p. 287)

Indeed, crimes related to epileptic seizures (and other so-called automatism defenses) are quite rare (Barnard, 1998; Melton et al., 1997). Occasionally, however, criminal defendants experience a neurological condition either severe enough, or proximal to the crime such, that it can hinder recall of events around the time of the alleged offense (Wynkoop & Denney, 1999). It is also possible that individuals conducting criminal activity while intoxicated may subsequently not recall these events due to alcoholic blackouts. Other examples could include individuals who experience a TBI during the crime or arrest or suffer a neurological insult, such as cerebrovascular stroke or hemorrhage, after the arrest but before legal proceedings are concluded (Denney & Wynkoop, 2000). Under such circumstances, it is not unreasonable to find loss of memory for events preceding the arrest, including the offense behavior. Criminal defendants' ability to recall events sufficiently to reconstruct their activities for the period of time around the offense is an important aspect of their ability to assist in their own defense. In this regard, amnesia for past events has the potential to limit a criminal defendant's competency to proceed.

Criminal case law has specifically addressed the issue of memory loss as it pertains to competency to stand trial. In a federal case in the Western District of Missouri (*Wieter v. Settle*, 1961), the court concluded that a criminal defendant needed to have memory sufficient to relate his or her recollections of events relevant to the time of the offense. In a more authoritative case, the U.S. Court of Appeals for the District of Columbia addressed the issue as well (*Wilson v. United States*, 1968). Defendant Wilson sustained a TBI when his "get-away car" crashed into a tree at the end of a high-speed chase. He was unconscious at the scene and was later determined to have "fractured his skull and ruptured several blood vessels in his brain" (p. 461). He was unconscious for 3 weeks and later denied recollection of five counts of assault with a deadly weapon and robbery. Supposedly, there were no observable mental difficulties beyond his claimed memory loss for the events of the crime. He was found competent to stand trial and convicted. On appeal to the U.S. Court of Appeals, the court concluded that amnesia, in and of itself, did not necessarily eliminate Wilson's competency to proceed with his case, although it could potentially play a part in the determination of competency. While *Wilson* does not have wide jurisdictional authority, it was decided by the U.S. Court of Appeals for the District of Columbia, and this district often leads the way in a precedent-setting manner for other jurisdictions regarding mental health issues in criminal law (Melton et al., 1997). Given these concerns, it is not surprising then that courts have an interest in determining the legitimacy of a criminal defendant's claimed amnesia.

Symptom Validity Testing for Remote Memory

Identifying feigned memory loss for a specific period of time, or for a specific event, is not an easy task. There have been a number of methods presented to evaluate claimed amnesia (see Rubinsky & Brandt, 1986; Schacter, 1986; Wiggins & Brandt, 1988), but most do not avail themselves to the detection of specific criminal events. However, classical symptom validity testing (SVT) has been adapted to address this very issue.

Originally designed to assess sensory complaints, SVT was modified to detect psychogenic learning and retention deficits (Haughton, Lewsley, Wilson, & Williams, 1979; Pankratz, 1979; Pankratz, Fausti, & Peed, 1975; Theodor & Mendelcorn, 1973). Frederick and Carter (1993; Frederick, Carter, & Powel, 1995) further adapted this technique to assess memory for events surrounding an alleged offense for which a criminal defendant was claiming amnesia. Several two-alternative, forced-choice questions were developed for events reported in criminal investigative records. These questions were presented to the defendant, and he performed statistically below expectations for an individual who has no memory for those events.

SVT is based on the binomial theorem which purports that when two possibilities of equal probability exist, results will fall around the mean in an expected pattern consistent with the bell-shaped curve (Siegel, 1956). Similarly, when an individual with no ability/knowledge is asked a number of questions with only two possible answers of equal probability, results should likewise fall in a random range around the mean. Knowledge is demonstrated to a particular level of statistical certainty when results fall outside the random range. Customarily, individuals with knowledge of events in question score well above the random range. Likewise, results falling below random range also demonstrate knowledge. Appendix 19.1 provides examples of such questions.

When applied in a criminal context, SVT questions are derived from investigative materials, medical records, or interviews of witnesses, family members, or law enforcement personnel. Often, the facts of the case are well described in the indictment and supportive information. This information is combed to create questions about events and facts which the defendant would have known or experienced during the period of claimed amnesia. Enough data are required in order to generate an ample number of questions (> 24 questions); increased number of items will increase sensitivity and overall accuracy. In addition, the information on which the questions are based must be salient enough that an individual without significant memory loss would likely have remembered it. Questions should be developed to include the correct answer and an equally plausible alternative. Frederick et al. (1995) noted the difficulty in creating reasonably plausible alternative answers. Subsequent research has demonstrated that unequal answers actually increase the conservative nature of the procedure (Frederick & Denney, 1998); however, it is important that the alternative answers not systematically present more likely possibilities. Biasing the test in this manner would inappropriately increase the possibility that a truly amnestic individual could select wrong answers more often than what would occur by chance. In this regard, it is helpful to have a colleague review the questions before administration. Questions should also be worded in such a manner that they avoid direct admissions of guilt, such as "investigative records allege . . . " or "the prosecution claims . . . ," as the procedure is designed to identify false claims of memory loss rather than identify guilt.

Defendants are instructed that because of their memory concerns, they will be tested regarding their memory for those specific events in order to more clearly understand their memory problem. Each item is prefaced with the query of whether they remember this information or not. Items for which they claim recall of the information or "reason out" the solution are discarded because the test is designed to measure their lack of recollection (Denney, 1996). Items not recalled or invalidated through deductive logic are administered with the instruction to choose the correct answer or simply to guess to the best of their ability if they cannot remember. Subjects are told whether they are correct or incorrect, and the correct answer is noted. Often, the task is constructed so that succeeding queries are a more specific variant of the preceding question (e.g., Investigative records allege you did what, rob a bank or perform a drug deal?; No, it alleges you robbed a bank; Was it First Interstate Bank or Seattle First Bank?; Was it on 2nd Avenue or 4th Avenue?, etc.). In this manner, an efficient and fluid analysis of the claimed amnesia can occur. Correct answers are totaled and applied to this formula from Siegel (1956):

$$z = [(x \pm 0.5) - NP]/\sqrt{NPQ}$$

where z is the test statistic; x is the number of correct responses; N is the number of questions administered; p is the probability of a correct discrimination given no true ability (0.5); and Q represents $1 - p$ (probability of an incorrect discrimination). The correction (adding 0.5 when $x < NP$; subtracting 0.5 when $x > NP$) is made to adjust for continuity as the binomial distribution involves discrete variables. A one-tail test is used to identify the exact probability using the Unit Normal Table (z table). The one-tail test is considered appropriate given the intent to identify suppressed performance (Larrabee, 1992; Siegel, 1956). A z-score of -1.65 is significant at $p = 0.05$ and -2.33 is significant at $p = .01$.

Denney (1996) and Frederick and Denney (1998) demonstrated that individuals with no knowledge of the events in question perform predominantly within the random range with scores clustering around the mean (50%). However, the mean was actually slightly better than 50% as the research subjects appeared to be able to identify a high number of correct responses. Results demonstrated that the procedure was actually slightly more conservative than that spelled out by the binomial distribution. Further, Frederick and Denney (1998) performed computer simulations in which P and Q were equal to 0.5 and demonstrated that instances in which item answers were equally plausible caused the test statistic to perform even more conservatively. The increased variability led to a decrease in sensitivity thereby lessening the likelihood of labeling a true amnestic as a malingerer. Denney (1996) and Frederick and Denney (1998) also provide case examples demonstrating the developed questions and the effectiveness of the procedure.

While the SVT procedure can be time-intensive in terms of acquiring investigative material and developing questions, it has proven itself an effective tool in identifying feigned claims of remote memory loss. Similarly, the procedure can also be adapted to claims of remote memory loss (e.g., ignorance regarding commonly known aspects of the criminal justice system as they relate to competency to stand trial). Appendix 19.2 presents examples of this type of questioning.

FUTURE DIRECTIONS IN MALINGERING DETECTION WITHIN THE CRIMINAL FORENSIC SETTING

Identifying exaggerated neurocognitive dysfunction in the criminal forensic setting is a critical issue. Society has a constitutional mandate to provide appropriate medical and mental health care to the incarcerated population, and it is important to criminal defendants who have legitimate neuro-cognitive and psychiatric disorders to have appropriate treatment. It is also important for judges to have an accurate understanding regarding a criminal defendant's mental health needs, not only to provide appropriate referral for care but also to maintain justice. In fact, case law has demonstrated how seriously the courts take this responsibility. The U.S. Court of Appeals for the Fifth Circuit upheld the trial court's decision to enhance the sentence of a feigning criminal defendant as a punishment for willfully obstructing justice by feigning incompetence (*United States v. Greer*, 1998; Knoll & Resnick, 1999). Neuropsychologists are well suited to address the legitimacy of criminal defendant's claims of neurocognitive dysfunction if they incorporate appropriate diagnostic methods and appreciate the significance of an elevated prevalence of symptom exaggeration in this unique population.

Unfortunately, little research exists regarding the prevalence of exaggeration and malingering in the criminal setting. Rates are certainly higher than in nonforensic settings, and preliminary results suggest that the rate is even higher in the criminal forensic setting than it is in the civil forensic arena. Further, rates of malingering may differ within the correctional setting, depending on such variables as the nature of the crimes defendants are charged with; for example, there is evidence that inmates charged with murder and who are undergoing competency evaluations may show a TOMM failure rate of 80% in contrast to the 25% rate observed in defendants facing lesser charges (Weinborn et al., 2003). Additional research is needed to replicate these findings.

Further research is also needed to determine the relative sensitivity and specificity rates of neurocognitive exaggeration detection methods in the criminal forensic setting, as there is no reason to expect all cognitive effort procedures to perform similarly in the criminal setting as they do in the civil forensic setting (Wynkoop & Denney, 1999), a contention supported by preliminary data. For example, some studies have found higher sensitivity rates in a correctional population as compared to a civil litigant sample for such effort measures as the Dot Counting Test (DCT) (i.e., 100% at a cutoff of ≥ 15; Boone et al., 2002) and the Rey 15-Item Memorization Test (i.e., 86% at a cutoff of < 9; Simon, 1994), although sensitivity rates comparable to those observed in civil litigants have been reported for Reliable Digit Span (RDS) (i.e., 57% at a cutoff of ≤ 6; Duncan & Ausborn, 2002). Also, given the impetus to accurately identify the presence of mental retardation given the recent U.S. Supreme Court decision banning execution of mentally retarded individuals (*Atkins v. Virginia*, 2002), special attention to the determination of actual versus feigned mental retardation is critical. There is evidence that specificity rates may be unacceptably low on many effort indicators in a mentally retarded population (see Victor & Boone, Chapter 14, this volume), and that within an incarcerated population, false-positive identifications on measures such as the TOMM can potentially occur in mildly to moderately mentally retarded individuals and in persons with treatment-resistent schizophrenia (Weinborn et al., 2003).

Additional research is also needed regarding the use of SVT for remote memory, particularly in the area of sensitivity and specificity. As with other SVT procedures, it may prove valuable to identify criterion-related cutoffs that increase sensitivity without losing meaningful specificity. For example, researchers could derive questions regarding events covered during the period of retrograde amnesia for head injury rehabilitation patients not in litigation and compare their performances with that of criminal defendants believed to be feigning remote memory loss. In this manner cutoffs higher than below-random performance could be derived that would potentially demonstrate significantly improved sensitivity without a great loss of specificity. Given the finding of Denney (1996) and Frederick and Denney (1998) that information-naïve experimental participants tended to guess slightly higher than the 50% mark, cutoffs higher than below random could be effective.

Finally, very little is known about how criminal defendants exaggerate on existing competency-to-stand trial measures and how those with actual versus exaggerated neurocognitive compromise perform on competency assessment tools. Further, no data are available regarding the relationship between feigned performance on cognitive effort tests and scores on competency measures.

Continued empirical focus on the neurocognitive functioning of criminal defendants will improve evaluation effectiveness and quality of mental health care for one of the most underserved populations in society.

REFERENCES

Adatto, C. P. (1949). Observations on criminal patients during narcoanalysis. *Archives of Neurology and Psychiatry*, *62*, 82–92.

Allen, L. M., Conder, R. L., Green, P., & Cox, D. (1997). *CARB '97 Manual for the Computerized Assessment of Response Bias*. Durham, NC: Cognisyst.

American Psychiatric Association. (2000). *Diagnostic and statistical manual of mental disorders* (4th ed., text rev.). Washington, DC: Author.

Ardolf, B. R., Denney, R. L., & Houston, C. M. (in press). Base rates of negative response bias and malingered neurocognitive dysfunction among criminal defendants referred for neuropsychological evaluation. *The Clinical Neuropsychologist*.

Atkins v. Virginia, 153 L. Ed 2d 335 (2002).

Baldesserini, R. J., Finkelstein, S., & Arona, G. W. (1983). The predictive power of diagnostic tests and the effects of prevalence of illness. *Archives of General Psychiatry*, *40*, 569–573.

Barnard, P. G. (1998). Diminished capacity and automatism as a defense. *American Journal of Forensic Psychology*, *16*, 27–62.

Bassarath, L. (2001). Neuroimaging studies of antisocial behaviour. *Canadian Journal of Psychiatry, 46,* 728–732.

Bolter, J. F., Picano, J. J., & Zych, K. (1985, October). *Item error frequencies on the Halstead Category Test: An index of performance validity.* Paper presented at the annual meeting of the National Academy of Neuropsychology, Philadelphia.

Boone, K. B., Lu, P., Back, C., King, C., Lee, A., Philpott, L., et al. (2002). Sensitivity and specificity of the Rey Dot Counting Test in patients with suspect effort and various clinical samples. *Archives of Clinical Neuropsychology, 17,* 625–642.

Boone, K. B., Salazar, X., Lu, P., Warner-Chacon, K., & Razani, J. (2003). The Rey 15-Item recognition trial: A technique to enhance sensitivity of the Rey 15-Item Memorization Test. *Journal of Clinical and Experimental Neuropsychology, 24,* 561–573.

Bradford, J. W., & Smith, S. M. (1979). Amnesia and homicide: The *Padola* case and a study of thirty cases. *Bulletin of the American Academy of Psychiatry and Law, 7,* 219–231.

Cohen, R. A., Rosenbaum, A., Kane, R. L., Warnken, W. J., & Benjamin, S. (1999). Neuropsychological correlates of domestic violence. *Violence Victims, 14,* 397–411.

Cornell, D. G., & Hawk, G. L. (1989). Clinical presentation of malingerers diagnosed by experienced forensic psychologists. *Law and Human Behavior, 13,* 357–383.

Denney, R. L. (1996). Symptom Validity Testing of remote memory in a criminal forensic setting. *Archives of Clinical Neuropsychology, 11,* 589–603.

Denney, R. L. (1999). A brief symptom validity testing procedure for Logical Memory of the Wechsler Memory Scale–Revised which can demonstrate verbal memory in the face of claimed disability. *Journal of Forensic Neuropsychology, 1,* 5–26.

Denney, R. L., & Wynkoop, T. F. (2000). Clinical neuropsychology in the criminal forensic setting. *Journal of Head Trauma Rehabilitation, 15,* 804–828.

Duncan, S. A., & Ausborn, D. L. (2002). The use of Reliable Digits to detect malingering in a criminal forensic pretrial population. *Assessment, 9,* 56–61.

Frederick, R. I. (2000a). A personal floor effect strategy to evaluate the validity of performance on emmroy tests. *Journal of Clinical and Experimental Neuropsychology, 22,* 720–730.

Frederick, R. I. (2000b). Mixed group validation: A method to address the limitations of criterion group validation in research on malingering detection. *Behavioral Sciences and the Law, 18,* 693–718.

Frederick, R. I. (2004). *Validity Indicator Profile manual, revised.* Minnetonka, MN: NCS Assessments.

Frederick, R. I., & Carter, M. (1993, August). *Detection of malingered amnesia in a competency evaluee.* Paper presented at the annual convention of the American Psychological Association, Toronto, Canada.

Frederick, R. I., Carter, M., & Powel, J. (1995). Adapting symptom validity testing to evaluate suspicious complaints of amnesia in medicolegal evaluations. *The Bulletin of the American Academy of Psychiatry and the Law, 23,* 227–233.

Frederick, R. I., & Denney, R. L. (1998). Minding your "*p*s and *q*s" when using forced-choice recognition tests. *The Clinical Neuropsychologist, 12,* 193–205.

Frederick, R. I., Sarfaty, S. D., Johnston, J. D., & Powel, J. (1994). Validation of a detector of response bias on a forced-choice test of nonverbal ability. *Neuropsychology, 8,* 118–125.

Frierson, R. L., & Finkenbine, R. D. (2004). Psychiatric and neurological characteristics of murder defendants referred for pretrial evaluation. *Journal of Forensic Science, 49*, 604–609.

Galski, T., Thornton, K. E., & Shumsky, D. (1990). Brain dysfunction in sex offenders. *Journal of Offender Rehabilitation, 16*, 65–80.

Gervais, R. O., Rohling, M. L., Green, P., & Ford, W. (2004). A comparison of WMT, CARB, and TOMM failure rates in non-head injury disability claimants. *Archives of Clinical Neuropsychology, 19*, 475–487.

Green, P. (2003). *Green's Word Memory Test for Windows user's manual.* Edmonton, Alberta, Canada: Author.

Greiffenstein, M. F., Baker, W. J., & Gola, T. (1994). Validation of malingered amnesia measures with a large clinical sample. *Psychological Assessment, 6*, 218–224.

Greiffenstein, M. F., Baker, W. J., & Gola, T. (1996). Comparison of multiple scoring methods for Rey's malingered amnesia measures. *Archives of Clinical Psychology, 53*, 757–766.

Greve, K. W., Bianchini, K. J., Mathias, C. W., Houston, R. J., & Crouch, J. A. (2003). Detecting malingered performance on the Wechsler Adult Intelligence Scale: Validation of Mittenberg's approach in traumatic brain injury. *Archives of Clinical Neuropsychology, 18*, 245–260.

Guilmette T. J., Hart, K. J., Giuliano, A. J., & Leininger, B. E. (1994). Detecting simulated memory impairment: Comparison of the Rey 15-Item Test and the Hiscock Forced-Choice Procedure. *The Clinical Neuropsychologist, 8*, 283–294.

Guttmacher, M. S. (1955). *Psychiatry and the law.* New York: Grune & Stratton.

Hannay, H. J., Howieson, D. B., Loring, D. W., Fischer, J. S., & Lezak, M. D. (2004). Neuropathology for neuropsychologists. In M. D. Lezak, D. B. Howieson, & D. W. Loring (Eds.), *Neuropsychological Assessment* (4th ed., pp. 157–285). New York: Oxford University Press.

Hare, R. D. (1983). Diagnosis of antisocial personality disorder in two prison populations. *American Journal of Psychiatry, 140*, 887–890.

Haughton, P. M., Lewsley, A., Wilson, M., & Williams, R. G. (1979). A forced-choice procedure to detect feigned or exaggerated hearing loss. *British Journal of Audiology, 13*, 135–138.

Hemphill, J. F., & Hart, S. D. (2003). Forensic and clinical issues in the assessment of psychopathy. In I. B. Weiner (Series Ed.) & A. M. Goldstein (Vol. Ed.), *Handbook of psychology, Vol. 11: Forensic psychology* (pp. 87–107). Hoboken, NJ: Wiley.

Hopwood, J. S., & Snell, H. K. (1933). Amnesia in relation to crime. *Journal of Mental Science, 79*, 27–41.

Killgore, W. D., & Dellapietra, L. (2000). Using the WMS-III to detect malingering; Empirical validation of the Rarely Missed Index (RMI). *Journal of Clinical and Experimental Neuropsychology, 22*, 761–771.

Knoll, J. L., IV, & Resnick, P. J. (1999). *U. S. v. Greer*: Longer sentences for malingerers. *Journal of the American Academy of Psychiatry and the Law, 27*, 621–625.

Langlois, J. A., Rutland-Brown, W., & Thomas, K. E. (2004). *Traumatic Brain Injury in the United States: Emergency department visits, hospitalizations, and deaths* [Online}. Atlanta, GA: U.S. Department of Health & Human Services, Centers for Disease Control & Prevention, National Center for Injury Prevention & Control. Retrieved November 8, 2005, from *www.cdc.gov/ncipc/pub-res/TBI_in_US_04/TBI-USA_Book-Oct1.pdf.*

Larrabee, G. J. (1992). On modifying recognition memory tests for detection of malingering. *Neuropsychology, 6*, 23–27.

Larrabee, G. J. (2003). Detection of malingering using atypical performance patterns on standard neuropsychological tests. *The Clinical Neuropsychologist, 17*, 410–425.

Lees-Haley, P. R. (1992). Efficacy of MMPI-2 validity scales and MCMI-II modifier scales for detesting spurious PTSD claims: F, F-K, Fake Bad scale, Ego Strength, Subtle-Obvious subscales, DIS and DEB. *Journal of Clinical Psychology, 48*, 681–689.

Leitch, A. (1948). Notes on amnesia in crime for the general practitioner. *Medical Press, 219*, 459–463.

Lewis, J. L., Simcox, A. M., & Berry, D. T. R. (2002). Screening for feigned psychiatric symptoms in a forensic sample by using the MMPI-2 and Structured Inventory of Malingered Symptomology. *Psychological Assessment, 14*, 170–176.

Lezak, M. D. (1995). *Neuropsychological Assessment* (3rd ed.). New York: Oxford University Press.

Lynch, B. E., & Bradford, J. M. W. (1980). Amnesia: Its detection by psychophysiological measures. *Bulletin of the American Academy of Psychiatry and the Law, 8*, 288–297.

Martell, D. A. (1992). Estimating the prevalence of organic brain dysfunction in maximum-security forensic psychiatric patients. *Journal of Forensic Sciences, 37*, 878–893.

Martell, D. A. (1996). Organic brain dysfunctions and criminality. In L. B. Schlesinger (Ed.), *Explorations in criminal psychopathology: Clinical syndromes with forensic implications* (pp. 170–186). Springfield, IL: Charles C Thomas.

Mathias, C. W., Greve, K. W., Bianchini, K. J., Houston, R. J., & Crouch, J. A. (2002). Detecting malingered neurocognitive dysfunction using the reliable digit span in traumatic brain injury. *Assessment, 9*, 301–308.

Melton, G. B., Petrila, J., Poythress, N. G., & Slobogin, C. (1997). *Psychological evaluations for the courts* (2nd ed.). New York: Guilford Press.

Meyers, J. E., & Meyers, K. (1995). *Rey Complex Figure and Recognition Trial: Professional manual*. Odessa, FL: Psychological Assessment Resources.

Mittenberg, W., Azrin, R., Millsaps, C., & Heilbronner, R. (1993). Identification of malingered head injury on the Wechsler Memory Scale–Revised. *Psychological Assessment, 5*, 34–40.

Mittenberg, W., Patton, C., Canyock, E. M., & Condit, D. C. (2002). Base rates of malingering and symptom exaggeration. *Journal of Clinical and Experimental Neuropsychology, 24*, 1094–1102.

Mittenberg, W., Rotholc, A., Russell, E., & Heilbronner, R. (1996). Identification of malingered head injury on the Halstead–Reitan Battery. *Archives of Clinical Neuropsychology, 11*, 271–281.

Mittenberg, W., Theroux, S., Aguila-Puentes, G., Bianchini, K., Greve, K., & Rayls, K. (2001). Identification of malingered head injury on the Wechsler Adult Intelligence Scale 3rd edition. *The Clinical Neuropsychologist, 15*, 440–445.

Mittenberg, W., Theroux-Fichera, S., Zielinski, R. E., & Heilbronner, R. L. (1995). Identification of malingered head injury on the Wechsler Adult Intelligence Scale–Revised. *Professional Psychology: Research and Practice, 26*, 491–498.

Nitch, S., Boone, K. B., Wen, J., Arnold, G., & Alfano, K. (2006). The utility of the

Rey Words Recognition Test in the detection of suspect effort. *The Clinical Neuropsychologist, 20,* 873–887.

O'Connell, B. A. (1960). Amnesia and homicide. *British Journal of Delinquency, 10,* 262–276.

Pankratz, L. (1979). Procedures for the assessment and treatment of functional sensory deficits. *Journal of Consulting and Clinical Psychology, 47,* 409–410.

Pankratz, L., Fausti, S., & Peed, S. (1975). A forced-choice technique to evaluate deafness in the hysterical or malingering patient. *Journal of Consulting and Clinical Psychology, 43,* 421–422.

Parwatikar, S. D., Holcomb, W. R., & Menninger, K. A., II. (1985). The detection of malingered amnesia in accused murderers. *Bulletin of the American Academy of Psychiatry and the Law, 13,* 97–103.

Power, D. J. (1977). Memory, identification and crime. *Medicine, Science, and the Law, 17,* 132–139.

Price, G. E., & Terhune, W. B. (1919). Feigned amnesia as a defense reaction. *Journal of the American Medical Association, 72,* 565–567.

Robins, L. N., Tipp, J., & Przybeck, T. (1991). Antisocial personality. In L. N. Robins & D. Regier (Eds.), *Psychiatric disorders in America: The Epidemiologic Catchment Area study* (pp. 258–290). New York: Free Press.

Rogers, R. (1986). *Conducting insanity evaluations.* New York: Van Nostrand Reinhold.

Rogers, R. (1990). Models of feigned mental illness. *Professional Psychology, 21,* 182–188.

Rogers, R., Bagby, R. M., & Dickens, S. E. (1992). *SIRS Structured Interview of Reported Symptoms: A professional manual.* Odessa, FL: Psychological Assessment Resources.

Rosenbaum, A., Hoge, S. K., Adelman, S. A., Warnken, W. J., Fletcher, K. E., & Kane, R. L. (1994). Head injury in partner-abusive men. *Journal of Consulting and Clinical Psychology, 62,* 1187–1193.

Rubinsky, E. W., & Brandt, J. (1986). Amnesia and criminal law: A clinical overview. *Behavioral Sciences and the Law, 4,* 27–46.

Schacter, D. L. (1986). Amnesia and Crime: How much do we really know? *American Psychologist, 41,* 286–295.

Siegel, S. (1956). *Nonparametric statistics for the behavioral sciences.* New York: McGraw Hill.

Simon, M. J. (1994). The use of the Rey Memory Test in assess malingering in criminal defendants. *Journal of Clinical Psychology, 50,* 913–917.

Slaughter, B., Fann, J. R., & Ehde, D. (2003). Traumatic brain injury in a county jail population: Prevalence, neuropsychological functioning and psychiatric disorders. *Brain Injury, 17,* 731–741.

Slick, D. J., Hopp, G., Strauss E., & Thompson, G. B. (1997). *Victoria Symptom Validity Test. Professional manual.* Odessa, FL: Psychological Assessment Resources.

Slick, D. J., Sherman, E. M. S., & Iverson, G. L. (1999). Diagnostic criteria for malingered neurocognitive dysfunction: Proposed standards for clinical practice and research. *The Clinical Neuropsychologist, 13*(4), 545–561.

Swanson, D. A. (1985). Malingering and associated syndromes. *Psychiatric Medicine, 2,* 287–293.

Taylor, P. J., & Kopelman, M. D. (1984). Amnesia for criminal offences. *Psychological Medicine, 14,* 581–588.

Tenhula, W. N., & Sweet, J. J. (1996). Double cross-validation of the Booklet Category Test in detecting malingered traumatic brain injury. *The Clinical Neuropsychologist, 10*, 104–116.

Theodor, L. H., & Mendelcorn, M. S. (1973). Hysterical blindness: A case report and study using a modern psychophysical technique. *Journal of Abnormal Psychology, 82*, 552–553.

Tombaugh, T. N. (1996). *TOMM. Test of Memory Malingering.* North Tonawanda, NY: Multi-Health Systems.

Turkstra, L., Jones, D., & Toler, H. L. (2003). Brain injury and violent crime. *Brain Injury, 17*, 39–47.

Weinborn, M., Orr, T., Woods, S. P., Conover, E., & Feix, J. (2003). A validation of the Test of Memory Malingering in a forensic psychiatric setting, *Journal of Clinical and Experimental Neuropsychology, 25*, 979–990.

United States v. Greer, 158 F.3d 228 (5th Cir. 1998).

Wieter v. Settle, 193 F. Supp. 318 (W.D. Mo. 1961).

Westby, M. D., & Ferraro, F. R. (1999). Frontal lobe deficits in domestic violence offenders. *Genetic, Social, and General Psychology Monograph, 125*, 71–102.

Wiggins, E. C., & Brandt, J. (1988). The detection of simulated amnesia. *Law and Human Behavior, 12*, 57–78.

Wilson v. United States, 391 F.2d 460 (DC Cir. 1968).

Wynkoop, T. F., & Denney, R. L. (1999). Exaggeration of neuropsychological deficit in competency to stand trial. *Journal of Forensic Neuropsychology, 1*(2), 29–53.

APPENDIX 19.1. SAMPLE REMOTE MEMORY QUESTIONS

Sample items comprising a portion of the forced-choice, two-alternative test used in the illustrative case related to claims of amnesia for events surrounding the alleged assault. Details have been changed to protect privacy. Correct alternatives are marked with asterisks.

1. Investigative materials allege that you had problems with a gang, which gang was it?

   A. Texas Syndicate*

   B. Aryan Brotherhood

2. Those troubles allegedly occurred when?

   A. April 1993

   B. April 1994*

3. What did you supposedly do to make the TS angry at you?

   A. Provided information about a murder plot*

   B. Provided information about drug smuggling

4. Were you ever hit in the head with a pipe by another inmate?

   A. Yes*

   B. No

5. At what institution did this occur?

   A. Lewisburg

   B. Beaumont*

6. When did this occur?

   A. June 1989

   B. June 1988*

7. Why did the other inmate hit you?

   A. You and 5 other inmate had confronted him*

   B. He was trying to rob you

APPENDIX 19.2. SAMPLE COMPETENCY-RELATED QUESTIONS

Examples of two-alternative, forced-choice questions dealing with competency-to-stand-trial related information specific to the defendant's criminal case as well as commonly understood aspects of criminal judicial proceedings, both aspects of remote memory. Asterisks denote correct responses.

1. What is your charge?

    A. Possessing a weapon*

    B. Possessing drugs

2. What is a judge?

    A. He or she oversees court proceedings*

    B. He or she makes a record of what happens in court

3. Your attorney is called?

    A. Prosecuting attorney

    B. Defense attorney*

4. The prosecution attorney wants to do what?

    A. Set you free

    B. Put you in jail*

5. The defense attorney does what?

    A. Works for you*

    B. Works for the judge

6. Gulty means what?

    A. You did it*

    B. You did not do it.

CHAPTER 20

Future Directions in Effort Assessment

Martin L. Rohling
Kyle Brauer Boone

One challenge to drafting a manuscript that is designed to predict the future is that there is a high probability of "getting it wrong." If either of us were very good at predicting the future, we would likely be doing something that would lead to greater income than neuropsychology. In contrast to other chapters in this volume in which the authors have had the ability to appeal to known findings, our chapter is by definition prospective. At best, we can take the results of research that have recently been published and use them to "project out" into the future. We think we would be lucky if 20% of what we predict comes to pass. We leave it to the reader to determine which of the following 20% this will be.

Another dilemma we face in drafting a manuscript titled "Future Directions in Effort Assessment" is to determine whether we should predict the future or more ambitiously try to shape it. It is possible that whatever we write may in some way alter the future, making what we have written a self-fulfilling prophesy. This may ease our anxiety about soothsaying; on the other hand, it also brings added social responsibility to our writing. We would not want to generate a future that is less than might otherwise be achieved had we not made our predictions.

In response to these dilemmas, we have decided to hedge our bets a bit and mix together what we think is most likely to happen with what we might want to have happen. In preparing to write this chapter, we returned to the literature to view the history of symptom validity testing. By going backwards in time, we hoped to generate what might be analogous to a regression line that projects into the future. Furthermore, we thought we could create a band of error around our predictions, a "standard error of the estimate" if you will, that might help readers see what the range of possible outcomes are for the future. We did this to increase our comfort with writing a "subjective" manuscript, as our habit has been to rely on data to guide the direction of the text. In fact, a close colleague of ours once joked that Rohling's preferred method of writing an empirical research article is to list many summary statistics (e.g., descriptive and inferential statistics) in well-conceived tables and figures. The only text that is written would read "See tables and figures for details regarding our findings." Nevertheless, because the data for our "Future Directions" chapter is not yet in, we will have to wing it by actually providing the reader with text.

As Philip Tetlock (2005) noted in his book titled *Expert Political Judgment: How Good Is It? How Can We Know*, the more you get paid, the more confident you are in your predictions, but the less likely you are to make valid predictions. Experts rarely have the humility needed to couch their predictions in an appropriate level of uncertainty. We are bucking that trend by noting that we were paid (virtually) nothing to write this chapter and have much humility about our predictions.

GROWING ACCEPTANCE OF SYMPTOM VALIDITY TESTING

We have found that the vast majority of clinical psychologists, and even most clinical neuropsychologists, fail to fully appreciate the frequency with which patients provide us with invalid data either during our clinical evaluations or when participating in research (Essig, Mittenberg, Petersen, Strauman, & Cooper, 2001; Sharland, Gfeller, Justice, Ross, & Hughes, 2005; Slick, Tan, Straus, & Hultch, 2004). It is the "default setting" of most clinical psychologists to accept at face value patient test responses even in those contexts in which patients might be motivated to be less than forthright. As the research cited in this volume shows, however, such a stance at the current time is no longer tenable.

There has been an explosion of research on the issue of symptom validity since the 1990s (Sweet, King, Malina, Bergman, & Simmons, 2002). Rohling (MLR) can recall when he was approached over 15 years ago by a more senior colleague, Dr. Laurence Binder, to participate in meta-analyses on the influence of financial incentives on the experience and treatment of chronic pain and head injury. Rohling viewed this to be a pointless exercise, as he believed the effects would be negligible. However, the resulting articles (Binder & Rohling, 1996; Binder, Rohling, & Larrabee, 1997; Rohling, Binder, & Langhinrichsen-Rohling, 1995) have been so frequently cited that Rohling doubts that any subsequent manuscripts he publishes will approach the influence that these papers have had on the field. The effect sizes that were related to financial incentives were not only statistically significant but clinically meaningful. Since that time, all three of these meta-analyses have been replicated, some more than once (e.g., Belanger, Curtiss, Demery, Lebowitz, & Vanderploeg, 2005), with the original findings corroborated.

Further evidence of the importance of symptom validity testing for the field of neuropsychology is reflected in the recent position paper on the use of symptom validity tests (SVTs) in neuropsychological assessment by the National Academy of Neuropsychology (NAN; Bush et al., 2005). The NAN paper states that it should now be routine for neuropsychologists to include validity checks in nearly all clinical evaluations unless there are unusual circumstances (e.g., neuroimaging data of severe dementia or cerebrovascular accident) that might make it difficult or impossible.

Despite such recommendations, a recent survey by Slick et al. (2004) found that even for those who routinely practice in forensic settings, few use well-validated SVTs and most still significantly underestimate the base rate of malingering likely to occur in their practice. In particular, we have found that a significant majority of our colleagues who were trained before the 1990s have a limited awareness of the plethora of techniques and tests designed to determine the validity of cognitive test scores. In fact, many of these colleagues still do not seem to recognize the need to check the veracity of patients' symptom reports and cognitive test performances.

When we were educated, circa 1980s, the training of graduate students in clinical psychology rarely or barely touched on the issue of suboptimal effort or malingering. For example, Rohling's training involved no discussions of malingering during 4 years of graduate school and only a cursory introduction to the Rey 15-Item Test and Dot Counting Test on internship. These were the only two tests suggested for use when one wanted to assess for malingering and they were only to be used if suspicions emerged that a patient was not putting forth his or her best effort. Rohling was fortunate to have completed a postdoctoral fellowship at the Veterans Administration Medical Center in Portland, Oregon, where Drs. Pankratz and Binder were conducting research on measurement of effort. This resulted in an exposure to the topic that exceeded that of many trainees of the era. However, Rohling can still recall thinking, "Who would want to study malingering, it's not *real* neuropsychology?" Unfortunately, such views appear to remain in many training centers around the country, as well as for some journal editorial boards. For example, a quick literature search of the *Journal of the International Neuropsychological Society* (JINS) found only one article on the topic over a 10-year period from 1995 to 2005. In contrast, articles on the topic of forensic neuropsychology comprise a substantial percentage (5%) of the publications in several other mainstream neuropsychological journals from 1990 to 2000 (Sweet et al., 2002).

Certainly, the relatively recent requirement for psychologists to accrue continuing education units will lead to increased knowledge and skills in assessment for effort. Researchers and clinical experts in the area have a responsibility to ensure that continuing education courses offer this information. However, clinical practice will be slow to change until there is routine incorporation of didactic coursework on the base rate of symptom exaggeration or feigning, as well as the appropriate use of SVTs, in graduate-level coursework. In addition, students should also be socialized into the awareness that they have a professional responsibility to stay abreast of the research findings in this rapidly evolving area. Finally, students should be taught that effort indicators are powerful tools that should not be misused; the examiner's role is to be an open-minded, objective evaluator who interacts with all patients in a respectful manner.

ROLE IN THE FORENSIC ARENA

As with many health care providers, clinical neuropsychologists have seen dramatic changes in income and reimbursement over the past two decades (Sweet, Peck, Abramowitz, & Etzweile, 2003a, 2003b). Managed care has been the predominant influence, seeking to limit reimbursements and restrict access to neuropsychological testing in the service of limiting health and mental health care costs. This has resulted in many clinical neuropsychologists turning to other avenues of income, and forensic evaluations have rapidly become the most common "alternative source" of income to replace lost third-party reimbursement of clinical services (Larrabee, 2000; Purisch & Sbordone, 1997).

Forensic evaluations are associated with heightened scrutiny of assessment procedures, and, because forensic assessments typically occur in contexts in which there is motive to feign, these evaluations have highlighted the necessity of assessing for suboptimal performance or poor effort. Forensic evaluations have been the major impetus for the proliferation of research on instruments and methods that are designed to detect noncredible cognitive test scores (Nelson et al., 2003). Moreover, court rulings such as *Daubert* (*Daubert v. Merrell Dow*, 1993) and *Joiner* (*Joiner v. General Electric*, 1997) have pushed test designers to focus on reliability and validity issues of the instruments they have developed (Greiffenstein & Cohen, 2004; Lees-Haley, Iverson, Lange, Fox, & Allen, 2002). In particular, the *Daubert* ruling requires attention to the error rates of tests, and data regarding false-positive and false-negative rates are now more available for effort measures than for most other psychological tests.

We expect that neuropsychological testing, including verification of level of effort, will continue to gain prominence in the forensic arena. Our discipline has the most well-validated measures to verify veracity of symptom report, and it is likely that neuropsychologists will become even more relied on, and perhaps be viewed as the primary experts, in this area.

PSYCHOMETRIC DILEMMAS

There are several reasons why effort testing presents scientific challenges to the traditional psychometric approach to test development and construct validation (Nelson et al., 2003). Let us start with basic psychometric true score theory—specifically, the old adage that validity is bounded by reliability. That is, we learn little about an individual's true cognitive status if the instruments we use provide us with unreliable or inconsistent data. However, consistency of results is a necessary but not sufficient condition for one to assess a construct validly.

It is illustrative for us to consider the concept of malingering as an example of why construct validity is problematic in this area. The construct validity of malingering is dependent on the instruments we use to measure it. Many of these instruments rely on the responses of participants whose response frequency distributions are highly skewed and near ceiling. Such distributions present challenges to the traditional formulas that are used to determine reliability. In particular, the resulting restriction in range of scores makes it difficult to substantiate the consistency in the measurements. Therefore, because of reduced reliability, the construct validity of malingering becomes even more difficult to establish.

Further, to maintain consistent feigned impairment within several cognitive domains across sequential assessments is highly difficult. The challenge, however, is that inconsistency is both a sign of potential malingering (Rogers, 1997; Rohling, Langhinrichsen-Rohling, & Miller, 2003) and a hindrance to its detection. Consider that malingering is a hypothetical construct, a diagnosis that is similar to other psychiatric diagnoses, and is assessed using behavioral signs and symptoms. Most psychometric instruments require a high degree of consistency of an examinee's performance to minimize measurement error and maximize the percent of score variance that is related to variability in the hypothetical construct. In most cases, examinees are not able to intentionally alter their behavior and/or emotional experience to change the true score variance that is accounted for by their test scores. For example, one cannot be severely depressed one minute and nondepressed the next. Similarly, one cannot have superior intellect one minute and be mentally retarded the next. Therefore, in most contexts, the consistency of patients' behavior increases the examiner's ability to detect their true score on the constructs of interest. However, when we consider the construct of malingering in this manner, it is apparent that a patient can be faking one minute and perform genuinely the next. One is not a "malingerer" but rather one engages in "malingering" periodically, and at times, in rapidly alternating fashion. Many clinicians may experience this phenomenon as "now you see it, now you don't." Another possible outcome is that one clinician, who sees a patient one day, may observe the patient malingering, whereas another clinician who sees the patient on a different day may not. These two experts are then set up to debate in court whether or not the patient is a "malingerer."

Now imagine this type of inconsistency occurring when a test developer is attempting to establish the psychometric properties (i.e., reliability and validity) of SVTs. What one hopes for is consistency across the two episodes of measurement. The very nature of malingering as a construct makes such consistency more difficult to establish and thus more difficult to assess. However, this does not mean that the construct does not exist. Who among us has not "feigned" a bit as a child to stay home from school or has called in sick to work so that he or she might have a "mental health day." The "face validity" for malingering seems quite high.

An additional problem with construct validity raised by Faust and Ackley (1998), as well as Larrabee (2003), is the multidimensional nature of malingering. One is never a "malingerer" of all disorders. For example, one who feigns cognitive impairment may not feign physical symptoms (e.g., low back pain) or psychiatric disorders (e.g., schizophrenia). Similarly, one may feign depression, anxiety, or posttraumatic stress disorder, while simultaneously performing genuinely on tests of cognitive ability. Thus, feigning and malingering may not be a single construct but, rather, may have multiple domains.

One psychometric method of identifying various components of a construct is to use factor analysis. Yet, this statistical procedure is correlational in nature and rests on the assumptions that the measured variables are normally distributed, of equal variance, and independently sampled from one another. Failure to meet these assumptions makes the use of factor analysis at times dubious. Although parametric statistics can be rather robust to violations of assumptions, highly skewed variable distributions, such as that often seen using test validity measures, far exceeds what might be considered reasonable for the purposes of conducting a factor analysis. There are nonparametric methods of conducting factor analysis (see Sheskin, 2003, for a discussion of nonparametric factor analysis), but to date we are unaware of any researcher utilizing any of these to determine the domains of malingering based on a large sample of data with multiple measures of feigning, or whether the degree of skewness of the variables that are likely to be analyzed is sufficiently great enough to require such procedures. Thus, left unanswered is how many subtypes of malingering exist and how they relate to each other.

We recommend that these domain or factor structure problems be the focus of researchers in the field. Further, many clinicians continue to assume that measures of validity derived from personality tests (e.g., Minnesota Multiphasic Personality Inventory–2 [MMPI-2] Lees-Haley Fake Bad Scale) are of equal quality in detecting feigned expressions of pain or psychiatric illness as they are at detecting feigned cognitive deficits. This may or may not be a correct assumption that requires future investigation.

GENERALIZABILITY ACROSS SAMPLES

Another complex psychometric and research design issue is related to the operational definition of the experimental group (e.g., malingerers), as well as determining who should be in the control group. First, a researcher has to decide if simulated malingering is a suitable surrogate for actual malingering. To generalize findings from simulator studies, one has to assume that these two phenomenon are the same or at least roughly equivalent. However, the magnitude of the reinforcement provided in these two situations is rarely comparable, and groups typically differ on demographic variables (age, educational and occupational level, socioeconomic status), which brings the issue of generalization from simulator studies to the clinic into question. Employing real-world noncredible groups is preferable but has its own unique problems. For example, the use of real-world samples of litigants or disability seekers will underestimate the true effectiveness of effort indicators in identifying suspect effort because not all compensation seekers are feigning. On the other hand, composing noncredible groups with subjects who score significantly below chance on forced-choice measures will inflate the hit rate of the effect indicators under investigation because this subset of noncredible subjects is particularly "obvious" and unsophisticated in their feigning approach.

Second, should control participants be a group of "normal" individuals who have never had or ever claimed to have had the disorder that is being alleged by the malingering group? This is not desirable because discrimination between "normal" and malingering is not the differential faced by the clinician in actual practice. Rather, the clinician must distinguish between real versus feigned manifestations of clinical disorders. However, the practice in some studies of using as "controls" patients in litigation who pass an effort indicator results in underestimates of the true effectiveness of effort indicators because it is unlikely, given that individual effort indicators have sensitivity rates of $\leq 80\%$, that all noncredible subjects are in fact excluded from the comparison group. There are also questions as to what extent the results from one group of "clinical control participants" (e.g., moderate to severely head injured patients) can be generalized to another set of "clinical controls" (e.g., patients who experienced toxic exposure). Boone, Lu, and Herzberg (2002a, 2002b) and Arnold et al. (2005) have shown that cutoffs for effort indicators should be adjusted as a function of claimed diagnosis. This requires that effort measures be validated through comparing compensation-seeking noncredible subjects (as identified through independent effort and behavioral indices) against non-compensation-seeking credible patients (determined by passed independent effort indices) in discrete diagnostic groups (depression, psychosis, traumatic brain injury, learning disability, attention-deficit disorder, etc.). However, this is a very time-consuming and labor-intensive approach.

Third, most effort indices have been validated on mild head injury litigants, and there is some evidence that approaches to faking may vary depending on the alleged condition. For example, inmates feigning in prison psychiatric hospitals showed much more blatant faking on the Dot Counting Test than did civil litigants and disability-seeking individuals (Boone et al., 2002). In addition, noncredible head-injured individuals showed more evidence of feigning on a Rey Word Recognition combination score than individuals feigning in the context of other conditions (Nitch, Boone, Wen, Arnold, & Alfano, 2006), while the reverse was observed for Digit Span (Babikian, Boone, Lu, & Arnold, 2006) and finger tapping (Arnold et al., 2005). As discussed in several chapters in this book, noncredible cognitive symptoms can be found in the context of claimed chronic pain and chronic fatigue, exposure to toxins, learning disability/attention-deficit disorder, mental retardation, and seizures. Ideally, systematic information is needed regarding effort test performance in individuals feigning cognitive symptoms in the context of differing disorders.

It has been assumed that effort tests developed on native English-speaking, primarily Caucasian, mild head injury litigants can be imported for use in other populations, such as in ethnic minorities, in persons who speak English as a second language or not at all, and actual versus feigned mental retardation, psychosis, and dementia. However, as summarized by Goldberg, Back-Madruga, and Boone (Chapter 13), Victor and Boone (Chapter 14), and Salazar, Lu, Wen, and Boone (Chapter 18), high rates of false positive identifications on standard effort indicators may be present in these groups, necessitating that cutoffs be adjusted to preserve specificity. Further, whether existing effort tests paradigms are appropriate for these populations has not been questioned, despite the fact that there is little rationale for expecting that effort tests developed on, for example, a normal IQ population should be effective in individuals of low IQ. Marshall and Happe (in press, cited in Chapter 14) reported that mentally retarded individuals, who typically fail standard effort indicators, show a "yes" response bias on Wechsler Memory Scale—III (WMS-III) Logical Memory recognition that is not likely to be displayed by malingerers. These observations suggest that effort measures that capitalize on this characteristic of mentally retarded individuals might be particularly effective in discriminating actual versus feigned mental retardation.

Concerns have also been raised regarding the use of effort tests in children. Children may malinger, but it does not follow that the results of studies of malingering conducted on adults can be generalized to children (Donders, 2005; Rohling, 2004, 2005). Rohling suggested that using some SVTs with children to assess malingering is "invalid" when the child is too young, actually suffering from a significant degree of cognitive impairment (e.g., mentally retarded), or suffering from some types of psychopathology (e.g., attention-deficit/hyperactivity), a finding that is at least preliminarily supported by Donders (2005). If all three of these conditions exist simultaneously, there is a high degree of error introduced into the decision matrix and the probability of misdiagnosis is increased. On the other hand, the bright and suave youngster might well be able to feign symptoms of mental retardation and/or attention-deficit/hyperactivity disorder, such that a clinician would inaccurately conclude that the child performed genuinely, when he or she did not. This may lead to inappropriate treatment plans, such as the prescription of stimulant medication or concluding that the child should be exempt from certain academic requirements, when this is actually not in the patient's best interest. The issues of development of effort measures specifically designed for unique populations, as well as identification of subgroups with differing approaches to feigning of cognitive symptoms, are important areas for future research.

VALIDITY THREATS RELATED TO TEST SECURITY MAY DRIVE TEST DESIGN

An additional future concern is SVT security. Test security is threatened when psychologists release test materials and procedures (including test scores sheets and stenographic, audio, or visual recordings) to lawyers and their clients and others who do not have an ethical mandate to maintain test security as do psychologists. Attorneys may believe that it is their responsibility to educate their clients regarding the procedures a psychologist may use, as well as describing how their clients might respond to test items to maximize the chance that they will receive a favorable settlement (Wetter & Corrigan, 1995). Thus, uncontrolled release of test information potentially jeopardizes the validity of these procedures for future use.

Even if not provided by psychologists, researchers have found that it is relatively easy for patients to gain access to SVT materials (Coleman, Rapport, Millis, Ricker & Farchione, 1998; Wetter & Corrigan, 1995; Youngjohn, 1995; Youngjohn, Lees-Haley, & Binder, 1999). Considerable information regarding SVTs is now available via Internet, through which patients may actually be able to gain access to the test design, stimulus items, and cutoff scores used for diagnostic purposes (Bauer & McCaffery, 2006). Some of these patients may then use this information to alter their behavior to avoid being detected as feigning (Bauer & McCaffery, 2006; Essig et al., 2001; Youngjohn, 1995). Such knowledge, if widespread, will reduce a well-validated SVT's ability to detect suboptimal performance by examinees.

At the time we wrote this chapter, it appeared that widespread coaching or access to SVT information was on the increase. Furthermore, as found by Bauer and McCaffery (2006), the most frequently used and best known SVT (Sharland et al., 2005), the Test of Memory Malingering (TOMM), had the most information available on the Internet. We believe that the more popular (i.e., well-researched, biggest selling, most often used) SVTs are most prone to this liability. There will, of course, be a delay between a SVT's popularity and the point in time at which sufficient information is available to the public to make the test's sensitivity too diminished for use. How much time is required for this to be the case is unknown. However, it is our opinion that tests such as the TOMM, Computerized Assessment of Response Bias (CARB), and the Rey 15-Item Test have already lost some, if not much, of their sensitivity and clinical utility over the past few years (Gervais, Allen, & Green, 2001). In fact, a recent cross-validation of the Rey 15-Item plus recognition trial (Boone & Lu, 2007) showed a substantial and unexpected drop in sensitivity, from 71% on initial validation data collected between 1986 and 2000 to 56% on cross-validation data collected after 2000. However, this type of loss in sensitivity was not found on cross-validation in the same sample of the Dot Counting Test.

If, indeed, a loss of validity through coaching and education is occurring, our prediction is that neuropsychologists will be forced to rely on a continuous supply of new instruments, which David Berry (personal communication, April 27, 2002) has referred to as the "arms race" in clinical neuropsychology. However, this assumes that there are an infinite number of measures that can be developed and that there are resources available to validate adequately each new addition to the arsenal. Further, test development will require more creativity than simply applying forced-choice paradigms to new types of test stimuli. Substituting new forced-choice tests will not likely prevent coaching (e.g., all an unscrupulous attorney will need to advise a plaintiff is, "When you are given a test where you have to pick between two choices, do well on that test"). Novel but objectively easy paradigms may need to be utilized, such as continuous performance tests (e.g., b Test and Test of Variables of Attention) and recognition paradigms that are either not forced-choice (e.g., Rey Word Recognition) or more complicated then a binary choice (e.g., Amsterdam Short Term Memory Test; Schmand, de Sterke, Lindeboom, & Millis, 2002).

A second, and more attractive option that is being pursued is the development and validation of scores and algorithms derived from standard cognitive tests, individually or in combination with each other, to identify noncredible performance. These, many of which are described in chapters in this book, serve "double duty" (i.e., measure effort and specific cognitive skills) and thereby do not add to test administration time. As discussed by Arnold and Boone (Chapter 9), motor and sensory tasks appear to be particularly sensitive to suspect effort but have been underutilized in the assessment of effort. Some studies have found that not all test items are necessarily equal in their ability to detect noncredible performance, and equations involving items rarely missed or rarely endorsed by credible subjects (see Lu, Rogers, and Boone, Chapter 7) or double-weighting of items (see Nitch and

Glassmire, Chapter 5, and Lu, Rogers, and Boone, Chapter 7) appear to increase a measure's sensitivity.

An additional advantage of embedded algorithms over freestanding effort tests is that they provide direct, rather than inferred, information regarding adequacy of effort. Specifically, they circumvent the argument that just because a patient failed an effort test, this does not necessarily mean the patient was underperforming on a separate standard memory or other test. Some of the more successful advocates of these embedded procedures have been John Meyers (see Chapter 11) and Scott Millis (Millis & Volinsky, 2001). Ideally, virtually all standard neuropsychological measures will in the future have validated methods for extracting information regarding veracity of effort.

Finally, effort indices derived from standard cognitive tests are less likely to be "coachable" than freestanding forced-choice effort tests; for the latter an unscrupulous attorney could simply advise, "If you are asked to count dots, do it quickly and accurately." However, the patterns of the interrelationships between standard cognitive scores in truly brain-injured patients are complex, not commonly understood by attorneys, and therefore not easily taught to plaintiffs.

Several studies have shown that noncredible individuals perform more slowly than credible subjects (Babikian et al., 2006; Boone et al., 1999, 2002). No doubt, this is in part due to the fact that they believe a brain injury leads to marked slowing in thinking speed, but also because the process of deciding how to feign takes time (Victor & Abeles, 2004). Time scores are only modestly related to accuracy data (Boone et al., 2000; Boone et al., 2002) and thus provide nonredundant information. The incorporation of completion time into freestanding (i.e., Boone et al., 2000; Boone et al., 2002) and embedded (Babikian et al., 2006) effort indicators has been shown to increase test sensitivity, and it is recommended that time data, which are easy to collect, be systematically examined for all other effort measures.

Algorithms for embedded effort techniques may be best developed using logistic regression to distill the maximum benefit of multiple scores from the same or multiple tests (Millis & Volinsky, 2001). Procedures for generating such algorithms, which involve Bayesian Model Averaging (BMA), have been provided by Millis and Volinsky (2001), and which they illustrate using the California Verbal Learning Test. Bianchini, Mathias, and Greve (2001) have in fact predicted that such models are likely to become prominent in future SVT development.

In addition, as discussed by Boone (Chapter 3), it is preferable, for several reasons, to use multiple techniques, both freestanding and embedded, interspersed throughout the battery to assess for effort. First, the chance that patients can be successfully coached/educated on effort measures obviously declines with increasing numbers of effort tests employed (i.e., it is much easier to coach on 1 or 2 tests than 8 or 10). In addition, use of several techniques allows effort to be continuously sampled throughout the battery. Further, the use of multiple measures significantly raises specificity. As noted in Chapter 3, while failure on two effort tests is associated with optimal sensitivity, failure on increasing numbers of measures is associated with decreasing false-positive identifications in credible patients. For example, we have frequently observed noncredible patients to fail five, six, seven, eight, or more effort indicators, yet no patient in our clinical population with no motive to feign (and excluding patients with dementia, psychosis, and IQ < 70) failed more than four; thus, failures on ≥ five tests in our battery of effort indicators is associated with 100% specificity.

However, this simple tabulation of the number of effort indicators failed does not take into consideration that effort measures are not necessarily comparable in their ability to detect suspect effort (e.g., see Vickery, Berry, Inman, Harris, & Orey, 2001). Unfortunately, research directly comparing the relative sensitivity of various effort indicators, such as the work of Gervais, Rohling, Green, and Ford (2004), is sparse. Further, as discussed earlier, sensitivity of effort measures likely varies as a function of what condition is being feigned (traumatic brain injury, chronic pain, dementia/psychosis in a correctional setting) requiring that relative sensitivity of effort indicators be examined in discrete noncredible populations.

Use of factor analysis, cluster analysis, and other multivariate methods also shows promise in terms of identifying patterns of scores that are inconsistent with what is known about brain–behavior relationships (Nelson et al., 2003). Reports of symptoms and actual objective measures may show a pattern in truly brain-injured individuals that is not replicated by individuals who are attempting to feign injury. Such methods were used by Rohling, Allen, and Green (2002), who demonstrated that the factor structure generated from data obtained from both cognitive testing and self-report inventories from those who failed a SVT were different from those obtained by normal individuals as well as neurologically impaired patients. These latter two groups had similar factor structures, suggesting that neurological impairment does not alter the basic brain–behavior pattern of relationships.

Another method that may yet prove to be of some benefit is including measures of event-related potentials (ERPs) using electroencephalography (EEG). The P300 wave in particular has shown some potential in identifying examinees who claim to not recall information when the ERP measurements suggest that they do. This area has been investigated by Rosenfeld and colleagues (e.g., Ellwanger, Tenhula, Rosenfeld, & Sweet, 1999; Rosenfeld, Sweet, Chuang, Ellwanger, & Song, 1996; Rosenfeld, Soskins, Bosh, & Ryan, 2004), who have found that by using both SVT scores and ERPs the accuracy of classification as a malingerer could be increased substantially over the use of either ERPs or SVT scores alone. However, these results were obtained in a laboratory setting with an analog design, which limits the generalizability of these findings to clinic settings. Rohling is currently involved in a replication study of these findings and expects to expand this into the clinical setting with actual referred patients over the next year. Finally, as summarized by Kingery and Schretlen (Chapter 2), functional brain imaging may eventually have utility in detection of feigned symptoms.

EXPANDING OUR HORIZONS BEYOND GROUPS
WITH OBVIOUS INCENTIVE TO FEIGN

While it is becoming appreciated that effort tests should be administered in a clinical context, the idea of examining for effort in neuropsychological research on clinical disorders receives little attention. However, as discussed by McCaffrey and Yantz (Chapter 17), studies examining cognition in multiple chemical sensitivity and toxic mold have frequently not reported whether participants had motive to feign, and examination of test scores for individual subjects has shown substantial evidence of feigning. Reports from the 1970s and 1980s describing the 10–15% of mild head injury individuals who do not recover (e.g., Rutherford, Merrett, & McDonald, 1979; McLean, Temkin, & Dikmen, 1983), did not consider litigation status or administer effort tests. Typically, authors based their findings on patient self-report, raising clear questions regarding the veracity of those conclusions. Neuropsychological studies on conditions for which diagnosis is based solely on patient self-report and for which there might be monetary or other incentive to be symptomatic (e.g., mild head injury, chronic fatigue syndrome, fibromyalgia, multiple chemical sensitivity, chronic pain, and most toxic exposures) have all likely been contaminated by poor effort in at least a subset of participants, requiring that these studies be discarded and redone. In addition, we have encountered subjects feigning symptoms with no immediate motive to feign (e.g., in depression and Alzheimer's disease clinical trials), but who have shown nonsensical and noncredible cognitive performance. These observations suggest that virtually all neuropsychological research studies must screen for poor effort. Thus, the future of symptom validity research related to noncredible cognitive performance will likely expand into numerous psychiatric and medical conditions to ensure that our conclusions about the degree to which these conditions impact cognition are accurate.

Finally, as discussed in Chapter 3 (Boone), we have no objective methods for differentiating between malingering and somatoform conditions and the view that these are in fact dichotomous phenomena requires careful reexamination and potential reconceptualization. Unless clinical neuropsychologists somehow acquire "mind reading" capabilities, it will forever be impossible to determine "intention to feign," which is what would be necessary to differentiate these two types of disorders. It may be that either functional neuroimaging or ERP data will someday help to resolve the clinician's dilemma when faced with this difficult differential diagnosis, but to date these are investigational procedures and not ready for the real world of patient referrals.

So, what does the future hold for neuropsychologists and SVTs? We believe that future scientists will be creating assessment procedures that are less prone to diagnostic error and less likely to be hampered by coaching or exposure on the Internet. Some of these methods might be more time-consuming or expensive (e.g., P300). Most will require additional expertise on the part of the clinician. This will only be accomplished through changes in standard graduate school education, in conjunction with better methods of ensuring that practicing clinicians are incorporating new knowledge and technology into their assessment batteries.

REFERENCES

Arnold, G., Boone, K. B., Lu, P., Dean, A., Wen, J., Nitch, S., et al. (2005). Sensitivity and specificity of finger tapping scores for the detection of suspect effort. *The Clinical Neuropsychologist, 19*, 105–120.

Babikian, T., Boone, K. B., Lu, P., & Arnold, G. (2006). Sensitivity and specificity of various digit span scores in the detection of suspect effort. *The Clinical Neuropsychologist, 20*, 145–159.

Bauer, L., & McCaffery, R. J. (2006). Coverage of the Test of Memory Malingering, Victoria Symptom Validity Test, and Word Memory Test on the Internet: Is test security threatened? *Archives of Clinical Neuropsychology, 21*, 121–126.

Belanger, H. G., Curtiss, G., Demery, J. A., Lebowitz, B. K., & Vanderploeg, R. D. (2005). Factors moderating neuropsychological outcomes following mild traumatic brain injury: A meta-analysis. *Journal of the International Neuropsychological Society, 11*, 215–227.

Bianchini, K. J., Mathias, C. W., & Greve, K. W. (2001). Symptom validity tests: A critical review. *The Clinical Neuropsychologist, 15*, 19–45.

Binder, L., & Rohling, M. L. (1996). Money matters: A meta-analysis of the effect of financial incentives on recovery from closed-head injury. *American Journal of Psychiatry, 153*, 7–10.

Binder, L., Rohling, M. L., & Larrabee, G. (1997). A review of mild head trauma. Part I: A meta-analytic review of neuropsychological studies. *Journal of Clinical and Experimental Neuropsychology, 19*, 421–431.

Boone, K. B., & Lu, P. (2007). Non-forced choice effort measures. In G. Larrabee (Ed.), *Assessment of malingered neuropsychological deficits*. New York: Oxford University Press.

Boone, K. B., Lu, P., Back, C., King, C., Lee, A., Philpott, L., et al. (2002). Sensitivity and specificity of the Rey Dot Counting Test in patients with suspect effort and various clinical samples. *Archives of Clinical Neuropsychology, 17*, 625–642.

Bush, S., Ruff, R. M., Troster, A. I., Barth, J. T., Koffler, S. P., Pliskin, N. H., et al. (2005). Symptom validity assessment: Practice issues and medical necessity—

NAN Policy and Planning Committee. *Archives of Clinical Neuropsychology, 20*, 419–426.

Coleman, R. D., Rapport, L. J., Millis, S. R., Ricker J. H., & Farchione, T. J. (1998). Effects of Coaching on Detection of Malingering on the California Verbal Learning Test. *Journal of Clinical and Experimental Neuropsychology, 20*, 201–210.

Daubert v. Merrell Dow, 509 U.S. 579 (1993).

Donders, J. (2005). Performance on the Test of Memory and Malingering in a mixed pediatric sample. *Child Neuropsychology, 11*, 221–227.

Ellwanger, J., Tenhula, W. N., Rosenfeld, P., & Sweet, J. J. (1999). Identifying simulators of cognitive deficit through combined use of neuropsychological tests of performance and event-related potentials. *Journal of Clinical and Experiential Neuropsychology, 21*, 866–879.

Essig, S. M., Mittenberg, W., Peterson, R. S., Strauman, S., & Cooper, J. T. (2001). Practices in forensic neuropsychology: Perspectives of neuropsychologists and trial attorneys. *Archives of Clinical Neuropsychology, 16*, 271–291.

Faust, D., & Ackley, M. A. (1998). So you thought it was going to be easy. In C. R. Reynolds (Ed.), *Detection of malingering during head injury litigation* (pp. 261–286). New York: Plenum Press.

Gervais, R. O., Allen, L. M., & Green, P. (2001). Effects of coaching on symptom validity testing in chronic pain patients presenting for disability assessments. *Journal of Forensic Neuropsychology, 2*, 1–19.

Gervais, R. O., Rohling, M. L., Green, P., & Ford, W. (2004). A comparison of WMT, CARB, and TOMM failure rates in non-head injury disability claimants. *Archives of Clinical Neuropsychology, 19*, 475–488.

Greiffenstein, M. F., & Cohen, L. (2004). Neuropsychology and the law: Principles of productive attorney–neuropsychologist relations. In G. Larrabee (Ed.), *Forensic neuropsychology: A scientific approach* (pp. 29–91). New York: Oxford University Press.

Joiner v. General Electric, 522 U.S. 136 (1997).

Larrabee, G. (2000). Preface to the forensic neuropsychology issue. *Journal of Head Trauma Rehabilitation, 15*, v–viii.

Larrabee, G. (2003). Detection of malingering using atypical performance patterns on standard neuropsychological tests. *The Clinical Neuropsychologist, 17*, 410–425.

Lees-Haley, P. R., Iverson, G. L., Lange, R. T., Fox, D. D., & Allen, L. M. (2002). Malingering in forensic neuropsychology: *Daubert* and the MMPI-2. *Journal of Forensic Neuropsychology, 3*, 167–203.

McLean, A., Temkin, N. R., & Dikmen, S. (1983). The behavioral sequelae of head injury. *Journal of Clinical Neuropsychology, 5*, 361–376.

Millis, S. R., & Volinsky, C. T. (2001). Assessment of response bias in mild head injury: Beyond malingering tests. *Journal of Clinical and Experimental Neuropsychology, 23*, 809–828.

Nelson, N. W., Boone, K., Dueck, A., Wagener, L., Lu, P., & Grills, C. (2003). Relationship between eight measures of suspect effort. *The Clinical Neuropsychologist, 17*, 263–272.

Nitch, S., Boone, K. B., Wen, J., Arnold, G., & Alfano, K. (2006). The utility of the Rey Word Recognition Test in the detection of suspect effort. *The Clinical Neuropsychologist, 20*, 873–887.

Purisch, A., & Sbordone, R. (1997). Forensic neuropsychology: Clinical issues and practices. In A. Horton, Jr., D. Wedding, & J. Webster (Eds.), *The neuropsychology handbook, Volume 2: Treatment issues and special populations.* New York: Springer.

Rogers, R. (1997). Researching dissimulation. In R. Rogers (Ed.), *Clinical assessment of malingering and deception* (pp. 98–426). New York: Guilford Press.

Rohling, M. L. (2004). Who do they think they're kidding: A review of the use of symptom validity tests with children. *Clinical Neuropsychology Division 40 of APA Newsletter, 22,* 1–8.

Rohling, M. L. (2005). *Who do they think they're kidding–Use of the Word Memory Test with children: Follow-up results.* Symposium presented at the 25th annual convention of the National Academy of Neuropsychology, Tampa, FL.

Rohling, M. L., Allen, L. M., & Green, P. (2002). Who is exaggerating cognitive impairment and who is not? *CNS Spectrum, 7,* 387–395.

Rohling, M. L., Binder, L., & Langhinrichsen-Rohling, J. (1995). Money matters: A meta-analysis of the association between of financial compensation and the experience and treatment of chronic pain. *Health Psychology, 14,* 537–547.

Rohling, M. L., Langhinrichsen-Rohling, J., & Miller, L. S. (2003). Statistical methods for determining malingering. In R. Franklin (Ed.), *Prediction in forensic and neuropsychology: Sound statistical practices* (pp. 171–207). Mahwah, NJ: Erlbaum.

Rosenfeld, J. P., Soskins, M., Bosh, G., & Ryan, A. (2004). Simple, effective countermeasures to P300-based tests of detection of concealed information. *Society for Psychophysiological Research, 41,* 205–219.

Rosenfeld, J. P., Sweet, J. J., Chuang, J., Ellwanger, J., & Song, L. (1996). Detection of simulated malingering using forced choice recognition enhanced with event-related potentials recording. *The Clinical Neuropsychologist, 10,* 163–179.

Rutherford, W. H., Merrett, J. D., & McDonald, J. R. (1979). Symptoms at one year following concussion from minor head injuries. *Injury, 10,* 225–230.

Schmand, B., de Sterke, S., Lindeboom, J., & Millis, S. R. (2002). *Amsterdam Short Term Memory Test Manual.* Lutz, FL: Psychological Assessment Resources.

Sharland, M. J., Gfeller, J. D., Justice, L. M., Ross, M. J., & Hughes, H. M. (2005). *A survey of neuropsychologists beliefs and practices with respect to the assessment of effort.* Poster presented at the 25th annual convention of the National Academy of Neuropsychology, Tampa, FL.

Sheskin, D. J. (2003). *The handbook of parametric and nonparametric statistical procedures.* Boca Raton, FL: CRC Press.

Slick, D. J., Tan, J. E., Strauss, E. H., & Hultch, D. F. (2004). Detecting malingering: A survey of experts' practices. *Archives of Clinical Neuropsychology, 19,* 465–473.

Sweet, J. J., King, J. H., Malina, A. C., Bergman, M. A., & Simmons, A. (2002). Documenting the prominence of forensic neuropsychology at national meetings and in relevant professional journals from 1990 to 2000. *The Clinical Neuropsychologist, 16,* 481–494.

Sweet, J. J., Peck, E. A., Abramowitz, C., & Etzweile, S. (2003a). National Academy of Neuropsychology/Division 40 of the American Psychological Association Practice Survey of Clinical Neuropsychology in the United States, Part I: Practitioner and Practice Characteristics, Professional Activities, and Time Requirements. *Archives of Clinical Neuropsychology, 18,* 109–127.

Sweet, J. J., Peck, E. A., Abramowitz, C., & Etzweile, S. (2003b). National Academy of Neuropsychology/Division 40 of the American Psychological Association Practice Survey of Clinical Neuropsychology in the United States Part II: Reimbursement experiences, practice economics, billing practices, and incomes. *Archives of Clinical Neuropsychology, 18,* 557–582.

Tetlock, P. E. (2005). *Expert political judgment: How good is it? How can we know?* Princeton, NJ: Princeton University Press.

Vickery, C. D., Berry, D. T. R., Inman, T. H., Harris, M. J., & Orey, S. A. (2001). Detection of inadequate effort on neuropsychological testing: A meta-analytic review of selected procedures. *Archives of Clinical Neuropsychology, 16,* 45–73.

Victor, T., & Abeles, N. (2004). Coaching clients to take psychological and neuropsychological tests: A clash of ethical obligations. *Professional Psychology: Research and Practice, 35,* 373–379.

Wetter, M., & Corrigan, S. K. (1995). Providing information to clients about psychological tests: A survey of attorneys' and law students' attitudes. *Psychological Assessment, 26,* 474–477.

Youngjohn, J. R. (1995). Confirmed attorney coaching prior to neuropsychological evaluation. *Assessment, 2,* 279–283.

Youngjohn, J. R., Lees-Haley, P. R., & Binder, L. M. (1999). Comment: Warning malingerers produces more sophisticated malingering. *Archives of Clinical Neuropsychology, 14,* 511–515.

Index

"f" following a page number indicates a figure; "n" following a page number indicates a note; "t" following a page number indicates a table.